Evolution and Innovation in Parkinson's Disease Therapies in Under-Resourced Settings

Abraham Olufemi Asuku
https://orcid.org/0000-0003-0071-0531

National Biotechnology Research and Development Agency, Nigeria

Olaniyan Tope Olugbemi
https://orcid.org/0009-0006-0351-4666

Kwara State University, Nigeria & Korea University, South Korea

IGI Global
Scientific Publishing
Publishing Tomorrow's Research Today

Vice President of Editorial	Melissa Wagner
Director of Acquisitions	Mikaela Felty
Director of Book Development	Jocelynn Hessler
Production Manager	Mike Brehm
Cover Design	Jose Rosado

Published in the United States of America by
IGI Global Scientific Publishing
701 East Chocolate Avenue
Hershey, PA, 17033, USA
Tel: 717-533-8845 | Fax: 717-533-7115
Website: https://www.igi-global.com E-mail: cust@igi-global.com

Library of Congress Cataloging-in-Publication Data

LCCN: 2026934948 (CIP Data Pending)
ISBN13: 9798337374376
Isbn13Softcover: 9798337374383
EISBN13: 9798337374390
British Cataloguing in Publication Data
A Cataloguing in Publication record for this book is available from the British Library.

The book is in honor of the millions of people with Parkinson disease in the under-resourced settings across the globe, whose survival, bravery, and dignity despite inadequate access to care have been inspiring innovation and hope.

We celebrate patients and their families who are able to face everyday difficulties with strength and grace when they do not always have access to the advanced diagnostics, prescribed medications, and clinics. What you have experienced is the real basis of significant scientific growth.

We dedicate this work to the clinicians, the nurses, the therapists, the caregivers, and the community health workers who work on the front lines to improvise, advocate, and innovate within limited resources to provide compassionate care where it is needed the most.

To the researchers and policymakers who strive to close the gap in global inequality in neurological care: hopefully this book will aid the solutions that are not merely scientifically plausible but affordable, accessible, and sustainable.

And thirdly, to those who will come after us, scientists and healthcare leaders in the world of the low- and middle-income countries—may you keep turning the limitations into the opportunities of the locally grounded and globally relevant innovation.

With honor, unity, and optimism.

Table of Contents

Detailed Table of Contents

Christopher Oloruntoba Akintayo, Obafemi Awolowo University Teaching Hospital Complex, Ile-Ife, Nigeria
Samuel Obiosa Onyekweli, Lagos University Teaching Hospital, Idi-Araba, Nigeria
Gloria Osayamen Omoruyi, Obafemi Awolowo University Teaching Hospital Complex, Ile-Ife, Nigeria
Joseph Oluwatomi Akintayo, University of Ibadan, Nigeria
Ajoke Akinola, Achievers University, Nigeria

A chronic neurodegenerative disease, Parkinson's disease which manifests in a wide range of motor and non-motor symptoms. It can last anywhere from three to four decades, and its management is basically palliative. Age, family history, exposure to pesticides, and environmental pollutants (such as synthetic heroin use) are risk factors for Parkinson's disease. The reason or causes of it remain unknown at this time. Deep brain stimulation, the Apo morphine pump, and levodopa gel intestine infusion are examples of device-assisted therapies that have greatly enhanced the treatment of advanced Parkinson's disease. Non-motor symptoms, which are of great concern to both patients and their carers, might occur ten or two years before a diagnosis of Parkinson's disease. These symptoms include neuropsychiatric, gastrointestinal, urogenital, and sleep-related issues.

Parkinson's Disease (PD) diagnosis in developing and low-resource settings is hampered by a mix of clinical, structural, and sociocultural factors that produce late, missed, or incorrect diagnoses. This ambiguity is exacerbated in poor- and Middle-Income Countries (LMICs) by a lack of neurologists and movement-disorder experts, limited access to specialized diagnostics and confirmatory imaging, poor public and primary-care awareness, and sociocultural obstacles that cause delays in presentation. The diagnostic gap is further exacerbated by poor referral systems, transportation and financial obstacles, and the misattribution of symptoms at the community level to aging or non-neurological reasons. Emerging solutions include task-shifting to trained primary-care workers, telemedicine, simplified clinical screening tools, and novel low-cost biomarkers such as blood-based assays. However, these require further validation and context-sensitive implementation.

Parkinson's disease (PD) is a progressive neurodegenerative disorder characterized by diminished striatal dopamine levels resulting from the degeneration of dopaminergic neurons in the substantia nigra. About 10 million people around the world are affected by this disease. Levodopa was first used in the 1960s as a symptomatic cure for the disease and it is still the mainstay or PD treatment. Levodopa is not always available in low- and middle-income countries (LMICs) because of problems with the supply chain, high costs, and a lack of diagnostics. In rural areas without pharmacovigilance, doctors use cheaper alternatives like Mucuna pruriens or Vicia faba beans. The Parkinson's Disease and Movement Disorder Society in India is an example of a

side effects. Several research on the role of neuromodulation and deep brain stimulation in Parkinson's disease have revealed much more beneficial properties. Neuromodulation and deep brain stimulation is an innovative and safe therapeutic approach in neurodegenerative diseases that can effectively improve neuroimaging, structure and functions of the brain to enhance movement functions. The approach can enhance electrophysiological markers as feedback signals mechanism within the brain highlighting the potential of integrating and making an informed decision on selecting non-invasive and invasive neuromodulation techniques for the condition. This book chapter is to give an overview on the recent advances in the novel application of deep brain stimulation and neuromodulation technology in the therapeutic treatment of Parkinson's disease.

Parkinson's disease has been described as a neurodegenerative disease characterized by non-motor and motor symptoms that impact negatively on individual's lifestyle. Due to the nature of this condition, it requires constant monitoring to evaluate the progress of treatment, clinical assessment and therapeutic interventions. Consequently, wearable and digital technologies are emerging advances in artificial intelligence that are now recently being mobilized to provide real-time, promising solutions, personalized intervention and objective data collection for neurodegenerative diseases. These technologies are very specific and highly sensitive in tracking non-motor and motor variations, tremors and gait abnormalities. Furthermore, many of these devices are able to provide feedback mechanisms, cognitive impairment, sleep/autonomic and gastrointestinal comorbidities. The aim of the book chapter is to give an overview on the recent advances in the novel application of digital and wearable technology in the therapeutic monitoring of Parkinson's disease.

also focused on the ethical considerations and complications associated with these interventions, while also examining future directions for surgical innovation aimed at overcoming current limitations. This review article underscores the significance of a multifaceted approach in treating PD, combining surgical, pharmacological, and rehabilitative therapies to enhance patient outcomes.

Parkinson's disease (PD) is the second most common neurological disorder in India. Accurate diagnosis of PD is limited due to the unavailability of sufficient resources. In this research, an IoT-based Parkinson's Smart Watch System that combines both the motion and voice analysis models to attain a real-time PD detection is being proposed. This system uses ESP32 microcontroller along with MEMS inertial sensors and microphones to capture and analyze the motor and voice patterns. The acquired voice data was evaluated using tuned K-Nearest Neighbor and Random Forest classifiers to achieve a prediction accuracy of 97.40% and 95%, respectively. The proposed watch also has the capability to detect falls based on the IMU sensor threshold values and gives SOS alerts powered by GSM modules and Twilio messaging systems to achieve immediate response during emergencies. This system also has additional features like individualized medication and meal reminders along with remote monitoring capacity to enhance patient care.

This study describes a framework utilizing fuzzy soft sets for the automatic classification of the severity of Parkinson's disease from voice telemonitoring data. The framework achieved an accuracy of 78.4% for the classification of mild, moderate, and severe disease while providing greater explainability than black box models. The analysis was based on 5875 voice recordings from 42 patients. Fuzzy membership functions were used to model the gradual voice deterioration and the correlation-based weighting was used to clinically informative features passes (shimmer, HNR: r = 0.45 - 0.51). Confidence scoring calibrated to the classifiers allowed the implementation of risk-stratified workflows, achieving 91.4% accuracy on high confidence predictions. The fuzzy method was 4.2% better than crisp soft sets s (p < 0.001). The framework also demonstrated the ability to handle naturally occurring patterns of missing data and the unexplainable classification made a case for the fuzzy soft sets to be used preferentially for clinical workflows.

The neurological disorder with the fastest rate of increase in the world, Parkinson's disease (PD), poses serious management challenges due to its progressive deterioration and debilitating nature, which significantly affects quality of life. The process of creating novel medical treatments, especially for neurodegenerative diseases, is drawn out and includes several testing stages before a medication is authorised for use in a clinic. As the condition worsens, treatment gets more complicated, and it is essential to have objective, straightforward instruments to identify changes in patients' motor status and closely track how they respond to treatment. The available treatment aims

Preface

INTRODUCTION

Parkinson's disease (PD) is one of the most serious neurodegenerative disorders of the 21st century. Initially recognized in 1817 by James Parkinson in his paradigm essay on the shaking palsy, the disease has transformed from a medical interest to a health concern in the world. Although extraordinary progress has been achieved in the development and treatment of PD within high-income nations, tremendous inequities exist in the under-resourced setting in which a lack of infrastructure, lack of skilled professionals, cultural views on neurological disease, and financial limitations largely influence the process of diagnosis, treatment, and long-term care.

The book, *Evolution and Innovation in Parkinson Disease Therapies in Under-Resourced Settings*, is a result of the belief that scientific innovation is supposed to be a global endeavor. The therapeutic breakthroughs have a true meaning when they are available, flexible, and sustainable in the varying socioeconomic environments. Chapters within this book are all relevant to exploring the biological basis of PD and the transformative innovations that have the potential to help close the treatment gap in the world, including technological, pharmacological, digital, and rehabilitative innovations.

CHAPTER OVERVIEW

Pathophysiology and Symptoms of PD is the first chapter, and it creates a biological and clinical framework of the disease. It examines the dopaminergic neuronal degeneration in the basal ganglia, alpha-synuclein pathology, neuroinflammation, and mitochondrial dysfunction, as well as motor and non-motor manifestations with a significant impact on the quality of life. It is imperative to have a clear understanding of the disease so as to put therapeutic innovations discussed in the following chapters in perspective.

The second chapter, Diagnostic Challenges of PD in Under-Resourced Settings, focuses on the realities that exist in diagnosing PD in a potentially unfamiliar setting where advanced imaging, specialists in movement disorders, and biomarker assays may be scarce. This chapter suggests that culturally sensitive clinical assessment instruments, task-shifting, and inexpensive screening technologies are necessary to improve early diagnosis.

Chapter three, Dopaminergic Therapies of PD in Under-Resourced Settings, reviews the persistence of levodopa-based treatments, dopamine agonists, MAO-B inhibitors, and combination regimens in the context of the cost-effectiveness, availability, and rational use of these treatments in limited health care systems.

Chapter four, Herbal Remedies in the Under-Resourced Settings, discusses the ethnopharmacological practices based on the traditional knowledge framework. It critically analyzes plant-derived compounds, safety, and integration routes by the traditional healers and formal healthcare systems.

Chapter five, Stem Cell Therapy of PD in Under-Resourced Settings, discusses the potential and issues of regenerative medicine and evaluates—specifically—whether cell-based therapies can be scaled to areas lacking adequate laboratory facilities.

Chapter six, Immunotherapy and Targeted Molecular Therapies for Parkinson Disease in Under-Resourced Settings discusses disease-modifying interventions against alpha-synuclein aggregation and neuroinflammation and their potential applicability in different global settings.

Chapter seven, Deep Brain Stimulation and Neuromodulation Advances in PD in Under-Resourced Settings discusses how the miniaturization of hardware and increased battery life and tele-programming capabilities can enhance the access to high-level neuromodulation therapies.

Chapter eight, Digital and Wearable Technology in Therapeutic Monitoring of PD in Under-Resourced Settings and Smart Watch-Based Motion and Voice Signal Analysis for PD Detection and Management show how inexpensive wearable sensors, mobile health applications, and remote operations of monitoring can democratize healthcare delivery.

Chapter nine, Transcranial Magnetic Stimulation as a novel therapeutic strategy for PD in under-resourced settings evaluates the non-invasive brain stimulation method, especially in motor and cognitive outcomes, with regard to portability and cost.

Chapter ten, Surgical Interventions for PD in Under-Resourced Settings examines procedures involving lesioning and other operative approaches with the view of their feasibility and risk-benefit profile in under-resourced neurosurgical settings.

Chapter eleven, Smart Watch-Based Motion and Voice Analysis for Parkinson's Disease in Under-Resourced Settings presents a low-cost, IoT-enabled wearable system that integrates motion and voice analytics for real-time detection and monitoring of Parkinson's disease. It highlights how accessible digital tools can support early diagnosis, emergency response, and continuous patient care in resource-limited environments.

Chapter twelve, A Soft Set-Theoretic Framework for the Prediction and Personalization of Parkinson's Disease Management in Under-Resourced Settings introduces an interpretable predictive framework that uses voice data to classify disease severity and support personalized management strategies. The chapter emphasizes explainable analytics and data-efficient methods suited to clinical decision-making in under-resourced settings.

Lastly, The Road Ahead: Current Clinical Trials and Research, Challenges, and Recommendations for PD Therapies summarizes some of the new evidence, which points at current trials globally, as well as some practical guidelines that can help make sure the innovation is paired with equity.

This book is not a list of treatments; it is a wake-up call. It compels researchers, clinicians, policymakers, engineers, and community stakeholders to reconstruct the concept of care in Parkinson disease with the prism of accessibility, sustainability, and global unity.

As things become increasingly faster in the field of scientific discovery, the moral aspect of it is rather evident: advancement should not increase the gap but rather make it smaller. Through the convergence of the most advanced innovation with contextual implementation, we will be steps closer to the future where people with Parkinson's disease will be able to receive good, dignified, and personalized care, no matter where they live or how much money they have.

We hope this book can be a guide to more academic knowledge as well as a source of the transformative change.

Chapter 1
Pathophysiology and Symptoms of Parkinson's Disease in Under-Resourced Settings

Christopher Oloruntoba Akintayo
http://orcid.org/0009-0008-3446-466X
Obafemi Awolowo University Teaching Hospital Complex, Ile-Ife, Nigeria

Samuel Obiosa Onyekweli
http://orcid.org/0000-0002-4715-7932
Lagos University Teaching Hospital, Idi-Araba, Nigeria

Gloria Osayamen Omoruyi
Obafemi Awolowo University Teaching Hospital Complex, Ile-Ife, Nigeria

Joseph Oluwatomi Akintayo
University of Ibadan, Nigeria

Ajoke Akinola
Achievers University, Nigeria

ABSTRACT

A chronic neurodegenerative disease, Parkinson's disease which manifests in a wide range of motor and non-motor symptoms. It can last anywhere from three to four decades, and its management is basically palliative. Age, family history, exposure to pesticides, and environmental pollutants (such as synthetic heroin use) are risk factors for Parkinson's disease. The reason or causes of it remain unknown at this time. Deep brain stimulation, the Apo morphine pump, and levodopa gel intestine

DOI: 10.4018/979-8-3373-7437-6.ch001

infusion are examples of device-assisted therapies that have greatly enhanced the treatment of advanced Parkinson's disease. Non-motor symptoms, which are of great concern to both patients and their carers, might occur ten or two years before a diagnosis of Parkinson's disease. These symptoms include neuropsychiatric, gastrointestinal, urogenital, and sleep-related issues.

INTRODUCTION

Parkinson's disease is a progressive neurodegenerative disease that affects millions of people all over the world. The second most common neurodegenerative disease is Alzheimer's disease, affecting an estimated 1 million in the U.S. and 10 million worldwide (DeMaagd & Philip, 2015). James Parkinson first described it in 1817 in his seminar book An Essay on the Shaking Palsy. "In addition to PD, the acute effects on motor and non-motor functioning have also been identified as among the most serious neurological disorders in history" (Marino et al., 2020), which by 2050 will increase in LMICs in low- and middle-income countries due to demographic development and industrialization, particularly in Sub-Saharan Africa. This disease affects the central nervous system and causes a series of symptoms that impact one's quality of life. Parkinson's disease is caused by the destruction of dopaminergic neurons in the substantia nigra pars compacta, the area of the brain that controls motor activities. But, as age grows, PD becomes increasingly evident as more than motor impairment alone. Other non-motor symptoms, such as depression, mood disorders, and autonomic dysfunction, are emerging as examples of the disease's clinical manifestation (Magrinelli et al., 2016). The non-motor symptoms are often symptomatic of motor symptoms, complicating diagnosis and treatment for PD. But PD pathophysiology does not involve dopaminergic mechanisms, and is mediated via genes, environment and cell mechanisms (Aubignat et al., 2021). This variety provides another dimension to the disease for better outcomes. While there have been some improvements in Parkinson's disease treatment, many questions remain. But, one of the questions still relevant to research and clinical practice is "What are the mechanisms of Parkinson's disease, and how do they manifest themselves as symptoms in under-sourced settings?" This is particularly relevant given that PD is being seen as more of a syndrome than a disease. Vázquez-Vélez and Zoghbi (2021) conclude that PD is a pathological co-occurring entity because the accumulation of alpha-synuclein in Lewy bodies binds these two pathways. But it is not clear how these changes will take effect in overlapping PD symptoms. This is an obvious question, and I am asking it for several reasons. First, it could go to work for earlier, more accurate diagnosis of patients with non-motor symptoms that are too often ignored in the low- and middle-income population. Second, it could contribute to developing disease-modifying therapies that are a huge gap in PD management for low-income countries. Finally, one might be able to learn about other neurodegenerative conditions that may be of benefit to a wider population (Akinyemi & Owolabi, 2023). Pathophysiology and symptoms of PD are not pre-universitarian activities but direct applications to the practice. The speed of symptoms and their overlap with other neurological conditions complicate early diagnosis. For example, the signs of sensory impairment, such as hypersmia or pain, are common in patients but not generally considered to be early signs of PD (Zhu et al., 2016). Knowing what drives these symptoms allows clinicians to understand the risk factors and prevent intervention. Also, PD symptoms should trend to help tailor treatment. Other treatments for motor symptoms, such as dopamine replacement therapy are more often used than nonmotor symptoms (Kaur et al., 2019). This is a limitation that needs to be addressed in a broadening, integrated understanding of all possible PD manifestations. On top of that, the ubiquity of current knowledge regarding the pathophysiology of PD may lead to new therapies such as gene therapy or an anti-protein aggregation and neuroinflammation (Bloem et al., 2021). Such innovations may be of value to PD patients and their families, particularly within the home. This disease is characterized by complex neurodegenerative processes that include dopaminergic and non-dopaminergic treatments that produce motor and non-motor symptoms which progressively worsen over time. This surely requires more complex knowledge on pathophysiology and symptomatology of PD in order to devise an optimal diagnosis and treatment strategy for low-sourced contexts. This chapter examines the mechanisms through which PD propagates from neurodegeneration to accumulation of alpha-synuclein and to a role in non-dopaminergic systems. This also explains the effect of these mechanisms on motor and nonmotor symptoms associated with clinical presentation of the disease. Finally, the last section summarizes PD and provides recommendations for study and clinical application in low and middle-income countries. Discussion of progress in pathophysiology research, difficulty with managing symptoms and the potential for disease-modifying treatments are more detailed. This is in addition to the overall goal of this chapter to give an international perspective on Parkinson's disease and the need for multi-disciplinary understanding and treatment of this elusive disease. In general, Parkinson's disease poses an enormous problem for researchers and clinicians due to its plethora of pathologies and diverse symptoms. Yet, the constant changes in the understanding of this disease do open up new ways to identify and treat it. This paper aims to add to the literature of knowledge about how Parkinson's Disease works by discussing mechanisms of the condition and its clinical manifestations, and by identifying and demonstrating the mechanism. In doing so, this chapter also aims to highlight the importance of persistent research and innovation in fighting one of the most debilitating neurodegenerative diseases of our time.

Parkinson's disease impacts the majority of motor functions because the dopaminergic neurons lose synaptic activity in the brain, leading to impaired motor function. This loss is mainly sustained in the substantia nigra pars compacta, which is important for the control of movement (Olugbemi et al., 2023). But many other factors contribute to this degeneration, including mitochondrial dysfunction, oxidative stress, neuroinflammation and genetic mutations. These processes are important for evaluating new therapeutic interventions intended to slow or prevent disease progression.

Parkinson's is associated with neurodegeneration of dopaminergic neurons in the substantia nigra pars compacta. These neurons act as important motor action determinants and produce dopamine that induces the basal ganglia to initiate communication with them. Dopamine is one of the main regulators of voluntary movement, which is needed to initiate and control movement. Thus, motor symptoms such as bradykinesia, rigidity, tremor, and postural instability are caused by PD (Marino et al., 2020). Dopaminergic neuron loss is positively related to motor symptoms. For example, when motor performance is noted, 50% - 80% of dopaminergic neurons have reportedly already fueled (DeMaagd & Philip, 2015). This was not possible immediately, but could be attributable to brain compensatory mechanisms such as suppressing dopamine secretion or receptor sensitivity. But these mechanisms may collapse later if neuronal loss persists and leads to progressive motor impairment. Parkinson's disease suffers from mitochondrial dysfunction, which is involved in the loss of dopaminergic neurons. The mitochondria are sometimes referred to as the "powerhouses" of the cell, and they produce ATP, which is the energy currency of cells. Plus, mitochondrial dysfunction blocks the production of ATP and leads to energy deficits that disrupt neuronal function and survival in PD (Zhu et al., 2016). Complex I changes during the transport of electrons to produce ATP, one of the most common causes of mitochondrial dysfunction in PD. These failings produce a stronger ROS and oxidative stress. ROS are highly reactive compounds that can corrode lipids, proteins and DNA. Dopaminergic neurons are particularly vulnerable to oxidative stress due to their high metabolic demands and the fact that dopamine is so easily oxidized to produce toxic byproducts (Ishiguro et al., 2021; Jaiswal et al., 2021; Vázquez-Vélez & Zoghbi, 2021). In addition, PARKIN and PINK1, two mitochondrial quality control genes, have been implicated in PD-induced mutations. These changes also impact mitophagy, the cellular process of removing damaged mitochondria and permit deficient mitochondria to accumulate and increase oxidative stress (Aubignat et al., 2021). Oxidative stress is strongly associated with neuroinflammation, a second major neuronal death in Parkinson's Disease. Injured or diseased, the neuroinflammation leads to the microglia, the immune cells of the central nervous system. Atypically high levels of alpha-synuclein are released by microglia in the brain of PD sufferers (Bloem et al., 2021). Inflammatory cytokines and ROS, secreted by activated microglia, deplete neurons and contribute to higher levels of oxidative stress. This leads to a vicious circle: oxidative stress and neuroinflammation collide, and brain damage is worsened. Among patients with PD, inflammatory mediators were significantly elevated in the substantia nigra after postmortem examination suggesting neuroinflammation is implicated in disease progression (Sveinbjornsdottir, 2016). Among the physiological mechanisms of Parkinson disease, the majority of the pathogenesis is genetic, and is primarily familial. PD has been described as the result of several genetic mutations including one in the SNCA gene, the LRRK2 gene and the PARKIN gene. These changes affect cell functions such as aggregation of proteins, mitochondrial function and autophagy, and can eventually cause neuronal damage and death. SNCA is the SNCA gene, and it is a highly expressed neurohormone involved in the formation of synaptic communication. Mutations in SNCA and genes that overlap, double, or triple the gene may be responsible for the lack of production of alpha-synuclein, which can then be absorbed into Lewy bodies, a pathology in PD (Magrinelli et al., 2016). These aggregates destabilize normal cell processes and cause neuronal toxicity. PD is a non-specific genetic disorder, most often caused by LRRK2 mutations, and is associated with both familial and out-of-pocket cases. LRRK2, is a kinase that regulates many cell processes, including vesicle trafficking and cytoskeletal regulation. Mutations in LRRK2 have been shown to increase the kinase activity, resulting in dephosphorylation of substrates and loss of cell function (Kaur et al., 2019).

PARKIN is another PD gene that encodes an E3 ubiquitin ligase critical for mitophagy. PARKIN mutations affect mitochondria and oxidize these damaged mitochondria. These types of mutations are also implicated specifically in early PD and provide evidence of mitochondrial dysfunction in PD (Dirkx & Bologna, 2022). Parkinson's is not a single neurodegenerative disease with specific neurodegenerative mechanisms, but has multiple mechanisms that harm neurons more severely. Also, mitochondrial disease and oxidative stress can bind alpha-synuclein, and genetic mutations that affect mitochondrial quality control may increase exposure to oxidative stress. Also, inactivation of alpha-synuclein increases neuroinflammation that can interfere negatively with mitochondrial function and increase oxidative damage. These interactions reflect the multifactorial nature of PD pathogenesis and the need for multiple pathways to be treated simultaneously. Clinical research in these two domains has been being conducted currently to find ways of addressing disease progression, and has thus far provided evidence of a slow or even no response to Parkinson's Disease progression (Marino et al., 2020). Parkinson's Disease is associated with loss of dopaminergic neurons, mitochondrial dysfunction, oxidative stress, neuroinflammation, and gene mutation. They block the regenerative effects of neuronal damage and cause disease progression. A better understanding of these mechanisms is essential to developing novel treatments that will address the real cause of PD rather than relapse. The pathophysiology of Parkinson's Disease has been thoroughly researched, and many studies are producing lagging data. Future research should continue to investigate the exact interactions between these processes and help identify therapeutic approaches that may be targeted at multiple fronts at once. This will essentially allow researchers to design treatments that can improve the quality of life for people with this terminal illness.

Figure 1. Integrated Cascade of Neurodegenerative Mechanisms in Parkinson's Disease

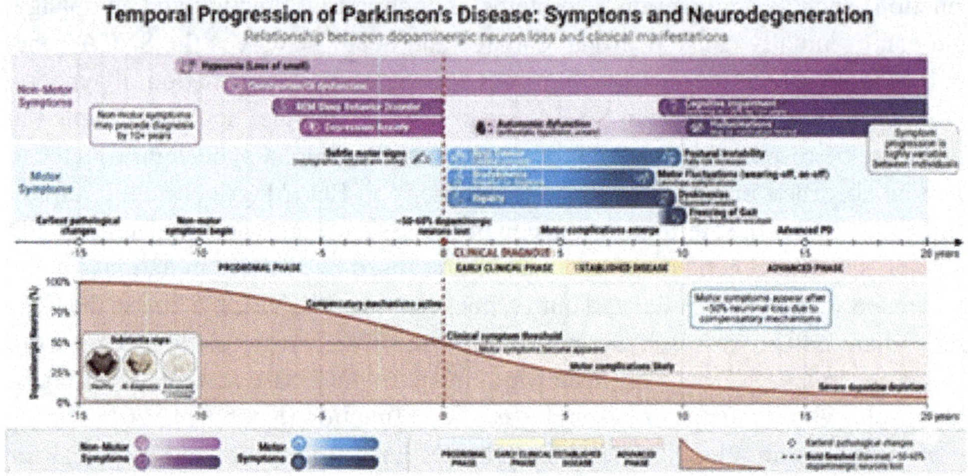

Alpha-Synuclein Aggregation

Alpha-synuclein, a presynaptic neuronal protein that regulates the synaptic vesicle and releases neurotransmitter, is well known to be involved in the synthesis of this apresynaptic neuronal protein in Parkinson's, a chronic neurodegenerative disease. It is known as one of the most common PD pathologies and an important mediator of Lewy bodies, the intracellular inclusion that accompanies the disease. These aggregates are not just asymptomatic but are critical in promoting PD symptoms and causing symptoms. Alpha-synuclein is an alpha strand of the SNCA gene expressed in the brain. Alpha-synuclein is an asoluble monomer that maintains synaptic and neuronal health in normal conditions. But, PD is pathologically altered when alpha-synuclein is misfolded and solublefibrillated. These fibrils accumulate in neurons, resulting in Lewy bodies and Lewyneurites that are ubiquitously expressed in the central and peripheral nervoussystems of PD patients (Marino et al., 2020). During the early 20 century, Lewy bodies were recovered from Friedrich Lewy. But the predominant protein present in these inclusions was only alpha-synuclein later. These lewy bodies are uncommon in the substantia nigra pars compacta, one of the most crucial sites for motorcontrol. They are highly associated with the loss of dopaminergicneurons that is characteristic of PD pathophysiology (Zhu et al., 2016). A further benefit is that PDsymptoms represent the entirety of PD symptoms, including non-motor conditions such as cognitive decline and autonomic dysfunction, which are increasingly considered by Lewybodies to be an important factor. First, astrogenetic and environmental factors initiate a misfolding process, resulting in amplification of alpha-synuclein. Mutations in SNCAgenes are A53T, A30P, and E46K, which all strongly implicate familial PD and have been shown to enhance the aggregation process. These changes also affect the structure of the protein, resulting in a beta-sheet-rich fibril rather than a normal alpha-helical type (DeMaagd & Philip, 2015). Other environmental factors, such as pesticides and heavymetals, are more likely to misfoldalalpha-synuclein. Oxidativestress, a manifestation of mitochondrialdysfunction and neuroinflammation is also important in this pathology. The oxidation of alpha-synuclein is due to the bynitration and phosphorylation of the protein, which combusts with the aggregation (Vázquez-Vélez & Zoghbi, 2021). These oligomers are toxic to neurons and were also shown to be more harmful than mature fibrils present in Lewy bodies. Oligomers are toxic to cells by inhibiting membraneintegrity, mitochondrial function and protein degradation. Theseoligomers take form, are re-formed into larger fibrils, and produce Lewy bodies (Dirkx & Bologna, 2022). One of the most interesting features of alpha-synucleinpathology is the tendency to spread over the nervous system, suggesting an aprion mechanism. Some studies have found misfoldedalpha-synuclein can also be spread across neurons and from one part of the brain to another. This propagation would perhaps explain the progressive nature of PD, since it is closely connected to the sequential action of many neurons in the pathology process (Aubignat et al., 2021). As alpha-synuclein is prionlike, aggregates are pumped out of affected neurons into the extracellular space. They also mingle with toneighboring neurons and grow into seed cells that amplification of endogenous alpha-synuclein. It is followed by endocytosis and other cellular transporters. Other neuralpathways have been hypothesized to include alpha-synucleinaggregates such as the vagus nerve that connects the gut to the brain. This leads to the hypothesis that PD could start in the gastrointestinal tract and spread to the central nervous system (Bloem et al., 2021). This is also the case for glial cells, such as astrocytes and microglia. These cells can transport the ainapha-synuclein together, causing neuroinflammation and pathology.

This role of glial cells corresponds also to the complex interaction between alpha-synuclein and the generalcellular environment of PD (Sveinbjornsdottir,

2016). This accumulation ofalpha-synuclein aggregate is thus directly associated with neuronal toxicity and results in the neurodegeneration of PD. Alpha-synuclein causes neuronal death through several hypothesized mechanisms, including indirect and direct mechanisms. Unsurprisingly, one of the major toxic effects of alpha-synuclein aggregates is the repression of membrane. Alpha-synuclein oligomers may also exhibit pore-like structures in lipid bilayers that help membrane permeability and absorption of calcium. It produces a degeneracy of cells, an apoptosis and, eventually, neuronal death (Magrinelli et al., 2016). Alpha-synuclein aggregates inhibit the function of the mitochondria, an essential organ for neuronal survival. They slow the metabolization of the mitochondria, causing less energy production and more ROS. This means that oxidative stress increases the accumulation of alpha-synuclein and leads to a vicious circle of toxicity (Kaur et al., 2019). In addition to direct toxicities, alpha-synuclein aggregates can produce indirect neuronal death through activation of the neuroinflammatory response. These alpha-synuclein aggregates activate the brain's immune cells, the microglialcells. This leads to the release of pro-inflammatory cytokines and chemokines that kill neurons as well as accelerate pathology growth. Chronic neuroinflammation is a major contributor to PD development, and the predominant mediator is alpha-synuclein (Marino et al., 2020). But many of these questions remain unanswered, despite substantial research efforts to investigate alpha-synuclein aggregation. For example, it remains to be understood what triggers alpha-synuclein misfolding and how this may explain the prion-like behaviour of this compound. Further investigation of the association between phosphorylated adiposities and non-motor PD symptoms, such as cognitive impairment and mood disorders, is warranted. Recent studies have focused on attempting to develop therapy to prevent alpha-synuclein aggregation. There are ways to keep it from misfolding, spreading or clearing. Immunotherapy with alpha-synuclein antibodies has been successful in preclinical trials and is in clinical trials. The development of a new therapy may also involve the development of small molecules that either stabilize or further degrade alpha-synuclein (Zhu et al., 2016). Thus, the role of alpha-synucleinaggregation is one of the pillars of PD pathophysiology and therefore involved in the formation of Lewy bodies, pathology propagation and neuronal toxicology. Understanding these processes could help to guide the appropriate course of treatment and outcome for PD patients. But, since we are now aware of alpha-synucleinaggregation, strategies can be implemented that slow or even reverse PD progression.

Dopaminergic Neuron Degeneration

This is an autoimmune neurodegeneration that causes neuronal inflammation. SNpc is a form ofParkinson's disease where dopaminergic neurons are selectively degenerated and are associated with motor symptoms. Inhibitors of dopaminergic neurons in the SNpc are at high risk of oxidative stress, mitochondrial dysfunction and protein misfolding. These neurons are implicated in the development and regulation of dopamine, a motor neurotransmitter necessary for smooth and coordinated motor function. The new study from the BBB (Marino et al., 2020) posits that loss of these neurons will increase the motor symptoms of PD such as bradykinesia, rigidity andtremor. Indeed, selectivevulnerability is part of intrinsicproperties of dopaminergic neurons in the SNpc. These neurons are highly metabolically dependent because they contain large axonal arborizations that require significant energy to maintainssynaptic activity. These two metabolisms have a higher risk for cytokine deficiency, a pathological trait of PD. These neurons are also more sensitive to oxidative stress as they are dependent upon the dopamine metabolism, which produces ROS in the form of byproducts. ROS enlargement can oversaturate DNA, lipids and proteins and thus destabilize neurons and the function and survival of neurons (DeMaagd & Philip, 2015). Another important contributor to the selective degeneration is a component of alpha-synuclein that aggregates and binds to Lewy bodies in dopaminergic neurons. In fact, adenosine amplification has been associated with disruption of processes such as protein degradation, mitochondrial function, and synapticcommunication. Plus, the spread of alpha-synuclein aggregates across brain regions also magnifies the vulnerability of such neurons and results in a gradual loss over time (Vázquez-Vélez & Zoghbi, 2021). It shows that removal of dopaminergic neurons from the SNpc leads to loss of dopaminergic neurons and affects basal ganglia circuits controlling motor functions. As the striatum, globus pallidus, subthalamic nucleus, and substantianigra are formed within the basal ganglia, they can begin to perform voluntary movements. Dopamine is a key mediator of these circuits as it regulates excitatory and inhibitory signaling pathways (Dirkx & Bologna, 2022). In PD this decrease in dopamine robs the balance of both the direct and indirect pathways in basalganglia. The direct path to movement is mutated and the indirect path to movement is overactive. Thisimbalance results in more inhibition of the thalamus that inhibits motor cortex stimulation and impairs motor functioning. This disturbance is also clinically documented as bradykinesia, rigidity and tremor, the most common motor symptoms of PD (Marino et al., 2020). Plus, basal ganglia are less plastic with a lack of dopamine. Low levels of dopamine have been shown to inhibit potentiation and worsen long-run depressive symptoms that are associated with motorlearning and adaptation. This limitation is also a reason for difficulties in initiating and performing movements among PD patients (Magrinelli et al., 2016). In the early stages of PD, the brain develops compensatory mechanisms to counter the effects of dopamine depletion and aid in maintaining motor function. These processes include increases in dopamine levels, increased release of dopamine from other neurons, and upregulation of dopamine receptors in the striatum. These adaptive mechanisms make basal ganglia circuits relatively normal, even when dopaminergic neurons lose their neurons slowly (Kaur et al., 2019), but not sufficient to account for persistent neurodegeneration associated with PD. Dopaminergic neurons dwindle while the brain is too adaptable, leading to excessive dopamine depletion and motor symptoms. This was confirmed by imaging and indicates that symptoms of motor function occur at the end of the period, when on average 50-60% of dopaminergic neurons in the SNpc are lost and thestriatum levels below threshold (Aubignat et al., 2021). This failure also stems from the progressive nature of alpha-synuclein aggregation and its detrimental effects on neuronal functioning. The pathology of the disease is also increased by the encoding of alpha-synuclein in brainstem and cortex which can produce both motor symptoms and nonmotor symptoms. This trend also demonstrates the importance of early intervention in preservedopaminergic neurons and the prevention of breakdown of compensatory mechanisms (Bloeme et al., 2021). Many studies have shown that dopaminergic neurons are selectively sensitive and their actions have effects on basal ganglia circuits. For example, post-mortem analyses of PD patients have reported similar dramatic reduction in dopaminergic neurons in the SNpc as well as decreased alpha-synuclein aggregates and Lewy bodies. PET and SPECT have also shown that dopamine depletion in the striatum is associated with a higher prevalence of motor symptoms but are not readily available in low or under-resourced settings. In addition, animal models with PD, such as models with PD caused by genetic mutations or neurotoxins, have shown that mitochondrial dysfunction, oxidative stress, and alpha-synuclein aggregation are associated with the destruction of dopaminergic neurons. These studies also identify potential therapeutic targets for stopping or preventing PD development, such as promoting mitochondrial function or reducing oxidative stress (Zhu et al., 2016). Parkinson's disease results in motor symptoms and pathophysiology controlled by the degeneration of dopaminergic neurons in the substantia nigra, or pars compacta. The fragility of these neurons, and the effect of dopamine depletion on the basal ganglia circuits, show PD complexity, and difficult to coordinate PD pathogenesis.

Compensation systems fail at first sign, but failure itself becomes a sign that early intervention and therapy can be beneficial. Future research should focus on mechanisms of dopaminergic neuron degeneration and on ways to maintain neuronal function and improve patient quality of life.

Involvement of Non-Dopaminergic Systems

Some indications of a faster role of non-dopaminergic systems in the role of PD have multiple forms. In addition to dopamine, other neurotransmitters including dopamine are also important markers in clinical presentation of the disease, including nonmotor symptoms. These systems are also liable for many sorts of problems including cognitive impairment, mood disorders, autonomic dysregulation, and sensory impairment.

In particular, PD is associated with a high concentration of acetylcholine in the basal forebrain cholinergic system, specifically the nucleus basalis of Meynert. This region of loss of cholinergic neurons has been implicated in impairment of executive function, attention and memory in PD patients (Marino et al., 2020). Some authors have concluded that this age at diagnosis is over 10 days prior to motor symptoms, suggesting cholinergic system involvement in early PD (Magrinelli et al., 2016). Cholinergic fusion is associated with gait, postural stability and cognitive decline. Various developmental PDs tend to exhibit gait disorders and freeze when the cholinergic neurons of the PPN, a brainstem structure, fall out. More specifically, imaging with cholinergic markers such as PET and radioligands targeting acetylcholinesterase has shown that cholinergic deficits are directly associated with PD. These results suggest that cholinergic activity decreases in the basal forebrain and brainstem, with consequences for cognition and motor function (DeMaagd & Philip, 2015). Serotonin (5-hydroxytryptamine or 5-HT) regulates mood, sleep and other autonomic functions. The raphe nucleus of the brain, the dorsal dorsal nucleus, is strongly degenerationally expressed in PD and implicated in several non-motor symptoms. Depression and anxiety are two of the most common non-motor PD symptoms and can affect 50% or more of the patients (Zhu et al., 2016). These symptoms appear to be a result of serotonergic dysfunction and/or decreased availability of serotonin transporter in the raphe nuclei and other areas of the brain. Serotonergic degeneration is also implicated in sleep disorders such as RBD or rapid eye movement disorder, which tend to precede motor symptoms. RBD causes vivid dreams and loss of muscle atonia during REM sleep that results in physical acting out of dreams. Imaging results show that serotonin transporter is not binding to serotonin as frequently in the brainstem of PD patients with RBD and that serotonergic dysfunction may be a contributing factor to this sleep disorder (Vázquez-Vélez & Zoghbi, 2021). This implies that, among PD patients, pain and deficient olfaction may be sensory manifestations of serotonergic deficits. These symptoms may be mediated by a change in the serotonergic pathways of pain and sensory processing. These results seem to agree with pathological observations that the raphe nuclei contain very low numbers of serotonergic neurons (Dirkx & Bologna, 2022). A second important pathway implicated in PD is the noradrenergic system, located in the brainstem at locus coeruleus. It produces a neurotransmitter known as norepinephrine, which regulates arousal, attention, stress response and autonomic functions. Noradrenergic degeneration in the locus coeruleus has long been known to cause PD and is associated with a number of non-motor symptoms including motor symptoms, fatigue and cognitive impairment (Aubignat et al., 2021). PD is an autonomic disease with orthostatic hypotension, constipation and urinary incontinence as well as frequently noradrenergic deficits. For example, orthostatic hypotension, which causes low blood pressure when standing, reduces norepinephrine release and decreases arterial tone. In similar fashion, a loss of noradrenergic communication with the enteric nervous system can lead to diarrhea and constipation (Bloem et al., 2021). Fatigue is a complication of many PD patients and is also associated with noradrenergic dysfunction. This reduction of arousal and motivation may be explained by lowered levels of norepinephrine in the prefrontal cortex and other brain areas. Imaging confirms reduced binding of locus coeruleus and other regions of the norepinephrine transporter radiotracers and reveals a second role for noradrenergic action in PD (Sveinbjornsdottir, 2016). PD decreases not only if there is no specific pathway but also when there is a complex relationship between cholinergic, serotonergic and noradrenergic dysfunction. This multigeneration also explains the heterogeneity of non-motor symptoms amongst PD patients and may be of interest to them in their quality of life. PD is one of the most common nonmotor symptoms and is more likely to develop dementia later in life. Although dopaminergic dysfunction of frontostriatal circuits is also associated with executive dysfunction, cholinergic degeneration of the basal forebrain is one of the most common causes of memory and attention deficits. Second, it seems that serotonergic and noradrenergic dysfunction may further impair cognitive development by impairing mood, sleep, and arousal, all key aspects of good cognitive performance (Magrinelli et al., 2016). Depression and anxiety are also multifactorial and contain the serotonergic and dopaminergic systems. The pathophysiology of PD has been shown to increase serotonin levels in the limbic system, one of the main brain regions involved in regulating emotions. On top of that, high levels of norepinephrine in the locus coeruleus can alter response to stress and therefore affect emotional stability resulting in the appearance of anxiety (Vázquez-Vélez & Zoghbi, 201). Another study indicates that non-dopaminergic degeneration mediates autonomous dysregulation in PD. Also, dysregulation of noradrenergic and cholinergic dysfunction reduces the ability to perform motor functions, resulting in orthostatic hypotension, gastroenteritis, and impaired thermoregulation. These symptoms have a huge impact on everyday life and general wellbeing, and can influence specific interventions to improve quality of life (DeMaagd & Philip, 2015). Neuroimaging and other imaging methods have uncovered new insights into the role of non-dopaminergic systems in PD.

Spectroscopy, PET imaging, including cholinergic, serotonergic and noradrenergic markers and some radioligands, have found that PD patients exhibit high levels of deficit in these systems as assessed by tactile and immunohistochemical methods. For example, acetylcholinesterase inhibitors have been shown to be less effective in the basal forebrain and brainstem, and have been shown to inhibit cognitive and gait function (Marino et al., 2020). Imaging studies have also shown that serotonin transporters are less readily present in the raphe nucleus and in the limbic system suggesting that mood disorders and sleep disorders might be associated with PD, radiotracers targeting the norepinephrine transporter have been used to detect noradrenergic deficits, and the locus coeruleus and other brain regions associated with autonomous and cognition activities have been less active (Aubignat et al., 2021). Pathology was used to support the imaging data. Postmortem examination of PD brains has revealed a significant loss of cholinergic neurons in the basal forebrain and PPN, serotonergic neurons in the raphe nuclei, and noradrenergic neurons in the locus coeruleus. These data also support the multifactorial nature of neurodegeneration in PD beyond the dopaminergic system (Bloem et al., 2021). Other pathologies and clinical presentations are noted for PD involvement with non-dopaminergic systems. This is counter-intuitive to cholinergic, serotonergic and noradrenergic degeneration, which can trigger lots of non-motor disorders, including cognitive decline, mood disorders, and autonomic dysfunction that have a powerful impact on patient outcomes. Imaging and pathology have provided information that could be used to further explore the role of these systems in PD and thus for more targeted therapy. Understanding the roles of non-dopaminergic systems in PD is important to selecting targeted treatment strategies to reduce the risk of motor and non-motor symptoms. Although dopaminergic drugs are still the gold standard for PD prevention, non-dopaminergic therapies are increasingly important to improve the quality of life in PD patients. Next steps are to learn more about the mechanisms of non-dopaminergic degeneration and a new treatment regimen for all PD symptoms. The focus on the interplay of neurotransmitter systems can only bring good change to the lives of PD patients. The symptoms of Parkinson's Disease are of crucial, vital significance when diagnosing the disease condition as it works in practice. Parkinson's disease possesses neuropsychiatric symptoms including mental disorders, anxiety and depression. Generally, undiagnosed Parkinson's patients are anxious and depressed; therefore they are misdiagnosed as having impaired motor activity and hence, do not develop the disease (Lee et al., 2022). In addition, 67% of patients with Parkinson's disease suffer from motor impairment, anxiety, depression and approximately 80% of patients with Parkinson's Disease suffer from cognitive impairment/impairment, and this is related to neuropathological cholinergic depletion, cortical dysfunction, and frontostriatal dysfunction (Elefante et al., 2021). Sexual dysfunction, constipation, hypotension (orthostatic), bradycardia, arrhythmia, and urinary incontinence, and the most recent antipsychotics such as dopamine agonist, dopamine replacement therapy, have been reported to cause hallucinations, psychosis, and impulse control disorders. Other antiretroviral medications that treat the human immunodeficiency virus include antiretroviral therapies and neurological conditions associated with AIDS, which have been known to have symptoms similar to those of Parkinson's disease (cognitive dysfunction and bradykinesia), and should not be interpreted as mimicry of Parkinson's disease symptoms (Denaro et al., 2022). These features can be achieved by altering the action mechanism of Levodopa's pharmacokinetic activity, mitochondrial dysfunction, reactive oxygen species/oxidative stress, and through interference with dopamine metabolism (Marino et al., 2020).

MOTOR SYMPTOMS

Primary Motor Symptoms: Akinesia/ Bradykinesia, Rigidity, and Tremor

Akinesia and bradykinesia are motor symptoms of Parkinson's disease. Akinesia is when there is less spontaneous movement and the ability to move freely; bradykinesia is when movement is slow. Other major motor symptoms commonly referred to as muscle stiffness, in patients, is stiffness that is clinically assessed as resistance to passive limb motion. Ironically, the stiffness index has been associated with the length and extent of the long-latent stretch reflex (Berardelli et al., 1983). PD tremor is identified as resting, postural and kinetic. The most common tremor for those with PD is resting tremor, in which the affected leg is supported rather than active. Rather, primary tremor is more common in postural tremor, i.e., at the point when the body cannot sit on a fixed surface in the face of gravity, than in kinetic or action tremor, when the body moves involuntarily (Bhidayasiri, 2005; Toth et al., 2004). But, clinically, the difference between PD and essential tremor is difficult to distinguish (Thenganatt & Louis, 2012). On top of that, intention tremor in PD has been noted to increase with the approaching target visualised, although minimal evidence has been provided for this effect (Fahn, 2011; Zakaria et al., 2013). Tremors are most likely to occur in the hands and feet, but may also occur in other parts of the body and are felt at low (4-6) or high (8-11 Hz). About 70% of PD suffer from tremors sometime in their lifetime (Helmich et al., 2012). Other motor symptoms of PD are tremor, rigidity, akinesia, bradykinesia and postural instability. This leaves the possibility that different motor symptoms may be experienced by individual patients (Hughes et al., 1992). Thus PD is also commonly classified into the tremor-dominant, akinesia-dominant or akineto-rigid motor classes (Jankovic et al. 1990; Lewis et al. 2005; Mure et al. 2011). Although it is a difficult to identify the particular subtype of tremor, this subtype of classification has also been used to examine clinical associations and pathways with different motor functions. But there are no further findings linking tremor-dominant patients with akinesia-dominant patients as significantly in age, duration of disease, levodopa dose, or motor severity in the UPDRS-III Unified Parkinson's Disease Rating Scale motor section (Eggers et al., 2011). But the differences in motor subtypes appear to be correlated with certain diseases. Many longitudinal studies have shown that akinesia-dominant PD is more likely to accelerate than tremor-dominant PD (Eggers et al., 2012; Louis et al., 1999). Also, bradykinesia has been described as a marker of early onset patients (Jankovic et al. 1990). One of the most important aspects here is that motor phenotypes are not constant. The tremor-dominant patients continue to be associated with the akinesia-dominant, but these pathologies also persist in subtypes as reported in longer-run analysis. Recent studies have also shown that both akinesia and bradykinesia severity do not necessarily correlate with each other (Evarts et al., 1981) and that resting tremor intensity correlates with other motor symptoms (Louis et al. 2001). Other variables that affect the presentation of motors are also related to different non-motor outcomes (Aarsland et al., 2003; Williams-Grey et al., 2007; Poletti et al., 2012).

Bradykinesia: patients who have loud tremors are more likely than those who have no tremors to develop dementia. Rather, there have been some studies that show the magnitude of tremors declines over time in some patients (Helmich et al., 2012; Toth et al., 2004), and this may at least partially explain the fact that tremor-dominant individuals are more likely to survive than nontremor PD individuals (Forsaa et al., 2010; Lo et al., 2009). These results show an association between dominant motor symptoms of PD and clinical courses.

The most common neuropathology of PD is the loss of dopaminergic neurons in the basal ganglia and particularly in the dorsal striatum (Kish et al., 1988). It is strongly suggested that akinesia and rigidity are caused by the loss of dopamine from the circuits of the cortico-striato-thalamo-cortical motor. The association between tremor and dopaminergic dysfunction is less clear, but (Albin, Young & Penney, 1989; Helmich et al., 2011; Rodriguez-Oroz et al., 2009). Some have argued that resting tremor appears to be somewhat unrelated to dopamine loss and that postural and kinetic tremors appear to be more dopamine-responsive, as a result of several pharmacological agents (Spiegel et al., 2007; Rossi et al., 2010). In addition to dopaminergic pathways, rigidity has been linked with changes in distributed neural networks. Functional imaging suggests that rigidity may be associated with a lack of functional connectivity between the cerebellum, motor, temporal, and occipital cortices, and the caudate nucleus in moderate to severe PD patients who had been off medication for motor activities that depend on external signals as well as internal signals (Baradaran et al., 2013). They find that rigidity correlated with dysfunction beyond the STN and large cortical-subcortical networks. The neural mechanism of tremor in PD is quite heterogeneous. Likewise, tremor has been described in subthalamic, thalamic, and cerebellar anomalies (Helmich et al., 2012; Kassubek et al., 2002). Neuronal tremor-frequency oscillation is observed in electrophysiological recordings from intraoperatively induced STN neurons, but functional MRI does not exhibit consistent activation of STN via tremor expression (Helmich et al., 2011). On top of that, structural imaging studies show that tremor-dominant PD patients lose less grey matter than non-tremor individuals (Rosenberg-Katz et al., 2013), and functional studies show that tremor-dominant individuals activate more prefrontal cortical nerves (Prodoehl et al., 2013). Nevertheless, the neural mechanisms that govern kinetic and postural tremor in PD remain poorly understood. Future research directing the neural activation response of both types of tremor, as well as those that interact between PD and essential tremor may also help clarify.

Some researchers have hypothesised that increased cerebellar activity in moving is a compensatory mechanism of decreased functions in the cortico-striatal motor circuit (Wu & Hallett, 2013; Yu et al., 2007). For example, PD and essential tremor have demonstrated that cerebellar networks can also play a role in resting and kinetic tremor (Brittain et al., 2015). Non-Motor Symptoms. Parkinson's disease causes tremor, rigidity and bradykinesia in the motor parts. Some people believe that non-motor symptoms are part of the disease, but can develop well before motor symptoms. Such symptoms have a major adverse effect on quality of life and can even contribute to poorer daily functioning than motor impairment. Therefore, for an accurate diagnosis, surveillance, and treatment plan, it is important to understand the frequency, clinical relevance, and pathophysiology of non-motor symptoms. Non-motor symptoms are extremely common in PD, and almost every patient exhibits at least one non-motor manifestation of PD (Marino, de Souza & Sousa, 2020). And most importantly, these symptoms occur in the early stages of the disease and can be early indications. Anosmia, constipation, and REM sleep behaviour disorder are common signs of motor dysfunction that appear years prior to the development of motor neurons (Zhu et al., 2016). These features may have been early identified and will offer an opportunity for action in the future, and may have implications for prevention. Non-motor symptoms have clinical relevance as they have profound effects on patients' ability to function and general well-being. The presence of cognitive decline, affective disorders and motor deficit may be associated with lower quality of life, caregiver burden and higher access to medical services (DeMaagd & Philip, 2015). Nonmotor symptoms are important but often underrecognized in practice, where direct motor deficits are the most common nonmotor symptom. This calls for the coordinated management of all forms of PD symptoms **(Figure 2).** Cognitive impairment is one of the most frustrating non-motor symptoms of PD and affects many patients as the disease progresses. A range of mild cognitive impairment to Alzheimer's disease dementia is experienced by as many as 80 per cent of PD patients. (Vázquez-Vélez & Zoghbi, 2021). Executive dysfunction in the early years is also a cause of depression, cognitive flexibility, and working memory. These limitations are likely to reflect dopaminergic impairment of frontostriatal circuitry and cortical amplification of alpha-synuclein pathology (Aubignat et al., 2021). Cognitive decline impairs memory and visual perception. Patients may have difficulty recalling, organizing or navigating information, which can lead to PD. PD is a neuropathological subunit that is highly adaptive in dopaminergic and cholinergic neurons and forms an excessive corpus of Lewy body deposits (Bloem, Okun, & Klein, 2021). PD also produces neuropsychiatric symptoms, including depression, anxiety and apathy. Depression is the characteristic trait of around 40% of PD patients and is thought to be a combination of neurochemical disorders, including suppression of dopamine, serotonin, and norepinephrine, and psychological challenges associated with a chronic neurodegenerative disorder (Sveinbjornsdottir, 2016). Other anxiety disorders, including generalised anxiety, panic disorder or social anxiety, are also common and often accompany depression (Magrinelli et al., 2016). Such symptoms may be multiple, including motor symptoms, and may occur during "off-time" from the medication. Apathy is another affective disorder resulting from PD associated with lower motivation and lower goal setting. This is a consequence of impairment in the dopaminergic pathways of the mesolimbic system, and this is unlike depression, though it is rarely mutually exclusive (Dirkx & Bologna, 2022). Collectively, PD mood disorders significantly increase withdrawal symptoms, affect treatment outcomes and result in poor quality clinical outcomes. Therefore, it is important to find out early and to respond early. PD is not only associated with motor symptoms but is also associated with sleep and affects up to 90% of patients (Kaur, Mehan & Singh, 2019). These symptoms include insomnia, excessive night sleepiness, REM sleep behaviour disorder, and restless legs syndrome. Sometimes the cause is a combination of nocturnal motor symptoms and psychopathology, including depression and anxiety. For example, excessive sleeping during the day has been linked to neurodegenerative changes in the areas of the brain involved in the regulation of arousal activity, such as the hypothalamus (Aubignat et al., 2021). The REM sleep behaviour disorder is particularly relevant because it has been shown to have a long association with motor symptoms, having been reported for years before and as a possible predictor of PD (Vázquez-Vélez & Zoghbi, 2021). Restless legs syndrome is common because legs are not mobile when they are wet, and it can also refer to basal ganglia and spinal cord dopaminergic dysfunction. Sleep disorder is not only detrimental to everyday life, but also contribute to cognitive and emotional deficits, which require attention and therapy frequently. A second non-motor manifestation of PD is a malfunction of the motor nervous system that affects cardio, digestion, urinary, and thermoregulation. These symptoms are hypothesised to be associated with autonomic neurodegeneration and α-synuclein accumulation in the central and peripheral autonomic networks (DeMaagd & Philip, 2015). Orthostatic hypotension leads to lower blood pressure when standing and can be associated with dizziness, syncope and falls. Gastrointestinal problems and constipation are the first non-motor symptoms reported and may be spotted at least ten years before the appearance of motor symptoms. These symptoms are associated with decreased enteric nervous system function and alpha-synuclein pathology affecting gut motility (Zhu et al.,

2016). Urinary conditions like urgency, frequency, and nocturia are also common and are associated with decreased bladder control.

More recently, changes in thermoregulation, such as excessive sweating or heat intolerance, are also noted to contribute to the burden of inflammatory symptoms in PD (Marino et al., 2020). Another important and overlooked side effect of PD is sensory symptoms. These include pain, paresthesia, and sensory processing delays, especially olfaction. One of the more common early symptoms of PD is that anosmia is thought to be more than 90% prevalent among early PD cases (Zhu et al., 2016). Essentially, this impairment is explained by an association between synuclein in the olfactory bulb and other neural structures. Pain, too, seems to be extremely common in PD, often in large proportions among patients, and is of many kinds, including musculoskeletal pain, neuropathic pain or dystonic pain (Magrinelli et al., 2016). Pain mechanisms in PD are complex and can be related to changes in the central processing of pain, dopaminergic deficits and motor features such as rigidity and dystonia. Sensory disorders, in particular, create discomfort and impairment of functions that worsen quality of life. Finally, non-motor symptoms are one of the most acute and often underdiagnosed symptoms of Parkinson's disease. These four dimensions – cognitive, psychiatric, sleep-related, motor, and sensory – typically precede motor symptoms and can affect the burden of disease and patient outcome. Ultimately, the objective is to learn about their interactions and to encourage early detection and targeted interventions. Integrated PD management for motor and nonmotor patients with PD reduces the risk of death and enhances the quality of life of patients suffering from this complex neurodegenerative disease.

Figure 2. Temporal Progression of Parkinson's Disease Symptoms and Neurodegeneration.

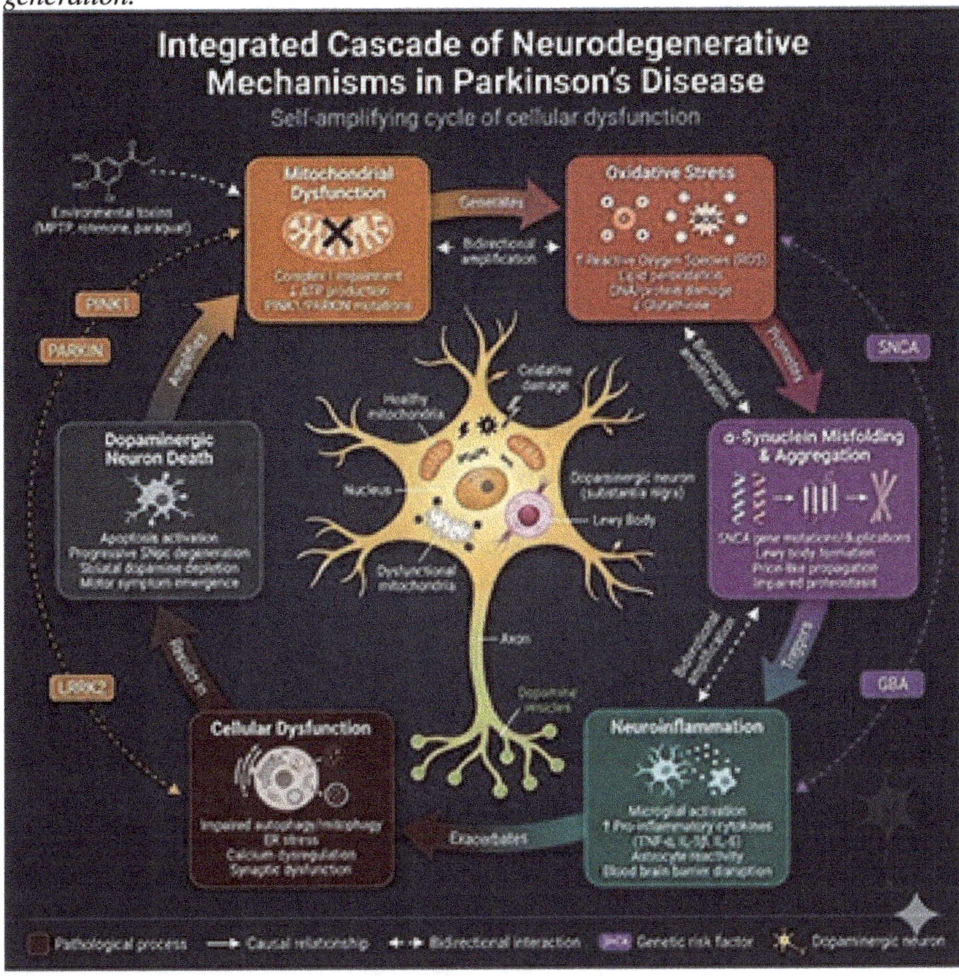

Progression of Symptoms Over Time

Parkinson's Disease is a slow-moving neurodegenerative disorder with motor and non-motor symptoms. This progression is often portrayed in clinicalstaging systems such as the Hoehn and Yahr scale that plots the disease severity over time. This knowledge of progress in symptoms can be used to better serve patients since it allows doctors to anticipate change, tailor treatment and support the patient over time. PD symptoms may differ greatly among individuals due to genetic predispositions, environmental factors and genetic variability in pathophysiology. This scale, designed by Hoehn and Yahr in 1967, continues to be one of the most widely used tools for identifying PD stages. There are five categories of symptoms from mild symptoms on one side of the body in Stage 1 to severe disability requiring assistance in Stage 5. Early motor symptoms, such as tremor or rigidity in Stage 1, are usually unilateral and may be so subtle that they do not strike the patient immediately. At the end of Stage 2, symptoms of motor symptoms include postural changes and facial expressive deprivation. These patients are relatively independent, as the daily tasks are a bit of a mystery. Stage 3 exhibits significant postural instability, which increases the risk of falls and injuries. Balance problems are worse, and some tasks require patient help. Stage 4 generates other motor symptoms and leads to severe disability. Walking, standing, and dressing are hard work; patients may also need caretaker assistance. Lastly, Stage 5 is the most severe phase and exhibits severe motor impairment and immobility. Patients often require a wheelchair or bed, and caregivers are involved in everything of the day. While the Hoehn and Yahr scale is a generalised model, the route is pushed back by individualvariability. Some patients may have high symptoms in absorption, while others may be young for decades. Also, non-motor symptoms that cannot be reported by the Hoehn and Yahr scale are often cited to complicate the progression. But these types of cognitive decline and motor dysfunction can also play important roles in the quality of life, even when motor impairments are relatively minor (Marino et al., 2020).

Nonmotor symptoms are usually second to motor symptoms and therefore early warning signs of PD. Such signs of constipation, sleep problems and smell loss are not found, or assigned another condition. Anosmia or loss of taste, for example, is a prodromal marker of PD that may occur years prior to symptoms of motor functions (Zhu et al., 2016). As noted, RBD and depression and anxiety are all early, suggesting dopaminergic pathways are involved in pathophysiology. But, non-motor symptoms are exacerbated and decompose over time into cognitive deficits, psychotic disorders and psychotic dystrophy. This cognitive decline may occur within a few episodes of executive dysfunction and may progress to PPD later. This shift is often associated with neurodegeneration beyond the substantia nigra, the cortical and limbic regions. They can also be hallucinations and delusions related to dopaminergic drugs that evade motor symptoms (DeMaagd & Philip, 2015).

Temporal disability leads to motor problems that typically include tremor, rigidity and bradykinesia. Dopamine on movement is absent in the basal ganglia and causes PD. These types of postural instability are the most common in Stage 3, suggesting there might be other systems, other than the dopaminergic pathways, such as the cholinergic system. This is a proxy for increased falls among patients and their caregivers (Vázquez-Vélez & Zoghbi, 2021). The symptoms are similar between motor and non-motor, although these symptoms can sometimes be viewed as a vicious circle in which one improves the other. For instance, postural degeneration can inhibit movement, weaken the muscles, and reduce mobility. Similarly, cognitive dysfunction may delay treatment and complicate symptoms. This breadth of complexity indicates the need for integrated approaches to treatment for the motor and nonmotor aspects of PD. PD symptoms may occur at different times based on genetic predispositions, environmental exposure, and lifestyle. PD is associated with SNCA, LRRK2, and PARKIN for families with particular patterns of progression. For example, SNCA mutations accelerate onset, while LRRK2 mutations could also accelerate onset. These types of genetic factors can also contribute to the risk for certain symptoms such as dementia or dyskinesia (Dirkx & Bologna, 202). PD pathogenesis has been shown to contribute to the development of PD, and exposure to pesticides and heavy metals may be an underlying cause of symptoms. Some researchers have shown that those at high risk for environmental stress will die earlier, have earlier symptoms, and experience worse symptoms. Lifestyle factors such as exercise and diet have been shown to influence disease progression. Regular exercise, for example, has been shown to promote motor function and early cognitive decline among patients with PD (Aubignat et al., 2021). There is also a difference in neuroplasticity that explains the variation in frequency of symptoms. The brain may respond to dopamine depletion at an early age with a higher spike in sensitivity to receptors or by adding pathways that can enhance movement coordination. Such compensatory mechanisms are not always effective in the progression of disease and can create obvious symptoms. The failure time and intensity can vary depending on the individual and, therefore, may vary with respect to timing and severity of progression of PD (Bloem et al., 2021). I have found that imaging studies of variability in symptom patterning have provided a vast amount of information. PET and fMRI, two new imaging techniques, show differences in the distribution of neurodegeneration among patients. For example, some individuals may exhibit considerable cortical atrophy in relation to serious cognitive impairment, and others may have relatively intact cortical structures in relation to more severe motor symptoms (Sveinbjornsdottir, 2016). Parkinson's disease is a complex, multi-year process, and different for every person. Clinical models such as the Hoehn scale and Yahr scale can be useful in predicting the stage of disease, but do not cover the entire spectrum of motor and non-motor symptoms. Anasmia and RBD are nonmotor symptoms that predate motor impairment and are important in identifying motor impairment earlier. As the disease progresses, patients and their caretakers are unable to differentiate between motor and non-motor symptoms. Personalised medicine in PD care also provides a way to account for the individual's pathology. The degree to which pathogenesis differs is also tied to genetic factors, environmental factors and lifestyle that indicate an indication of a need for targeted treatment. This is supported by the advancement of imaging and biomarker studies, which can also aid in predicting symptoms and improving treatment. Finally, understanding the progression of symptoms in PD is of critical importance to improving outcomes for patients. Providing a more holistic, patient-centered approach is possible when clinicians measure the motor and non-motor mechanisms of the disease as well as individual preferences. Future research should explore the mechanisms of variability in progression in order to develop targeted therapies to slow progression and increase the quality of life for patients with Parkinson's Disease. Problems with Symptom Management: But, treatment of PD symptoms and related motor and nonmotor symptoms is still somewhat complex and sometimes incomplete, despite significant therapy advances. Although improvements in PD care have raised some questions about limitations of existing approaches, incorrect diagnosis and non-treatment of symptoms other than motor impairment and personalised medicine recommendations. Since the 1960s, PD treatment has been a dopamine replacement drug, usually levodopa, for motor symptoms. But levodopa is the gold standard for the treatment of motor dysfunction such as bradykinesia, rigidity and tremor because it directly compensates for the loss of dopamine in the basal ganglia circuits (DeMaagd & Philip, 2015). It is not easy, but it is. The prolonged exposure to levodopa results in an impairment of motor control, dyskinesia, and thus lowers life expectancy for the sufferers (Kaur et al., 2019). Similarly, the success of levodopa therapy in preventing disease suggests that treatment must address the mechanisms that lead to neurodegenerative disease. Alternatives to levodopa include dopamine agonists or monoamine oxidase B inhibitors that can induce hallucinations, impulse control disorders and orthostatic hypotension (Kaur et al., 2019). Plus, DBS, as well as other non-pharmacological agents, have been shown to reduce motor symptoms such as tremor and dyskinesia (Magrinelli et al., 2016). But DBS is not for all patients, and the consequences on non-motor symptoms are complex. PD burden is increasingly identified as an association between cognitive impairment, mood disorders, sleep disorders and autonomic dysfunction. These symptoms are but are often overlooked by current treatments (Bloem et al., 2021). For example, two commonly occurring PD symptoms, depression and anxiety, are often undertreated since no PD-specific antidepressants are available, and psychotropic effects are likely. Like autonomic conditions such as orthostatic hypotension and constipation, specific strategies need to be taken to treat these conditions, although a number of these are either unhelpful or do not work well in practice (Sveinbjornsdottir, 2016). Non-motor PD symptoms are most commonly associated with or precede the motor symptoms, but are rare and are poorly targeted for and treated. Dementia is a major non-motor disorder, affecting daily functioning and caregiver burden. For example, "Dopaminergic deficits are associated with cholinergic, serotonergic, and noradrenergic system development". PD-associated cognitive decline is pathogenic to both neurons (Magrinelli et al., 2016). This is complex but few treatments are able to treat cognitive symptoms and cholinesterase inhibitors, along with other drugs, are completely effective. Depression and anxiety are among the most common mood disorders in relation to PD and have a large influence on patients' lives. Such symptoms are not screened for in clinical trials because they overlap with motor symptoms and mental health stigma. PD's mood disorders can be treated with many types of drugs and psychotherapies, and a plan can be developed with the help of a therapist and caregiver (Bloem et al., 2021). Yet PD patients have not received specialized mental health care. Other non-motor conditions are insomnia, nighttime sleepiness and sleep behaviour disorder that relates to REM (rapid eye movements). These conditions, in turn, negatively affect patients' quality of life and can even contribute to other PD symptoms, creating a vicious cycle of symptoms. Zhu et al. (2016) note that the neuromuscular system is involved in the initiation of sleep. These strategies generally fail; to treat such symptoms, they may need targeted therapies like melatonin or dopamine agonists. Other PD problems are autonomic, including diarrhoea, urinary tract infections, and cardiovascular disease. Constipation is a common PD cause associated with alpha-synuclein aggregation in the enteric nervous system (Vázquez-Vélez & Zoghbi, 2021). Diet changes and laxatives are symptomatic, but not antipathophysiologic. Likewise, orthostatic hypotension, a debilitating consequence of impaired motor function, is a serious condition that must be controlled for falls and patient safety. Unfortunately, orthostatic hypotension is not well-reported in PD. And the variability in the appearance, progression, and response to treatment of PD points to the value of personalized medicine. Plus, recent research has shown that PD is not just a condition but a family of diseases that cause undesirable pathophysiology including alpha-synucleinaggregation, mitochondrial dysfunction, and neuroinflammation (Vázquez-Vélez & Zoghbi, 2021). This variability indicates the need for treatments tailored to the individual patient's genetic, clinical and environmental background. Mutations in SNCA, LRRK2 and PARKIN have been described as influencing the formation of PD (Bloem et al., 2021). Genetic testing will identify those at risk and make appropriate therapeutic choices based on findings. For example, patients with LRRK2 mutations may require targeted therapies to inhibit kinase activity, and patients with PARKIN mutations may need targeted therapies to inhibit mitochondrial dysfunction. Biomarkers such as Alpha-synuclein in cerebrospinal fluid or imaging of dopaminergic degeneration may help to distinguish and control disease. Adding biomarker data to the practice may enable an accurate diagnosis and the development of individual treatment plans (Vázquez-Vélez & Zoghbi, 2021). Other diagnostic tools, such as SPECT and PET may be used to identify individual variability in pathology and response to treatment for PD. Newer tools, such as single-cell transcriptomics, can be used to characterize the molecular basis of PD and to determine potential therapeutic targets (Dirkx & Bologna, 2022). Understanding the molecular signature of a particular patient allows for targeted therapeutic interventions based on a particular pathology. For instance, patients at high risk for neuroinflammatory disorders may benefit from anti-inflammatory medicines, and those with mitochondrial dysfunction may need treatment to enhance the metabolism of cell energy. Personalised medicine does not entail pharmacological intervention but includes lifestyle modification, physical therapy and psychosocial care designed specifically for the individual. For example, aerobics and dance therapy have been shown to improve PD symptoms and overall well-being (Bloem et al., 2021). And also, diets like the Mediterranean diet may be neuroprotective and potentially less likely to cause cognitive decline. Adding these non-pharmacological interventions to the personalised care plan will support clinicians in managing PD in several areas. As noted above, treatment of ischallenging of Parkinson's Disease is difficult due to the limited therapies available, but non-motor symptoms are complex and not all patients are diagnosed the same way. Dopamine replacement therapy and other drugs have been proven to treat motor symptoms, but have been found to be very weak in the treatment of non-motor symptoms. The lack of information and treatment on nonmotor symptoms exacerbates PD, because the burden is heavier than it should be and therefore needs coordinated, multidisciplinary intervention. Customisation may be an alternative to address this rare form of epilepsy and to improve outcomes. Utilising genetic, biomarker, and molecular information, clinicians can tailor therapeutic interventions to the individual patient. PD patients have an increased quality of life by adding non-pharmacological treatments such as exercise and diet to the individual health care plan. Although these changes have made some progress, we still have a long way to go in terms of PD pathophysiology and symptom management. The cross-institutional research that spans the boundary between clinical and basic science is fundamental to creating disease-modifyingtherapies and enhancing patient care. The extension of personalised medicine into everyday practice is a significant step toward addressing symptoms and developing the field of neurodegenerative disease treatment as we continue to solve the mysteries of PD. Several promising new treatments have been developed, but many translational difficulties can prevent the full utilisation of new, disease-modifying treatments for Parkinson's disease. One of the clinical concerns is that there are no valid and robust biomarkers that can inform early PD and predict therapeutic responsiveness. This severely limits the pooling of patients and personalised interventions. Also, heterogeneity in PD often does not appear in current clinical trialplans and can lead to underpowered subgroup analyses and inconsistent efficacy outcomes. They call for a paradigm shift in precision neurology, to create personalised treatment plans based on genetic, molecular and digital markers where nonmotor therapy is not available. Future models need to charge forsymptoms relief and prevention, multi-omics profiling and longitudinal digital monitoring, and non-dopaminergic drug development. Outlook and Shortcomings PD is a rare neurodegenerative disorder with complicated pathophysiology. While much has been learned about the mechanisms and development of effective symptomatic treatments, there is a major gap to be filled in development of therapies that will change the disease, since such mechanisms are not available in the LMIC. This section features ways that new therapies may be pursued to combat alpha-synuclein aggregation, neuroinflammation, and mitochondrial dysfunction, shortcomings of existing literature and the importance of a multidisciplinary approach to address gaping clinical and basic research. The other promising research endeavor in PD is developing disease-modifying treatments to prevent or inhibit neurodegeneration. Today, dopamine replacement with levodopa ordopamine agonists is the most common treatment of symptoms, including motorimpairment. But these medications overlook the pathology at work, and therapies that address the roots of PD are largely unsupported. Current Information and Perspectives Parkinson's disease is a multicellular neurodegenerative disease that has complex genetic, molecular and cellular mechanisms. Recently, new research has exposed several important areas, including new ways in which gene mutations, protein aggregation and neuroinflammation increase ease of growth.

Genetics have dramatically changed the way we think about PD, such as the finding that mutations in SNCA, LRRK2, PARKIN and PINK1 are ubiquitous in the development of disease (Marino et al., 2020). SNCA encodes alpha-synuclein, which is of particular significance because the mutation leads to abnormal protein aggregation, a hallmark of PD pathology (Vázquez-Vélez & Zoghbi, 2021). These lunes are toxic, and cells form lipid molecules that inflate and accumulate alpha-synuclein, which is metabolized and the normal cell function is denatured. Another discovery is that mitochondrial dysfunction is mediated primarily by mutations in PARKIN and PINK1. These genes are necessary for the maintenance of mitochondrial quality and mutations in these genes lead to decreased energy production and oxidative stress. Oxidative stress contributes to neurodegeneration and may also account for the selective vulnerability of dopaminergic neurons in the substantia nigra pars compacta (Sveinbjornsdottir, 2016). Also, LRRK2 mutations induce increased neuroinflammation that worsens neurodamage by activating microglia and astrocytes (Aubignat et al., 2021). The protective effect recurs, becomes irreversible over time, and induces a loop of neuronal damage and inflammation. Other studies also point to the interplay of these mechanisms, which is interesting because they are interlinked. For example, mitochondrial dysfunction and oxidative stress may promote the accumulation of alpha-synuclein while neuroinflammation may cause protein misfolding and neuronal death (Bloem et al., 2021). Understanding these linked pathways is important because it provides a more accurate account of the pathogenesis of PD and its potential therapeutic target. Biomarkers have become an important diagnostic and surveillance tool for early detection of Parkinson's disease. Identifying reliable biomarkers is a vital condition to understanding the infectious nature and slow progression of the disease. A biomarker candidate has been described because alpha-synuclein is associated with pathophysiology of PD. High levels of alpha-synuclein in CSF and blood plasma are associated with atypical diseases (Zhu et al., 2016). They are unable to be standardized to differentiate PD from other alpha-synucleinopathies such as multiple system atrophy. Image biomarkers are another promising avenue. PET and SPECT imaging can capture the transient disadsorption of dopaminergic neurons and shedding of alpha-synuclein in vivo (MF Dirkx & M Bologna, 2022). These methods, along with early detection, allow for easy tracking of disease progression by monitoring brain metabolism and structural connectivity. For example, PET images of dopamine transporter binding indicate the prevalence of dopaminergic degeneration and hence direct association between DAT binding and the severity of motor symptoms. Among biomarkers are also alpha-synuclein, cytokines and chemokines. Interleukin-6 and TNF- are extremely high in PD patients suggesting that neuroinflammatory processes could be involved in the progression of disease (DeMaagd & Philip, 2015).

Also, mitochondrial biomarkers such as changes in mitochondrial DNA and respiratory chain enzyme activity may also reveal the metabolic dysfunction of PD (Magrinelli et al., 2016). There are few barriers to the use of biomarkers in clinical practice, including variation in the expression of biomarkers across populations and noninvasive sampling. But, existing methods and methods to analyze the data of multiplex biomarker panels as well as machine learning algorithms could be adapted to further improve diagnostics and re-assess drug efficacy (Kaur et al., 2019). Recent research has significantly improved our knowledge of Parkinson's Disease, particularly single-cell transcriptomics and use of new imaging techniques. Single-cell transcriptomics can study individual genes and thus reveal the heterogeneity of cellular components within the affected brain regions (Marino et al., 2020). These approaches have identified various subpopulations of dopaminergic neurons from the substantia nigra which are both highly resistant to PD-mediated stressors, including oxidative damage and alpha-synuclein toxicity. Plus, non-neuronal cells, such as microglia and astrocytes, that express neuroinflammation have been identified through single-cell transcriptomics. These results confirm the role of glial cell dysfunction in the pathophysiology of PD, and suggest novel anti-inflammatory drug targets (Zhu et al., 2016). Transcriptomic research, for one, has also helped explain the genetic and epigenetic processes that may be involved in determining risk for disease, and has opened up the door to personalized medicine. Large-scale imaging complements transcriptomic research because it provides spatial and temporal information on molecular evolution. DTI and fMRI inform the structure and functional connectivity of the PD brain. DTI also found that white matter tract microstructure differences, including between the basal ganglia and motor cortex, were associated with motor symptoms (Vázquez-Vélez & Zoghbi, 2021). Similarly, fMRI studies have indicated network-activation changes in the default mode network and the sensorimotor network that are likely to be responsible for non-motor symptoms of cognitive decline and mood disorders. New techniques, such as optogenetics and chemogenetics, are also being tested because they can reconstruct neural circuits that govern PD. These techniques enable us to observe and characterize the neuronal activity, as well as to investigate the causal relationship between circuit dysfunction and symptoms (Sveinbjornsdottir, 2016). Finally, cryo-electron microscopy for high resolution images has facilitated a clear understanding of the molecular structure of alpha-synuclein aggregation and new drug targets (Dirkx & Bologna, 2022).

Yet translating research results into practice is still a challenging task. Because they are expensive, technically complex, but not readily available, they can't be used; it's time to create cheap and usable platforms. Further, analyzing data from several technologies, such as transcriptomics and imaging, demands complex analysis and cross-disciplinary cooperation (Aubignat et al., 2021). New evidence on gene mutation, protein aggregation and neuroinflammation is changing the pathology of Parkinson's Disease. Currently available therapies, such as single-cell transcriptomics and imaging, allow for earlier diagnosis, improved tracking of progression, and targeted therapy. The road to convergence is not clear; the struggle for commonality among biomarkers, to reduce the costs of research, and to combine lots of types of data is constant. To address heterogeneity in PD, further studies will need to focus on collaboration between the researchers and personalized medicine interventions. The gap between clinical and basic science enables researchers to create new means of improving patient outcomes and, finally, a way out of this terrible disease. We hope that the efforts made in this regard will contribute not only to a better understanding of PD but will also lead to new approaches to neurodegeneration. Future Perspectives should also include innovations in the design of clinical trials, including adaptive trials, digital endpoints and health system research based on biological discoveries to provide equitable care. A well-conceived and objective study of disease-modification in PD is needed, including the phase II study, which will be the largest of the next wave. Phase II studies should examine the notion of safe use and appropriate doses, and phase III studies should be generalizable in size of sample and longitudinal follow-up (McGhee et al., 2016). On top of that, clinical parameters such as progression of MDS-UPDRS, time to event, and ad hoc biomarkers should be assessed for targetedness (Vijiaratman & Foltynie, 2023). Long intervals of trial and non-sensitive endpoints, such as simple UPDRS slopes, have historically been shown to imply clinically meaningful slowing of progression (Alhauda & Foltynie, 2016). This becomes even more complicated by the heterogeneity of the patient, and difficult to predict the effects of disease modification.

Neuroprotective effects are especially prominent in pre-symptomatic and early drug-naive populations, and amplification or late-stage populations also have particularly high levels of confounding effects, including motor fluctuations, dementia, and hallucinations (Lang & Espay, 2018). To avoid bias, the comparator must be selected carefully and blinding the true anti-inflammatory effects should be done, usually on a placebo. A biological target is required as well as a clear means of action. Preliminary clinical trials should include rigorous animal models and biomarker validation in order to show the translational relevance of these markers (Schapira, 2009). To avoid side effects, drug interactions that inhibit signalling should be addressed carefully. Most failures in the past were attributable to incorrectly planned targeting or off-target effects, which explains why priority should be extended pharmacokinetically and pharmacodynamically (Alhauda & Foltynie, 2016). The right statistics, enough time should be spent in studying the subject, and the right investigators at the best centres are all necessary operational conditions for success (Barber et al., 2025). The patient selection process is used to identify clinical trial participants through inclusion and exclusion criteria. These types of criteria ensure that the study participants will be suited to the research objectives, and they also improve the internal validity by minimising confounding effects (Friedman et al., 2015). On top of that, the patient selection is also subject to the design of the trial, as logistical variables such as the number of visits, distance from home or office, and specific patient participation needs, such as CSF collection, overnight stay, or off-state evaluation, can affect willingness and feasibility to participate in the trial (Getz & Campo, 2018). Recruitment and alignment to current care plans are operational but also important to ensuring maximum enrollment and minimal waiting time. Retention should also be characterised between scientific accuracy and practical access, as well as optimal generalizability (Treweek et al., 2018).

CONCLUSION

The involvement of the patient and caregiver in the low-income setting is relevant for the management of PD as it is relevant for the treatment of PD. The patients' experiences and experiences may contribute to the perception of PD in lived experience and to guidance for research priorities. Education programs that seek to educate patients and their families about PD and reduce stigma can be one way of making patients' lives more comfortable in low and middle-income communities. There is optimism regarding potential pathophysiologic therapies in the LMIC, including therapies addressing alpha-synuclein, neuroinflammation, and mitochondrial dysfunction among patients with PD. But to realize this potential, factors such as disease heterogeneity, lack of appropriate biomarkers, and limitations of existing/modern research models that are either not in or are not available in low and middle income or low-resourced communities, as well as medical professionals and facilities that can undertake screening exercises to diagnose and treat PD, are important in this context. Such gaps require collaboration and creative solutions based on scientific discoveries and applied in clinical applications. Understanding PD and the concerns it brings will help us to create a world in which treatment that can change lives for millions of people across the globe is a reality.

REFERENCES

Aarsland, D., Andersen, K., Larsen, J. P., Lolk, A., & Kragh-Sørensen, P. (2003). Prevalence and characteristics of dementia in Parkinson disease: An 8-year prospective study. *Archives of Neurology, 60*(3), 387–392. PMID: 12633150

Akinyemi, R. O., & Owolabi, M. O. (2023). Neurology in Africa: Bridging the gap between burden and resources. *The Lancet. Global Health, 11*(7), e1125–e1134. PMID: 37349038

Albin, R. L., Young, A. B., & Penney, J. B. (1989). The functional anatomy of basal ganglia disorders. *Trends in Neurosciences, 12*(10), 366–375. PMID: 2479133

Aubignat, M., Tir, M., & Krystkowiak, P. (2021). Non-motor symptoms of Parkinson's disease from pathophysiology to early diagnosis. *Revue de Médecine Interne, 42*(4), 251–257. DOI: 10.1016/j.revmed.2020.06.019 PMID: 32680717

Baradaran, N., Tan, S. N., Liu, A., Ashoori, A., Palmer, S. J., Wang, Z. J., Oishi, M. M., & McKeown, M. J. (2013). Parkinson's disease rigidity: Relation to brain connectivity and motor performance. *Frontiers in Neurology, 4*, 67. PMID: 23761780

Barber, D., Wijeratne, T., Singh, L., Barnham, K., & Masters, C. L. (2025). The search for disease modification in Parkinson's disease: A review of the literature. *Life (Chicago, Ill.), 15*. Advance online publication. DOI: 10.3390/life15081169 PMID: 40868817

Berardelli, A., Sabra, A. F., & Hallett, M. (1983). Physiological mechanisms of rigidity in Parkinson's disease. *Journal of Neurology, Neurosurgery, and Psychiatry, 46*(1), 45–53. DOI: 10.1136/jnnp.46.1.45 PMID: 6842199

Bhidayasiri, R. (2005). Differential diagnosis of common tremor syndromes. *Postgraduate Medical Journal, 81*(962), 756–762. PMID: 16344298

Bloem, B. R., Okun, M. S., & Klein, C. (2021). Parkinson's disease. *Lancet, 397*(10291), 2284–2303. DOI: 10.1016/S0140-6736(21)00218-X PMID: 33848468

DeMaagd, G., & Philip, A. (2015). Parkinson's disease and its management: Part 1—Disease entity, risk factors, pathophysiology, clinical presentation, and diagnosis. *P&T : a Peer-Reviewed Journal for Formulary Management, 40*(8), 504–532. PMID: 26236139

Denaro, F., Worthington, M., Williams, S., Benedetti, E., Zealand, D., & Davis, H.. (2022). Identification of increased blood–brain barrier permeability in the substantia nigra of HIV-1 transgenic rat. *Microscopy and Microanalysis*, *28*, 3214–3215. DOI: 10.1017/S1431927622011953

Dirkx, M., & Bologna, M. (2022). The pathophysiology of Parkinson's disease tremor. *Journal of the Neurological Sciences*, *435*, 120196. DOI: 10.1016/j.jns.2022.120196 PMID: 35240491

Eggers, C., Kahraman, D., Fink, G. R., Schmidt, M., & Timmermann, L. (2011). Akinetic-rigid and tremor-dominant Parkinson's disease patients show different patterns of FP-CIT single photon emission computed tomography. *Movement Disorders*, *26*(3), 416–423. PMID: 21264942

Eggers, C., Pedrosa, D. J., Kahraman, D., Maier, F., Lewis, C. J., Fink, G. R., Schmidt, M., & Timmermann, L. (2012). Parkinson subtypes progress differently in clinical course and imaging pattern. *PLoS One*, *7*(10), e46813. PMID: 23056463

Elefante, C., Brancaster, G. E., Bacciardi, S., Mazzucchi, S., Del Prete, E., & Palermo, G.. (2021). Prevalence and clinical correlates of comorbid anxiety and panic disorders in patients with Parkinson's disease. *Journal of Clinical Medicine*, *10*, 2302. PMID: 34070549

Evarts, E. V., Teräväinen, H., & Calne, D. B. (1981). Reaction time in Parkinson's disease. *Brain*, *104*(1), 167–186. PMID: 7470841

Fahn, S. (2011). Classification of movement disorders. *Movement Disorders*, *26*(6), 947–957. PMID: 21626541

Forsaa, E. B., Larsen, J. P., Wentzel-Larsen, T., & Alves, G. (2010). What predicts mortality in Parkinson disease? A prospective population-based long-term study. *Neurology*, *75*(14), 1270–1276. PMID: 20921512

Friedman, L. M., Furberg, C. D., DeMets, D. L., Reboussin, D. M., & Granger, C. B. (2015). *Fundamentals of clinical trials*. Springer.

Getz, K. A., & Campo, R. A. (2018). New benchmarks characterizing growth in protocol design complexity. *Therapeutic Innovation & Regulatory Science*, *52*, 22–28. DOI: 10.1177/2168479017713039 PMID: 29714620

Helmich, R. C., Hallett, M., Deuschl, G., Toni, I., & Bloem, B. R. (2012). Cerebral causes and consequences of parkinsonian resting tremor: A tale of two circuits? *Brain*, *135*(Pt 11), 3206–3226. PMID: 22382359

Helmich, R. C., Janssen, M. J. R., Oyen, W. J. G., Bloem, B. R., & Toni, I. (2011). Pallidal dysfunction drives a cerebellothalamic circuit into Parkinson tremor. *Annals of Neurology*, *69*(2), 269–281. PMID: 21387372

Hughes, A. J., Daniel, S. E., Kilford, L., & Lees, A. J. (1992). Accuracy of clinical diagnosis of idiopathic Parkinson's disease: A clinico-pathological study of 100 cases. *Journal of Neurology, Neurosurgery, and Psychiatry*, *55*(3), 181–184. PMID: 1564476

Ishiguro, M., Li, Y., & Yoshino, H.. (2021). Clinical manifestations of Parkinson's disease harboring VPS35 retromer complex component p.D620N with long-term follow-up. *Parkinsonism & Related Disorders*, *84*, 139–143. PMID: 33611076

Jaiswal, V., Alquraish, D., & Sandra, Z.. (2021). The influence of COVID-19 on Parkinson's disease: An updated systematic review. *Journal of Primary Care & Community Health*, *12*, 21501327211039708. PMID: 34404266

Jankovic, J., McDermott, M., Carter, J., Gauthier, S., Goetz, C., Golbe, L., Huber, S., Koller, W., Olanow, C., Shoulson, I., Stern, M., Tanner, C., & Weiner, W. (1990). Variable expression of Parkinson's disease: A base-line analysis of the DATATOP cohort. *Neurology*, *40*(10), 1529–1534. PMID: 2215943

Kassubek, J., Juengling, F. D., Hellwig, B., Spreer, J., & Lücking, C. H. (2002). Thalamic gray matter changes in unilateral Parkinsonian resting tremor: A voxel-based morphometric analysis of 3-dimensional magnetic resonance imaging. *Neuroscience Letters*, *323*(1), 29–32. PMID: 11911983

Kaur, R., Mehan, S., & Singh, S. (2019). Understanding multifactorial architecture of Parkinson's disease: Pathophysiology to management. *Neurological Sciences*. PMID: 30267336

Kish, S. J., Shannak, K., & Hornykiewicz, O. (1988). Uneven pattern of dopamine loss in the striatum of patients with idiopathic Parkinson's disease: Pathophysiologic and clinical implications. *The New England Journal of Medicine*, *318*(14), 876–880. PMID: 3352672

Lang, A. E., & Espay, A. J. (2018). Disease modification in Parkinson's disease: Current approaches, challenges, and future considerations. *Movement Disorders*, *33*, 660–677. DOI: 10.1002/mds.27360 PMID: 29644751

Lee, Y., Chang, Y. Y., Chen, Y. F., Lin, T. K., Hung, C. F., & Chiou, Y. J.. (2022). Prevalence and risk factors of depression between patients with Parkinson's disease and their caregivers: A one-year prospective study. *Health Care*, *10*, 1305. PMID: 35885832

Lewis, S. J. G., Foltynie, T., Blackwell, A. D., Robbins, T. W., Owen, A. M., & Barker, R. A. (2005). Heterogeneity of Parkinson's disease in the early clinical stages using a data driven approach. *Journal of Neurology, Neurosurgery, and Psychiatry, 76*(3), 343–348. PMID: 15716523

Lo, R. Y., Tanner, C. M., Albers, K. B., Leimpeter, A. D., Fross, R. D., Bernstein, A. L., McGuire, V., Quesenberry, C. P., Nelson, L. M., Van Den Eeden, S. K., & Tanner, C. M. (2009). Clinical features in early Parkinson disease and survival. *Archives of Neurology, 66*(11), 1353–1358. PMID: 19901166

Louis, E. D., Levy, G., Côte, L. J., Mejia, H., Fahn, S., & Marder, K. (2001). Clinical correlates of action tremor in Parkinson disease. *Archives of Neurology, 58*(10), 1630–1634. PMID: 11594921

Louis, E. D., Tang, M. X., Cote, L., Alfaro, B., Mejia, H., & Marder, K. (1999). Progression of parkinsonian signs in Parkinson disease. *Archives of Neurology, 56*(3), 334–337. PMID: 10190824

Magrinelli, F., Picelli, A., & Tocco, P. (2016). Pathophysiology of motor dysfunction in Parkinson's disease as the rationale for drug treatment and rehabilitation. *Parkinson's Disease, 9832839*. Advance online publication. DOI: 10.1155/2016/9832839 PMID: 27366343

Marino, B. L. B., de Souza, L. R., Sousa, K. P. A., Ferreira, J. V., Padilha, E. C., & da Silva, C. H. T. P.. (2020). Parkinson's disease: A review from pathophysiology to treatment. *Mini-Reviews in Medicinal Chemistry, 20*, 754–767. DOI: 10.2174/1389557519666191104110908 PMID: 31686637

McGhee, D. J. M., Ritchie, C. W., Zajicek, J. P., & Counsell, C. E. (2016). Clinical trial designs used to detect disease-modifying effects in Alzheimer's and Parkinson's disease. *BMC Neurology, 16*, 92. DOI: 10.1186/s12883-016-0606-3 PMID: 27312378

Mure, H., Hirano, S., Tang, C. C., Isaias, I. U., Antonini, A., Ma, Y., Dhawan, V., & Eidelberg, D. (2011). Parkinson's disease tremor-related metabolic network: Characterization, progression, and treatment effects. *NeuroImage, 54*(2), 1244–1253. PMID: 20851193

Olugbemi, T., Olaniyan, C. O., Adetunji, A. D., Olorunsola, A., Mayowa, J., & Adeniyi, A. E. (2023). Prevention and diagnosis of neurodegenerative diseases using machine learning models. In *Artificial Intelligence for Neurological Disorders* (pp. 289–304). Academic Press.

Poletti, M., Frosini, D., Pagni, C., Baldacci, F., Nicoletti, V., Tognoni, G., Lucetti, C., Del Dotto, P., Ceravolo, R., & Bonuccelli, U. (2012). Mild cognitive impairment and cognitive-motor relationships in newly diagnosed drug-naive patients with Parkinson's disease. *Journal of Neurology, Neurosurgery, and Psychiatry*, *83*(6), 601–606. PMID: 22492216

Prodoehl, J., Planetta, P. J., Kurani, A. S., Comella, C. L., Corcos, D. M., & Vaillancourt, D. E. (2013). Differences in brain activation between tremor- and nontremor-dominant Parkinson disease. *JAMA Neurology*, *70*(1), 100–106. PMID: 23318516

Rodriguez-Oroz, M. C., Jahanshahi, M., Krack, P., Litvan, I., Macias, R., Bezard, E., & Obeso, J. A. (2009). Initial clinical manifestations of Parkinson's disease: Features and pathophysiological mechanisms. *Lancet Neurology*, *8*(12), 1128–1139. PMID: 19909911

Rosenberg-Katz, K., Herman, T., Jacob, Y., Giladi, N., Hendler, T., & Hausdorff, J. M. (2013). Gray matter atrophy distinguishes between Parkinson disease motor subtypes. *Neurology*, *80*(16), 1476–1484. PMID: 23516323

Rossi, C., Volterrani, D., Nicoletti, V., Mugnaini, M., Frosini, D., Kiferle, L., Unti, E., De Feo, P., Bonuccelli, U., & Ceravolo, R. (2010). "Parkinson-dementia" diseases: From pathogenetic mechanisms to possible treatment strategies. *Journal of Alzheimer's Disease*, *21*(1), 3–23. PMID: 20378955

Schapira, A. H. (2009). Neurobiology and treatment of Parkinson's disease. *Trends in Pharmacological Sciences*, *30*(1), 41–47. PMID: 19042040

Spiegel, J., Hellwig, D., Samnick, S., Jost, W., Fassbender, K., Kirsch, C. M., & Dillmann, U. (2007). Striatal FP-CIT uptake differs in the subtype of early Parkinson's disease. *Journal of Nuclear Medicine*, *48*(3), 359–364. PMID: 17332612

Sveinbjornsdottir, S. (2016). The clinical symptoms of Parkinson's disease. *Journal of Neurochemistry*, *139*, 318–324. PMID: 27401947

Thenganatt, M. A., & Louis, E. D. (2012). Distinguishing essential tremor from Parkinson's disease: Bedside tests and laboratory evaluations. *Expert Review of Neurotherapeutics*, *12*(6), 687–696. PMID: 22650171

Toth, C., Rajput, A., & Rajput, A. H. (2004). Anomalies of asymmetry of clinical signs in parkinsonism. *Movement Disorders*, *19*(3), 151–157. PMID: 14978669

Treweek, S., Pitkethly, M., & Cook, J.. (2018). Strategies to improve recruitment to randomized trials. *Cochrane Database of Systematic Reviews*, *2*, MR000013. PMID: 29468635

Vázquez-Vélez, G. E., & Zoghbi, H. Y. (2021). Parkinson's disease genetics and pathophysiology. *Annual Review of Neuroscience*, *44*(1), 87–108. PMID: 34236893

Williams-Gray, C. H., Foltynie, T., Brayne, C. E. G., Robbins, T. W., & Barker, R. A. (2007). Evolution of cognitive dysfunction in an incident Parkinson's disease cohort. *Brain*, *130*(Pt 7), 1787–1798. PMID: 17535834

Zakaria, R., Lenz, F. A., Hua, S., Avin, B. H., Liu, C. C., & Mari, Z. (2013). Thalamic physiology of intentional essential tremor is more like cerebellar tremor than postural essential tremor. *Brain Research*, *1529*, 188–199. PMID: 23856324

Zhu, M., Li, M., Ye, D., Jiang, W., Lei, T., & Shu, K. (2016). Sensory symptoms in Parkinson's disease: Clinical features, pathophysiology, and treatment. *Journal of Neuroscience Research*, *94*(8), 685–692. PMID: 26948282

Chapter 2
Diagnostic Challenges of Parkinson Disease in Under-Resourced Settings

U. Subhalakshmi
http://orcid.org/0009-0007-8989-5486
Department of Microbiology, Sacred Heart College, Tirupattur, India

G. Vithiya
http://orcid.org/0009-0001-0729-4318
Department of Microbiology, Sacred Heart College, Tirupattur, India

P. Saranraj
http://orcid.org/0000-0002-5052-6532
Department of Microbiology, Sacred Heart College, Tirupattur, India

B. Lokeshwari
http://orcid.org/0009-0005-6612-5134
Department of Microbiology, Sacred Heart College, Tirupattur, India

S. Kanshiya
Department of Microbiology, Sacred Heart College, Tirupattur, India

M. Manigandan
http://orcid.org/0000-0002-8115-2713
Department of Microbiology, Sacred Heart College, Tirupattur, India

ABSTRACT

Parkinson's Disease (PD) diagnosis in developing and low-resource settings is hampered by a mix of clinical, structural, and sociocultural factors that produce late, missed, or incorrect diagnoses. This ambiguity is exacerbated in poor- and Middle-Income Countries (LMICs) by a lack of neurologists and movement-disorder experts, limited access to specialized diagnostics and confirmatory imaging, poor public and primary-care awareness, and sociocultural obstacles that cause delays in presentation. The diagnostic gap is further exacerbated by poor referral systems, transportation and financial obstacles, and the misattribution of symptoms at the

DOI: 10.4018/979-8-3373-7437-6.ch002

community level to aging or non-neurological reasons. Emerging solutions include task-shifting to trained primary-care workers, telemedicine, simplified clinical screening tools, and novel low-cost biomarkers such as blood-based assays. However, these require further validation and context-sensitive implementation.

INTRODUCTION

Parkinson's disease is the second most prevalent neurological condition, affecting more than six million people worldwide. Research studies are currently being carried out to investigate drugs that are specific to various subtypes. Parkinson's disease has a complex neuropsychiatric condition that is now mostly identified by motor symptoms, while neuropsychiatric markers are increasingly being recognized as being important in a range of contexts (Shang et al., 2023). The clinical indicators are the same as those of other neurodegenerative disorders, therefore existing diagnostic methods and biomarkers cannot definitively diagnose the disease in its early stages. Even when the disease is fully evident, the clinical diagnosis is therefore inaccurate. Identification of prodromal sickness is a critical issue that remains unresolved. This is due to the fact that now is the best moment for future disease-modifying medicines to produce positive. Parkinson's disease affects a variety of demographics. Each group's causes, signs, and chances for recovery are different. This is treatment plans need to be customized. Parkinson's disease that is monogenic is the most obvious example. Studies are now being conducted to look into medications that are unique to certain subtypes (Antonini et al., 2003).

The three primary categories of symptoms are mood (such as depression and anxiety), perception and reasoning (such as psychosis), and motivation (such as apathy and difficulty subduing cravings). PD aims to advance translational medicine in African nations by introducing state-of-the-art genetic technologies (Kalluri & LeBleu, 2020). It will also demonstrate focusing on the distinct genetic composition of those who are excluded could contribute to a healthier world. The latter ultimately deteriorates. It may from cell death in the area of the brain that produces dopamine and regulates balance and movement. This sickness affects more than 10 million people worldwide. By 2050, 20 million people worldwide are predicted to have Parkinson's disease (Matsui et al., 2005). There is no known cure, although there are treatments and drugs that can reduce the symptoms.

The main symptoms are tense muscles, shaking, and difficulty speaking, one of the primary causes of dependency and disability is this illness (Gomperts et al., 2012). Dementia is another frequent consequence of Parkinson's disease. Parkinson's Disease (PD) can damage cognitive abilities such as memory and language. Parkinson's Disease (PD) can cause dementia and concomitant conditions. Recent research indicates that Parkinson's disease can be more accurately diagnosed using enhanced clinical diagnostic criteria (Dorsey et al., 2018). Due to its clinical symptoms might be confused with those of other neurodegenerative diseases, the illness is more challenging to diagnose. Moreover, there are yet no trustworthy biomarkers or diagnostic methods that could facilitate a prompt, conclusive diagnosis. The accuracy of the clinical diagnosis is still subpar even after the disease has fully advanced (Ling et al., 2016). However, detecting prodromal disease is an important unmet need, as this stage provides the best opportunity for future disease-modifying drugs to be effective. Since the many subgroups of Parkinson's disease have distinct underlying pathophysiology's, clinical presentations, and prognostic outcomes, it is imperative to characterize them (Petrou et al., 2012). This calls for individualized treatment plans. In clinical trials, subtype-specific treatment is currently being tried for monogenic Parkinson's disease, the most prevalent occurrence. Patients should see a doctor at least once because Parkinson's disease can cause fatal severe acute and subacute symptoms. One only. Either the disease process itself or the way it interacts with different medical and surgical procedures in an emergency. some diseases can be difficult to identify and treat (Fereshtehnejad et al., 2017).

EPIDEMIOLOGY CAUSES AND MODIFIED FACTORS

Parkinson's disease worsens with age, yet its incidence and prevalence increase as people age (Asuku et al., 2022; Asuku et al. 2024). Parkinson's disease does not, however, primarily affect the elderly. Over a quarter of persons with the illness experience symptoms before the age of sixty-five, and five to ten percent experience symptoms before the age of fifty (Sperling et al., 2018). The term "early onset" was created to describe individuals with Parkinson's disease whose symptoms started before they turned forty or even fifty years old. Despite the fact that the illness is widespread around the world, China has a remarkably high rate of new cases, and high-income European nations are growing quickly (Beach et al., 2010). Parkinson's disease can affect both men and women, but women may have certain advantages over males because it usually manifests earlier in life and is less frequent in women, particularly in older people (Oertel et al., 2014). Three key elements are examined in the research of Parkinson's disease etiology: environment, heredity, and the interaction of these elements.

It is impossible to assess environmental influences that might have affected a person ten years ago or that have built up over time, perhaps in combination with inherited characteristics. Further limiting ethiological study is the brain's inaccessibility (Meloni et al., 2023). Interestingly, the only method to determine what makes Parkinson's disease worse is to do long-term research. These factors are typically different from those that increase the likelihood of getting the illness (He et al., 2017). Table 1 depicting the etiology of Parkinson's disease was developed based on the information above in order to highlight the primary elements affecting the onset and course of the disease. The primary risk factor mentioned is age, along with significant genetic alterations and biological contaminants. The primary effects of biologic sex are listed in the table along with other preventive variables like exercise. It is important because it offers details on the intricate relationships between environmental and biologic elements, with an emphasis on those that affect development and those that affect progression.

Table 1. Comprehensive Summary of Parkinson's Disease: Epidemiology, Etiology, and Modifying Factors

Category	Specific Factor/ Example	Mechanism / Evidence	Associated Risk/ Effect	Notes & Implications	Reference
Primary Epidemiology	Age	The strongest risk factors. Neuronal resilience declines, and cellular repair mechanisms become less efficient with age.	Risk increases exponentially after age 60; majority of cases are sporadic and late-onset.	While aging is not the cause, it creates a permissive environment for other factors to trigger neurodegeneration.	(Rossi et al., 2009)
Genetic Factors	Monogenic Forms **(e.g., SNCA, LRRK2, PARKIN mutations)**	Mutations cause autosomal dominant or recessive inheritance, leading to protein aggregation, mitochondrial dysfunction.	High penetrance; accounts for ~5-10% of cases, especially in early-onset and familial PD.	Provides crucial insights into disease pathways (e.g., alpha-synuclein pathology) relevant to sporadic PD.	(Swallow & Counsell, 2023)
Environmental Exposures	Pesticides & Herbicides **(e.g., Rotenone, Paraquat)**	In animal models, inhibit mitochondrial complex I, raise oxidative stress, and encourage alpha-synuclein aggregation.	Strong epidemiological link; rural living and well-water use are associated risks.	Suggests a "multiple-hit" hypothesis where toxins interact with genetic susceptibility over time.	(He et al., 2017)
Protective & Modifiable Factors	Physical Activity & Exercise	Promotes neurotrophic factors (BDNF), reduces neuroinflammation, and may enhance mitochondrial health and synaptic plasticity.	Regular correlation with a lower chance of getting Parkinson's disease and a slower rate of disease development.	A non-pharmacological intervention for motor and non-motor symptoms in diagnosed patients.	(Mahlknecht et al., 2015)
Sex Differences	Biological Sex **(Lower incidence in women)**	Potential protective effects of estrogen, differences in immune response, and X-linked genetic factors.	Women have a ~1.5 times lower lifetime risk and often a later age of onset compared to men.	Influences symptom presentation (e.g., more tremor dominant in women) and response to treatment.	(Shahed & Jankovic, 2007)

continued on following page

Table 1. Continued

Category	Specific Factor/ Example	Mechanism / Evidence	Associated Risk/ Effect	Notes & Implications	Reference
Age-Related Mechanisms	Cellular Senescence & Inflammation	Accumulation of senescent cells and "inflammaging" (chronic, low-grade inflammation) in the brain microenvironment.	Creates a pro-degenerative milieu that may accelerate the loss of dopaminergic neurons.	A growing research focus for novel therapeutic targets aimed at modifying the disease process.	(Andersson et al., 2018)
Gene-Environment Interaction	GBA Mutations & Toxin Exposure	Neurons that carry GBA mutations, a significant genetic risk factor, may have compromised lysosomal function, which increases their susceptibility to environmental pollutants.	Synergistic effect significantly increases risk beyond either factor alone.	Highlights the complex interplay explaining why only some exposed individuals develop PD.	(Shahed & Jankovic, 2007)
Progression vs. Onset	Smoking & Caffeine	Inverse association with **disease risk** (protective for onset), but mixed or negligible evidence for slowing **disease progression**.	Protective for **risk of developing PD**; not a confirmed modifier after diagnosis.	A critical distinction for research: factors influencing initiation of pathology differ from those affecting its clinical course.	(Tolosa et al., 2020)

EXOSOME ISOLATION METHODS AND miRNA EXPRESSION CHARACTERIZATION

Despite the promising of Exosomal miRs in indicators and treatments of Parkinson's disease, there have been technical difficulties in obtaining exosomes and determining the expression levels of the miRs (Faghri et al., 2018). There are significant differences among the tiny vesicles called exosomes. Extremely precise techniques are needed to separate them since they usually need to be purified with other extracellular vesicles and impurities (Gilman et al., 2008). Even now, ultracentrifugation remains the most used method. Exosomes are separated by size and density using density gradients and high-speed centrifugation. One drawback of the method is that shear forces might cause vesicles to break apart and lose their miRNA content (Shah et al., 2016). SEC is a very powerful tool in miRNA analysis, as high recovery rates are achieved without compromising the integrity of the exosomal structure and RNA cargo. Techniques utilized for the extraction and analysis of exosomal microRNA in the study of Parkinson's disease (Marras & Lang, 2013). On the left panel, biofluids such as serum, plasma, urine, saliva, or cerebrospinal fluid (CSF) are collected by liquid biopsy. Techniques such as size exclusion chromatography, precipitation, ultracentrifugation, or immunoaffinity capture methods are used to separate or concentrate the exosomes; see center panel. Transmission

Electron Microscopy (TEM), Dynamic Light Scattering (DLS), or Nanoparticle Tracking Analysis (NTA) are used to analyze the size of the exosome, exosomal markers through Western Blotting, and ELISA, while Flow Cytometry is done on the surface markers of the exosomes (Tolosa et al., 2009). The idea is to isolate the exosomes for miRNA analysis in the later stages. A method for the detection and analysis of microRNAs associated with Parkinson's disease. Exosomal microRNA analysis in general. Findings in the left panel relate to the separation of RNA from the purified exosomes (Cilia et al., 2014). The middle panel demonstrates customized miRNA expression profiles with high resolution are determined using.

Figure 1. Exosome Isolation and miRNA Analysis in Parkinson's Disease

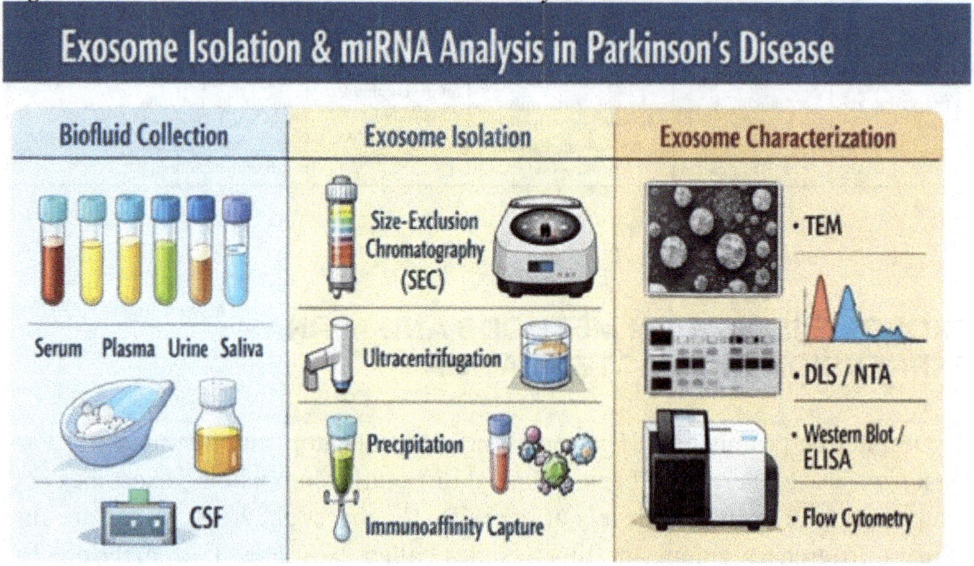

Exosomes

Exosomes are small vesicles with membranes measuring between 40 and 100 nm. The vesicles are used to deliver several types of biological cargo to the target cells; this includes proteins, lipids, and nucleic acids. Multivesicular bodies (MVBs) produce exosomes (Guevremont et al., 2023). Together, these vesicles create early sorting endosomes, which subsequently develop into late sorting endosomes, late sorting endosomal membranes invade and produce a large number of ILVs. Late-sorting endosomes as MVB (Shirvan et al., 2019). The MVB can then either break down these ILV by joining with lysosomes or release them as exosomes by interacting with the plasma membrane. Urine, saliva, blood, and CSF are some of the fluids in the body made up of exosomes. Neurons, immune cells, and MSCs are a few of the cells that release them (Dickson et al., 2009). Exosomes transport a vast array of substances, including proteins, lipids, and genetic material like DNA and RNA. Lipids are required for the synthesis and release of exosomes into the environment, much as they are for membrane.

Figure 2. miRNA Analysis Workflow

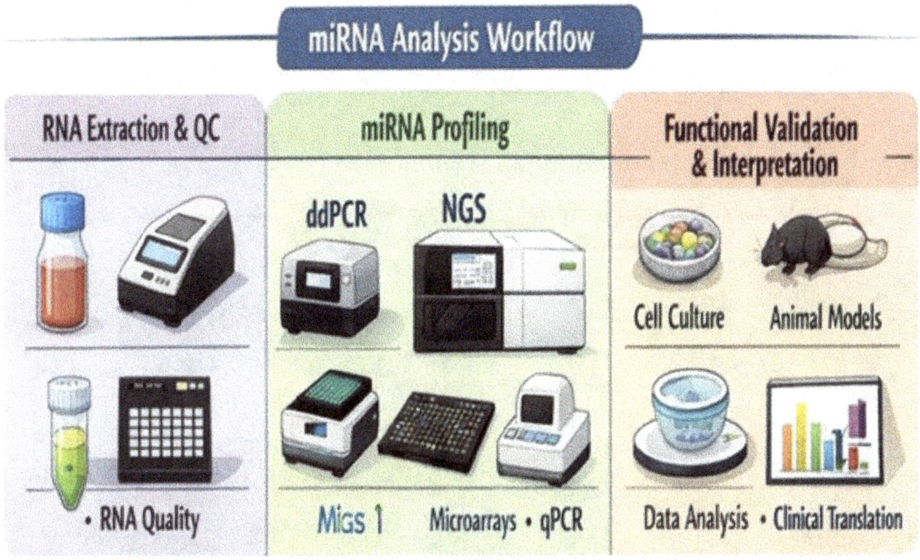

miRNA in Animal Models of Parkinson's Disease

Animal Models of Parkinson's Disease miRNA in together alongside the additional neuroprotective miRNAs, miR-7, miR-30e, and miR-124 in MPTP-caused Parkinson's disease mice, decreased neuroinflammation and maintained dopaminergic neurons (Jellinger, 2012). Two regulators of neuroinflammatory responses, miR-7 and miR-30e, both block the NLRP3 inflammasome. MiR-124, on the other hand, reduces inflammation by inhibiting microglial activation via the MEKK3/NF-κB signalling (Manna et al., 2021). Additionally, miR-190 enhances neuroprotection and delays neurodegeneration by lowering oxidative stress and inflammatory signaling. However, additional miRNAs appear to exacerbate the mechanisms (Rossi et al., 2009) behind Parkinson's disease. Neuronal damage and neuroinflammation are associated with ROCK1 signaling. Overexpression of miR-195 triggers the activation of microglia. In addition to controlling inflammatory pathways including the

SOCS1/Nrf2 signaling pathway and the NLRP3 in the flammasome, miR-29c-3p and miR-155-5p also alter immune system function and microglia activity (Shahed & Jankovic, 2007). By connecting STAT3, SOCS1, and PDK1/IFN, the JAK/STAT pathway provides regulatory input via TET2/autophagy and AKT (Kordower et al., 2013). It is possible that FoxO1 could provide regulatory input through these routes. The outcomes are in line with TET2's vital role in anti-inflammatory signaling via autophagy activation and SOCS1 overexpression. AKT and autophagy (via TET2 and FoxO1) provide additional layers of regulation to govern pro- and anti-inflammatory responses. These systems cooperate to control anti-inflammatory and pro-inflammatory reactions (Armstrong et al., 2013).

Figure 3. miRNA in Parkinson's Disease pathways

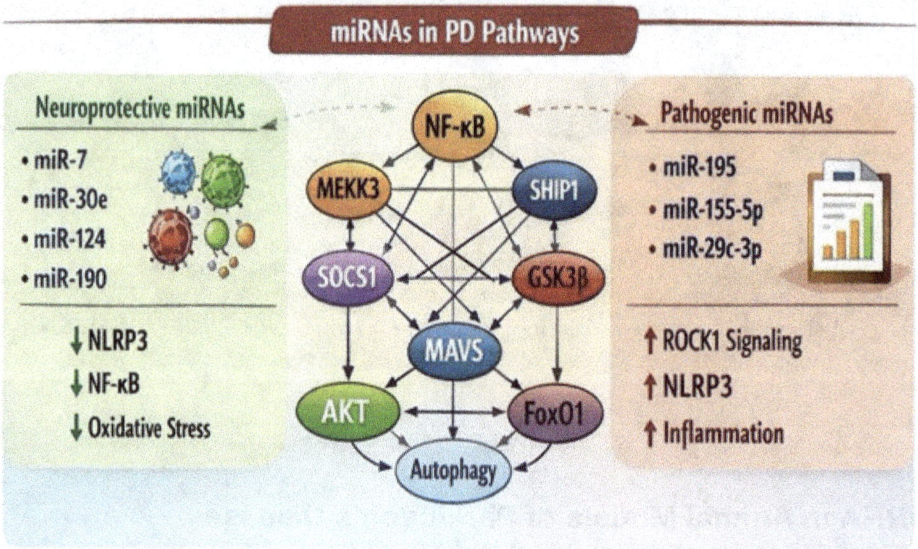

CARDINAL MOTOR SYMPTOMS IN PD IDENTIFICATION

Parkinson's disease is characterized by bradykinesia, rigidity, resting tremor, and loss of postural reflexes. Other clinical manifestations as the disease advances include neuro-ophthalmologic abnormalities, bulbar dysfunction, and respiratory issues. The majority of motor symptoms of PD are responsive to dopaminergic therapy (Maini Rekdal et al., 2019). This is one of the distinguishing signs that could differentiate PD from other parkinsonian disorders.

Tremor

The most obvious sign of Parkinson's disease is rest tremor. Although it can happen in the lips, chin, and mouth, it mainly happens in the arms and legs when there is a lot of muscle contraction and relaxation (Fanciulli & Wenning, 2015). Pronation and supination are the two main ways that rest tremors in the hands manifest, state that sleep or exercise may help with these tremors. People with Parkinson's disease have also been reported to experience postural tremor, which happens when a person lies down against gravity (Lobotesis et al., 2001). More noticeable than rest tremor, postural tremor could be one of the first indications of Parkinson's disease. In contrast to essential tremors, both kinds of tremors happen at the same frequency range (4–6 Hz) and can be treated with dopaminergic medications (Donaghy et al., 2020). Botulinum toxins, beta-blockers, and alcohol may all be useful therapy for essential tremor. However, they may have more frequent tremors in their head and voice. Parkinson's disease risk is increased in early childhood by essential tremor (Pringsheim et al., 2014).

Quick Eye Motion Disorders of Sleep Behavior

RBD, restless legs syndrome, and sleep apnea are the most prevalent nonmotor indicators of Parkinson's disease. Parkinson's disease, a prevalent cause of sleep issues, has been most strongly linked to RBD (Dilsiz, 2024). RBD is a form of insomnia that is linked to decreased muscle tone, REM sleep, and constantly replaying dreams (Li et al., 2018). Understanding the distinction between sleepwalking and dreaming is crucial since sleepwalking typically occurs during non-REM sleep. Muscle activation on the electromyogram channels during polysomnography indicates RBD (Harding & Halliday, 2001). It has been linked to many system atrophies, Parkinson's disease, Lewy body dementia, and other synucleopathies. RBD patients are expected to have a much higher risk of developing Parkinson's Disease (PD) than the general population (Martínez-Fernández et al., 2018). Once they do, their condition deteriorates more rapidly than it does for people without RBD. RBD is the best early sign for diagnosing sickness because of its high specificity and predictive value. However, this is not particularly helpful in clinical practice since it requires the use of electromyogram channels to represent muscle activity and polysomnography, which is a costly and time-consuming procedure (Gui et al., 2015). Certain synucleinopathies are associated with RBD. These include Parkinson's disease, Lewy body dementia, and other systemic atrophies. those with RBD are more likely than the general population to develop Parkinson's disease, and they learn how to move more quickly than those without RBD. Among the aforementioned, RBD is the most precise and predictive precursor; nevertheless, polysomnography is hardly employed in practice due to its high cost and time requirements (Irwin et al., 2012).

EVOLUTION OF DIAGNOSTIC PARKINSONIAN SYMPTOMS

Degenerative Parkinson's Disease can be in many forms, but it lacks a symptom by which it can be easily identified (Antonini et al., 2001). Therefore, in the last few decades, certain criteria have been established, which are mainly based on the efficacy of a drug and the appearance or absence of certain symptoms. These criteria have been formed to identify and classify individuals who are affected by it in such a manner that it may be enhanced and improve their quality of life (Poewe et al., 2020). The attempt to identify and understand Parkinson's disease was made by Hoehn and Yahr back in 1967, who found 77 characteristics based on what was collected during the two-year survey done on patients suffering from Parkinson's (Lees et al., 2009). The characteristics include Neurological symptoms, co-existing syndromes, medical history, characteristics of the disease, and the level of disability (Mahlknecht et al., 2015). The percentage of individuals suffering from Parkinson's was not based on age or gender factors, which is very surprising. The most common initial presentation of the disease was said to be stiffness and tremors; it was said to progress slowly and render movement difficult. The Activities of Daily Living (ADL) scale was created two years later by Schwab and England (Matsuda et al., 2010). This scale can be used by those with Parkinson's Disease (PD) as a measure of the extent of reduced mobility in their lives each day. This percentage of the patient's every day life rendered dysfunctional due to the disease's symptoms is measured on the scale; the first set of clinical diagnostic criteria for Parkinson's Disease (PD) was proposed by the United Kingdom Parkinson's Disease Society Brain Bank (UKPDSBB). The entire process of classification is composed of three parts, namely the diagnostic criteria, exclusion criteria, and supportive criteria (Firbank et al., 2005). Presence of Babinski sign, encephalitis, early severe autonomic involvement/dementia, a history of repeated stroke/head trauma, inadequate response to levodopa medication, exposure to MPTP (1-methyl-4-phenyl-1,2,3,6-tetrahydropyridine), and any one of the following: bradykinesia, Levodopa-induced dyskinesia, persistent symmetry not present, progressive course, unilateral onset, rest tremor present, good response to dopaminergic medications, good response to levodopa therapy for five years or longer, clinical course of the disease for ten years or longer are all the required features according to Dutta et al. (2021). As the levodopa medication, motor function improved. This led to a greater emphasis on the nonmotor characteristics of PD patients, demonstrating the limitations of the UKPDSBB and Gelb criteria. Due to their importance and influence on quality of life, better recommendations that take these attributes into account have been generated. In 2009, Lees and his associates enhanced the Queen Square Brain Bank's (QSBB) clinical diagnostic standards in order to solve this problem. Originally based on the UKPDSBB criteria, this proposal was later extended to include nonmotor characteristics such as hyposmia and hallucinations (Del Tredici et al., 2010). It assisted medical practitioners in diagnosing Parkinson's illness. Hallucinations may indicate that a different diagnosis was intended, according to the Gelb criteria. This is a major development. Parkinson's disease patients mostly experience problems with their autonomic nervous system, sleep, mental health, and smell. these symptoms were linked to MDS-PD, a distinct illness type that resembles Parkinson's disease. Table 2 shows the evolution of Parkinson's Disease (PD) criteria and diagnosis during the past 50 years. Structured clinical diagnosis criteria (UKPDSBB, Gelb) come after the motor-centric tests created by Hoehn and Yahr. The inclusion of non-motor symptoms (Queen Square modification) and the deliberate blending of excluding and supportive factors to differentiate Parkinson's Disease (PD) from other parkinsonisms (MDS Criteria) were important turning points. The pre-motor, prodromal phase (MDS Research Criteria), which aims to identify people who are at risk long before the usual motor symptoms arise, is highlighted at the end of the timeline. Future methods to avoid the illness from this (Foster et al., 2010).

Table 2. The Evolution of Diagnostic Criteria for Parkinson's Disease (1967-2015): From Motor Scales to Integrated Clinical Guidelines

Timeline / Milestone	Components & Symptoms	Purpose & Impact	Limitations & Evolution	Reference
Hoehn & Yahr Staging (1967)	Motor disability progression (Stages I-V). Early symptoms: tremor, rigidity, bradykinesia.	First standardized scale to describe disease severity and progression. Established a common language for clinicians.	Purely motor-based; did not account for non-motor symptoms or quality of life.	(van Meer et al., 2008)
Schwab & England ADL Scale (1969)	Percentage-based assessment of independence in daily activities (100% = normal, 0% = vegetative).	Provided a patient-centric measure of functional capacity and impact on quality of life.	Subjective measure; still focused on motor disability without addressing non-motor burden.	(Zervos et al., 2018)
UKPDSBB Criteria (1992)	Step 1: Postural instability, stiffness, or tremor plus bradykinesia. Step 2: Exclusion criteria (e.g., encephalitis history). Step 3: Supportive criteria (e.g., excellent levodopa response, unilateral onset).	Introduced a structured, multi-step diagnostic algorithm, increasing diagnostic specificity. Became the clinical gold standard for decades.	Over-reliance on motor response to levodopa; largely ignored non-motor symptoms (e.g., considered hallucinations an exclusion).	(Fanciulli & Wenning, 2015)

continued on following page

Table 2. Continued

Timeline / Milestone	Components & Symptoms	Purpose & Impact	Limitations & Evolution	Reference
Gelb et al. Criteria (1999)	Core feature: Bradykinesia. Supporting features: rest tremor, rigidity. Exclusionary features similar to UKPDSBB.	Aimed to simplify and operationalize diagnosis for clinical research studies.	Maintained strict exclusion of non-motor features, failing to reflect the full clinical spectrum of PD.	(Harding & Halliday, 2001)
Queen Square Brain Bank Revision (2009)	Added supportive non-motor criteria: hyposmia, visual hallucinations, REM sleep behavior disorder (RBD). Reclassified hallucinations as supportive, not exclusionary.	Incorporated crucial non-motor aspects into the diagnostic framework, recognizing them as intrinsic to PD.	A significant update, but still a modification of the motor-centric UKPDSBB framework rather than a full overhaul.	(Ortega-Pinazo et al., 2023)
MDS Clinical Diagnostic Criteria (2015)	Absolute Exclusion Criteria (such as anomalies in the cerebellum). Red flags, such as quick development. Supportive Criteria: **non-motor symptoms, positive levodopa response, dopaminergic deficit on imaging.**	First to formally integrate **"Red Flags"** to warn of atypical parkinsonism. More balanced evaluation of motor and non-motor evidence.	Complex but more accurate. Represented a paradigm shift from rigid lists to a probabilistic, clinically nuanced approach.	(Zhou et al., 2016)
MDS Research Criteria for Prodromal PD (2015)	Identifies risk markers (e.g., RBD, hyposmia, specific genetic mutations) and calculates probability of prodromal disease.	Shifts focus to **pre-motor diagnosis**, enabling research into disease prevention and neuroprotective therapies.	Not for clinical diagnosis; intended solely for research to identify at-risk populations for interventional trials.	(Matsuda et al., 2010)

PET Imaging of Neuroinflammation

Neuropathological analyses conducted after death verify that the 11C-PIB PET uptake correctly depicts amyloid buildup before death. A pathology-validated investigation identified the apparent gradient of increasing amyloidopathy detected by PET as follows, PD < PD-MCI < PDD < DLB (Jiang et al., 2021). The substantial pathogenic diversity of these diseases may lead to uneven. Over 50% of DLB patients had elevated 11C-PIB binding, which could be crucial for diagnosis. The majority of PDD patients and all PD patients showed no discernible variations in 11C-PIB binding. However, studies on DLB have revealed that compared to controls, there are greater amyloid deposits in the striatum, cingulum, and frontal and temporoparietal cortices. Increased amyloid pathology on PET scans is most consistently linked to reduced overall cognition in LBSD, despite inconsistent data about its association to the onset of dementia, motor capabilities, and the course of dementia. People with amyloid-positive PET scans did worse on mini-mental state and daily functioning assessments, according to a recent one-year study of DLB patients. Both striatal and cortical amyloidopathy are linked to increased cognitive dysfunction in Parkinson's Disease (PD) when compared to cortical amyloidopathy alone (Ren et al., 2019). This suggests that amyloid deposition has detrimental and cumulative effects on cognition. Although amyloid buildup in the brain due to PSP, MSA, and CBD/CBS disorders may be seen by 11C-PIB PET, this could be due to changes brought on by aging. When paired with cerebrospinal fluid examination that reveals decreased amyloid beta-42 and increased total tau/phospho-tau, a significant tracer retention on amyloid PET may indicate intrinsic Alzheimer's Disease (AD) pathology, ruling out the diagnoses of PSP and CBD/CBS (51,52) (Shang et al., 2023). Amyloid imaging is especially important in this aspect since patients with REM Sleep Behavior Disorder are substantially more susceptible to develop α-synucleinopathies (Galvin et al., 2001). These methods must be used to rule out Alzheimer's disease in future trials of possible tau-based disease-modifying therapies in individuals with PSP and CBS. Increased 11C-PK11195 binding was seen in the left substantia nigra and occipital lobe in polysomnography-validated cases of idiopathic RBD (probably indicating a higher risk of developing DLB); however, no significant changes in 11C-PK11195 binding were seen in the putamen or caudate, despite decreased 18F-dopa uptake in the putamen. To find biomarkers for RBD patients who are vulnerable to overt clinical synucleinopathy, such as dementia or parkinsonism, longitudinal research is required.

The blood flow in the brain Using a range of radiotracers, SPECT measures variations in blood flow in various brain regions to determine the metabolic status of brain tissue. Although occipital hypoperfusion is frequently seen in DLB, this is not always the case. The likelihood that DLB is the primary cause should increase when the illness manifests. When 99mTc-HMPAO was employed as a radiotracer, both AD and DLB subjects displayed varying degrees of temporal parietal hypoperfusion in comparison to controls. However, the primary distinction between AD and DLB was occipital hypoperfusion. Other SPECT radiotracers, such as 123I-IMP and 99mTc-ECD, have been used to record occipital hypoperfusion. In several studies, perfusion SPECT showed similar perfusion profiles; nonetheless, it was difficult to distinguish between cases with PDD and DLB (Théry et al., 2018).

Additionally, DLB patients without visual hallucinations may be distinguished from CBS at an earlier stage of the disease by hypoperfusion in the left occipital region and reduced episodic memory function. Frontal lobe blood flow is decreased in people with PD and MSA-P (Song et al., 2015). But according to SPECT scans, PD sufferers' occipital brains exhibited less blood flow than those of healthy individuals. Frontal lobe hypoperfusion was discovered during a one-year longitudinal study on Parkinson's illness. While MSA-C patients demonstrated localized cerebral atrophy in the pons and cerebellum in comparison to controls, MSA-P patients displayed hypoperfusion in the putamen, in contrast to PD. Few studies concentrating on MSA, PSP, and CBS, small sample sizes, and a dearth of pathology-validated trials are the main constraints on the current research on perfusion SPECT. Perfusion SPECT may also be inferior to other methods, such as DAT imaging or 123I-metaiodobenzylguanidine myocardial scintigraphy, when perfusion profiles overlap. When issues are unclear, multimodal imaging can assist medical professionals in identifying them.

CLINICAL PARKINSON'S DISEASE

A degenerative neurological disorder that affects both motor and non-motor abilities is Parkinson's Disease (PD) (Shaheen et al., 2024; Asuku et al., 2025). Particularly, dopaminergic neurons are destroyed early in the illness. Reduction of the substantia nigra pars compacta, which transmits vital signals to the basal ganglia, is especially apparent. The substantia nigra's ventrolateral and caudal layers, which reach the striatum's dorsal putamen, are typically the most severely injured. A progressive dopamine deficit specific to this region is most likely the cause of differential motor characteristics. Parkinson's Disease (PD) causes neuronal loss not only in the basal ganglia but also in the Hypothalamus, Amygdala, Locus Coeruleus, Raphe Nucleus, Pedunculopontine Nucleus, Nucleus Basalis of Meynert, and Dorsal Motor nucleus of the vague nerve. The external nervous system components containing Parkinson's disease genetic markers include the Spinal Cord, Vagus Confidence, Sympathetic Ganglia, Cardiac Plexus, Enteric Nervous System, Adrenal Medulla, and Cutaneous Nerves. Parkinson's Disease (PD) seems to affect both dopaminergic and non-dopaminergic pathways (Sun et al., 2019).

Figure 4. Clinical Parkinson's disease

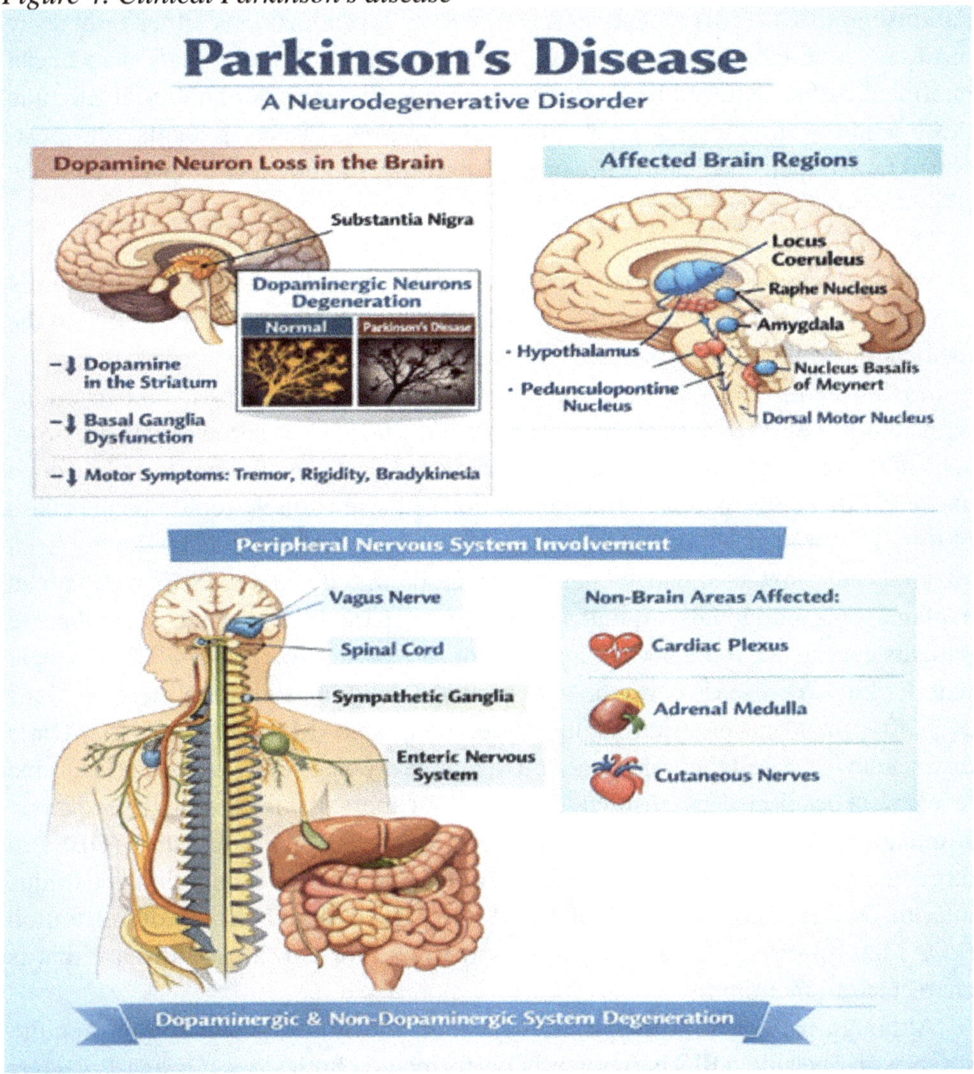

TREATMENT INITIATION IN PARKINSON'S DISEASE

The long-held notion that levodopa may be detrimental and hasten the disease's progression by raising oxidative stress, inducing levodopa phobia, and driving physicians and (Fumimura et al., 2007) Parkinson's patients to postpone therapy is one factor contributing to treatment delays. However, the delayed start designs of the LEAP study showed no evidence of neuroprotective effects or levodopa toxicity. Parkinson's disease participants in this trial were given levodopa either right away or after a nine-month placebo break. On the other hand, individuals who began treatment earlier reported fewer motor symptoms and a higher quality of life than those who began treatment later. African Parkinson's disease patients who postponed taking their medication because of disability did not have a lower incidence of motor issues or dyskinesias.

However, the fact that there are symptoms and no disability shouldn't be used as justification for starting pharmaceutical treatment. Individuals react differently to levodopa, and many Parkinson's disease patients who first react favorably to the medication eventually lose their receptiveness to it (Bond et al., 2017). Two important issues that are manageable are chronic constipation and forgetting to take levodopa with high-protein meals. Bacterial decarboxylases may be overproduced in the stomachs of people with Parkinson's disease. Bacterial overgrowth, long-term levodopa use, persistent constipation, or a combination of these variables could be the cause of this. The amount of dopamine in mouse blood can be decreased by the bacterial enzyme decarboxylase, which changes levodopa into dopamine. This mechanism explains some individuals respond poorly to levodopa and certain Parkinson's disease patients experience more severe and early on-off swings than others. Many people with Parkinson's disease continue to experience crippling swings in their reactions even after their oral medications have been optimized (Misch et al., 2019). Three distinct device-based therapies that aim to maintain consistently elevated dopamine levels were developed as a result of this. The first approach involves high-frequency stimulation, also referred to as Lesion Surgery or Deep Brain Stimulation (DBS), to target the basal ganglia. DBS can develop in the subthalamus and globus pallidus internus nuclei. Though it is rarely used, the US Food and Drug Administration (FDA) has approved thalamic DBS as a treatment for Parkinson's disease that is characterized by tremors.

Although patients whose symptoms are obviously unequal may only require surgery on one side, DBS is frequently performed on both sides (Ortega-Pinazo et al., 2023). Advantage of lesion therapy is that they are a long-term solution that eliminates the need for regular battery changes and the ensuing modifications to stimulation parameters. Lesion therapies are typically not administered to both sides of the body simultaneously since they can impair thinking, speaking, and swallowing. A technique known as unilateral focused ultrasound, which employs high frequencies and may harm the thalamus, was recently approved by the FDA. Even though it only affects one side of the body, this medication is excellent for tremors. The third technique that is permitted in Europe is pump therapy. While the patient is conscious, apomorphine is administered subcutaneously. A 12-week, double-blind RCT examined the effectiveness and safety of apomorphine infusion.

The findings showed that the medication was well tolerated and reduced off-time in a way that was clinically significant (Cao et al., 2017).

EXOSOMAL BIOMARKERS FOR PARKINSONIAN DIFFERENTIATION

MSA is a neurological disease that kills people and attacks them sporadically. It has no recognized cause. A neuropathological feature of MSA is the misfolding of oligodendrocyte α-synuclein. MSA-P, which mostly affects Parkinsonism, and MSA-C, which primarily affects the cerebellum, are the two types of MSA (Deuschl et al., 2020). It is associated with significant structural changes in both types of Olivopontocerebellar Atrophy (OPCA) and degeneration. The symptoms of PD and MSA may coexist early in the illness. Both find it challenging to get an early diagnosis at the clinic (Edison et al., 2008). A recent study investigated if α-syn in exosomes made from neurons and oligodendrocytes extracted from blood or plasma might distinguish between individuals with MSA, Parkinson's disease, and healthy individuals. The characteristics of Progressive Supranuclear Palsy (PSP), a common atypical parkinsonian illness, include frontal brain dysfunction, dysarthria, dysphagia, and vertical gaze palsy. When PD is still in its early stages, it might be challenging to distinguish PSP from PD (Lv et al., 2020). Eventually, larger series would be used for this (2019). Ren and other people. Asymmetric akinetic-rigid states, dystonia, dysfunction, and bad posture are signs of a developing neurological illness. In neurons and glial cells, tau protein inappropriately builds up, signifying the illness (Kalia & Lang, 2015). Some people are under the impression that degenerative diseases like Parkinson's Disease (PD) and others have early-stage CBD (Lachenal et al., 2011). Recently, extracted neural-derived exosomes from the blood of individuals with APS and PD, including those with CBD and PSP, to check if exosomal Tau and α-syn aggregates have a special diagnostic influence. Exosomal oligomeric α-syn is much higher in PD than in APS, which suggests that exosomal Tau aggregates may be significantly higher in APS than in PD. Exosomes from RBD, PD, and DLB were shown to have nearly three times as much α-syn than those from controls, MSA, or other proteinopathies. Clusterin levels in serum neuronal exosomes varied significantly between illness groups, as did α-syn Additionally, when paired with exosomal clusterin, 4-repeat tauopathy and Parkinson's disease may be discriminated more readily. state that this amazing discovery implies that clusterin should be employed as a marker to differentiate APS in future studies (Swallow & Counsell, 2023).

CONCLUSION

It has never been simple to treat Parkinson's disease (PD), but in underdeveloped areas, access to better imaging, biomarkers, and specialized neurology services is limited, which exacerbates delays and misdiagnosis. Although they are gradually beginning to incorporate non-motor symptoms and imaging markers, all current clinical diagnostic frameworks are focused on motor symptoms and response to dopaminergic treatment. This implies a severe lack of early and precise diagnosis, particularly during the prodrome. It may be possible to distinguish Parkinson's Disease (PD) from atypical parkinsonian disorders like Multiple System Atrophy (MSA), Corticobasal Degeneration (CBD), and progressive supranuclear palsy (PSP) by using recent studies on exosomal biomarkers, particularly microRNAs and a-synuclein aggregates. Nanoparticle tracking, size-exclusion chromatography, and next-generation sequencing are some of the technologies that have made it easier to extract and characterize exosomes. Both sensitivity and specificity are high in these approaches for identifying disease-specific protein profiles and miRNA signatures. By examining cerebral perfusion patterns, amyloid deposition, and neuroinflammation, neuroimaging methods such as PET and SPECT can also assist in distinguishing between the many causes of parkinsonian diseases. However, due to their high cost, complexity, and stringent regulations, many current diagnostic tools are really difficult to employ, particularly in underdeveloped nations.

REFERENCES

Antonini, A., Benti, R., De Notaris, R., Tesei, S., Zecchinelli, A., Sacilotto, G., Meucci, N., Canesi, M., Mariani, C., Pezzoli, G., & Gerundini, P. (2003). 123I-Ioflupane/SPECT binding to striatal dopamine transporter (DAT) uptake in patients with Parkinson's disease, multiple system atrophy, and progressive supranuclear palsy. *Neurological Sciences, 24*(3), 149–150. DOI: 10.1007/s10072-003-0103-5 PMID: 14598060

Antonini, A., De Notaris, R., Benti, R., De Gaspari, D., & Pezzoli, G. (2001). Perfusion ECD/SPECT in the characterization of cognitive deficits in Parkinson's disease. *Neurological Sciences, 22*(1), 45–46. DOI: 10.1007/s100720170039 PMID: 11487194

Armstrong, M. J., Litvan, I., Lang, A. E., Bak, T. H., Bhatia, K. P., Borroni, B., Boxer, A. L., Dickson, D. W., Grossman, M., Hallett, M., Josephs, K. A., Kertesz, A., Lee, S. E., Miller, B. L., Reich, S. G., Riley, D. E., Tolosa, E., Tröster, A. I., Vidailhet, M., & Weiner, W. J. (2013). Criteria for the diagnosis of corticobasal degeneration. *Neurology, 80*(5), 496–503. DOI: 10.1212/WNL.0b013e31827f0fd1 PMID: 23359374

Asuku A.O., Adeyemo M.B., Adeyemo R.O., Agoro S.A., Odugbesan O.A., & Ayoola S.A. (2022). Applications of stem cell therapy in neurodegenerative diseases. European Journal of Biotechnology and Bioscience. 10 (2): 17-24, 2321-9122

Asuku, A. O., Ayinla, M. T., Aransiola, S. A., Ajibare, A. J., Adeyemo, M. B., & Adeyemo, R. O. (2024). Chitosan-Based Nanoparticles to bypass the Blood-Brain Barrier for the Treatment of Neurological Diseases: A Review. *Pakistan Journal of Medical Sciences, 25*(1), 2072–1625.

Asuku, A. O., Ogungbangbe, G. O., & Fajemidagba, G. A. (2025). Gene therapy for Parkinson's disease: A new frontier in neurodegenerative diseases. *Exploration of Neuroprotective Therapy, 5*, 1004119. DOI: 10.37349/ent.2025.1004119

Beach, T. G., Adler, C. H., Sue, L. I., Vedders, L., Lue, L., White, C. L.III, Akiyama, H., Caviness, J. N., Shill, H. A., Sabbagh, M. N., & Walker, D. G.Arizona Parkinson's Disease Consortium. (2010). Multi-organ distribution of phosphorylated alpha-synuclein histopathology in subjects with Lewy body disorders. *Acta Neuropathologica, 119*(6), 689–702. DOI: 10.1007/s00401-010-0664-3 PMID: 20306269

Bond, A. E., Shah, B. B., Huss, D. S., Dallapiazza, R. F., Warren, A., Harrison, M. B., Sperling, S. A., Wang, X.-Q., Gwinn, R., Witt, J., Ro, S., & Elias, W. J.International Essential Tremor Stereotactic Radiofrequency Ablation (ESTRA) Study Group. (2017). Safety and efficacy of focused ultrasound thalamotomy for patients with medication-refractory, tremor-dominant Parkinson disease: A randomized clinical trial. *JAMA Neurology, 74*(12), 1412–1418. DOI: 10.1001/jamaneurol.2017.3098 PMID: 29084313

Cao, X.-Y., Lu, J.-M., Zhao, Z.-Q., Li, M.-C., Lu, T., An, X.-S., & Xue, L.-J. (2017). MicroRNA biomarkers of Parkinson's disease in serum exosome-like microvesicles. *Neuroscience Letters, 644*, 94–99. DOI: 10.1016/j.neulet.2017.02.045 PMID: 28223160

Cilia, R., Akpalu, A., Sarfo, F. S., Cham, M., Amboni, M., Cereda, E., Fabbri, M., Adjei, P., Akassi, J., Bonetti, A., & Pezzoli, G. (2014). The modern pre-levodopa era of Parkinson's disease: Insights into motor complications from sub-Saharan Africa. *Brain, 137*(10), 2731–2742. DOI: 10.1093/brain/awu195 PMID: 25034897

Del Tredici, K., Hawkes, C. H., Ghebremedhin, E., & Braak, H. (2010). Lewy pathology in the submandibular gland of individuals with incidental Lewy body disease and sporadic Parkinson's disease. *Acta Neuropathologica, 119*(6), 703–713. DOI: 10.1007/s00401-010-0665-2 PMID: 20229352

Deuschl, G., Beghi, E., Fazekas, F., Varga, T., Christoforidi, K. A., Sipido, E., Bassetti, C. L., Vos, T., & Feigin, V. L. (2020). The burden of neurological diseases in Europe: An analysis for the Global Burden of Disease Study 2017. *The Lancet. Public Health, 5*(10), e551–e567. DOI: 10.1016/S2468-2667(20)30190-0 PMID: 33007212

Dickson, D. W., Braak, H., Duda, J. E., Duyckaerts, C., Gasser, T., Halliday, G. M., Hardy, J., Leverenz, J. B., Del Tredici, K., Wszolek, Z. K., & Litvan, I. (2009). Neuropathological assessment of Parkinson's disease: Refining the diagnostic criteria. *Lancet Neurology, 8*(12), 1150–1157. DOI: 10.1016/S1474-4422(09)70238-8 PMID: 19909913

Dilsiz, N. (2024). A comprehensive review on recent advances in exosome isolation and characterization: Toward clinical applications. *Translational Oncology, 50*, 102121. DOI: 10.1016/j.tranon.2024.102121 PMID: 39278189

Donaghy, P. C., Firbank, M. J., Thomas, A. J., Lloyd, J., Petrides, G., Barnett, N., Olsen, K., Taylor, J.-P., & O'Brien, J. T. (2020). Amyloid imaging and longitudinal clinical progression in dementia with lewy bodies. *The American Journal of Geriatric Psychiatry, 28*(5), 573–577. DOI: 10.1016/j.jagp.2019.12.009 PMID: 31953009

Dorsey, E. R., Sherer, T., Okun, M. S., & Bloem, B. R. (2018). The emerging evidence of the Parkinson pandemic. *Journal of Parkinson's Disease*, *8*(s1), S3–S8. DOI: 10.3233/JPD-181474 PMID: 30584159

Dutta, S., Hornung, S., Kruayatidee, A., Maina, K. N., del Rosario, I., Paul, K. C., Wong, D. Y., Duarte Folle, A., & Bitan, G. (2021). α-Synuclein in blood exosomes immunoprecipitated using neuronal and oligodendroglial markers distinguishes Parkinson's disease from multiple system atrophy. *Acta Neuropathologica*, *142*(3), 495–511. DOI: 10.1007/s00401-021-02324-0 PMID: 33991233

Edison, P., Rowe, C. C., Rinne, J. O., Ng, S., Ahmed, I., Kemppainen, N., Villemagne, V. L., O'Keefe, G., Någren, K., Chaudhury, K. R., Masters, C. L., & Brooks, D. J. (2008). Amyloid load in Parkinson's disease dementia and Lewy body dementia measured with [11C]PIB positron emission tomography. *Journal of Neurology, Neurosurgery, and Psychiatry*, *79*(12), 1331–1338. DOI: 10.1136/jnnp.2007.127878 PMID: 18653550

Faghri, F., Hashemi, S. H., Leonard, H., Scholz, S. W., Campbell, R. H., Nalls, M. A., & Singleton, A. B. (2018). Predicting onset, progression, and clinical subtypes of Parkinson disease using machine learning [Preprint]. *bioRxiv*. https://doi.org/ DOI: 10.1101/338913

Fanciulli, A., & Wenning, G. K. (2015). Multiple-system atrophy. *The New England Journal of Medicine*, *372*(3), 249–263. DOI: 10.1056/NEJMra1311488 PMID: 25587949

Fereshtehnejad, S.-M., Zeighami, Y., Dagher, A., & Postuma, R. B. (2017). Clinical criteria for subtyping Parkinson's disease: Biomarkers and longitudinal progression. *Brain*, *140*(7), 1959–1976. DOI: 10.1093/brain/awx118 PMID: 28549077

Firbank, M. J., Molloy, S., McKeith, I. G., Burn, D. J., & O'Brien, J. T. (2005). Longitudinal change in 99mTcHMPAO cerebral perfusion SPECT in Parkinson's disease over one year. *Journal of Neurology, Neurosurgery, and Psychiatry*, *76*(10), 1448–1451. DOI: 10.1136/jnnp.2004.058685 PMID: 16170094

Foster, E. R., Campbell, M. C., Burack, M. A., Hartlein, J., Flores, H. P., Cairns, N. J., Hershey, T., & Perlmutter, J. S. (2010). Amyloid imaging of Lewy body-associated disorders. *Movement Disorders*, *25*(15), 2516–2523. DOI: 10.1002/mds.23393 PMID: 20922808

Fumimura, Y., Ikemura, M., Saito, Y., Sengoku, R., Kanemaru, K., Sawabe, M., Arai, T., Ito, G., Iwatsubo, T., Fukayama, M., & Hattori, N. (2007). Analysis of the adrenal gland is useful for evaluating pathology of the peripheral autonomic nervous system in lewy body disease. *Journal of Neuropathology and Experimental Neurology*, *66*(5), 354–362. DOI: 10.1097/nen.0b013e3180517454 PMID: 17483692

Galvin, J. E., Lee, V. M.-Y., & Trojanowski, J. Q. (2001). Synucleinopathies: Clinical and pathological implications. *Archives of Neurology*, *58*(2), 186–190. DOI: 10.1001/archneur.58.2.186 PMID: 11176955

Gilman, S., Wenning, G. K., Low, P. A., Brooks, D. J., Mathias, C. J., Trojanowski, J. Q., Wood, N. W., Colosimo, C., Dürr, A., Fowler, C. J., Kaufmann, H., Klockgether, T., Lees, A., Poewe, W., Quinn, N., Revesz, T., Robertson, D., Sandroni, P., Seppi, K., & Vidailhet, M. (2008). Second consensus statement on the diagnosis of multiple system atrophy. *Neurology*, *71*(9), 670–676. DOI: 10.1212/01.wnl.0000324625.00404.15 PMID: 18725592

Gomperts, S. N., Locascio, J. J., Marquie, M., Santarlasci, A. L., Rentz, D. M., Maye, J., Johnson, K. A., & Growdon, J. H. (2012). Brain amyloid and cognition in Lewy body diseases. *Movement Disorders*, *27*(8), 965–973. DOI: 10.1002/mds.25048 PMID: 22693110

Guevremont, D., Roy, J., Cutfield, N. J., & Williams, J. M. (2023). MicroRNAs in Parkinson's disease: A systematic review and diagnostic accuracy meta-analysis. *Scientific Reports*, *13*, 16272. DOI: 10.1038/s41598-023-43463-6 PMID: 37770507

Gui, Y., Liu, H., Zhang, L., Lv, W., & Hu, X. (2015). Altered microRNA profiles in cerebrospinal fluid exosome in Parkinson disease and Alzheimer disease. *Oncotarget*, *6*(35), 37043–37053. DOI: 10.18632/oncotarget.6158 PMID: 26497684

Harding, A. J., & Halliday, G. M. (2001). Cortical Lewy body pathology in the diagnosis of dementia. *Acta Neuropathologica*, *102*(4), 355–363. DOI: 10.1007/s004010100390 PMID: 11603811

He, Q., Wang, Q., Yuan, C., & Wang, Y. (2017). Downregulation of miR-7116-5p in microglia by MPP+ sensitizes TNF-alpha production to induce dopaminergic neuron damage. *Glia*, *65*(8), 1251–1263. DOI: 10.1002/glia.23153 PMID: 28543680

Irwin, D. J., White, M. T., Toledo, J. B., Xie, S. X., Robinson, J. L., Van Deerlin, V., Lee, V. M.-Y., Leverenz, J. B., Montine, T. J., Duda, J. E., Hurtig, H. I., & Trojanowski, J. Q. (2012). Neuropathologic substrates of Parkinson disease dementia. *Annals of Neurology*, *72*(4), 587–598. DOI: 10.1002/ana.23659 PMID: 23037886

Jellinger, K. A. (2012). Neuropathology of sporadic Parkinson's disease: Evaluation and changes of concepts. *Movement Disorders, 27*(1), 8–30. DOI: 10.1002/mds.23795 PMID: 22081500

Jiang, C., Hopfner, F., Berg, D., Hu, M. T., Pilotto, A., Borroni, B., Davis, J. J., & Tofaris, G. K. (2021). Validation of alpha-synuclein in L1CAM-immunocaptured exosomes as a biomarker for the stratification of parkinsonian syndromes. *Movement Disorders, 36*(11), 2663–2669. DOI: 10.1002/mds.28591 PMID: 33826157

Kalia, L. V., & Lang, A. E. (2015). Parkinson's disease. *Lancet, 386*(9996), 896–912. DOI: 10.1016/S0140-6736(14)61393-3 PMID: 25904081

Kalluri, R., & LeBleu, V. S. (2020). The biology, function, and biomedical applications of exosomes. *Science, 367*(6478), eaau6977. Advance online publication. DOI: 10.1126/science.aau6977 PMID: 32029601

Kordower, J. H., Olanow, C. W., Dodiya, H. B., Chu, Y., Beach, T. G., Adler, C. H., Halliday, G. M., & Bartus, R. T. (2013). Disease duration and the integrity of the nigrostriatal system in Parkinson's disease. *Brain, 136*(8), 2419–2431. DOI: 10.1093/brain/awt192 PMID: 23884810

Lachenal, G., Pernet-Gallay, K., Chivet, M., Hemming, F. J., Belly, A., Bodon, G., Blot, B., Haase, G., Goldberg, Y., & Sadoul, R. (2011). Release of exosomes from differentiated neurons and its regulation by synaptic glutamatergic activity. *Molecular and Cellular Neurosciences, 46*(2), 409–418. DOI: 10.1016/j.mcn.2010.11.004 PMID: 21111824

Lees, A. J., Hardy, J., & Revesz, T. (2009). Parkinson's disease. *Lancet, 373*(9680), 2055–2066. DOI: 10.1016/S0140-6736(09)60492-X PMID: 19524782

Li, D., Yang, H., Ma, J., Luo, S., Chen, S., & Gu, Q. (2018). MicroRNA-30e regulates neuroinflammation in MPTP model of Parkinson's disease by targeting Nlrp3. *Human Cell, 31*(2), 106–115. DOI: 10.1007/s13577-017-0187-5 PMID: 29274035

Ling, H., Kovacs, G. G., Vonsattel, J. P. G., Davey, K., Mok, K. Y., Hardy, J., Morris, H. R., Warner, T. T., Holton, J. L., & Revesz, T. (2016). Astrogliopathy predominates the earliest stage of corticobasal degeneration pathology. *Brain, 139*(12), 3237–3252. DOI: 10.1093/brain/aww256 PMID: 27797812

Lobotesis, K., Fenwick, J. D., Phipps, A., Ryman, A., Swann, A., Ballard, C., McKeith, I. G., & O'Brien, J. T. (2001). Occipital hypoperfusion on SPECT in dementia with Lewy bodies but not AD. *Neurology, 56*(5), 643–649. DOI: 10.1212/wnl.56.5.643 PMID: 11245717

Lv, R., Du, L., Zhou, F., Yuan, X., Liu, X., & Zhang, L. (2020). Rosmarinic Acid Alleviates Inflammation, Apoptosis, and Oxidative Stress through Regulating miR-155-5p in a Mice Model of Parkinson's Disease. *ACS Chemical Neuroscience, 11*(20), 3259–3266. DOI: 10.1021/acschemneuro.0c00425 PMID: 32946211

Mahlknecht, P., Seppi, K., & Poewe, W. (2015). The Concept of Prodromal Parkinson's Disease. *Journal of Parkinson's Disease, 5*(4), 681–697. DOI: 10.3233/JPD-150685 PMID: 26485429

Maini Rekdal, V., Bess, E. N., Bisanz, J. E., Turnbaugh, P. J., & Balskus, E. P. (2019). Discovery and inhibition of an interspecies gut bacterial pathway for Levodopa metabolism. *Science, 364*(6445), eaau6323. Advance online publication. DOI: 10.1126/science.aau6323 PMID: 31196984

Manna, I., De Benedittis, S., Quattrone, A., Maisano, D., Iaccino, E., & Quattrone, A. (2021). Exosomal miRNA as peripheral biomarkers in Parkinson's disease and progressive supranuclear palsy: A pilot study. *Parkinsonism & Related Disorders, 93*, 77–84. DOI: 10.1016/j.parkreldis.2021.11.020 PMID: 34839044

Marras, C., & Lang, A. (2013). Parkinson's disease subtypes: Lost in translation? *Journal of Neurology, Neurosurgery, and Psychiatry, 84*(4), 409–415. DOI: 10.1136/jnnp-2012-303455 PMID: 22952329

Martínez-Fernández, R., Rodríguez-Rojas, R., Del Álamo, M., Hernández-Fernández, F., Pineda-Pardo, J. A., Dileone, M., Alonso-Frech, F., Foffani, G., Obeso, I., Gasca-Salas, C., de Luis-Pastor, E., Vela, L., & Obeso, J. A. (2018). Focused ultrasound subthalamotomy in patients with asymmetric Parkinson's disease: A pilot study. *Lancet Neurology, 17*(1), 54–63. DOI: 10.1016/S1474-4422(17)30403-9 PMID: 29203153

Matsuda, H., Imabayashi, E., Kuji, I., Seto, A., Ito, K., Kikuta, D., & Yamada, M. (2010). Evaluation of both perfusion and atrophy in multiple system atrophy of the cerebellar type using brain SPECT alone. *BMC Medical Imaging, 10*, 17. DOI: 10.1186/1471-2342-10-17 PMID: 20701753

Matsui, H., Udaka, F., Miyoshi, T., Hara, N., Tamura, A., Oda, M., Kubori, T., & Nishinaka, K. (2005). Brain perfusion differences between Parkinson's disease and multiple system atrophy with predominant parkinsonian features. *Parkinsonism & Related Disorders, 11*(4), 227–232. DOI: 10.1016/j.parkreldis.2005.01.001 PMID: 15878583

Meloni, M., Agliardi, C., Guerini, F. R., Zanzottera, M., Bolognesi, E., Picciolini, S., Marano, M., Magliozzi, A., Di Fonzo, A., Arighi, A., Fenoglio, C., Scarpini, E., Parnetti, L., & Clerici, M. (2023). Oligomeric alpha-synuclein and tau aggregates in NDEVs differentiate Parkinson's disease from atypical parkinsonisms. *Neurobiology of Disease*, *176*, 105947. DOI: 10.1016/j.nbd.2022.105947 PMID: 36481435

Misch, M. R., Mitchell, S., Francis, P. L., Sherborn, K., Meradje, K., McNeely, A. A., Chen, J. J., & Tang-Wai, D. F. (2019). Differentiating between visual hallucination-free dementia with Lewy bodies and corticobasal syndrome on the basis of neuropsychology and perfusion single-photon emission computed tomography. *Alzheimer's Research & Therapy*, *11*(1), 9. DOI: 10.1186/s13195-018-0456-x PMID: 30658705

Oertel, W. H., Depboylu, C., Krenzer, M., Vadasz, D., Ries, V., Sixel-Döring, F., & Mayer, G. (2014). REM sleep behavior disorder as a prodromal stage of alpha-synucleinopathies: Symptoms, epidemiology, pathophysiology, diagnosis and therapy. *Der Nervenarzt*, *85*(1), 19–25. DOI: 10.1007/s00115-013-3870-0 PMID: 24399499

Ortega-Pinazo, J., Pacheco-Rodríguez, M. J., Serrano-Castro, P. J., Martínez, B., Pinto-Medel, M. J., Gómez-Zumaquero, J. M., Lago-Sampedro, A., García-Díaz, B., Estivill-Torrús, G., & Emilio Ferro Gallego, P. (2023). Comparing RNA extraction methods to face the variations in RNA quality using two human biological matrices. *Molecular Biology Reports*, *50*(11), 9263–9271. DOI: 10.1007/s11033-023-08809-3 PMID: 37812354

Petrou, M., Bohnen, N. I., Müller, M. L. T. M., Koeppe, R. A., Albin, R. L., & Frey, K. A. (2012). Aβ-Amyloid deposition in patients with Parkinson disease at risk for development of dementia. *Neurology*, *79*(11), 1161–1167. DOI: 10.1212/WNL.0b013e3182698d4a PMID: 22933741

Poewe, W., Seppi, K., Marini, K., & Mahlknecht, P. (2020). New hopes for disease modification in Parkinson's Disease. *Neuropharmacology*, *171*, 108085. DOI: 10.1016/j.neuropharm.2020.108085 PMID: 32298705

Pringsheim, T., Jette, N., Frolkis, A., & Steeves, T. D. (2014). The prevalence of Parkinson's disease: A systematic review and meta-analysis. *Movement Disorders*, *29*(13), 1583–1590. DOI: 10.1002/mds.25945 PMID: 24976103

Ren, Y., Li, H., Xie, W., Wei, N., & Liu, M. (2019). MicroRNA-195 triggers neuroinflammation in Parkinson's disease in a Rho-associated kinase 1-dependent manner. *Molecular Medicine Reports*, *19*(6), 5153–5161. DOI: 10.3892/mmr.2019.10178 PMID: 31059087

Rossi, C., Volterrani, D., Nicoletti, V., Manca, G., Frosini, D., Kiferle, L., Palumbo, B., Bonuccelli, U., & Ceravolo, R. (2009). "Parkinson-dementia" diseases: A comparison by double tracer SPECT studies. *Parkinsonism & Related Disorders, 15*(10), 762–766. DOI: 10.1016/j.parkreldis.2009.05.012 PMID: 19553153

Shah, N., Frey, K. A., Müller, M. L. T. M., Petrou, M., Kotagal, V., Koeppe, R. A., Scott, P. J. H., Albin, R. L., & Bohnen, N. I. (2016). Striatal and cortical β-amyloidopathy and cognition in Parkinson's disease. *Movement Disorders, 31*(1), 111–117. DOI: 10.1002/mds.26369 PMID: 26380951

Shahed, J., & Jankovic, J. (2007). Exploring the relationship between essential tremor and Parkinson's disease. *Parkinsonism & Related Disorders, 13*(2), 67–76. DOI: 10.1016/j.parkreldis.2006.05.033 PMID: 16887374

Shaheen, N., Shaheen, A., Osama, M., Nashwan, A. J., Bharmauria, V., & Flouty, O. (2024). MicroRNAs regulation in Parkinson's disease, and their potential role as diagnostic and therapeutic targets. *npj. Parkinson's Disease, 10*(1), 186. DOI: 10.1038/s41531-024-00810-2 PMID: 39369002

Shang, R., Lee, S., Senavirathne, G., & Lai, E. C. (2023). microRNAs in action: Biogenesis, function and regulation. *Nature Reviews. Genetics, 24*(12), 816–833. DOI: 10.1038/s41576-023-00611-y PMID: 37380761

Shirvan, J., Clement, N., Ye, R., Katz, S., Schultz, A., Johnson, K. A., Gomez-Isla, T., Frosch, M. P., Growdon, J. H., & Gomperts, S. N. (2019). Neuropathologic correlates of amyloid and dopamine transporter imaging in Lewy body disease. *Neurology, 93*(5), e476–e484. DOI: 10.1212/WNL.0000000000007855 PMID: 31243072

Song, I.-U., Yoo, I.-R., Chung, Y.-A., & Jeong, J. (2015). The value of brain perfusion SPECT for differentiation between mildly symptomatic idiopathic Parkinson's disease and the Parkinson variant of multiple system atrophy. *Nuclear Medicine Communications, 36*(10), 1049–1054. DOI: 10.1097/MNM.0000000000000354 PMID: 26087241

Sperling, S. A., Shah, B. B., Barrett, M. J., Bond, A. E., Huss, D. S., Costa, M. G. L., & Elias, W. J. (2018). Focused ultrasound thalamotomy in Parkinson disease: Nonmotor outcomes and quality of life. *Neurology, 91*(14), e1275–e1284. DOI: 10.1212/WNL.0000000000006279 PMID: 30158160

Sun, Q., Wang, S., Chen, J., Cai, H., Huang, W., Zhang, Y., Wang, L., & Xing, Y. (2019). MicroRNA-190 alleviates neuronal damage and inhibits neuroinflammation via Nlrp3 in MPTP-induced Parkinson's disease mouse model. *Journal of Cellular Physiology, 234*(12), 23379–23387. DOI: 10.1002/jcp.28907 PMID: 31232472

Swallow, D. M. A., & Counsell, C. E. (2023). The evolution of diagnosis from symptom onset to death in progressive supranuclear palsy (PSP) and corticobasal degeneration (CBD) compared to Parkinson's disease (PD). *Journal of Neurology, 270*(8), 4065–4076. DOI: 10.1007/s00415-023-11629-x PMID: 36971841

Théry, C., Witwer, K. W., Aikawa, E., Alcaraz, M. J., Anderson, J. D., Andriantsitohaina, R., Antoniou, A., Arab, T., Archer, F., Atkin-Smith, G. K., Ayre, D. C., Bach, J.-M., Bachurski, D., Baharvand, H., Balaj, L., Baldacchino, S., Bauer, N. N., Baxter, A. A., Bebawy, M., & Zuba-Surma, E. K. (2018). Minimal information for studies of extracellular vesicles 2018 (MISEV2018): A position statement of the International Society for Extracellular Vesicles and update of the MISEV2014 guidelines. *Journal of Extracellular Vesicles, 7*(1), 1535750. DOI: 10.1080/20013078.2018.1535750 PMID: 30637094

Tolosa, E., Gaig, C., Santamaría, J., & Compta, Y. (2009). Diagnosis and the premotor phase of Parkinson disease. *Neurology, 72*(7, Suppl), S12–S20. DOI: 10.1212/WNL.0b013e318198db11 PMID: 19221308

Tolosa, E., Vila, M., Klein, C., & Rascol, O. (2020). LRRK2 in Parkinson disease: Challenges of clinical trials. *Nature Reviews. Neurology, 16*(2), 97–107. DOI: 10.1038/s41582-019-0301-2 PMID: 31980808

van Meer, G., Voelker, D. R., & Feigenson, G. W. (2008). Membrane lipids: Where they are and how they behave. *Nature Reviews. Molecular Cell Biology, 9*(2), 112–124. DOI: 10.1038/nrm2330 PMID: 18216768

Zervos, T. M., Hamani, C., & Schwalb, J. M. (2018). MRIgFUS in tremor-dominant PD does not lead to substantial cognitive adverse events. *Neurology, 91*(14), 641–642. DOI: 10.1212/WNL.0000000000006241 PMID: 30158164

Zhou, Y., Lu, M., Du, R.-H., Qiao, C., Jiang, C.-Y., Zhang, K.-Z., Ding, J.-H., & Hu, G. (2016). MicroRNA-7 targets Nod-like receptor protein 3 inflammasome to modulate neuroinflammation in the pathogenesis of Parkinson's disease. *Molecular Neurodegeneration, 11*, 28. DOI: 10.1186/s13024-016-0094-3 PMID: 27084336

Chapter 3
Dopaminergic Therapies for Parkinson's Disease in Under-Resourced Settings

Vibhas Mittra
http://orcid.org/0009-0003-6238-4708
Panjab University, India

Alka Bali
http://orcid.org/0000-0002-8034-3518
Panjab University, India

Bhawna
Panjab University, India

ABSTRACT

Parkinson's disease (PD) is a progressive neurodegenerative disorder characterized by diminished striatal dopamine levels resulting from the degeneration of dopaminergic neurons in the substantia nigra. About 10 million people around the world are affected by this disease. Levodopa was first used in the 1960s as a symptomatic cure for the disease and it is still the mainstay or PD treatment. Levodopa is not always available in low- and middle-income countries (LMICs) because of problems with the supply chain, high costs, and a lack of diagnostics. In rural areas without pharmacovigilance, doctors use cheaper alternatives like Mucuna pruriens or Vicia faba beans. The Parkinson's Disease and Movement Disorder Society in India is an example of a community-based model that stresses multidisciplinary care to fill

DOI: 10.4018/979-8-3373-7437-6.ch003

in the gaps by teaching carers about levodopa timing, voice therapy, and physiotherapy. Wearables for monitoring, telemedicine, changes to registries, and generic medication policies all help promote equity.

INTRODUCTION

Parkinson's disease (PD) is a progressive neurodegenerative disorder that causes comprehensive motor and non-motor symptoms, the accumulation of misfolded α-synuclein in Lewy bodies, and the selective degeneration of dopaminergic neurons in the substantia nigra pars compacta (SNpc) which is a crucial midbrain structure which contains densely packed dopaminergic neurons. Levodopa-based regimens remain the cornerstone of symptomatic management; however, an increasing number of PD patients reside in low- and middle-income countries (LMICs), where access to standard dopaminergic therapies and advanced device-assisted interventions is hindered by delayed diagnosis, a shortage of specialists, fragile drug supply chains, and significant out-of-pocket costs. Interest has increased in cost-effective strategies such as telemedicine-enabled models designed to deliver more equitable dopaminergic care despite structural resource limitations, community-centered multidisciplinary care, natural levodopa sources like *Mucuna pruriens* and *Vicia faba*, and repurposed medications like amantadine.

Dopaminergic neurons in the substantia nigra pars compacta die too soon in PD, which is a long-lasting, progressive neurodegenerative disease (Radhakrishnan & Goyal, 2018). People with PD have a lot of the intracellular protein alpha synuclein (Ajagun et al., 2024; Asuku et al., 2024). Global prevalence of this disease is estimated to be more than 10 million people (Zafar & Yaddanapudi, 2025). Around 2-3% of population in age group of more than 65 years is afflicted by it and this is considered to be the fastest growing disorder worldwide. In 2016, it affected about 6.1 million people around the world (Bloem et al., 2021). As the number of elderly people living in low- and middle-income countries (LMICs) is increasing due to improved healthcare systems, this number is expected to grow quickly in the next few decades (Caronni et al., 2024). Even though we don't know exactly what causes Parkinson's disease (PD), most people think that a mix of genetic and environmental factors is to blame for most cases. About 10% of people with Parkinson's disease (PD) are thought to have genetic causes (Hauser et al., 2025).

Figure 1. Symptoms of Parkinson's disease

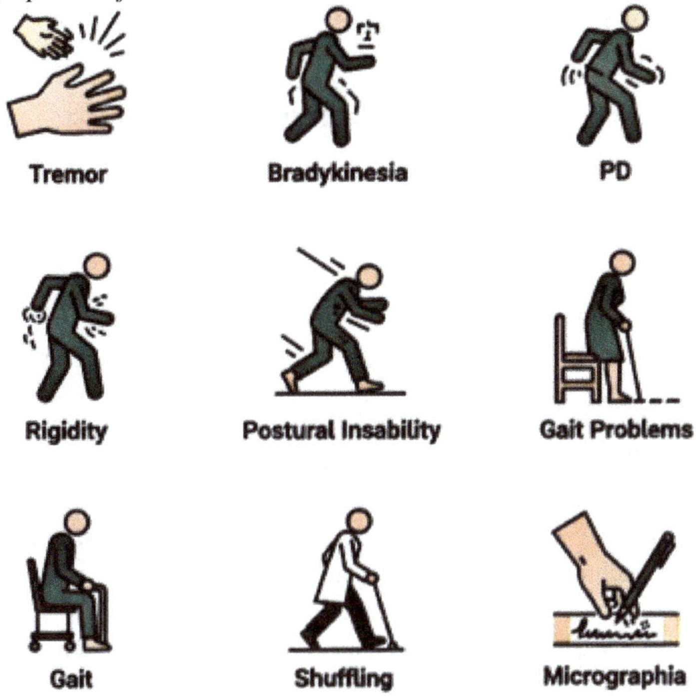

Figure 1 illustrates the key motor symptoms of Parkinson's disease, which include tremors, bradykinesia (slow movement), muscular rigidity, postural instability, gait problems with shuffling steps, and micrographia (small, cramped handwriting), all of which impair daily activities and mobility.

Some researchers think that dopaminergic neurons are more likely to get sick because they need a lot of energy to keep sending signals through their long axonal arborizations (Mitchell et al., 2024). The symptoms get worse over time as the disease progresses, even though it starts with mild symptoms like tremors. Bradykinesia and rigidity get progressively linked to tremors with time. Postural instability, which usually happens in late stages of the disease, can have a big effect on quality of life (Zafar et al., 2023). Most cases of Parkinson's disease are probably caused by a mix of genetic and environmental factors (Asuku et al., 2025a). The risk of getting PD can be lowered in a few ways; however, exposure to toxic chemicals and head injuries may make your risk higher. Genetic susceptibility can change how environmental exposures affect people. While identifiable mutations in specific genes account for 5 to 10% of PD cases, the majority of PD patients do not possess these mutations. Moreover, the observation that the predominant genetic mutations linked to Parkinson's disease do not invariably induce the condition implies the potential involvement of additional genetic or environmental factors (Simon et al., 2020).

THE EVOLUTION OF DOPAMINERGIC THERAPIES

The treatment of PD with dopamine-basis started in the 1960s and is still considered the best today amongst the limited approaches available. There is an urgent need to find not only therapies that change the disease but also better symptomatic and regenerative dopaminergic treatments (Barker et al., 2024). A lot has changed in the treatment of Parkinson's disease since levodopa therapy was introduced for the purpose fifty years back. In 1913, Marcus Guggenheim took L-dopa, which is a naturally occurring isomer of the amino acid 3,4-dihydroxyphenylalanine, out of legumes (seedlings of *Vicia faba*). In the Wellcome Labs in London, England, two years earlier, Casimir Funk made D, L-dopa (Ovallath et al., 2017). Scientists discovered in the early 1970s that using a dopa decarboxylase inhibitor in treatment had advantages such as fewer side effects and better symptom control.

In 1975, the first combination of levodopa and carbidopa was sold in stores (Tolosa et al., 1998). Since the late 1970s, L-DOPA has been taken with carbidopa, which is an inhibitor of dopa decarboxylase, an enzyme responsible for peripheral degradation of levodopa. It can prolong its half-life in the blood by up to ninety minutes. To prolong the effects of L-DOPA, physicians have recently incorporated inhibitors of both enzymes responsible for dopamine degradation (i.e., catechol-O-methyltransferase (COMT) and monoamine oxidase MAO), into the treatment protocol (Abbott, 2010). To combat Parkinson's disease (PD), DA receptor agonists were subsequently developed as either monotherapies or adjunct therapies in conjunction with L-DOPA.

Dopaminergic approaches mainly rely on the synthesis, release or reuptake of dopamine by dopaminergic neurons. L-DOPA is considered the primary drug treatment which replenishes the depleted dopamine levels in nigrostriatal regions of the CNS. This is brought about by its enzymatic conversion to dopamine by L-aromatic acid decarboxylase (commonly called as DOPA decarboxylase (Wickens et al., 2007). However, the long-term treatment with L-DOPA has been shown to result in dyskinesias in several cases. DAT inhibitors including bupropion are known to cause inhibition or blockage of dopamine transporter, resulting in extension of the dwell time of levodopa. Further, monoamine oxidase–B inhibitors (MAO-B inhibitors) such as selegiline, rasagiline, etc. prevent its intraneuronal metabolic degradation whereas, COMT inhibitors like entacapone block the metabolism at extra-neuronal sites (Sonne et al., 2024). There are five different types of DA receptors in the brain: D1, D2, D3, D4, and D5. D2-like receptors are D2, D3, and

D4 receptors because they stop cAMP from working. Conversely, the D1 and D5 receptors are categorized as D1-like receptors due to their stimulatory impact on adenylyl cyclase (cAMP) (Mao et al., 2020).

Selegiline, a selective MAO-B inhibitor, was examined in Parkinson's disease (PD) as early as the 1970s (Riederer et al., 1978). A plethora of studies have evidenced symptomatic improvement with minimal to moderate effects. Rasagiline selectively and irreversibly inhibits MAO-B, akin to selegiline, but at doses five to ten times lower (Finberg et al., 1996). MAO-B is completely stopped after a few days of treatment, but some people may not see a clinical response for up to four weeks (Mao et al., 2020).

Figure 2. Evolution of therapies for Parkinson's disease

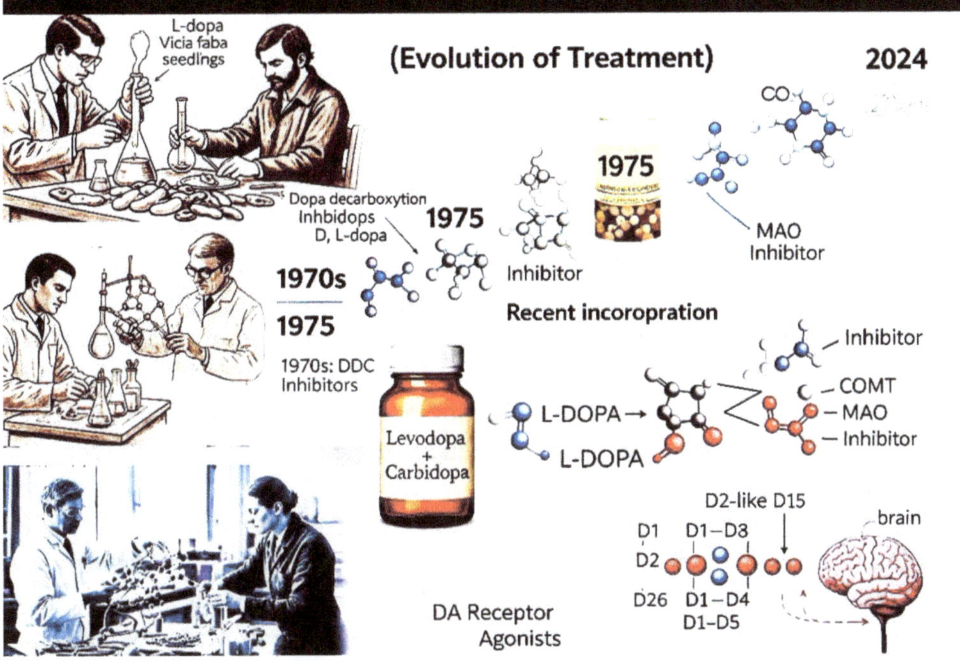

Figure 2 illustrates how L-DOPA therapy was improved with the addition of peripheral dopa decarboxylase inhibitors like carbidopa and benserazide to therapy in early 70s, followed by introduction of other drugs like monoamine oxidase (MAO) and catechol-O-methyltransferase (COMT) inhibitors to keep dopamine levels high for longer amount of time. Further, some newer strategies are being explored that use dopamine receptor agonists to boost dopaminergic signaling in the brain and give longer-lasting control of symptoms.

DISPARITIES IN ACCESS TO CONVENTIONAL TREATMENTS

Health equity is a very important goal for public health, even though it is not often reached. The quality of life and overall well-being of individuals with neurological disorders are profoundly affected by the prevalence of inequities across multiple health domains, including the neurological field (Fornari et al., 2025). The WHO Intersectoral Global Action Plan on Epilepsy and Other Neurological Disorders 2022-2031 (WHOiGAP), released in 2024, seeks to enhance awareness regarding the challenges and deficiencies in neurological disorders, while highlighting the presence of health disparities in nearly every nation and region (Fornari et al., 2025). From June 2020 to June 2024, a retrospective chart review of patients newly diagnosed with Parkinson's disease was conducted at Thammasat University Hospital, a tertiary care institution located on the northern outskirts of Bangkok. The Movement Disorder Society Parkinson's Disease (MDS-PD) diagnostic criteria were applied retroactively to ensure diagnostic consistency following a probable diagnosis of Parkinson's disease by neurologists, movement disorder specialists, or referral physicians (Lolekha et al., 2025).

L-DOPA is not available to everyone with Parkinson's disease around the world, and the amount of it available varies greatly from country to country. Africa is probably the best example of this inequality (Merello et al., 2018). According to the World Health Organization's (WHO) 2nd Edition Neurology Atlas, only 3% of the countries in the WHO African Region had levodopa/carbidopa available at the primary care level all the time. The initial report regarding L-DOPA utilization in Africa emerged in 1972, shortly following its introduction. It talked about a five-year study of 30 PD cases treated at an outpatient clinic in Nairobi, Kenya (Merello et al., 2018).

Surveys of pharmacies in Kenya, Nigeria, and Ghana, along with a survey of neurologists across Africa, have indicated that PD medications are both inaccessible and excessively costly (Fothergill-Misbah et al., 2024). Because health insurance programs don't cover PD medications very well in sub-Saharan Africa, people have to pay for them out of their own pockets. One of the biggest problems is that there aren't enough healthcare facilities, like pharmacies and health centers in remote and rural areas. People with Parkinson's disease (PD) have a hard time getting an accurate diagnosis, quick treatment, and ongoing care because of this lacuna. Moreover, another fact of the matter is that there aren't enough qualified medical professionals too to cater in remote and under-resourced areas (Zewde, 2020). Further, affordability, which is based on the cost of medications and the ability to pay for them for the length of the illness or for the rest of one's life, becomes a key part of accessibility to quality healthcare (Fothergill-Misbah et al., 2024). Functional neurosurgery (FNS) is a non-invasive and highly effective neurosurgical subspeciality utilizing deep brain stimulation (DBS) and it has created new perspectives for the surgical management of PD patients, due to the low morbidity, reversibility and improvement of both motor function and quality of life as compared to the lesioning techniques. However, the technique is still not accessible to majority of patient population, particularly in lower middle-income countries (LMICs) (Asija et al., 2024).

THE FUNCTION OF AFFORDABLE NATURAL LEVODOPA SOURCES

Mucuna pruriens (Velvet bean; Kaunch) and *Vicia faba* (Broad Bean or Fava Bean; Bakla) are two inexpensive natural sources of levodopa that can help people with Parkinson's disease (PD) move better, especially in places where there aren't many resources (Cilia et al., 2017).

Mucuna pruriens (MP) seeds are rich in levodopa. For example, 7 g of roasted MP powder can give you about 400 mg of levodopa, which is about the same as 100/25 mg of levodopa/carbidopa (Cilia et al., 2017).

In Sub-Saharan Africa, it costs about 10–15 USD per patient per year, while standard levodopa/DDCI costs about 365 USD per year which makes it an ultimate option. MP is a good choice when pharmaceutical levodopa is hard to get or not always available because it is much cheaper, easy to make, and widely available in tropical areas (Hammoud et al., 2025).

Vicia faba (broad beans) contains pharmacologically active levels of levodopa (Caronni et al., 2024). Consuming cooked broad beans has been demonstrated to elevate plasma levodopa levels and enhance motor performance in patients with Parkinson's disease. This indicates that locally cultivated food crops can temporarily enhance dopaminergic therapy (Chaudhuri & Batzu, 2023). In the initial phases of Parkinson's disease or during mild symptomatology, these food-based sources may serve as a culturally acceptable and readily accessible means to compensate for insufficient medication or the necessity to await standard treatment (Rabey et al., 1992).

Randomized crossover trials comparing MP preparations with levodopa/DDCI have shown that single doses of MP can produce similar or even faster onset of motor benefits, along with longer "on" time and a decrease in dyskinesias in some patients with advanced Parkinson's disease (Aureli et al., 2025). One study found that high-dose MP caused a longer "on" period (about 45 minutes longer) and fewer dyskinesias than standard levodopa/benserazide. This indicates that natural levodopa sources may be equally effective for motor control in the short term (Soumyanath et al., 2012). Long-term data are more limited: in an observational study of daily MP intake in advanced PD, about half of the patients stopped taking it because of gastrointestinal side effects or worsening motor performance which is the downside of MP. However, those who could handle MP had motor outcomes similar to those who took levodopa/carbidopa (Cilia et al., 2017). However, existing studies are constrained by their limited size, heterogeneity, and often short duration, rendering long-term efficacy and safety indeterminate (de Heer et al., 2024).

Eating *Vicia faba* has been associated with significant enhancements in motor function and substantial elevations in plasma levodopa concentrations. Some patients, however, experienced severe dyskinesias, indicating that natural sources can yield clinically significant doses that require adjustment and monitoring (Rabey et al., 1993). Case reports and small studies suggest that the motor benefits following broad bean consumption may be comparable to a standard dose of levodopa/carbidopa, especially in individuals with mild to moderate disease (Botello-Villagrana & Martinez-Ramirez, 2021).

Plant-based levodopa has a big problem: its pharmacokinetics change a lot depending on the plant genotype, growing conditions, processing methods, and the fact that DDCI is not given at the same time (Katzenschlager et al., 2004). Kinetic-dynamic studies show that MP capsules with analytically verified levodopa have much lower peak plasma concentrations and overall exposure than the same amount of levodopa/carbidopa. This means that some patients may not respond at all or respond less strongly to the drug (Hammoud et al., 2025).

Tests on commercial MP supplements and natural L-dopa products have shown that some products contain less than 10% of the stated dose. Environmental and botanical factors influence seed levodopa concentrations. MP plants that are grown closer to the equator tend to have more levodopa, and the levels differ in different parts of the plant. This makes it even harder to standardise doses (Soumyanath et al., 2012). In environments with constrained resources and the absence of routine laboratory testing, this variability complicates the formulation of consistent dosing regimens (Aureli et al., 2025).

In controlled trials, acute MP administration has demonstrated a safety profile that may be better than that of pharmaceutical levodopa, as evidenced by a decrease in short-term adverse events (Caronni et al., 2024). In real life, long-term MP therapy has had different effects on patients, and many have stopped the treatment because of stomach problems and worsening motor function. Excessive or poorly timed consumption of Vicia faba can lead to severe dyskinesias in patients already receiving levodopa treatment, and individuals with glucose-6-phosphate dehydrogenase deficiency may be vulnerable to favism, thereby increasing safety concerns in specific populations (de Heer et al., 2024). Toxicological tests reveal that MP seed preparations may be detrimental to the liver, kidneys, and reproductive system in addition to the typical negative effects of dopamine.There are also reports of poisoning after eating raw, unprocessed MP seeds, which can cause serious digestive and possibly neurological problems (Rabey et al., 1992).

Many low-income communities lack adequate pharmacovigilance systems, if any exist at all. Accordingly, it is likely that those who experience adverse reactions to herbal levodopa products are not adequately identified or reported (Soumyanath et al., 2012). When relying on community anecdotes and small case series, it is challenging to weigh the perceived benefits against the rare but significant harms in the absence of formal post-marketing surveillance (Ramírez-Moreno et al., 2015).

Patients must be informed of the uncertainties surrounding long-term safety and efficacy, and these interventions should be viewed as context-specific responses to medical scarcity rather than simply superior or more natural treatments (Botello-Villagrana & Martinez-Ramirez, 2021). The main goals are still to make standard levodopa supply chains stronger and to build basic pharmacovigilance skills. Using natural levodopa sources can be a short-term or long-term fix for health systems that don't have a lot of money (Chaudhuri & Batzu, 2023). Hence, these natural supplements can't be used on a long-term basis due to variability in levodopa content, effectiveness in different cases, documented problems with tolerability, and lack of strong systems for regulation and pharmacovigilance (Caronni et al., 2024). These preparations can therefore be considered as alternatives or additions to standard levodopa-decarboxylase inhibitor (DDCI) therapy that is specific to the situation, and not as full replacements. This means that careful clinical supervision and local policies for quality assurance and monitoring are needed (Katzenschlager et al., 2004).

OBSTACLES TO DIAGNOSIS AND THE BURDEN OF NON-MOTOR SYMPTOMS

In low- and middle-income countries (LMICs), Parkinson's disease (PD) is often diagnosed late because early symptoms are misconstrued as typical manifestations of ageing, arthritis, or general musculoskeletal issues rather than a neurodegenerative condition (Van Laar & Jain, 2004).Non-specific neuromuscular symptoms (NMS), such as depression, anxiety, sleep disturbances, and autonomic complaints, are frequently managed independently from the underlying Parkinson's disease, resulting in postponed disease-specific treatment (Li et al., 2024).Primary care providers may have insufficient neurology training and limited knowledge of early Parkinson's disease characteristics, resulting in misdiagnosis and underdiagnosis, especially when motor symptoms are mild and non-motor symptoms are more prominent (Tibar et al., 2018).

Optimal dopaminergic therapy in LMICs is obstructed by various systemic barriers, such as restricted formularies, inconsistent drug supply, and substantial costs, even when Parkinson's disease is diagnosed (Van Laar & Jain, 2004). Advanced formulations, levodopa, and dopamine agonists may not always be available in public systems, necessitating that patients pay privately or endure inadequate or inconsistent dosing schedules, leading to poorly managed motor and non-motor symptoms (Aslam et al., 2025). Instead of being proactively modified based on shifting NMS like mood, sleep, and cognitive function, dopaminergic therapy is frequently started late, underdosed, or only increased when there is obvious motor decline (Yang et al., 2024).

Household income has a major impact on long-term adherence because families who are unable to pay for chronic medications frequently experience treatment interruptions due to financial limitations and inadequate insurance coverage. Most LMICs still lack access to sophisticated device-aided therapies (such as deep brain stimulation and infusion therapies) that can help with recalcitrant motor and some non-motor issues because of a lack of personnel, infrastructure, and funding (Koehn et al., 2025).

Regular follow-up with specialists is often less possible because of things such as long travel distances, high transportation costs and low income, especially for patients who live in rural areas or are in below poverty line (Bloem et al., 2021). Because of this, a lot of people only go to the doctor when their symptoms are so bad that they can't work, or they only go to tertiary centers once in a while, which makes a reactive model of care even stronger.

For non-motor complications that change over time, like cognitive decline, psychosis, impulse-control disorders, and autonomic dysfunction, systematic screening and long-term assessment are important. However, they are not often part of routine visits in systems with limited resources (Aslam et al., 2025). Multidisciplinary teams are not common, so physiotherapy, speech therapy, occupational therapy, mental health support, and social care are not often available or coordinated. Consequently, the broader functional and psychosocial ramifications of NMS remain predominantly unaddressed (Van Laar & Jain, 2004).

NMS are now known to be important parts of PD, and they often show up years before motor signs. They greatly affect the quality of life, disability, and the stress on carers. Common domains include neuropsychiatric symptoms (depression, anxiety, apathy, and psychosis), sleep and circadian disturbances, pain and sensory symptoms, fatigue, gastrointestinal, urinary, and sexual dysfunction, as well as cognitive impairment or dementia (Yang et al., 2022). Extensive cohort and questionnaire-based studies have shown that nearly all people with Parkinson's Disease (PD) have one or more non-motor symptoms (NMS) as the disease gets worse. The burden of NMS is often greater than that of motor symptoms on health-related quality of life (Radad et al., 2023).

In low- and middle-income countries (LMICs), healthcare providers and patients may focus on visible motor impairments while disregarding or normalising non-motor symptoms, particularly mood changes or issues related to sexual function and bowel and bladder control, which may be stigmatised or difficult to address (Van Laar & Jain, 2004). Validated NMS screening tools are rarely utilised in standard practice, and structured cognitive assessment is generally limited to advanced stages, leading to unrecorded and untreated early cognitive deficits, mild depression, REM sleep behaviour disorder, and autonomic symptoms (Li et al., 2024).

Depression and anxiety are among the best signs of a low quality of life and affect a large number of people with Parkinson's disease. However, they are still not diagnosed or treated enough around the world, and the problem is even worse in low- and middle-income countries where mental health resources are scarce. Mood symptoms are often addressed, if at all, by non-specialists who have limited time and training, primarily due to stigma, the shortage of psychiatrists and psychologists, and the financial burden of antidepressants or counselling (Singh et al., 2025). There is a paucity of systematic reviews regarding psychotropic-dopaminergic interactions or tailored regimens for depression and anxiety linked to Parkinson's disease (PD), attributable to insufficient integration between neurology and mental health services (Koehn et al., 2025). Psychosis, characterised by visual hallucinations and delusions, often occurs in advanced neurodegenerative diseases and may be exacerbated by dopaminergic medications (Aslam et al., 2025). Safer alternatives for PD psychosis are often inaccessible or excessively costly, and antipsychotic options in resource-limited environments may be restricted to medications with an elevated risk of extrapyramidal side effects. To prevent stigma, carers may refrain from disclosing psychotic symptoms, while clinicians may focus on motor control, potentially leading to prolonged distress and an increased risk of institutionalisation (Radad et al., 2025).

Autonomic dysfunction is one of the most common NMS clusters in PD and is a major cause of disability, falls, and hospital stays (Van Laar & Jain, 2004). It can show up as orthostatic hypotension, constipation, needing to urinate often or not being able to hold it, problems with sex, and problems with regulating body temperature. In LMICs, diagnostic work-up for autonomic symptoms is often restricted due to the unavailability or lack of coverage for specific pharmacologic options, compression garments, or dietary supplements within public systems. Consequently, management may be confined to fundamental advice or symptomatic over-the-counter remedies (Tibar et al., 2018). These symptoms may also make it hard to stick to the plan. For example, patients may discontinue dopaminergic therapy without informing clinicians if they encounter significant constipation, nausea, or postural hypotension (Bloem et al., 2021).

Cognitive impairment can range from mild executive and attentional deficits to severe dementia (Asuku et al., 2025b). It affects up to three-quarters of people with long-standing PD, making carers' jobs much harder and people with PD much more dependent. Neuropsychological services are limited in many low- and middle-income countries (LMICs), and cholinesterase inhibitors or other cognitive enhancers may not be easily accessible or affordable. This forces families to deal with progressive changes in behavior and cognition with little help from professionals (Yang et al., 2022). System-level issues include weak referral pathways, poor coordination between primary and specialist care, lack of national PD guidelines adapted to resource constraints (Singh et al., 2025). In many countries, PD is not prioritized in health-policy agendas despite rapidly rising prevalence and disability, so investments in workforce training, medication supply chains, and multidisciplinary services remain inadequate (Aslam et al., 2025).The high, unrelieved burden of NMS in LMICs has substantial implications for quality of life, disability, and societal costs, with many patients becoming dependent earlier and carers experiencing marked physical, emotional, and financial stress (Radad et al., 2025).

Figure 3. PDMDS rehabilitation model of care for Parkinson's disease

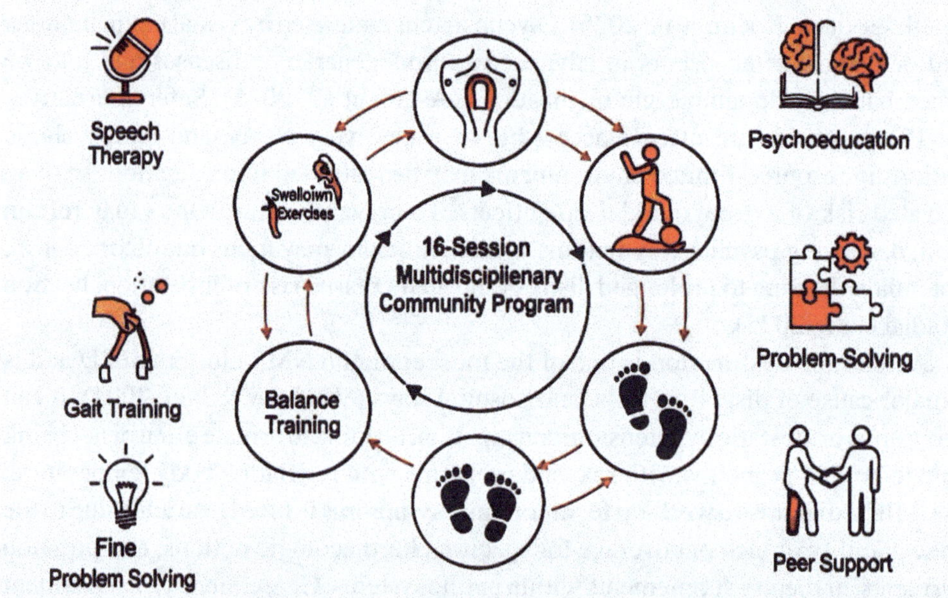

It illustrates a 16-session multidisciplinary community rehabilitation program created by the Parkinson's Disease and Movement Disorder Society (PDMDS) in India for individuals with Parkinson's disease and their carers. It emphasizes important parts like speech therapy, exercises for swallowing, training for walking and balance, psychoeducation, structured problem-solving, fine motor problem-solving, and peer support. Most of these services are provided through community-based Parkinson's support centers to make group-based care easy to get and cheap.

Community-based rehabilitation (CBR), which is supported by the WHO as a way to manage chronic diseases and disabilities in LMICs, combines health, education, work, and social inclusion within local communities (Barretto & D'souza, 2023). CBR principles for Parkinson's disease are used in group therapy settings, community support centres, and locally run rehabilitation programmes that address both motor and non-motor symptoms as well as social engagement and carer support (Goldman et al., 2024).

The WHO technical brief on Parkinson's disease says that community-delivered models are very important for filling treatment gaps because most people in LMICs don't have access to neurologists, structured rehabilitation, or long-term follow-up (Lemmi et al., 2017). These models should be cheap, easy to repeat, and adaptable to different sociocultural settings, especially in rural and peri-urban areas where specialized services are hard to find (Barretto & D'souza, 2023).

The PDMDS rehabilitation "model of care" in India is a standardized, 16-session, multidisciplinary community program for people with Parkinson's disease (PwP) and their carers. It is mostly offered through community-based Parkinson's Support Centers (PSCs). The model includes evidence-based group exercises for speech, swallowing, balance, gait, fine motor skills, and problem-solving, as well as locally specific psychoeducation, problem-solving, and peer support components (Goldman et al., 2024). This program was specifically designed to be low-cost, feasible for non-specialist facilitators, and sustainable through collaboration with local stakeholders such as community organizations, non-governmental organizations (NGOs), and lay volunteers (Weise et al., 2024). The PSC network has grown across India, including rural and tribal areas, demonstrating the model's replicability and ability to function in resource-constrained environments when supported by community partnerships (Iemmi et al., 2017).

The task-shifting literature supports the notion that, with proper training and supervision, community health workers can safely deliver chronic disease care components such as screening, basic counselling, lifestyle support, and follow-up, thereby expanding specialist reach (Watson et al., 2023). Diabetes and physical activity interventions in low- and middle-income countries have demonstrated that trained frontline workers can improve adherence, early detection, and continuity of care by using digital tools and simple checklists to guide decision-making and referrals (Weise et al., 2024).

Multidisciplinary Parkinson's disease care models prioritize physiotherapy, occupational therapy, and speech-language pathology as essential interventions for sustaining function and participation throughout the disease trajectory (Goldman et al., 2024). Community group classes, emphasizing gait training, balance exercises, amplitude-based movements, dual-task practice, and fine-motor activities, can be conducted in local centers or halls, reducing travel expenses and facilitating peer motivation. Voice and communication therapy, encompassing loudness and articulation exercises, can be administered in group or home environments under the supervision of trained therapists or community facilitators, occasionally augmented by mHealth tools. These sessions provide education on medication adherence and the timing of dietary intake in relation to pharmacological regimens, such as spacing levodopa from high-protein meals to enhance absorption, thereby aiding individuals with Parkinson's disease and their families in integrating pharmacological treatments into their daily routines (Bonnechère et al., 2023).

Multidisciplinary and community-based teams ensure continuity by coordinating between neurologists, primary care providers, therapists, and community workers, reducing fragmentation that occurs in traditional care (Pirtošek et al., 2024). Regular group sessions and follow-up contacts help to establish predictable routines, allowing for early detection of problems like falls, dysphagia, mood changes, or carer overload, as well as timely adjustments and referrals (Weise et al., 2024).

Practical training (safe transfers, cueing, and environmental modifications), emotional support, and peer exchanges in support groups all help to reduce carer burden, making carers feel more competent and less isolated (Goldman et al., 2024). Multidisciplinary Parkinson's disease teams and community rehabilitation studies have shown that when carers actively participate in goal-setting, education, and shared decision-making, their quality of life and distress improve (Pirtošek et al., 2024).

Community-centred models reframe people with Parkinson's as active partners instead of passive recipients. They focus on self-management skills like setting goals, pacing activities, sticking to home exercises, and keeping an eye on symptoms (Goldman et al., 2024). Structured programmes often teach patients how to add walking, posture exercises, voice practice, and cognitive strategies to their daily tasks, using written or digital resources and regular feedback (Watson et al., 2023).

Evidence from multidisciplinary and telehealth-enhanced Parkinson's disease rehabilitation indicates that empowering patients to manage both motor and non-motor symptoms, alongside education and coaching, can enhance functional outcomes and decrease unplanned healthcare utilisation. Community-based CBR frameworks prioritise social participation, fostering engagement in family, work, and community roles, thereby promoting psychological well-being and resilience in patients with chronic neurological conditions (Iemmi et al., 2017).

Models like the PDMDS approach can be used in a lot of different places because they are cheap per person, use community spaces, rely on trained non-specialists, and have flexible group formats. The World Health Organization and other experts on Parkinson's disease around the world support integrated, community-based services as part of national plans for noncommunicable diseases and rehabilitation, especially in areas with few specialists (Barretto & D'souza, 2023).

Future directions proposed in multidisciplinary Parkinson's disease care literature include integrating tele-rehabilitation, mobile apps, and remote monitoring to support rural centers; creating clear referral pathways between community and specialist services; and developing guidelines for MDT structures in various resource settings (Weise et al., 2024). Overall, community-centered multidisciplinary care models offer a practical way to increase Parkinson's disease care coverage, improve functional outcomes, and support families in low- and middle-income countries through locally anchored, task-shared, and culturally informed strategies (Pirtošek et al., 2024).

TELEMEDICINE AND DIGITAL HEALTH ADVANCES

Tele-neurology for PD utilizes video consultations to conduct a substantial portion of the motor examination visually, which corresponds effectively with the evaluation of bradykinesia, tremor, and dyskinesia (Chirra et al., 2019).

Randomised and cohort studies on "virtual house calls" for PD reveal that high patient satisfaction and clinical outcomes are comparable to in-person care, while reducing travel time and costs (Cubo et al., 2022).

In Brazil's public health system, direct-to-home video consultations using low-cost platforms like WhatsApp were possible, with more than 90% attendance. These consultations also improved sleep and physical activity in PD patients (Santos et al., 2022). Tele-neurology programs in areas with few resources have shown that neurologists can change dopaminergic medications and keep an eye on complications from a distance, as long as there is some access to smartphones and the internet (Shalash et al., 2021).Telemedicine models allow clinicians to modify levodopa regimens through home-recorded video, structured symptom diaries, and carer reports, thus obviating the need for multiple in-person consultations (Shalash et al., 2021).

Research on tele-assisted titration of advanced dopaminergic therapies, including levodopa–carbidopa intestinal gel, indicates that home-based video-guided adjustment is technically viable, resource-efficient, and satisfactory for both patients and staff (Cubo et al., 2022). Continuous or frequent remote review can also help identify troublesome peak-dose dyskinesias or wearing-off phenomena sooner, which makes it possible to start fractionation or adjunct therapy sooner (Moreau et al., 2023).

Body-worn sensors (accelerometers and inertial measurement units) and smartwatches can objectively quantify tremor, bradykinesia, gait disturbances, and dyskinesias during daily life, complementing clinician observation during short consultations (Din et al., 2021). Reviews of wearable systems for PD show that they can collect motor data around the clock, create digital endpoints like step counts, gait variability, and dyskinesia burden, and help people make personalized treatment choices (Moreau et al., 2023).

The STAT-ON sensor, which is worn around the waist, can automatically detect on-off states, dyskinesia episodes, and freezing of gait. The results are shown on clinician dashboards to help with timing and dose adjustments of levodopa (Chirra et al., 2019). Research prototypes and remote monitoring platforms, like the Parkinson's Remote Interactive Monitoring System, are made to reduce the need for in-person neurology consultations in rural and resource-limited areas (Shalash et al., 2021).

Telerehabilitation programmes use video conferencing to provide physiotherapy, balance training, and gait exercises to people with Parkinson's disease at home (Ramos et al., 2023). According to physical therapists in Brazil and other middle-income countries, telerehabilitation can help people with Parkinson's disease (PD) and other neurological conditions to receive continued ecare. However, they point out problems like patients not being able to get to devices, inconsistent home space, and the need for both therapist and patient training. Telerehabilitation platforms that use wearable sensors can give patients immediate feedback and give clinicians' objective logs of motor performance and exercise compliance (Din et al., 2021).

Inconsistencies also exist in policy and reimbursement frameworks. E.g., emergency telemedicine authorisations granted during the COVID-19 pandemic in Brazil increased healthcare access, but national guidelines for remote neurological care, funding mechanisms, and long-term integration into routine care are still lacking (Ramos et al., 2023). Reviews of telemedicine in Parkinson's disease highlight that clear regulations data privacy safeguards, and infrastructure investments in broadband and devices particularly for older adults and rural populations are necessary for sustainable models (Cubo et al., 2022).

DRUG REPURPOSING AND COST-EFFECTIVE PHARMACOTHERAPY

Amantadine was initially developed as an antiviral agent before its NMDA receptor-modulating and dopaminergic properties were discovered (Metman et al., 1998). Randomised controlled trials have shown that adding amantadine to levodopa can reduce the severity of levodopa-induced dyskinesia (LID) by 50-60% without compromising the benefit of levodopa, supporting its role as an antidyskinetic agent for motor complications (Pahwa et al., 2017). However, these proprietary products are typically more expensive than immediate-release generics. In under-resourced settings, immediate-release generic amantadine remains the more realistic option (Mendoza, 2022). Its long-term antidyskinetic effect has been documented, providing a relatively inexpensive way to manage LID when device-assisted therapies are unavailable (Metman et al., 1999).

Another layer of low-dose, frequently well-tolerated dopaminergic support is provided by selective MAO-B inhibitors like rasagiline and selegiline, which inhibit central dopamine breakdown and somewhat alleviate motor symptoms or shorten "OFF" time. While rasagiline is pharmacologically appealing as a once-daily, second-generation MAO-B inhibitor, economic and prescribing-pattern analyses show that its branded formulations can be significantly more expensive than selegiline and many dopamine agonists, raising concerns about its affordability in everyday practice (Esposti et al., 2016). Because it delays levodopa use and lowers dyskinesia-related costs, cost-effectiveness modelling from high-income settings indicates that rasagiline may still be cost-effective when compared to some branded dopamine agonists and levodopa initiation. If pricing and reimbursement are in line with local budgets, generic rasagiline and locally produced MAO-B inhibitors could become significant low-cost adjuncts (Farkouh et al., 2012). Prioritising generic selegiline or generic rasagiline and using levodopa in a logical stepwise manner can help prolong the dopaminergic benefit while minimising financial toxicity in LMIC settings where patients frequently pay out of pocket (Fothergill-Misbah et al., 2025).

Flexible combination regimens utilising inexpensive adjuncts, such as amantadine, MAO-B inhibitors, and, when practical, generic dopamine agonists or catechol-O-methyltransferase (COMT) inhibitors, enable clinicians to tailor treatment based on symptom profile, tolerability, and cost when levodopa monotherapy proves inadequate (Metman et al., 1999). Addition of amantadine and adjusting levodopa dosage can improve function in a patient with problematic peak-dose dyskinesias. Early use of an inexpensive MAO-B inhibitor may delay the onset of levodopa or permit lower dosages, which could reduce the long-term risk of motor complications (Farkouh et al., 2012). This is particularly helpful when management is given in primary or secondary care and specialist follow-up is infrequent. Customisation must consider not only clinical criteria but also the patient's financial situation and any limitations imposed by local formularies or essential medicines lists, as these regimens are often assembled using generics with different price points and availability profiles (Fothergill-Misbah et al., 2025).

PD medications, such as levodopa, amantadine, MAO-B inhibitors, and dopamine agonists, are often unavailable or too expensive in public facilities, according to data from Kenya and other LMICs. These force patients to either forego treatment entirely or buy medications from private pharmacies at a high out-of-pocket expense (Zewde, 2020). Numerous people receive subtherapeutic doses or interrupted courses of levodopa, and very few have access to adjunctive agents or device-assisted therapies due to stock-outs, fragmented procurement, and weak financing mechanisms, according to surveys of neurologists and patients (Gavidia et al., 2020). Numerous

Parkinson's medications are included in the 2023 World Health Organization essential medicines list (EML). However, analyses of national essential medicines lists have revealed that dopaminergic therapies, particularly more recently developed agents, are frequently omitted or listed in a restricted manner, which restricts their uptake into publicly funded care (Misbah et al., 2025). The availability of low-cost pharmacotherapy options at the point of care is determined by policy decisions regarding inclusion on national lists, procurement priorities, and pricing regulation. In this context, the theoretical affordability of generics does not necessarily translate into equitable access (Oertel et al., 2017).

Although they continue to be a structural weakness in many low-income countries, robust medicine supply chains are essential for achieving the advantages of drug repurposing and generic-based PD pharmacotherapy (Fothergill-Misbah et al., 2025). While more direct "cross-docking" models that connect central warehouses to frontline clinics can significantly reduce stock-out duration and improve availability, traditional multi-tier distribution systems are linked to frequent and prolonged stock-outs, according to large-scale evaluations of essential drug logistics, such as randomized trials in Zambia (Metman et al., 1999). It is difficult for clinicians to maintain stable, combination-based regimens for chronic conditions like Parkinson's disease (PD), where symptom control depends on ongoing dopaminergic stimulation, because such stock-outs not only exacerbate motor and non-motor symptoms but also have the potential to cause dangerous withdrawal syndromes and compromise adherence (Gavidia et al., 2020). In addition to national and international advocacy to secure reliable supplies of essential generics like levodopa, amantadine, selegiline, and rasagiline, it is imperative to improve forecasting, cold-chain-independent storage, last-mile distribution, and data systems for tracking PD medicine availability in order to translate pharmacotherapeutic possibilities into tangible benefits (Mendoza, 2022).

EDUCATION, ADVOCACY, AND LOCALIZATION OF CARE

The majority of people with Parkinson's disease currently live in low- and middle-income nations, where education, advocacy, and localizing care are thought to be essential elements for achieving equitable dopaminergic access (Schiess et al., 2022). Future strategies stress early diagnosis, smart use of levodopa, culturally appropriate education, rehabilitation based on lifestyle, and structural measures to make sure that cheap, generic dopaminergic drugs are available on a national scale (Leon-Rojas, 2025). In light of the rapidly growing global burden, especially in places with limited resources, traditional "passive" models of care, in which health systems wait for patients to show up with advanced motor symptoms, are becoming less and less viable (Trinh et al., 2025).

National protocols that prioritize early detection through digital screening tools and primary-care training argue that intervening earlier is both clinically more effective and more cost-efficient than treating late-stage disability, while critical analyses of the global rise in Parkinson's disease highlight that under-diagnosis in older adults and misattribution of symptoms to ageing or musculoskeletal disease delay levodopa initiation and contribute to preventable functional loss. In this context, levodopa is still the most important drug (Bhidayasiri et al., 2024). Mechanistic and health-system studies indicate that in numerous low-income environments, patients either do not receive levodopa or face frequent stock-outs and dose interruptions, which compromise adherence and clinical stability (Kwok et al., 2019). This emphasizes how important it is to plan at the system level for the sensible distribution and prescription of levodopa. Simultaneously, examinations of unequal access to healthcare underscore that cultural beliefs, stigma, and inadequate health literacy influence the timing of patient care-seeking and the consistency of dopaminergic medication adherence (Schiess et al., 2022).

Exercise, yoga, and dietary changes are examples of lifestyle-based interventions that are increasingly being recognised as essential supplements to medication that can be incorporated into community initiatives. Frequent resistance and aerobic exercise may enhance quality of life and motor function, and it may even alter the course of disease (Sharma et al., 2015). Beyond resistance training and stretching, mindfulness-based yoga offers additional psychological benefits (Misbah et al., 2024). Through the integration of basic dietary guidelines, sleep education, and physical activity promotion with screening and follow-up, the "eat, move, sleep" models show how lifestyle-centered community programs can improve medication adherence by integrating dopaminergic regimens within comprehensive self-management frameworks (Pochigaeva et al., 2023).

Effective dopaminergic medications, including cost-effective generics, are already available, but treatment gaps surpass 75% in numerous low-income nations, rendering access a fundamental justice concern (Leon-Rojas, 2025). They advocate for unified advocacy from patients, clinicians, and professional organizations to urge governments and donors to fund essential dopaminergic medications and to reform procurement, supply chains, and coverage systems (Kwok et al., 2019). Empirical work from African settings demonstrates how weak supply systems translate into prolonged stock-outs of levodopa and lack of access to adjunct therapies, resulting in "off" periods, reduced mobility, loss of employment, and carer strain, and these case studies are presented as models for understanding the disparities that must be addressed through policy reform, better procurement practices, and partnerships with global and regional stakeholders. Policy- and industry-orientated reports compile expert recommendations for enhancing access to high-quality generics in low- and middle-income countries (Trinh et al., 2025). These measures are directly relevant to stabilising national supplies of generic levodopa and other dopaminergic medications, and they align with broader noncommunicable disease access frameworks aimed at improving the availability of essential medicines, diagnostics, and technologies for chronic conditions, including neurological disorders (Pochigaeva et al., 2023). This can be achieved by combining digital screening in primary care, training community health workers to recognise Parkinson's disease, and embedding "eat, move, sleep" lifestyle packages into local clinics and community centers (Janssen Daalen et al., 2022).

All of these analyses states that fair access to dopamine cannot be achieved through drugs alone; it requires early detection, prudent levodopa use, culturally sensitive education, lifestyle-improving community programs, strong support for generic manufacturing and sustainable funding, and international partnerships that help nations build robust health care systems and local rehabilitation capacity so that pharmaceutical innovations translate into real improvements for Parkinson's patients in low-resource settings (Bhidayasiri et al., 2024).

TOWARDS FAIR, COMMUNITY-BASED DOPAMINERGIC CARE

ParkinsonNet was founded to improve Parkinson's disease treatment by establishing geographically organised networks of allied health professionals with specialised training, such as physiotherapists, occupational and speech therapists, and PD nurses, around nearby hospitals (Keus et al., 2012). This network has expanded to include approximately 3,000 professionals and 70 regional networks, demonstrating how focusing PD expertise on community-based providers can improve quality while keeping costs low (Bloem et al., 2017).

The Indian PDMDS model has a similar community focus, but it adapts its delivery to the needs of low- and middle-income areas. It offers free, multidisciplinary services through more than 60 support groups and centers in 24 Indian states. These centers are located in accessible, disability-friendly community spaces like schools, churches, and nonprofit organizations, so people with Parkinson's disease (PD) and their carers can get education, counselling, speech therapy, physiotherapy, and other services near their homes without having to pay a lot of money out of pocket (Gary et al., 2016).

The global shortage of movement-disorder neurologists has led to a growing recognition of PD nurses and other allied health professionals as key coordinators of dopaminergic care in both high- and low-resource settings. Evaluations of PD nurse specialist roles (Bloem et al., 2017) show that nurse-led, community-based interventions can improve symptom control, patient satisfaction, and continuity of care while encouraging medication optimization and self-management over time.

To standardize dopaminergic prescribing and follow-up across primary and secondary care, ParkinsonNet's local coordinators—usually nurses or physiotherapists—organise regional education, encourage communication between different fields, and serve as points of contact for patients and families (Dash et al., 2025). In India, PDMDS teams made up of physiotherapists, speech therapists, psychologists, and social workers provide voice therapy, group exercise, and counselling sessions in regional languages, incorporating dopaminergic management into peer support networks and culturally appropriate routines (Keus et al., 2012).

iCARE-PD is an evolution of all these ideas. It is a home-based, community-centered integrated care network that uses telemedicine and digital tools to support dopaminergic care trajectories. The model combines technology-enabled monitoring, remote consultations, and structured self-management support within a personalised care plan to meet the complex needs of people with PD at different stages of the disease and in different health-system contexts (Thomas et al., 2024).

Qualitative research with nurses providing telemedicine care under iCARE-PD also shows that video visits and remote education can bring specialized knowledge into patients' homes. However, it also shows that low-resource areas are especially affected by problems with digital literacy, connectivity, and reimbursement policies (Gary et al., 2016).

ParkinsonNet in the Netherlands uses information and communication technology (ICT) platforms to share guidelines, teach patients, and get feedback on the quality of care. This creates a learning network that can help with service planning and registry-type data collection over time. In India, online support groups and virtual sessions are becoming more common as a way to provide education, exercise classes, and counselling to people who can't physically visit centers. This effectively creates informal registries and communities that can be used for advocacy and health-system reform (van Munster et al., 2022).

To enhance mobility and social participation alongside medication management, ParkinsonNet and PDMDS integrate regular exercise, physiotherapy, and group-based activities such as dance, art, and movement sessions into their community programs (van den Bergh et al., 2021).

Policymakers created incentives that stabilised and expanded community-based dopaminergic care across the country by formalising training requirements, recognising network participation, and linking care procedures to quality reporting and reimbursement (Thomas et al., 2024).

These networks, in conjunction with telemedicine platforms offer low- and middle-income countries a model to progress beyond conventional specialist-focused approaches (Keus et al., 2012). This encompasses the training of nurses and allied health professionals, the establishment of community education and exercise programs, and the creation of registries to document unmet dopaminergic needs as a basis for equity-driven reform (Dash et al., 2025).

CONCLUSION

Dopaminergic treatments are the oldest approach for management of PD and these still form the keystone of contemporary PD treatment. However, the under-resourced settings must contend with the increasing prevalence of the disease, ongoing disparities in access to multidisciplinary care, accurate diagnosis, ongoing levodopa supply, and adjunctive medication. Context-specific solutions, such as community-based rehabilitation models, tele-neurology and telerehabilitation platforms, carefully supervised use of natural levodopa sources, and repurposed agents like amantadine for levodopa-induced dyskinesia, can help fill treatment gaps, according to emerging evidence. In general, attaining equitable dopaminergic therapy for Parkinson's disease (PD) is not only a pharmacological challenge but also a health justice issue, necessitating concurrent action at the clinical, infrastructure, and policy levels to guarantee that treatment advancements result in significant benefits for patients regardless of location or income.

FUTURE DIRECTIONS

Future research should focus on increasing the capacity of the national and international health systems to handle PD by incorporating PD into non-communicable disease strategies, increasing training in neurology and rehabilitation, obtaining reasonably priced, high-quality levodopa and its adjuncts, and growing community-centered multidisciplinary programs that are tailored to local resources and cultures. To improve telemedicine and wearable-sensor platforms that facilitate remote titration and monitoring in LMICs, standardize and optimize natural levodopa preparations like *Mucuna pruriens* for safe, monitored use in situations where pharmaceutical levodopa is scarce, and produce implementation science evidence on the most effective ways to implement these innovations in fragile health systems, parallel research is required. Globally, registries, coordinated advocacy, and WHO-aligned action plans should monitor disparities, direct reimbursement and regulatory reforms, and cultivate collaborations to ensure that dopaminergic therapies—as well as the digital and community infrastructures that support them—are sustainably available to the increasing number of people with Parkinson's disease around the world.

REFERENCES

Abbott, A. (2010). Levodopa: The story so far. *Nature*, *466*(7310), S6–S7. PMID: 20739934

Ajagun, E. J., Asuku, A. O., Ayinla, M. T., Abdulsalam, T. A., Ajibare, A. J., Olajide, T. S., Hamza, Y. O., & Ganiyu, K. O. (2024). Pharmacotherapy of Parkinson's Disease and their Limitations. In: Zebrafish as a Model for Parkinson's Disease. Taylor and Francis, CRC, https://doi.org/DOI: 10.1201/9781003402893-17

Asija, S., Pahwa, B., Agarwal, A., Patil, Y., & Chaurasia, B. (2024). Status of functional neurosurgery in lower middle-income countries (LMICs): A multinational cross sectional survey based analysis of exposure, utilization and perceived barriers. *Clinical Neurology and Neurosurgery*, *245*, 108411. PMID: 39089202

Aslam, S., Sharrief, A. Z., Holden, S. K., Fullard, M., Holtrop, J. S., Maw, A. M., & Amara, A. W. (2025). The future of Parkinson's care: A need to expand access. *Frontiers in Neurology*, *16*, 1622283. PMID: 40612798

Asuku, A. O., Ajagun, E. J., & Oyinlola Ogungbangbe, G. (2025b). *Non-Pharmacological Interventions for Dementia: A Comprehensive Approach* (1st ed.). CRC Press., DOI: 10.1201/9781003516033

Asuku, A. O., Ayinla, M. T., Olajide, T. S., Ajagun, E. J., Ganiyu, K. O., Hamza, Y. O., Ajibare, A. J., & Abdulsalam, T. A. (2024). Diagnosis and Biomarkers of Parkinson's Disease. In: Zebrafish as a Model for Parkinson's Disease. Taylor and Francis, CRC, https://doi.org/DOI: 10.1201/9781003402893-15

Asuku, A. O., Ogungbangbe, G. O., & Fajemidagba, G. A. (2025a). Gene therapy for Parkinson's disease: A new frontier in neurodegenerative diseases. *Exploration of Neuroprotective Therapy*, *5*, 1004119. DOI: 10.37349/ent.2025.1004119

Aureli, F., Gaudiano, M. C., Raimondo, M., Maccelli, A., Di Giorgio, D., Gramazio, M., & Bartolomei, M. (2025). Quality assessment of" naturally occurring" high percentage L-dopa commercial products proposed as dietary supplements by Internet: From labelling to analytical findings. *Frontiers in Chemistry*, *13*, 1597784. PMID: 41169659

Barker, R. A., Björklund, A., & Parmar, M. (2024). The history and status of dopamine cell therapies for Parkinson's disease. *BioEssays*, *46*(12), 2400118. PMID: 39058892

Barretto, M., & D'souza, N. (2023). Conceptualizing a Rehabilitation 'Model of Care' for Improving the Quality of Life of People with Parkinson's in India. *Annals of Indian Academy of Neurology*, *26*(4), 387–394. PMID: 37970321

Bhidayasiri, R., Sringean, J., Phumphid, S., Anan, C., Thanawattano, C., Deoisres, S., & Bunnag, T. (2024). The rise of Parkinson's disease is a global challenge, but efforts to tackle this must begin at a national level: A protocol for national digital screening and "eat, move, sleep" lifestyle interventions to prevent or slow the rise of non-communicable diseases in Thailand. *Frontiers in Neurology*, *15*, 1386608. PMID: 38803644

Bloem, B. R., Okun, M. S., & Klein, C. (2021). Parkinson's disease. *Lancet*, *397*(10291), 2284–2303. PMID: 33848468

Bloem, B. R., Rompen, L., Vries, N. M. D., Klink, A., Munneke, M., & Jeurissen, P. (2017). ParkinsonNet: A low-cost health care innovation with a systems approach from the Netherlands. *Health Affairs*, *36*(11), 1987–1996. PMID: 29137501

Bonnechère, B., Kossi, O., Mapinduzi, J., Panda, J., Rintala, A., Guidetti, S., Spooren, A., & Feys, P. (2023). Mobile health solutions: An opportunity for rehabilitation in low- and middle income countries? *Frontiers in Public Health*, *10*, 1072322. DOI: 10.3389/fpubh.2022.1072322 PMID: 36761328

Botello-Villagrana, F., & Martinez-Ramirez, D. (2021). Mucuna pruriens as adjunct therapy to levodopa in advanced Parkinson's disease. Revista mexicana de neurociencia, 22(5), 180-183.

Caronni, S., Del Sorbo, F., Barichella, M., Fothergill-Misbah, N., & Denne, T., Laguna, & Cilia, R. (2024). Mucuna pruriens to treat Parkinson's disease in low-income countries: Recommendations and practical guidelines from the farmer to clinical trials. Paving the way for future use in clinical practice. *Parkinsonism & Related Disorders*, *124*, 106983. PMID: 38797572

Chaudhuri, K. R., & Batzu, L. (2023). Can continuous levodopa delivery be achieved in the absence of Intrajejunal Levodopa Infusion? Implications for India and Underserved Countries. *Movement Disorders Clinical Practice*, *11*(1), 21–29. PMID: 38291849

Chirra, M., Marsili, L., Wattley, L., Sokol, L. L., Keeling, E., Maule, S., & Merola, A. (2019). Telemedicine in neurological disorders: Opportunities and challenges. *Telemedicine Journal and e-Health*, *25*(7), 541–550. PMID: 30136898

Cilia, R., Laguna, J., Cassani, E., Cereda, E., Pozzi, N. G., Isaias, I. U., & Pezzoli, G. (2017). Mucuna pruriens in Parkinson disease: A double-blind, randomized, controlled, crossover study. *Neurology*, *89*(5), 432–438. PMID: 28679598

Cubo, E., & Delgado-López, P. D. (2022). Telemedicine in the management of Parkinson's disease: Achievements, challenges, and future perspectives. *Brain Sciences*, *12*(12), 1735. PMID: 36552194

de Heer, J. A., Buijtenhuijs, D., & de Wit-Bos, L. (2024). Risk assessment of herbal preparations containing seed extracts of Mucana pruriens.

Degli Esposti, L., Piccinni, C., Sangiorgi, D., Nobili, F., & Buda, S. (2016). Prescribing pattern and resource utilization of monoamine oxidase-B inhibitors in Parkinson treatment: Comparison between rasagiline and selegiline. *Neurological Sciences*, *37*(2), 227–234. PMID: 26474874

Del Din, S., Kirk, C., Yarnall, A. J., Rochester, L., & Hausdorff, J. M. (2021). Body-worn sensors for remote monitoring of Parkinson's disease motor symptoms: Vision, state of the art, and challenges ahead. *Journal of Parkinson's Disease*, *11*(s1), S35–S47. PMID: 33523020

Farkouh, R. A., Wilson, M. R., Tarrants, M. L., Castelli-Haley, J., & Armand, C. (2012). Cost-effectiveness of rasagiline compared with first-line early Parkinson disease therapies. *The American Journal of Pharmacy Benefits*, *4*(3), 99–107.

Finberg, J. P. M., Lamensdorf, I., Commissiong, J. W., & Youdim, M. B. H. (1996). Pharmacology and neuroprotective properties of rasagiline. In Deprenyl—Past and Future [Vienna: Springer Vienna.]. *Journal of Neural Transmission. Supplementum*, *48*, 95–101. PMID: 8988465

Fornari, A., Lanza, M., Guastafierro, E., Marcassoli, A., Sismondo, P., Curatoli, C., & Leonardi, M. (2025). Inequities in neurological care: Access to services, care gaps, and other barriers—A systematic review. *European Journal of Neurology*, *32*(1), e16553. PMID: 39582360

Fothergill-Misbah, N., Cataldi, R., Stothard, M., Chowdhary, N., Okubadejo, N., Cappello, B., & Dua, T. (2025). Parkinson disease treatments on national essential medicines lists, African Region. *Bulletin of the World Health Organization*, *103*(10), 626–634. PMID: 41035551

Fothergill-Misbah, N., Hooker, J., Kwasa, J., & Walker, R. (2024). Access to medicines for Parkinson's disease in Kenya: A qualitative exploration. *Movement Disorders Clinical Practice*, *11*(11), 1373–1378. PMID: 39166895

Goldman, J. G., Volpe, D., Ellis, T. D., Hirsch, M. A., Johnson, J., Wood, J., & Wallock, K. (2024). Delivering multidisciplinary rehabilitation care in Parkinson's disease: An international consensus statement. *Journal of Parkinson's Disease, 14*(1), 135–166. PMID: 38277303

Golovanova, K. A., Skorokhodov, A. P., & Torubarova, I. I. (2013). Patients with neurological disorders: Specifics of communication. *Youth Innovation Bulletin, 2*(1), 251.

Hammoud, F., Ismail, A., Zaher, R., El Majzoub, R., & Abou-Abbas, L. (2025). Mucuna pruriens Treatment for Parkinson Disease: A Systematic Review of Clinical Trials. *Parkinson's Disease, 2025*(1), 1319419. PMID: 40860042

Hauser, R. A., Skarpaas, T. C., Merriam, A., Rivera, J., Hoxhaj, V., Barbato, L. M., & Baladi, M. (2025). Burden of tremor in Parkinson's disease: A survey study. *Journal of Parkinson's Disease, 15*(3), 541–551. PMID: 40123351

Iemmi, V., Blanchet, K., Gibson, L. J., Kumar, K. S., Rath, S., Hartley, S., & Kuper, H. (2016). Community-based rehabilitation for people with physical and mental disabilities in low-and middle-income countries: A systematic review and meta-analysis. *Journal of Development Effectiveness, 8*(3), 368–387.

Iemmi, V., Kumar, K. S., Blanchet, K., Gibson, L., Hartley, S., Murthy, G. V., & Kuper, H. (2017). Community-based rehabilitation for people with physical and mental disabilities in low-and middle-income countries. *Cochrane Database of Systematic Reviews, 2017*(3), CD010617.

Janssen Daalen, J. M., Schootemeijer, S., Richard, E., Darweesh, S. K., & Bloem, B. R. (2022). Lifestyle interventions for the prevention of Parkinson disease: A recipe for action. *Neurology, 99*(7), 42–51. PMID: 35970584

Katzenschlager, R., Evans, A., Manson, A., Patsalos, P. N., Ratnaraj, N., Watt, H., & Lees, A. J. (2004). Mucuna pruriens in Parkinson's disease: A double blind clinical and pharmacological study. *Journal of Neurology, Neurosurgery, and Psychiatry, 75*(12), 1672–1677. PMID: 15548480

Keus, S. H. J., Oude Nijhuis, L. B., Nijkrake, M. J., Bloem, B. R., & Munneke, M. (2012). Improving Community Healthcare for Patients with Parkinson′ s Disease: The Dutch Model. *Parkinson's Disease, 2012*(1), 543426. PMID: 22496990

Koehn, S., Drummond, N., Jasper, L., Pham, A. N., Leung, K., Cloutier, D., & Jones, C. A. (2025). Mechanisms of inequitable access to Parkinson's disease care: A critical interpretive synthesis. *International Journal for Equity in Health, 24*(1), 250. PMID: 41039438

Kwok, J. Y., Kwan, J. C., Auyeung, M., Mok, V. C., Lau, C. K., Choi, K. C., & Chan, H. Y. (2019). Effects of mindfulness yoga vs stretching and resistance training exercises on anxiety and depression for people with Parkinson disease: A randomized clinical trial. *JAMA Neurology, 76*(7), 755–763. PMID: 30958514

Leon-Rojas, J. E. (2025). The global rise in Parkinson's disease: A critical analysis of causes and future directions. *Frontiers in Public Health, 13*, 1606732. PMID: 40535452

Lim, S. Y., Moro, E., & Lang, A. E. (2009). *Non-motor symptoms of Parkinson's disease and the effects of deep brain stimulation. Non Motor Symptoms of Parkinson's Disease*. Oxford University Press.

Lolekha, P., & Jieamanukulkit, P. (2025). Diagnostic Delays in Parkinson's Disease in Thailand: Clinical Pitfalls and Health System Barriers. *Life (Chicago, Ill.), 15*(10), 1513. PMID: 41157185

Mao, Q., Qin, W. Z., Zhang, A., & Ye, N. (2020). Recent advances in dopaminergic strategies for the treatment of Parkinson's disease. *Acta Pharmacologica Sinica, 41*(4), 471–482. PMID: 32112042

Mendoza, M. M. (2022). Is Extended-Release Amantadine Effective at Treating Levodopa-Induced Dyskinesia in Parkinson's Disease Patients?.

Merello, M. (2018). The dark side of globalization: Lack of universal levodopa availability. *Movement Disorders Clinical Practice, 6*(1), 7–8. PMID: 30746409

Metman, L. V., Del Dotto, P., LePoole, K., Konitsiotis, S., Fang, J., & Chase, T. N. (1999). Amantadine for levodopa-induced dyskinesias: A 1-year follow-up study. *Archives of Neurology, 56*(11), 1383–1386. PMID: 10555659

Metman, L. V., Del Dotto, P., Van Den Munckhof, P., Fang, J., Mouradian, M. M., & Chase, T. N. (1998). Amantadine as treatment for dyskinesias and motor fluctuations in Parkinson's disease. *Neurology, 50*(5), 1323–1326. PMID: 9595981

Mitchell, C. L., & Kurouski, D. (2024). Novel strategies in Parkinson's disease treatment: A review. *Frontiers in Molecular Neuroscience, 17*, 1431079. PMID: 39183754

Moreau, C., Rouaud, T., Grabli, D., Benatru, I., Remy, P., Marques, A. R., & Fabbri, M. (2023). Overview on wearable sensors for the management of Parkinson's disease. *NPJ Parkinson's Disease, 9*(1), 153. PMID: 37919332

Mughal, H., Javed, A. R., Rizwan, M., Almadhor, A. S., & Kryvinska, N. (2022). Parkinson's disease management via wearable sensors: A systematic review. *IEEE Access : Practical Innovations, Open Solutions*, *10*, 35219–35237.

Oertel, W., Eggert, K., Pahwa, R., Tanner, C. M., Hauser, R. A., Trenkwalder, C., & Stempien, M. J. (2017). Randomized, placebo-controlled trial of ADS-5102 (amantadine) extended-release capsules for levodopa-induced dyskinesia in Parkinson's disease (EASE LID 3). *Movement Disorders*, *32*(12), 1701–1709. PMID: 28833562

Ovallath, S., & Sulthana, B. (2017). Levodopa: History and therapeutic applications. *Annals of Indian Academy of Neurology*, *20*(3), 185–189. PMID: 28904446

Pahwa, R., Tanner, C. M., Hauser, R. A., Isaacson, S. H., Nausieda, P. A., Truong, D. D., & Stempien, M. J. (2017). ADS-5102 (amantadine) extended-release capsules for levodopa-induced dyskinesia in Parkinson disease (EASE LID study): A randomized clinical trial. *JAMA Neurology*, *74*(8), 941–949. PMID: 28604926

Pastana Ramos, L. F., Vilacorta-Pereira, T. D. C. S., Duarte, J. D. S., Yamada, E. S., & Santos-Lobato, B. L. (2023). Feasibility and effectiveness of a remote individual rehabilitation program for people with Parkinson's disease living in the Brazilian Amazon: A randomized clinical trial. *Frontiers in Neurology*, *14*, 1244661. PMID: 37693755

Pirtošek, Z. (2024). Breaking barriers in Parkinson's care: The multidisciplinary team approach. *Journal of Neural Transmission (Vienna, Austria)*, *131*(11), 1349–1361. PMID: 39417880

Rabey, J. M., Vered, Y., Shabtai, H., Graff, E., Harsat, A., & Korczyn, A. D. (1993). Broad bean (Vicia faba) consumption and Parkinson's disease. *Advances in Neurology*, *60*, 681–684. PMID: 8420210

Rabey, J. M., Vered, Y., Shabtai, H., Graff, E., & Korczyn, A. D. (1992). Improvement of parkinsonian features correlate with high plasma levodopa values after broad bean (Vicia faba) consumption. *Journal of Neurology, Neurosurgery, and Psychiatry*, *55*(8), 725–727. PMID: 1527547

Radad, K., Moldzio, R., Krewenka, C., Kranner, B., & Rausch, W. D. (2017). Pathophysiology of non-motor signs in parkinson's disease: Some recent updating with brief presentation. Explor Neuroprotective Ther 2023; 3: 24-46. *Journal of Neurology, Neurosurgery, and Psychiatry*, *88*(8), 653–662. PMID: 28554959

Radad, K., Moldzio, R., Krewenka, C., Kranner, B., & Rausch, W. D. (2023). Pathophysiology of non-motor signs in Parkinsons disease: Some recent updating with brief presentation. *Exploration of Neuroprotective Therapy*, *3*(1), 24–46.

Radad, K., Moldzio, R., Krewenka, C., Kranner, B., & Rausch, W. D. (2023). Pathophysiology of non-motor signs in Parkinsons disease: Some recent updating with brief presentation. *Exploration of Neuroprotective Therapy*, *3*(1), 24–46.

Radhakrishnan, D. M., & Goyal, V. (2018). Parkinson's disease: A review. *Neurology India*, *66*(Suppl 1), S26–S35. PMID: 29503325

Ramírez-Moreno, J. M., Bodes, I. S., Romaskevych, O., & Duran-Herrera, M. C. (2015). Broad bean (Vicia faba) consumption and Parkinson's disease: A natural source of L-dopa to consider. *Neurologia (Barcelona, Spain)*, *30*(6), 375–376. PMID: 24332774

Ramírez-Moreno, J. M., Bodes, I. S., Romaskevych, O., & Duran-Herrera, M. C. (2015). Broad bean (Vicia faba) consumption and Parkinson's disease: A natural source of L-dopa to consider. *Neurologia (Barcelona, Spain)*, *30*(6), 375–376. PMID: 24332774

Regensburger, M., Ip, C. W., Kohl, Z., Schrader, C., Urban, P. P., Kassubek, J., & Jost, W. H. (2023). Clinical benefit of MAO-B and COMT inhibition in Parkinson's disease: Practical considerations. *Journal of Neural Transmission (Vienna, Austria)*, *130*(6), 847–861. PMID: 36964457

Riederer, P., Youdim, M. B. H., Rausch, W. D., Birkmayer, W., Jellinger, K., & Seemann, D. (1978). On the mode of action of L-deprenyl in the human central nervous system. *Journal of Neural Transmission (Vienna, Austria)*, *43*(3), 217–226. PMID: 745014

Santos, D. T., Camelo, D. M. F., Strelow, M. Z., Silva, M. T. S., Führ, P., Marins, L. W., & Schumacher-Schuh, A. F. (2022). Feasibility of telemedicine for patients with parkinsonism in the Brazilian public health system. *Arquivos de Neuro-Psiquiatria*, *80*(09), 914–921. PMID: 36261128

Schiess, N., Cataldi, R., Okun, M. S., Fothergill-Misbah, N., Dorsey, E. R., Bloem, B. R., & Dua, T. (2022). Six action steps to address global disparities in Parkinson disease: A World Health Organization priority. *JAMA Neurology*, *79*(9), 929–936. PMID: 35816299

Shalash, A., Spindler, M., & Cubo, E. (2021). Global perspective on telemedicine for Parkinson's disease. *Journal of Parkinson's Disease*, *11*(s1), S11–S18. PMID: 33579872

Sharma, N. K., Robbins, K., Wagner, K., & Colgrove, Y. M. (2015). A randomized controlled pilot study of the therapeutic effects of yoga in people with Parkinson's disease. *International Journal of Yoga*, *8*(1), 74–79. PMID: 25558138

Simon, D. K., Tanner, C. M., & Brundin, P. (2020). Parkinson disease epidemiology, pathology, genetics, and pathophysiology. *Clinics in Geriatric Medicine*, *36*(1), 1–12. PMID: 31733690

Sonne, J., Reddy, V., & Beato, M. R. (2024). Neuroanatomy, substantia nigra. In *StatPearls* [Internet]. StatPearls Publishing.

Soumyanath, A., Denne, T., Peterson, A., & Shinto, L. (2012). Assessment of commercial formulations of Mucuna pruriens seeds for Levodopa (L-DOPA) content. [Abstract from the International Research Congress on Integrative Medicine and Health]. *BMC Complementary and Alternative Medicine*, *12*(Suppl 1), 36.

Sushama, A. P., Onkar A, A., Shripad N, S., & Jyoti P, J. (2013). Biological sources of L-DOPA: An alternative approach. *Advances in Parkinson's Disease, 2013.*

Thomas, S., Edwards, E., & Kobylecki, C. (2024). Parkinson's Nurses Are Crucial for the Management of Parkinson's Disease: 2007–2024. *Journal of Parkinson's Disease*, *14*(s1), S209–S217. PMID: 38578901

Tibar, H., El Bayad, K., Bouhouche, A., Ait Ben Haddou, E. H., Benomar, A., Yahyaoui, M., & Regragui, W. (2018). Non-motor symptoms of Parkinson's disease and their impact on quality of life in a cohort of Moroccan patients. *Frontiers in Neurology*, *9*, 170. PMID: 29670566

Tolosa, E., Martí, M. J., Valldeoriola, F., & Molinuevo, J. L. (1998). History of levodopa and dopamine agonists in Parkinson's disease treatment. *Neurology*, *50*(6), S2–S10. PMID: 9633679

van den Bergh, R., Bloem, B. R., Meinders, M. J., & Evers, L. J. (2021). The state of telemedicine for persons with Parkinson's disease. *Current Opinion in Neurology*, *34*(4), 589–597. PMID: 33990100

Van Laar, A. D., & Jain, S. (2004). Non-motor symptoms of Parkinson disease: Update on the diagnosis and treatment. *The Neurologist*, *10*(4), 185. PMID: 15245584

van Munster, M., Stümpel, J., Clemens, T., Czabanowska, K., Pedrosa, D. J., & Mestre, T. A., & iCare-Pd Consortium. (2022). Telemedicine as an untapped opportunity for Parkinson's nurses training in personalized care approaches. *Journal of Personalized Medicine*, *12*(7), 1057. PMID: 35887553

Watson, E. D., Moosa, S., Janse Van Rensburg, D. C., Schwellnus, M., Lambert, E. V., & Stoutenberg, M. (2023). Task-shifting: Can community health workers be part of the solution to an inactive nation? *International Journal of Environmental Research and Public Health*, *20*(17), 6675. PMID: 37681815

Weise, D., Claus, I., Dresel, C., Kalbe, E., Liepelt-Scarfone, I., Lorenzl, S., & Urban, P. P. (2024). Multidisciplinary care in Parkinson's disease. *Journal of Neural Transmission (Vienna, Austria), 131*(10), 1217–1227. PMID: 39039238

Wickens, J. R., Horvitz, J. C., Costa, R. M., & Killcross, S. (2007). Dopaminergic mechanisms in actions and habits. *The Journal of Neuroscience : The Official Journal of the Society for Neuroscience, 27*(31), 8181–8183. PMID: 17670964

Zafar, S., Lui, F., & Yaddanapudi, S. S. (2025). Parkinson Disease. NLB, https://www.ncbi.nlm.nih.gov/books/NBK470193/ Accessed Dec 26 2025.

Zafar, S., & Yaddanapudi, S. S. (2023). Parkinson disease. In *StatPearls* [Internet]. StatPearls Publishing.

Zewde, Y. (2020). Health related quality of life of Ethiopian Parkinson's disease patients in Addis Ababa, Ethiopia. *Parkinsonism & Related Disorders, 79*, e82. Gavidia M. (2020). Access to Parkinson Disease Medication Affected in Low-Income Countries. [AJMC]. *The American Journal of Managed Care*.

Chapter 4
Herbal Remedies for Parkinson's Disease in Under-Resourced Settings

Asiat Na Allah
http://orcid.org/0000-0002-0251-5492
Department of Biochemistry, Faculty of Pure and Applied Sciences, Kwara State University, Malete, Nigeria

Abraham Olufemi Asuku
http://orcid.org/0000-0003-0071-0531
Bioresources Development Centre, National Biotechnology Research and Development Agency, Nigeria

ABSTRACT

This chapter delivers an overview of the potential of medicinal plants in managing Parkinson's disease in under-resourced settings where access to conventional therapies is limited. Beginning with PD pathophysiology and inadequacies of conventional therapies, it establishes the rationale for herbal multi-target mechanisms, including oxidative stress, neuroinflammation, and dopaminergic neuron loss. Key medicinal plants, such as Mucuna pruriens, Ginkgo biloba, Withania somnifera, Curcuma longa, and Panax ginseng, were referenced for their anti-inflammatory, neuroprotective, and antioxidant properties, in conjunction with emerging candidates and their associated phytochemical mechanisms. Historical applications in Ayurvedic and Traditional Chinese Medicine systems, their relevance and multi-target therapeutic potential are highlighted. The chapter further addresses indications from

DOI: 10.4018/979-8-3373-7437-6.ch004

preclinical studies using experimental PD models alongside findings from clinical trials, highlighting promising outcomes and challenges related to safety, dosage, and standardization of herbal formulations.

INTRODUCTION

Parkinson disease (PD) is a progressive neurodegenerative disorder of dopamine-producing neurons of the substantia nigra of the central nervous system, which gradually degenerates over time with the result of hallmark motor signs such as tremor, rigidity, bradykinesia (slowness of movement), and postural instability (Kouli et al., 2018; Asuku et al., 2024). In low- and middle-income countries (LMIC) especially sub-Saharan Africa, its prevalence is underreported, and the ageing population along with the risk of diagnosis contributes to the identification and management gaps. This creates a significant burden on the healthcare systems, especially when the low-resourced setting is in place and the accessibility of the latest therapies and levodopa (L-DOPA) is hindered by both cost and disruption of the supply chain and insufficient infrastructure (Oluwole et al., 2019). Culturally relevant in the LMICs, where PD prevalence is increasing with ageing populations, herbal remedies based on traditional systems such as Ayurveda and Traditional Chinese Medicine can act as an economical intermediating factor between these two countries (Zhao et al., 2025).

CURRENT THERAPEUTIC INTERVENTIONS

An established therapeutic strategy to prevent or reverse neurodegeneration in PD is yet to be developed, so the only available treatment options are directed to control the symptoms. The most essential element of pharmacological treatment is L-DOPA which is usually used together with carbidopa to restore the level of dopamine in the brain and enhance motor status to a great extent. These adjuncts and alternatives include dopamine agonists, monoamine oxidase B (MAO-B) inhibitors, amantadine and catechol-O-methyltransferase (COMT) inhibitors among others, especially when the disease is in its early stages (Rascol et al., 2003). Examples of non-pharmacological methods that facilitate but do not change the course of disease include physiotherapy, speech therapy, and occupational therapy (El-Shorbagi et al., 2020).

Despite their efficacy, existing treatments face significant limitations and are unable to halt neurodegeneration, including dopa-resistance. Dyskinesias (involuntary movements) and motor fluctuations, commonly referred to as "on-off" phenomena, are two major complications associated with long-term use of L-DOPA (Ajagun et al., 2024). Additionally, dopaminergic therapy responds poorly to many non-motor symptoms, such as cognitive decline, autonomic dysfunction, and mood disorders (Rascol *et al.*, 2003). In resource-poor regions, (<1 per million) about 50-70% of PD patients are left untreated due to L-DOPA shortages, counterfeit drugs, and neurologist scarcity, necessitating affordable herbal alternatives (Kumar *et al.*, 2024).

RATIONALE FOR EXPLORING HERBAL REMEDIES: PATHOPHYSIOLOGY OF PARKINSON'S DISEASE

PD is caused by the advancing degeneration of dopaminergic neurons in the substantia nigra pars compacta, with dopamine deficiency in the striatum and motor dysfunction as a consequence (Asuku et al., 2025). Alpha-synuclein aggregation into Lewy bodies, mitochondrial dysfunction, oxidative stress, neuroinflammation, and impaired protein clearance via the ubiquitin-proteasome and autophagy systems are the principal pathological mechanisms. Existing pharmacological therapies do not halt the self-perpetuating cycle of neuronal damage and death caused by these processes (Yin *et al.*, 2021). Herbal remedies' multi-target therapeutic potential, which addresses several pathophysiological mechanisms at once, is the rationale for exploring them in PD disease. Unlike conventional drugs that primarily focus on dopamine replacement, many herbal compounds exhibit neuroprotective, anti-inflammatory, antioxidant, and anti-apoptotic properties (Bhusal *et al.*, 2023). For instance, the natural L-DOPA is found in *Mucuna pruriens* that has been used in treating motor symptoms, and *Withania somnifera* (Ashwagandha) and *Ginkgo biloba* exhibit antioxidant activity, which can reduce oxidative stress in dopaminergic neurons (Yan et al., 2022) (Figure 1). Also, the traditional systems such as Chinese medicine suggest that PD is caused by the pathogenic factors such as wind and phlegm, as well as the imbalances in the organ systems (e.g., deficiency of liver and kidney). This whole-person model of treatment is a supplement to the current pathophysiological knowledge (Hamood et al., 2024). The herbal medicine *Astragalus, Bacopa monnieri,* and *Acanthopanax* have been shown to possess protective properties by changing signaling pathways, including PI3K/Akt, NF- 6B, and AMPK, which control cell survival and inflammation. Nevertheless, the promising results do not eliminate the problems of extract standardization, bioavailability, drug-herb interaction, and the absence of clinical large-scale trials. Consequently, even if herbal remedies offer a compelling adjunctive or alternative strategy, their integration into mainstream PD therapy necessitates rigorous scientific validation and medical supervision (Kim *et al.*, 2012; Kaur and Gupta, 2025).

HERBAL REMEDIES WITH POTENTIAL IN PARKINSON'S DISEASE

The existing therapies for PD are largely symptomatic and do not stop neurodegeneration.

Plant-derived substances with neuroprotective potential or adjunctive symptomatic benefit have garnered the interest of PD patients. Highlighted are some widely explored medicinal herbs, their major bio-actives, and evidence.

Mucuna pruriens seed (velvet bean) has been proven to be naturally high in L-DOPA, the metabolic precursor of dopamine, and has been studied as a botanical source of dopamine replacement therapy. A prepared standardized *Mucuna* seed, while supporting symptomatic benefit, has been clinically proven to improve PD symptoms when compared to synthetic L-DOPA in a randomized, double-blind pharmacological study (Katzenschlager *et al.*, 2004).

Ginkgo biloba leaf screening reveals the presence of flavonoids and terpenoids with antioxidant and mitochondrial-stabilizing activity. In preclinical PD models, the mode of action of *Ginkgo biloba* leaf includes reactive oxygen species scavenging, neuroprotection, anti-inflammatory effects, improved mitochondrial function, and modulation of neurovascular function, with some inconsistent findings on core motor symptoms. Although improved cognitive and non-motor symptoms were reported in some clinical studies (Yu *et al.*, 2021).

An adaptogen with neuroregenerative potential, *Withania somnifera,* commonly known as Ashwagandha, has been proven to exhibit improved cognitive function, oxidative stress reduction, anti-inflammatory, neurotrophic activities, antioxidant, and memory improvement, attributed to its bioactive withanolides. Animal PD models revealed neuronal repair mechanisms, attenuation of oxidative markers, and better motor function. According to Wongtrakul *et al.* (2021), Withanolide A has also been reported to assist with dopaminergic tone enhancement, upregulation of neurotrophic factors, synaptic regeneration, reduction of oxidative stress, and neuroinflammation in PD models. Human clinical trials, specifically in PD, remain sparse, with robust preclinical evidence. Standardized extracts and dose-finding studies are needed (Lerose *et al.*, 2024).

The metal-chelating, mitochondrial-protective, antioxidant, and anti-inflammatory properties of *Curcuma longa* are important to PD pathogenesis. Although there is a lack of high-quality clinical trial data, preclinical studies emphasize minimization of α-synuclein aggregation and oxidative neuronal damage with current reviews emphasizing its promise as an adjuvant (Yu *et al.*, 2021). There are few human trials, and persistent issues with curcumin bioavailability but robust mechanistic and animal evidence revealed that it has the ability to protect the mitochondria, initiate free radical scavenging, prevent protein aggregation, modulate NF-κB and other inflammatory pathways while emphasizing safety and monitoring at high pharmacological doses (Yu *et al.*, 2021).

Panax ginseng and its bioactive (ginsenosides) has also proven neuroprotective actions (decrease in the loss of dopaminergic cells and modulation of neuroinflammation) in PD models. Research on animal models point to conserved motor function and lessened α-synuclein pathology (Van Kampen *et al.*, 2014), with antioxidants, mitochondrial support, anti-inflammatory, autophagy regulation, and protein clearance mechanisms documented. Clinical translation requires the discovery and standardization of active ginsenosides (Cho, 2012).

MULTI-TARGET POTENTIAL OF PHYTOCHEMICALS IN PARKINSON'S DISEASE

Phytochemicals exhibit a multi-target potential in PD by concurrently modulating several interconnected pathophysiological pathways, offering a notable advantage over conventional single-target therapies that mainly address dopamine deficit. Unlike synthetic drugs like L-DOPA that can decrease the motor symptoms but do not stop the neurodegeneration, phytochemicals of medicinal plants can interfere with different pathways, including oxidative stress, neuroinflammation, mitochondrial dysfunction, protein misfolding, and apoptosis (Balakrishnan et al., 2021) (Figure 2). The activation of the nuclear factor erythroid 2-related factor 2 (Nrf2)/antioxidant response element (ARE) is one of the best-studied mechanisms, and it regulates the expression of antioxidant enzymes, including heme oxygenase-1 (HO-1) and NAD(P)H quinone dehydrogenase 1 (NQO1). Phytochemicals that activate Nrf2 are curcumin, epigallocatechin gallate(EGCG) and baicalein, which enhance protection against oxidative damage that is a primary cause of dopaminergic neuron loss in the substantia nigra. At the same time, these molecules inhibit the nuclear factor kappa B (NF- κB) pathway which reduces the synthesis of pro-inflammatory cytokines like TNF- 6 and IL- 6 which enhance chronic neuroinflammation in PD (Tkaczenko et al., 2025). Other ones, including apigenin, hesperidin, etc., play an essential role in major cellular processes, including the neurotransmitter systems (GABA, serotonin), neurogenesis through brain-derived neurotrophic factor, and down-regulation of oxidative stress and neuro-inflammation (Tkaczenko et al., 2025).

Additionally, numerous phytochemicals stop monoamine oxidase B (MAO-B), the enzyme accountable for dopamine metabolism and the generation of reactive oxygen species (ROS). For instance, quercetin and hesperidin have been shown to exhibit MAO-B inhibitory activity, thus preserving dopamine levels while minimizing oxidative stress. Others, such as resveratrol and epigallocatechin gallate (EGCG), support mitochondrial biogenesis and autophagy by activating pathways like sirtuin

1/ peroxisome proliferating-activated receptor gamma coactivator 1-alpha (SIRT1/ PGC-1α) and phosphatidyinositol-3-kinase/ protein kinase B (PI3K/Akt), improving energy metabolism, damaged genes and protein aggregates clearance (Kumar, 2023). Crucially, phytochemicals also interfere with α-synuclein aggregation, a hallmark of PD pathology. EGCG has been shown to redirect α-synuclein into non-toxic, off-pathway oligomers, while naringenin and salidroside reduce its fibrillization and associated neurotoxicity.

Furthermore, compounds such as curcumin and quercetin improve proteasomal and lysosomal degradation systems, thereby assisting protein homeostasis (Tkaczenko *et al.*, 2025). This polypharmacological profile allows phytochemicals to deliver neuroprotection, symptom mitigation, and potentially disease modification, making them likely candidates for integrative PD management, especially in under-resourced settings where access to advanced pharmaceuticals is limited. However, challenges related to bioavailability, standardization, and clinical validation remain critical barriers to their widespread therapeutic application (Balakrishnan *et al.*, 2021).

Figure 1. Multitarget Mechanisms of Medicinal Herbs in Neurodegeneration

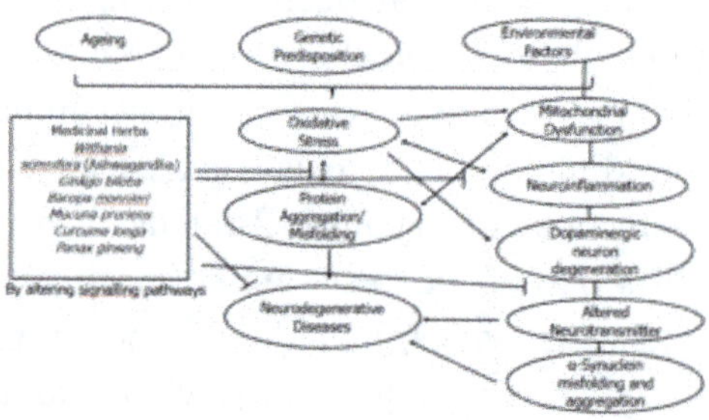

Figure 2. Phytochemicals derived from Medicinal Plants and their interventions on PD

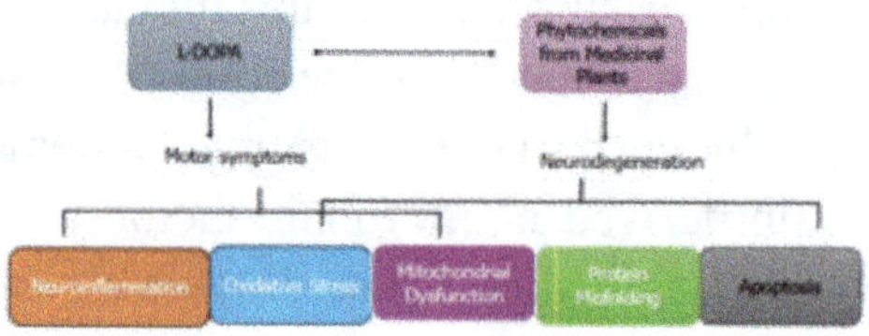

HISTORICAL USE IN TRADITIONAL SYSTEMS

Prior to modern biomedical definitions of PD, Ayurvedic medicine and Traditional Chinese Medicine (TCM) have been used traditionally as herbal remedies to treat symptoms that appear similar to PD. Symbolic PD-like symptoms are referred to as Kampavata, a condition that follows an imbalance of the Vata dosha that governs movement and neurological functions. The key treatment goal would be to replenish Vata balance by using herbal preparations, dieting, and detoxification, in other words, Panchakarma procedures in Ayurveda. Mucuna pruriens Ayurvedic treatment is a cornerstone containing L-DOPA (the gold-standard pharmacological agent of PD) in high levels. It has been shown to be efficient in clinical studies and preclinical studies and has been shown to be equally effective in improving motor functions as compared to synthetic L-DOPA. Withania somnifera, recommended because of its neuroprotective, anti-inflammatory, and adaptogenic effects, and Centella asiatica, which promotes neuronal regeneration and cognitive functions, are other important herbs (Lyu et al., 2024).

In Traditional Chinese Medicine, PD is explained by patterns of disharmony among the liver, kidney and spleen with symptoms attributed to internal wind, liver yang rising, deficiency of yin and obstruction of phlegm. The key treatment measures include calming the liver, extinguishing wind, nourishing the yin, and tonifying deficiencies. Some of the popular herbal prescriptions are Chaihu-Jia-Longgu-Muli-Tang (CJLMT) taken to treat mood and motor symptoms and Ma-Zi-Ren-Wan (MZRW) to treat constipation, a common non-motor symptom of PD. It uses Shao-Yao-Gan-Cao-Tang (SYGCT) which alleviates muscle rigidity and cramps due to its spasmolytic properties. Individual herbs like Gastrodia elata (Tian Ma) are commonly used to calm internal wind and have shown neuroprotective effects through the inhibition of oxidative stress and the prevention of L-DOPA induced dyskinesias in animals. Uncaria rhynchophylla (Gou Teng) is another important herb, which regulates the glutamate receptors and dopaminergic pathways, providing symptomatic improvement and possible disease modification (Lin et al., 2021).

Both systems place emphasis on the use of individualized treatment and holistic care, which is consistent with the modern concern of multi-target therapies. Evidence in the real-life experience of China as demonstrated indicates that more than 60 percent of PD patients seek TCM treatment following diagnosis and usually combine it with conventional treatment, which is an indication of its adoption in modern care. The most common TCM herbs include Astragalus membranaceus (Huang Qi) which supports energy, immunity, and neurological functioning, Rehmannia glutinosa (Di Huang), and Poria cocos (Fu Ling) which are ingredients of Bu Zhong Yi Qi Tang, a formula that promotes energy, immunity and neurological functioning. Such historical activities offer a rich source of scientific research on the scientific study of phytochemicals in PD by connecting the traditional knowledge with the contemporary neuropharmacology (Yin et al., 2021).

OTHER EMERGING HERBAL CANDIDATES AND MECHANISMS OF ACTION

Some of the phytochemicals and herbal candidates have proved to be promising in PD since they have multifaceted mechanisms of action against major pathophysiological events. Such phytochemicals will provide neuroprotection related to reducing oxidative stress, neuroinflammation, mitochondrial dysfunction, protein aggregation, and apoptosis, which play a central role in PD development (Balakrishnan et al., 2021). Nevertheless, clinical translation is still inadequate, and an equal weightage should be given to human trial evidence rather than the preclinical evidence.

Such noticeable finalizations are baicalein of *Scutellaria baicalensis*, which has antioxidant, anti-inflammatory, and anti-apoptotic properties. It has been shown that baicalein can lower oxidative damage, enhance mitochondrial dysfunction, and prevent the aggregation of α-synuclein in PD models, which produces an improvement in motor symptoms and neuronal survival. On the same note, epigallocatechin-3-gallate (EGCG), one of the most common green tea polyphenols, induces the Nrf2/ARE antioxidant pathway and inhibits neuroinflammation by inhibiting the NF-kB signaling. EGCG also regulates autophagy, which clears toxic α-synuclein aggregates (Haxhiu et al., 2025). Nanodelivery systems are under development to enhance the bioavailability and therapeutic efficacy of these phytochemicals to allow them to be better targeted in the brain and remains active in combating PD pathology. Further, such plants as Moringa oleifera are becoming promising neuroprotectants via antioxidant and anti-apoptotic pathways, contributing to its chances as an adjunct therapy (Saji et al., 2025). These results highlight the potential of these natural products as multi-target agents that have a potential of slowing neurodegeneration, relieving symptoms, and as adjunctive PD treatments. Nevertheless, additional clinical trials are necessary to establish safety and the most effective dose and efficacy in humans (Balakrishnan et al., 2025).

PRECLINICAL EVIDENCE IN EXPERIMENTAL MODELS

Preclinical evidence of herbal remedies in PD using experimental models supports their therapeutic potential, especially in rodents treated with neurotoxins such as 6-hydroxydopamine (6-OHDA) and Parkinsonian toxin, 1-methyl-4-phenyl-1,2,3,6-tetrahydropyridine (MPTP), that mimic PD pathology (Zhao *et al.*, 2025). Among the most studied herbs, *Mucuna pruriens* seed extract contains natural L-DOPA, and when used for treatment at a dose of 2.5–5 g/kg/day in rat models induced by 6-OHDA, it elevates dopamine levels in the substantia nigra and striatum, improving motor function and reducing PD-like symptoms more effectively than synthetic L-DOPA alone. Also, HP-200, a traditional Ayurvedic preparation from *M. pruriens* similarly increased brain dopamine concentrations and showed neuroprotective effects beyond L-DOPA replacement (Khazdair *et al.*, 2021). Other benefits of TCM herbal formulations are seen in Ping-wei-san plus herbal decoction, known for it motor and emotional behaviors improvement in PD mice via gut microbiota, protein expression, and metabolism modulation while revealing multi-system actions that extend beyond neural protection. In rat PD models, Tianma Gouteng Yin has been proven to alleviate motor deficits and conserve dopaminergic neurons through lipid peroxidation suppression. Huangqin decoction on the other hand protects mitochondria, reduces oxidative stress, and supports neuron survival. Additional decoctions like Bushen Jianpi and SiJunZi asisted metabolic functions, enhanced motor coordination, and supported neuronal survival through signaling pathways such as PI3K/AKT (Zhao *et al.*, 2025). In animal PD models, bio-actives such as resveratrol and berberine used individually showed neuroprotection via neuronal survival support and anti-oxidant effects. DA-9805, known as triple herbal extract, improved motor functions in PD models via mitochondrial protection and anti-apoptotic effects (Nahar *et al.*, 2025). Collectively, herbal therapies exert neuroprotective effects in PD models via multi-modal mechanisms as revealed by numerous preclinical studies. However, translation into human PD therapy awaits clinical validation (Nahar *et al.*, 2025).

IN VITRO AND ANIMAL STUDIES

Exploiting neurotoxin models like 6-OHDA and MPTP *in vitro* and animal studies for PD have been detailed for evaluating the efficacy of herbal remedies/ phytochemicals and supports assessment of neuroprotective interventions. These models mimics PD features such as selective dopaminergic neuron loss, oxidative stress, and motor deficits (Zhao *et al.*, 2025). In rodents, direct injection of 6-OHDA (the primary neurotoxin) into the nigrostriatal pathway, mimic symptoms of PD (dopaminergic neuron degeneration). *Mucuna pruriens*, when administered to 6-OHDA-lesioned rats revealed preservation of tyrosine hydroxylase-positive neurons, restoration of dopamine levels, and motor coordination improvement. Other TCM herbal decoctions, for example, Tianma Gouteng Yin showed reduced neuronal death and improved behavioral outcomes via antioxidant and anti-inflammatory effects (Khazdair *et al.*, 2021; Zhao *et al.*, 2025).

In the MPTP mouse model, dopaminergic cell death occurs via the induction of Parkinsonism through mitochondrial complex I inhibition. Bio-actives such as resveratrol, EGCG, and curcumin have shown promise in activating protective pathways, such as Nrf2-mediated antioxidant response and attenuating neuroinflammation. They achieve these via enhancing mitochondrial function, improving motor function, and reducing α-synuclein aggregation. Balakrishnan *et al.* (2021) and Tkaczenko *et al.* (2025) reported that the botanical formulations of Ping-wei-san showed reduction of systemic inflammation in MPTP-treated animals and modulation of gut microbiota, highlighting the multi-target effects of herbal therapies. Both models would be essential to decipher the mechanisms, such as oxidative stress, mitochondrial dysfunction, neuroinflammation, and protein misfolding in PD, and to provide preclinical proof-of-concept information to warrant the use of phytochemicals as neuroprotective agents. However, these are risky extrapolations to clinical use because of differences in species and human PD pathophysiology (Khazdair et al., 2021).

DOSE-RESPONSE RELATIONSHIPS AND SAFETY PROFILES

Dose-response associations of herbal remedies in PD play a significant role in defining the efficacy and safety effective therapeutic window. A significant number of herbal preparations, their bio-actives (including β-asarone, acteoside, curcumin) and numerous TCM decoctions have been identified to possess neuroprotective effects in dose-dependent fashion as disclosed by some studies. The optimal doses are beneficial to enhance motor performance and neuronal survival by enhancing the modulation of signaling pathways, reducing oxidative stress, and preventing neuroinflammation, whereas too high doses can be considered toxic or less effective (More et al., 2013). The safety profiles of these herbal remedies / treatments have generally been positive, and the well tolerated levels of these remedies in animal models and clinical observations at the recommended doses were good. The use of herbal medicines has fewer side effects as compared to conventional medicines, and there is hardly any resistance or dependency to drugs after long-term use. But safety is determined by a number of factors including dosage, herb quality and interaction with other drugs. As an illustration, herbal therapies when administered alongside standard PD treatments have shown better symptoms with minimal side effects, which support the possibility of using them as complementary therapies. However, to develop standard dosing schedules and provide safe clinical use, mechanistic, pharmacokinetic and toxicological research is still needed (Jin et al., 2022).

CLINICAL EVIDENCE AND HUMAN TRIALS

Although the evidence has yet to develop, clinical evidence and human trials of PD herbal remedies show an increasing amount of support on their effectiveness and safety.

In China predominantly, several randomized controlled trials (RCTs) and observational studies have tested multi-herbal formulations and individual herbs. For instance, some trials show that combining herbal medicine with conventional PD drugs improves symptom control, reduces medication dose, and decreases adverse events since numerous preclinical successes have failed clinically due to flawed trial design, patient heterogeneity, and symptomatic confounders (Kim *et al.*, 2022). CEP-1347 (protein kinase C inhibitor), promising in MPTP monkeys (TH+ neuron preservation 40%), but null in Phase II RCTs (n=200; UPDRS no change vs. placebo, p=0.45) due to poor CNS penetration. Herbs like *Glycyrrhiza uralensis* (licorice) have demonstrated symptom improvement and good safety in short-term RCTs without serious adverse events (Yin *et al.*, 2021; Lyu *et al.*, 2024; Zhao *et a*l., 2025).

SYMPTOM IMPROVEMENT AND BIOMARKER CHANGES

Herbal remedies for PD have shown notable improvements in symptom management and biomarker changes according to clinical evidence. The RCTs show that herbal formulation is a potent therapy to improve PD symptoms when administered with conventional medications but also lessens the doses of orthodox medications such as L-DOPA among others. Some of the successful herbal preparations that were used alongside anti-Parkinson medications were Fufangjangzhan wan, Kanapa granule, Pabing formula 2, and others, which demonstrated statistically significant changes in the general symptoms and Unified Parkinson disease rating scale (UPDRS) scores (Jun et al., 2023; Lyu et al., 2024).

Regarding biomarkers, there are herbs and formulations that decrease the oxidative stress markers and neuroinflammation as the most important factors of PD progression (Miller and O'Callaghan, 2015). These are through their antioxidative, anti-inflammatory and neuroprotective properties. Moreover, herbal adjunct therapy has also been linked to reduced side effects, which the researchers claim have safer side effects compared to traditional monotherapy drugs, and has shown an increased ability to reduce symptoms (Lyu et al., 2024). Herbs such as Ginkgo biloba have shown better delivery of dopamine and brain performance whereas Mucuna pruriens is a natural source of L-DOPA with motor symptom benefits. The study by Khazdair et al. (2020) demonstrates that the combination therapies in PD management are more likely to reflect the improvements in the symptom control and the quality of life. Nevertheless, the diversity of study design and herbal preparations emphasize the necessity to standardize the formulations and conduct more rigorous clinical trials aimed at maximizing the effects, ensuring the efficacy of the firm, and establishing its safety (Khazdair et al., 2020).

SAFETY, STANDARDIZATION, DOSAGE, CHALLENGES, AND REGULATORY LANDSCAPE

Various clinical studies and systematic reviews that have provided explicit clinical data have demonstrated the improvement of symptoms and biomarker variations in PD with the use of herbal remedies. Numerous studies regarding herbal interventions as supplements to conventional medications improve motor and non-motor symptoms besides decreasing doses and other side effects of medications.

Biomarkers analyses on the other hand demonstrated that herbal interventions provide biochemical evidence of neuroprotection and disease modification via modulation of inflammatory markers, and neurodegeneration-related proteins. For instance, some formulations, such as Ukgansan and Tianma Gouteng Yin, have shown improvements in clinical scores like the unified Parkinson's disease rating scale (UPDRS) and reductions in neuroinflammatory biomarkers, suggesting attenuation of disease progression. Jeong *et al.* (2023) reported that while results are promising and in order to definitively establish efficacy and safety in diverse patient populations, the variability in herbal formulations, dosing regimens, and trial methodologies requires the need for standardized protocols and larger randomized controlled trials. More importantly, the control of PD herbal remedies differs among the countries with low and middle income (LMICs) as the traditional use is being in competition with the safety/efficacy (Table 1).

Nigeria NAFDAC requires registration under the NAFDAC/HERB/001, which is GMP compliance, stability, and toxicity data of *Mucuna pruriens* products, but enforcement loopholes exist with 70 per cent unregistered sales. Malawi pharmacy and medicine regulatory authority (PMRA) does not have specific herbal frameworks since they have general drug laws resulting in poor labeling (90% non-compliant).

India's Ayurveda, Yoga and Naturopathy, Unani, Siddha, and Homoeopathy (AYUSH) ministry standardizes Ayurvedic PD formulations like *Mucuna*-based *Kapikacchu churna* via pharmacopoeial monographs. China's ational Medical Products Administration (NMPA) approves TCM patents (e.g., *Tianma Gouteng Yin*), with 60+ PD-related registrations (Eruaga *et al.*, 2024; Mponda *et al.*, 2025).

Table 1. Regulatory Landscape in Under-Resourced Regions

Region	Agency	Ker Requirements	Challenges	References
Nigeria	NAFDAC	GMP, Toxicology, L-DOPA assay	Unregistered products (70%), weak enforcement	World Bank, 2023; Mponda *et al.*, 2025
Malawi	PMRA	General drug laws	No herbal-specific rules, poor GMP	PMPB, 2018, World Bank, 2019
India	AYUSH/ CDSCO	Pharmacopoeial standards	Adulterations in export	Chen *at al.*, 2025
China	NMPA	Clinical trials for new TCM	Export standardization	Chen *at al.*, 2025

VARIABILITY IN HERBAL PRODUCT COMPOSITION

Lack of uniformity in the composition of herbal products is a major problem in using herbal remedies to PD. Since the bio-actives in medicinal herbs are highly variable, they vary with the species of plants, geographic location, environmental factors, time of harvest, and techniques of processing. Many herbal medicines involve the use of whole plants, and mixtures of various plant parts (roots, leaves, stems and seeds), and each is a complex mixture of numerous bio-active compounds and not all of these are completely characterized or standardized (Yin et al., 2021). This variability makes it more difficult to standardize the doses which influence the reproducibility of therapeutic results. As an illustration, most of the TCM PD preparations involve a combination of multiple herbs in different proportions, and each herb has different active compounds. The existence of these bio-active differences complicates the efforts to have consistency when it comes to potency and quality, affects the pharmacokinetics, efficacy and safety of the treatment. Determining key compounds and setting up a control mechanism to provide batch-to-batch consistency is a major driver of standardization without which, the variable composition may result in an unpredictable clinical efficacy, unexpected side effects, or interactions with other drugs. Hence, to effectively optimize the therapeutic potential and safety of herbal products in PD management, the quality control, chemical profiling, and validation protocols are required (Singh and Kumar, 2025; Wang et al., 2023).

RISK OF CONTAMINATION AND ADULTERATION

Contamination and adulteration in PD research are important issues that may undermine the integrity and validity of scientific results. The unintentional occurrence of extraneous substances, microorganisms, or impurities in biological samples, herbal extracts, or product is known as contamination. PD development has been linked to exposure to environmental toxicants (including pesticides), as well as chemicals, including trichloroethylene (TCE) (Posadzki et al., 2013; Opuni et al., 2023). The research that serves to test neuroprotective activities of herbal extracts or natural compounds contamination provides variable outcomes which impact reproducibility and reliability (Kanungo et al., 2024). Adulteration conversely addresses the intentional or unintentional modification of these products and this may result in erroneous conclusions. The deliberate interference or supply chain of impure natural products or chemicals affect the research results of PD, which present inappropriate information on neurotoxicity or protective capabilities (Smith and Zhang, 2021). Also deliberate contamination of herbal or chemical samples with impurities or otherwise inactive fillers usually skews the interpretation of the bio-active or toxicity of the bio-active(s) in question. Artificially obtained neurotoxic effects or a distortion of real disease processes can be created by impurities or microbial contamination that is introduced unintentionally in the course of handling the sample (Nims and Price, 2017; Bright-Ohaeri et al., 2024). To avoid such contamination, reagent purity, maintenance of sterile conditions and verification of sample sources are important processes. To alleviate these risks, strict quality control measures, such as chemical profiling, source verification and standardization, are necessary (Orhan et al., 2024).

HERBAL-DRUG INTERACTIONS AND CONTRAINDICATION

Contraindications and herbal-drug interactions are important factors to be considered in the management of PD wherein patients are most likely to take herbal supplements in addition to prescribed drug. In herbal products, there are several active compounds, which may influence the drug metabolism, transportation or activity in the body, thus altering its efficacy or causing a higher risk of adverse effects. As an illustration, the typical herbal supplement called St. Johns Wort can activate the enzymes of cytochrome P450 related to drugs metabolism and inhibit the efficiency of PD drugs like L-DOPA, potentially leading to worsening symptoms or treatment failure (Wilson and Maulik, 2019). Another commonly used cognitive and neuroprotective herb ginkgo biloba can interact with blood thinners and risk increasing the risk of bleeding, which is a significant issue in PD patients on anticoagulants (Wilson and Maulik, 2019). Patients taking L-DOPA, in form of Mucuna pruriens, should exercise caution because preparation concentrations vary across lot that could result in under- or over-dose in case they are used concomitantly with established L-DOPA treatment regimens. Certain herbal ingredients can also have an impact on dopamine metabolism or mitochondrial activity, which are vital radiation pathophysiology of PD, which should be carefully monitored (Srivastav et al., 2017).

CONCLUSION

In regions of low resource endowment where L-DOPA availability and innovative treatment is still limited with the constraints of health care facilities, supply chains, and affordability, herbal remedies are an unquestionable and culturally relevant way of treating Parkinson. Primarily, established phytochemicals with multi-target neuroprotective actions, including *Mucuna pruriens, Ginkgo biloba, Withania somnifera, Curcuma longa*, *Panax ginseng,* and emerging phytochemicals with multi-target actions on PD such as α-synuclein aggregation, neuroinflammation, oxidative stress, and dopaminergic degeneration are promising. Model preclinical data of MPTP and 6-OHDA models demonstrate dose-dependent activity and safety, and initial clinical trials show biomarker and motor symptom improvements, resembling centuries-old uses in Ayurvedic and Traditional Chinese Medicine.

However, by acknowledging such potential requirements, preventing contamination risks, compositional heterogeneity, significant obstacles, drug-herb interactions, and adulteration necessitate strong pharmacovigilance, setting of context-specific dosage, and standardization procedures. Community-based verification, training of traditional healers and hybrid models involving adjuncts of herbs and the existing pharmaceuticals are viable alternative ways of going in under-resource settings.

Finally, herbal remedies in the underserved areas close the therapeutic gap of PD patients and respect the knowledge of the Aborigines, transforming the evidence-based practice. Several strict, locally based, clinical trials, quality assurance regulatory frameworks, and interdisciplinary efforts are needed to turn promising ethnopharmacology into the possible accessible and safe interventions, which improves quality of life and equity in neurological care.

REFERENCES

Ajagun, E. J., Asuku, A. O., Ayinla, M. T., Abdulsalam, T. A., Ajibare, A. J., Olajide, T. S., Hamza, Y. O., & Ganiyu, K. O. (2024). Pharmacotherapy of Parkinson's Disease and their Limitations. In: Zebrafish as a Model for Parkinson's Disease. Taylor and Francis, CRC, https://doi.org/DOI: 10.1201/9781003402893-17

Asuku, A. O., Ayinla, M. T., Olajide, T. S., Ajagun, E. J., Ganiyu, K. O., Hamza, Y. O., Ajibare, A. J., & Abdulsalam, T. A. (2024). Diagnosis and Biomarkers of Parkinson's Disease. In: Zebrafish as a Model for Parkinson's Disease. Taylor and Francis, CRC, https://doi.org/DOI: 10.1201/9781003402893-15

Asuku, A. O., Ogungbangbe, G. O., & Fajemidagba, G. A. (2025). Gene therapy for Parkinson's disease: A new frontier in neurodegenerative diseases. *Exploration of Neuroprotective Therapy*, *5*, 1004119. DOI: 10.37349/ent.2025.1004119

Balakrishnan, R., Azam, S., Cho, D. Y., Su-Kim, I., & Choi, D. K. (2021). Natural Phytochemicals as Novel Therapeutic Strategies to Prevent and Treat Parkinson's Disease: Current Knowledge and Future Perspectives. *Oxidative Medicine and Cellular Longevity*, *6680935*. Advance online publication. DOI: 10.1155/2021/6680935 PMID: 34122727

Bhusal, C. K., Uti, D. E., Mukherjee, D., Alqahtani, T., Alqahtani, S., Bhattacharya, A., & Akash, S. (2023). Unveiling Nature's potential: Promising natural compounds in Parkinson's disease management. *Parkinsonism & Related Disorders*, *115*, 105799. DOI: 10.1016/j.parkreldis.2023.105799 PMID: 37633805

Bright-Ohaeri, F. C., Ihebuzo, N. G., Ejeta, K. O., Odimegwu, N., & Militus, I. O. (2024). Cell Culture and Laboratory Contaminants, Prevention and Recovery Strategy- A Review. *European Journal of Biology and Medical Science Research*, *12*(2), 32–51.

Chen, Q., Cheng, H. J., Bian, Z. X., Lyu, A. P., Yang, Y., & Chan, K. W. (2025). Regulatory frameworks and evidence requirements for traditional, complementary and integrative medicines. *Bulletin of the World Health Organization*, *103*(11), 696–707C. PMID: 41180280

Cho, I. H. (2012). Effects of Panax ginseng in Neurodegenerative Diseases. *Journal of Ginseng Research*, *36*(4), 342–353. DOI: 10.5142/jgr.2012.36.4.342 PMID: 23717136

El-Shorbagi, A.-N., Chaudhary, S., Alshemali, K. A., Alabdulrazzaq, R. F., & Alqahtani, F. Y. (2020). A comprehensive review on management of Parkinson's disease, inclusive of drug discovery and pharmacological approaches. *Journal of Applied Pharmaceutical Science*, *10*(10), 130–150.

Eruaga, M. A., Itua, E. O. and Bature, J. T. (2024). Exploring herbal medicine regulation in Nigeria: Balancing traditional practices with modern standards. GSC Advanced Research and Reviews. 18(3): 083–090.

Hamood, H. M., Alsaedi, M. A. Z., Al-Qrimli, A. F., & Jawad, A. Q. (2024). Parkinson Disease Pharmacological and Herbal Management: A Review. *South Asian Research Journal of Applied Medical Sciences.*, *6*(1), 1–9.

Haxhiu, H., Hoxha, M., Zela, I., & Zappacosta, B. (2025). An Overview of the Role of Medicinal Plants in Parkinson's Disease: A Semi-Systematic Review. *Biomedicines*, *13*(8), 2008. PMID: 40868260

Jeong, J. Y., Lee, H. J., Kim, N., Li, Y., Rah, J. C., & Oh, W. J. (2023). Impaired neuronal activity as a potential factor contributing to the underdeveloped cerebrovasculature in a young Parkinson's disease mouse model. *Scientific Reports*, *13*(1), 22613. PMID: 38114623

Jin, C., Cho, K.-H., Kwon, S., Lee, H.-G., Kim, T.-H., Jung, W.-S., Moon, S.-K., Cho, S.-Y., Kang, B.-K., Park, J.-M., Park, H.-J., & Ko, C.-N. (2022). Effectiveness and safety of herbal medicine Ukgansan for clinical symptoms in Parkinson's disease: A pilot, randomized, assessor-blinded clinical trial. *Frontiers in Neurology*, *13*, 1025269. DOI: 10.3389/fneur.2022.1025269 PMID: 36438946

Jun, P., Zhao, H., Jung, I. C., Kwon, O., Han, C. H., Won, J., & Jang, J. H. (2023). Efficacy of herbal medicine treatment based on syndrome differentiation for Parkinson's disease: A systematic review and meta-analysis of randomized placebo-controlled clinical trials. *Frontiers in Pharmacology*, *14*, 1108407. DOI: 10.3389/fphar.2023.1108407 PMID: 36925641

Kanungo, J., Sorkin, B. C., Krzykwa, J., Mitchell, C. A., Embry, M., Spencer, P., Harry, G. J., Cannon, J., Liu, F., McPherson, C. A., Gafner, S., & Westerink, R. H. S. (2024). Screening tools to evaluate the neurotoxic potential of botanicals: Building a strategy to assess safety. *Expert Opinion on Drug Metabolism & Toxicology*, *20*(7), 629–646. PMID: 38984683

Katzenschlager, R., Evans, A., Manson, A., Patsalos, P. N., Ratnaraj, N., Watt, H., Timmermann, L., Van der Giessen, R., & Lees, A. J. (2004). Mucuna pruriens in Parkinson's disease: A double blind clinical and pharmacological study. *Journal of Neurology, Neurosurgery, and Psychiatry*, *75*(12), 1672–1677. PMID: 15548480

Kaur, M., & Gupta, M. (2025). Role and mechanism of herbal bioactives in treatment of Parkinson's disease: A promising therapeutic approach. *South African Journal of Botany, 181*, 315–338.

Khazdair, M. R., Kianmehr, M., & Anaeigoudari, A. (2021). Effects of Medicinal Plants and Flavonoids on Parkinson's Disease: A Review on Basic and Clinical Evidence. *Advanced Pharmaceutical Bulletin, 11*(2), 224–232. PMID: 33880344

Kim, C. K., Lee, Y. R., Ong, L., Gold, M., Kalali, A., & Sarkar, J. (2022). Alzheimer's Disease: Key Insights from Two Decades of Clinical Trial Failures. *Journal of Alzheimer's Disease, 87*, 83–100. PMID: 35342092

Kim, T.-H., Cho, K.-H., Jung, W.-S., & Lee, M. S. (2012). Herbal Medicines for Parkinson's Disease: A Systematic Review of Randomized Controlled Trials. *PLoS One*, *7*(5), e35695. DOI: 10.1371/journal.pone.0035695 PMID: 22615738

Kouli, A., Torsney, K. M., & Kuan, W. L. (2018). Parkinson's Disease: Etiology, Neuropathology, and Pathogenesis. In: Stoker TB, Greenland JC, editors. Parkinson's Disease: Pathogenesis and Clinical Aspects [Internet]. Brisbane (AU): Codon Publications. Chapter 1.

Kumar, G. (2023). Editorial: Neuroprotective mechanisms by phytochemicals in neurological disorders. *Frontiers in Neuroscience, 17*, 1149639. DOI: 10.3389/fnins.2023.1149639 PMID: 37008215

Kumar, L., Malhotra, M., Singh, A., & Singh, A. P. (2024). Comprehensive Review on Parkinson's Disease: Insights into Prevalence, Pathophysiology, Diagnosis, and Multifaceted Treatment Approaches. *Journal of Drug Delivery and Therapeutics, 14*(6). Advance online publication. DOI: 10.22270/jddt.v14i6.6637

Lerose, V., Ponticelli, M., Benedetto, N., Carlucci, V., Lela, L., Tzvetkov, N. T., & Milella, L. (2024). *Withania somnifera* (L.) Dunal, a Potential Source of Phytochemicals for Treating Neurodegenerative Diseases: A Systematic Review. *Plants, 13*(6), 771. DOI: 10.3390/plants13060771 PMID: 38592845

Lin, C.-H., Chiu, H. E., Wu, S.-Y., Tseng, S.-T., Wu, T.-C., Hung, Y.-C., Hsu, C. Y., Chen, H.-J., Hsu, S.-F., Kuo, C. E., & Hu, W.-L. (2021). Chinese Herbal Products for Non-Motor Symptoms of Parkinson's Disease in Taiwan: A Population-Based Study. *Frontiers in Pharmacology, 11*, 615657. DOI: 10.3389/fphar.2020.615657 PMID: 33584294

Lyu, S., Zhang, C. S., Mao, Z., Guo, X., Li, Z., Luo, X., Sun, J., & Su, Q. (2024). Real-world Chinese herbal medicine for Parkinson's disease: A hospital-based retrospective analysis of electronic medical records. *Frontiers in Aging Neuroscience*, *16*, 1362948. DOI: 10.3389/fnagi.2024.1362948 PMID: 38756536

Miller, D. B., & O'Callaghan, J. P. (2015). Biomarkers of Parkinson's disease: Present and future. *Metabolism: Clinical and Experimental*, *64*(3, Suppl 1), S40–S46. PMID: 25510818

More, S. V., Kumar, H., Kang, S. M., Song, S. Y., Lee, K., & Choi, D. K. (2013). Advances in neuroprotective ingredients of medicinal herbs by using cellular and animal models of Parkinson's disease. *Evidence-Based Complementary and Alternative Medicine : eCAM*, *957875*. Advance online publication. DOI: 10.1155/2013/957875 PMID: 24073012

Mponda, J. S., Muula, A. S., Choko, A., Ajuwon, A. J., & Moody, J. O. (2025). Traditional medicine regulation status and challenges in Malawi and Nigeria. *BMC Complementary Medicine and Therapies*, *25*(1), 53. PMID: 39953523

Nahar, L., Charoensup, R., Kalieva, K., Habibi, E., Guo, M., Wang, D., Kvasnica, M., Onder, A., & Sarker, S. D. (2025). Natural products in neurodegenerative diseases: Recent advances and future outlook. *Frontiers in Pharmacology*, *16*, 1529194. DOI: 10.3389/fphar.2025.1529194 PMID: 40176910

Nims, R. W., & Price, P. J. (2017). Best practices for detecting and mitigating the risk of cell culture contaminants. *In Vitro Cellular & Developmental Biology. Animal*, *53*(10), 872–879. PMID: 29197027

Oluwole, O. G., Kuivaniemi, H., Carr, J. A., Ross, O. A., Olaogun, M. O. B., Bardien, S., & Komolafe, M. A. (2019). Parkinson's disease in Nigeria: A review of published studies and recommendations for future research. *Parkinsonism & Related Disorders*, *62*, 36–43. PMID: 30573414

Opuni, K. F. M., Kretchy, J-P., Agyabeng, K., Boadu, J. A., Adanu, T., Ankamah, S., Appiah, A., Amoah, G. B., Baidoo, M. and Kretchy, I. A. (2023). Contamination of herbal medicinal products in low-and-middle-income countries: A systematic review. Heliyon. 9: 9. e19370. https://doi.org/.DOI: 10.1016/j.heliyon.2023.e19370

Orhan, N., Gafner, S., & Blumenthal, M. (2024). Estimating the extent of adulteration of the popular herbs black cohosh, echinacea, elder berry, ginkgo, and turmeric – its challenges and limitations. *Natural Product Reports*, *41*(10). Advance online publication. DOI: 10.1039/d4np00014e PMID: 39108221

Posadzki, P., Watson, L., & Ernst, E. (2013). Contamination and adulteration of herbal medicinal products (HMPs): An overview of systematic reviews. *European Journal of Clinical Pharmacology*, *69*(3), 295–307. PMID: 22843016

Rascol, O., Payoux, P., Orym, F., Ferreira, J. J., Brefel-Courbon, C., & Montastruc, J. L. (2003). Limitations of Current Parkinson's Disease Therapy. *Annals of Neurology*, *53*(Suppl 3), S3–S12. PMID: 12666094

Saji, C. V., Mohanakumar, K. P., & Shenoi, R. A. (2025). Phytomedicine nanoformulations for Parkinson's disease. *Phytomedicine Plus : International Journal of Phytotherapy and Phytopharmacology*, *5*(1), 100704.

Singh, J., & Kumar, D. (2025). *In vivo* and *in vitro* perspectives in Parkinson's disease: Mechanisms and the role of phytomedicine. *Yao Wu Shi Pin Fen Xi*, *33*(3), 193–212. PMID: 41066749

Smith, J., & Zhang, L. (2021). Challenges in Natural Product Research: The Impact of Adulteration on Therapeutic Outcomes. *Phytotherapy Research*, *35*(5), 2437–2446.

Srivastav, S., Fatima, M., & Mondal, A. C. (2017). Important medicinal herbs in Parkinson's disease pharmacotherapy, Biomedicine & Pharmacotherapy, Volume 92, 2017, Pages 856-863, ISSN 0753-3322, https://doi.org/DOI: 10.1016/j.biopha.2017.05.137

Tkaczenko, H., Buyun, L., Kołodziejska, R., Kamiński, P., & Kurhaluk, N. (2025). Neuroactive Phytochemicals as Multi-Target Modulators of Mental Health and Cognitive Function: An Integrative Review. *International Journal of Molecular Sciences*, *26*(18), 8907. DOI: 10.3390/ijms26188907 PMID: 41009475

Van Kampen, J. M., Baranowski, D. B., Shaw, C. A., & Kay, D. G. (2014). Panax ginseng is neuroprotective in a novel progressive model of Parkinson's disease. *Experimental Gerontology*, *50*, 95–105. DOI: 10.1016/j.exger.2013.11.012 PMID: 24316034

Wang, H., Chen, Y., Wang, L., Liu, Q., Yang, S., & Wang, C. (2023). Advancing herbal medicine: Enhancing product quality and safety through robust quality control practices. *Frontiers in Pharmacology*, *14*, 1265178. PMID: 37818188

Wilson, V., & Maulik, S. K. (2019). Herb-Drug Interactions in Neurological Disorders: A Critical Appraisal. *Current Drug Metabolism*, *19*(5), 443–453. PMID: 29086684

Wongtrakul, J., Thongtan, T., Kumrapich, B., Saisawang, C., & Ketterman, A. J. (2021). Neuroprotective effects of *Withania somnifera* in the SH-SY5Y Parkinson cell model. *Heliyon*, *7*(10), e08172. DOI: 10.1016/j.heliyon.2021.e08172 PMID: 34765761

World Bank. Nigeria: Development News, Research, Data. World Bank. 2023. Available from: https://www.worldbank.org/en/country/nigeria

Yan, Y.-C., Xu, Z.-H., Wang, J., & Yu, W.-B. (2022). Uncovering the pharmacology of *Ginkgo biloba folium* in the cell-type specific targets of Parkinson's disease. *Frontiers in Pharmacology, 13*, 1007556. DOI: 10.3389/fphar.2022.1007556 PMID: 36249800

Yin, R., Xue, J., Tan, Y., Fang, C., Hu, C., Yang, Q., Mei, X., & Qi, D. (2021). The Positive Role and Mechanism of Herbal Medicine in Parkinson's Disease. *Oxidative Medicine and Cellular Longevity, 3*, 9923331. PMID: 34567415

Yu, D., Zhang, P., Li, J., Liu, T., Zhang, Y., Wang, Q., Zhang, J., Lu, X., & Fan, X. (2021). Neuroprotective effects of *Ginkgo biloba* dropping pills in Parkinson's disease. *Journal of Pharmaceutical Analysis, 11*(2), 220–231. PMID: 34012698

Zhao, W., Cui, H., Liu, J., Sun, H., Zhang, Z., & Ma, D. (2025). Herbal Interventions in Parkinson's Disease: A Systematic Review of Preclinical Studies. *Cellular and Molecular Neurobiology, 45*(1), 50. PMID: 40410612

Chapter 5

Stem Cell Therapy for Parkinson's Disease in Under-Resourced Settings

Mosunmola B. Oyeleke
http://orcid.org/0000-0001-5689-0936
Afe Babalola University, Ado-Ekiti, Nigeria

James O. Oluwafemi
Afe Babalola University, Ado-Ekiti, Nigeria

Ahmed Olalekan Bakare
Anaesthesiology and Critical Care Medicine, Johns Hopkins University School of Medicine, Baltimore, USA

ABSTRACT

Parkinson's disease is a neurological disorder that is characterized by the loss of dopaminergic neuron in the substantia nigra pars compacta of the basal ganglia. Its etiology is fully unknown; however, it could occur as a result of a mix of genetic predisposition, environmental factors and possibly aging. the build-up of alpha-synuclein protein into Lewy bodies is the major cause of the neuronal damage seen in PD. There drugs presently available are for managing the symptoms related with PD with no cure available, a lot of research is ongoing as far as PD drug discovery is concerned. Some treatments such as stem cell therapy, deep brain stimulation (DBS), herbal remedies among others have been suggested to have potentials of curing PD. Stem cell therapy involves the replacement of dopaminergic neurons

DOI: 10.4018/979-8-3373-7437-6.ch005

using either the induced pluripotent (iPSCs) or embryonic stem cells (ESCs). The use of this treatment strategy has shown promising effects in the reversal of PD. This chapter aims to explore the possibility of stem cell therapies in the treatment of PD.

INTRODUCTION

Parkinson's disease (PD) is a progressive neurodegenerative disorder driven mainly by the degeneration of nigrostriatal dopaminergic neurons, producing cardinal motor signs (bradykinesia, rigidity, resting tremor) and a broad array of non-motor symptoms that substantially reduce quality of life (Barker et al., 2024). Current pharmacological therapies, including levodopa and dopamine agonists, provide symptomatic benefit but do not replace lost neurons or arrest disease progression, motivating interest in regenerative approaches that restore dopaminergic circuitry (Chang, 2024).

Cell-replacement therapy using stem cell–derived midbrain dopaminergic progenitors is one of the most actively pursued regenerative strategies for PD. Preclinical work has advanced protocols to generate A9-type midbrain dopaminergic neurons from pluripotent stem cells under Good Manufacturing Practice (GMP) conditions, demonstrating robust survival, axonal outgrowth, and functional improvement in animal models (Park et al., 2024). These preclinical advances have allowed the clinical translation of both autologous induced pluripotent stem cell (iPSC)-derived grafts and standardized allogeneic embryonic stem cell (ESC)-derived cell products (Schweitzer et al., 2020; Tabar et al., 2025).

Early human studies and first-in-human case reports have confirmed feasibility and provided important safety signals. Autologous iPSC-derived midbrain progenitors were implanted in a patient with idiopathic PD and were tolerated with encouraging early readouts, marking a milestone for personalized cell therapy (Schweitzer et al., 2020). More recently, phase 1 trials of allogeneic hESCderived dopaminergic progenitor products have reported acceptable short-term safety and imaging evidence consistent with graft survival and dopaminergic reinnervation, supporting continued clinical evaluation (Tabar et al., 2025; Chang et al., 2024).

Although there is this moving forward, there are still major challenges in translation. These are to guarantee long term graft survival and functional integration under neurodegenerative host environment, establishing optimal cell dose and route of delivery, reducing immunogenicity and tumorigenic risk, and to show clinically significant and long term outcome (improvements) in a randomized trial (Barker, 2024; Chang, 2024). These gaps should be filled by standardizing manufacturing, conducting follow-up on a long-term basis, and alignment of outcome measures to capture both motor and non-motor benefits.

1 PARKINSON'S DISEASE

Parkinson disease (PD) is an advanced, multisystem neurodegenerative disorder with the primary characteristics of nigrostriatal dopaminergic neurons loss and misfolded α-synuclein accumulation, which causes both core motor (bradykinesia, rigidity, resting tremor) and a wide spectrum of non-motor symptoms (including cognitive impairment, autonomic dysfunction, sleep disorders, and neuropsychiatric manifestations) (Bloem et al., 2021; Aarsland et al., 2021). Clinical and pathological heterogeneity of PD is gaining more and more recognition: there is a wide variety of disease course, symptom profile, and pathological substrates in different patients, which are manifested through the complex interaction of aging, genetic vulnerability, and environmental exposures. According to epidemiological research, the prevalence of PD is increasing worldwide, which, in part, is due to the aging of populations and, perhaps, shifting environmental and diagnostic factors, which jointly pose an ever-increasing public-health, burden (Ben-Shlomo et al., 2024).

At the molecular level, advances since 2019 have refined understanding of pathogenic pathways implicated in neuronal vulnerability, including disturbances in proteostasis (α-synuclein aggregation), mitochondrial dysfunction, impaired autophagy–lysosomal flux (notably involving GBA), neuroinflammatory responses, and kinase signaling (e.g., LRRK2) — pathways that offer mechanistic targets for novel therapeutics (Sosero et al., 2023). Concurrently, the search for reliable biomarkers has accelerated. Recent work has evaluated multimodal biomarker panels combining neuroimaging, biofluid assays (including novel α- synuclein assays and other protein markers), and digital motor/behavioral measures to improve early diagnosis, stratify patients, and track progression in clinical trials (Yamashita et al., 2023; Das et al., 2024; Arya et al., 2024).

2 WHAT IS STEM CELL THERAPY?

Stem cell therapy encompasses a suite of biomedical approaches that use undifferentiated or lineage-committed cells to repair, replace, or modulate damaged tissues and organs. Broadly, therapeutic strategies rely on several cell types: hematopoietic stem cells (HSCs), mesenchymal stromal/stem cells (MSCs), embryonic stem cells (ESCs), and induced pluripotent stem cells (iPSCs) each with distinct biological properties, differentiation potentials, and translational trajectories (Hussen et al., 2024). These therapies act through direct cell replacement in some contexts and, importantly, through trophic, immunomodulatory, and paracrine effects that promote endogenous repair and modulate disease biology.

Stem cells can be grouped based on their ability to turn into different cell types and their stages of development.

Embryonic stem cells (ESCs), pluripotent cells produced by the inner cell mass of blastocysts, are the types of stem cell that can develop into any kind of cell in the body (Golchin et al., 2021). However, using ESCs is associated with some risks, such as tumor growth, and there are also ethical concerns because they involve the use of embryonic cells (Gage, 2000). Mesenchymal stem cells (MSCs) and Neural stem cells (NSCs) are examples of adult stem cells which are multipotent cells present in the bone marrow, fat tissues and the central nervous system (Wu et al., 2023, Uccelli et al., 2008). These cells are more often safer and less controversial than the ESCs but they can only differentiate into other cells types in a limited manner (Takahashi et al., 2007). In recent years, the reprogramming of adult somatic cells into a more primitive, pluripotent stem cell the induced pluripotent stem cells (iPSCs) using particular transcription factors was possible (Shi et al., 2017). Similar to ESCs, iPSCs are capable of differentiating into any type of cell, although the ethical considerations surrounding the use of ESCs do not exist with the former (Abbaszadeh et al., 2020). Other sources of stem cells are also perinatal tissues that have a diversity of multipotent stem cells like Umbilical cord blood and amniotic fluid.

3 MECHANISMS OF ACTION OF STEM CELLS IN TREATING NEUROLOGICAL DISEASES

These therapeutic potentials of stem cells to treat neurological disorders have a number of mechanisms, and they can be classified into four major categories. These are, cell replacement, paracrine signaling, immunomodulation and augmentation of the endogenous repair mechanisms.

1. Cell replacement: SC might be differentiated as certain types of neuronal and glial cells, which can substitute the damaged or lost neuronal cells in neurological diseases (Rodríguez-Pallares et al., 2023). To illustrate, in PD, the dopaminergic neurons differentiated out of SCs can be implanted to the striatum to restore the cells that have degenerated (Sonntag et al., 2018). Nevertheless, the efficacy of the cell replacement and functional incorporation may be different in the case of treating various neurological conditions, which needs additional studies to streamline the outcomes.
2. Paracrine signaling: Stem cells can release a variety of bioactive molecules such as growth factors, cytokines, and extracellular vesicles which promote

anti-inflammatory, neuroprotective, and regenerative effects on neural tissues (Liang et al., 2014, Zhang et al., 2015). These factors support the survival and regeneration of neural cells that are endogenous and help enhance immune response, synaptic plasticity, and angiogenesis (Xiong et al., 2017, Li et al., 2022). The mechanisms of action of paracrine signaling is thought to be very important in treating diseases where replacing cells alone might not be enough to restore function (Li et al., 2022).

Immunomodulation: Since neuroinflammation is a common pathological characteristic feature of most neurological disorders, giving rise to neuronal damage and impaired repair process (Zhang et al., 2023, Bátiz et al., 2016), Stem cells especially the MSCs have immunomodulatory effect, hence can interact with immune cells and create a favorable environment for neural repair and functional recovery (Xie et al., 2020). These cells can modulate the activities of immune cells such as T and B-lymphocytes, and microglia through direct cell to cell interactions (Brummer et al., 2022, Gugliandolo et al., 2019). Thus, there is a reduction of neuroinflammation, and enhancement of regenerative immune response, supporting neural function (Mao et al., 2019).

3. Stimulation of endogenous repair: Stem cells can activate and mobilize endogenous stem and progenitor cells in the brain to encourage their proliferation, differentiation, and integration into the injured neural tissue (Gilbert et al., 2022, Han et al., 2022). Growth factors and chemokines that draw endogenous stem cells to the injury site and promote their survival and differentiation can be secreted to achieve this (Geranmayeh et al., 2017). Moreover, stem cells can expand the brain's neurogenic and angiogenic areas, enhancing the conditions for endogenous repair mechanisms (Hess et al., 2017).

The way stem cells work in treating neurological diseases is complex and involves multiple factors working together.

The importance of each method can vary based on the specific disease, the type of stem cell used, and when and how the treatment is given. Understanding these processes is essential for developing more effective and targeted treatments for neurological conditions (Roda et al., 2022).

Each type of stem cell has its own different advantages and disadvantages when used for treating neurological conditions. Embryonic stem cells (ESCs) have a high capacity to differentiate into various cell types, but they may cause ethical issues and lead to tumour formation (Barker et al., 2018). On the other hand, adult stem cells, such as mesenchymal stem cells (MSCs) and neural stem cells (NSCs), are less versatile, i.e. they can develop into fewer types of cells, but they might be safer

(Thomson et al., 1998). Induced pluripotent stem cells (iPSCs) allow for the creation of cells that are specific to each individual, but they require detailed examination to ensure they are safe and effective (Uccelli et al., 2008). Therefore, choosing the right type of stem cell requires careful consideration of the specific neurological disease and the treatment goals (Lindvall & Kokaia, 2011).

4 CLINICAL APPLICATIONS OF STEM CELL THERAPIES

Clinical applications of stem cell therapy have expanded rapidly across specialties. HSC transplantation remains a standard, life-saving procedure for hematologic malignancies and certain genetic disorders, while MSCs have been widely investigated in inflammatory, autoimmune, and regenerative contexts for example, graft-versus-host disease (GVHD), Crohn's disease, osteoarthritis, and wound healing (Mousaei Ghasroldasht et al., 2022; Huynh et al., 2022). More recently, pluripotent stem cell–derived products (ESC- and iPSC-derived) have moved into interventional clinical trials for cardiac disease, ophthalmic disorders, spinal cord injury, and neurologic conditions, reflecting improved differentiation protocols, manufacturing under Good Manufacturing Practice (GMP) conditions, and strengthened preclinical efficacy/safety data. The advent of iPSC technology permitting patient-specific pluripotent lines and precise genetic engineering has accelerated personalized regenerative medicine, enabling disease modeling, drug screening and autologous or matched cell-replacement approaches that potentially reduce immunogenicity (Cerneckis et al., 2024). At the same time, regulatory milestones and commercial progress indicate clinical maturation: among them, the most recent approvals and regulatory reviews of cell-based products indicate that certain stem-cell therapeutics are leaving experimental clinical use and entering the approved clinical use (Mesoblast FDA action, 2024). Nonetheless, the profession has also been alerted with the dangers of safety in a poorly-regulated clinic, untested procedures, such as infections associated with off-label stem-cell treatments, the necessity of strict oversight and strict clinical evidence.

However, stem cell-based treatment of neurological diseases has a number of obstacles although their development is promising.

The risk of development of tumors especially with stem cells capable of becoming any form of cell is one. The other problem is that in the process of taking cells of another person the immune system can reject it. Stem cells might also fail to live and integrate well in the body tissues and they may also differentiate and migrate uncontrollably. The issues involving the use of embryonic stem cells are also ethically questionable. Lastly, there exist technical challenges in the generation of large quantities of high-quality stem cells that can be used in clinical applications (Riviere et al., 2017, Wood et al., 2016, Lindvall et al. and Kokaia et al., 2011).

The ethical and equitable access issues, i.e. the disparities in donor matches in allogeneic transplantation and the cost/scale of advanced cell products also need to be addressed deliberatively (Ghasroldasht et al., 2022; Kirkeby et al., 2025). The solution to these challenges will require joint work on the basic biology, manufacturing science, clinical trial design, and regulation policy.

Among the most promising directions in the future, it is a combination of stem cell biology innovations with complementary technologies-gene editing (i.e. CRISPR), 3D organoid systems, bio-materials to promote better engraftment, and digital biomarkers to detect sensitive outcomes to develop safer, more effective, and precisely targeted therapies. Strict randomized trials and longitudinal registries shall be necessary to provide solid proof of long-term clinical advantage as well as assist in conducting evidence-driven responsible clinical adoption.

5 UNDER-RESOURCED SETTING

Under-resourced settings refer to the settings where resources and vital materials, funding, infrastructure and trained personnel are scarce. The constraints are able to influence the quality and consistency of services which include education, healthcare, or community programs. Operating in these environments can be associated with a need to resolve problems creatively, utilize the available resources in an efficient way, and collaborate effectively. Nevertheless, rather than solely relying on the difficulties, under-resourced settings also allow innovation and resilience, as well as community-driven solutions that can contribute to sustainable and significant change.

6 REASONS FOR STEM CELL THERAPY

The term stem cell (SCs) refers to a type of unspecialized cell characterized by both the surface marker they recognize - also known as clusters of differentiation (CD) markers and by their degree of potency, or ability to form different highly specialized cell types. They can also be categorized based on their origin as it helps to reveal where they are at in terms of development e.g. embryonic stem cells or adult stem cells (Balzanelli et al, 2023). They are undifferentiated cells with the regeneration and repair of tissues and organs due to their amazing regenerative power, differentiation and self-renewal. By means of these properties they have therapeutic effects, which replace damaged cells or repair them; thus, helping the organs to heal and grow overall. Scientists have used their vital biological processes to create stem cell-based therapies that tap into the regenerative abilities of the stem cells that occur naturally (Mousaei Ghasroldasht et al, 2022).

Stem cells have the capability to proliferate, self-renew and differentiate into an extensive number of mature types of cells. These are distinguishable into a number of subtypes, such as embryonic stem cells (ESCs), induced pluripotent stem cells (iPSCs), mesenchymal stem cells (MSCs) and neural stem cells (NSCs). These categories are identified by the way they develop and ways of deriving. It is thus essential to know the defining characteristics of the different types of stem cells and how each type can be used therapeutically. The selection of stem cell to be used in a particular application is based on the target objectives and intended results since each type of the cell has its distinctive features and benefits (Sivandzade & Cucullo, 2021).

7 HISTORY OF STEM CELL BASED THERAPY FOR PARKINSON DISEASE

Stem cell therapy of Parkinson's disease has regained momentum in the late 2010s as developments in stem cell biology have rendered neuronal replacement a more realistic possibility. One of the main reviews of 2019 highlighted that embryonic stem cells, fetal derived cells and IPCs have extensive renewable sources that can differentiate into dopaminergic neurons lost in PD and overcoming the consideration of ethical issues and limited supply of fetal grafts (Fan et al, 2020).

In the subsequent years, preclinical studies consistently showed that stem cell derived and tissue cell derived neural grafts could survive, integrate into host circuits, and restore dopamine relate functions in animal models of parkinson's disease (Cueva et al, 2025). This progress paved the way for initial human applications. In 2018, a clinical trial employing autologous iPSC- derived dopaminergic neurons, created from patients' own reprogrammed somatic cells, commenced and represented a major step in bringing cell replacement strategies into clinical evaluation (Dong et al, 2024). From 2023 onward, clinical studies have increasingly focused on transplanting well characterized, homogenous cell populations, including dopaminergic progenitors derived from pluripotent stem cells, and systematic reviews and meta-analyses have started to evaluate their therapeutic potential and safety profile in PD patients (Wang et al, 2023). In summary, the field has progressed from early conceptual work using fetal-tissue grafts to a structured, carefully regulated framework in which patient derived or laboratory generated stem cells are investigated for neuronal replacement, representing the emergence of a new chapter in regenerative therapies for PD (Fan et al, 2020).

8 STEM CELLS CONSIDERED FOR STEM CELL BASED THERAPY FOR PARKINSON'S DISEASE

Mesenchymal Stem Cell, traditionally sourced from the bone marrow, umbilical cord, adipose tissue, and spleen, are adult self-renewing, multipotent stem cells capable of differentiating into a variety of cell types, including bone, cartilage, fat, and muscle (Sivandzade & Cucullo, 2021). The hallmark of MSCs is their ability to respond to stimuli by differentiating as well as their characteristic in vitro expression of a set of cell surface proteins. The enormous changes in gene and protein expression which occur in the course of culture expansion as well as stimulus-induced differentiation, hypoxic preconditioning, exposure to biological factors, trans differentiation, or coculture with other cell types yield useful information on the biological properties of MSCs. The changes can aid in understanding their anticipated physiological roles, roles in the pathophysiology of disease, and the possible mechanisms of therapeutic effect (Zhidu et al, 2024). MSC therapy has been proven to cure most of the diseases such as PD. Being low immunogenic, having no teratoma risk, minimal ethical issue, and having a low likelihood of becoming tumorigenic after being transplanted into the human body. Cell therapies and MSC based therapies have undergone preclinical and clinical trials with most results showing that they have the capability to repair diseased tissue by repopulating degenerating tissue with healthy and functional tissue.

However, the therapeutic effects are often not long lasting. This limitation is largely attributed to endogenous pathological proteins within the host environment, which can negatively influence or impair the transplanted cells (Liu & Cheung, 2020). MSCs possess a range of properties that make them strong candidates for cell-based regenerative therapies. They maintain stemness, can be readily isolated from multiple tissue sources, and can be efficiently expanded on a large scale for clinical use (Zhidu et al, 2024).

9 CLINICAL TRIALS FOR STEM CELL TREATMENT

In recent years, several pioneering clinical trials have advanced stem cell derived dopaminergic therapies from preclinical models to human testing. Notably, a phase I/II trial at Kyoto University Hospital transplanted iPSC-derived dopaminergic progenitors into seven patients with Parkinson's disease. At 24 months post transplantation, the study reported no serious adverse events, survival of the grafted cells, increased striatal dopamine production as measured by ^18F-DOPA PET and motor improvements in several participants, with a mean OFF-medication MDS-UPDRS-III score improvement of approximately 9.5 points (Sawamoto et al, 2025).

In 2023, the STEM-PD trial, led by Lund University and Skåne University Hospital in Sweden, initiated human transplantation of stem cell derived dopaminergic neurons. The low dose cohort, receiving 3.5 million cells per putamen, with plans to follow all participants for 36 months post-transplantation to evaluate safety, graft survival using dopamine PET imaging, and clinical outcomes (Lund University, 2024). In 2025, a novel autologous stem cell transplantation trial was initiated at the Mass General Brigham/McLean Hospital Neuroregeneration Research institute (NRI) in the United States. In this study, patients' own blood derived cells were reprogrammed into iPSCs, differentiated into midbrain dopaminergic neurons, and transplanted, thereby circumventing the immune rejection risk associated with donor derived grafts (Mass General Brigham, 2025).

Overall, these trials employing both allogenic (donor derived) and autologous (patient derived) iPSC-based approaches, at varying doses and in different countries represent the first wave of human applications of stem cell derived neuronal replacement therapy for Parkinson's disease. Early outcomes are reportedly positive and indicate safety, graft survival, and even motor benefit, but long-term efficacy and generalizability have yet to be determined (Barker & Parmar, 2025).

Figure 1. Schematic diagram showing the steps involved in clinical trials of stem cell therapy in Parkinson's disease

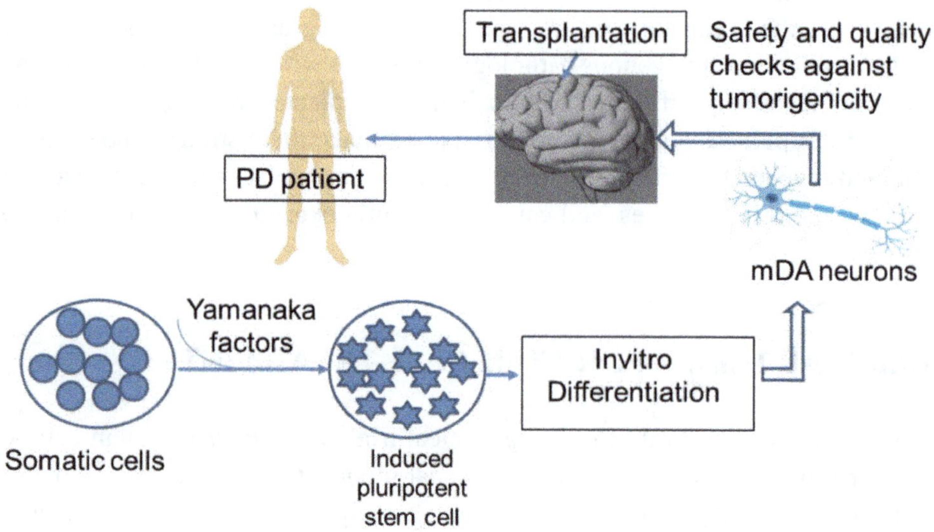

10 ADVANTAGES OF STEM CELL APPROACHES FOR PARKINSON DISEASE

1. Stem cells, in particular pluripotent stem cells (PSCs) and induced pluripotent stem cells (iPSCs) have the ability to differentiate into the neural cell types like midbrain dopaminergic (DA) neurons, and this presents a biologically plausible approach to replace the neuronal populations that degenerate in Parkinson's disease (Mokhtari et al, 2025). This potential leads to the prospect of tackling the symptoms as well as underlying pathology of neuronal loss with the possibility of restoring the synthesis of dopamine and functional synaptic connectivity (Cha et al, 2023)
2. Other cells like mesenchymal stem cells (MSCs) also show significant neuroprotective properties in part by secretion of neurotropic and growth factors that enhance neuron survival and potentially rescue vulnerable neurons against progressive degeneration (Heris et al, 2022).

MSCs also exert immunomodulatory and anti-inflammatory effects; through the release of cytokines and the modulation of immune activity such as reducing microglial activation, they may help attenuate the neuroinflammation implicated in Parkinson's disease pathology (Liu & Cheung, 2020). Beyond direct cell replacement, this "paracrine effect" (via secretion of bioactive factors, extracellular vesicles or exosomes) may support endogenous repair, reduce apoptosis, and promote a brain environment conducive to healing (Heris et al, 2022).

3. iPSCs are generated from reprogrammed adult cells (e.g., patient's own somatic cells). This avoids the ethical issues linked to embryonic stem cell (ESC) use (Dong et al, 2024). Use of autologous iPSCs (patient-derived) reduces risk of immune rejection and potentially eliminates the need for immunosuppression (Osborn et al, 2020).
4. According to a recent meta-analysis of controlled trials (up to July 2023), cell-therapy in PD showed beneficial effects on motor function and reduction in disease severity, in "off" state (i.e. when patients are off medication), with improvements lasting up to 36 months (Wang et al, 2023).
5. Modern PSC-based approaches allow generation of clinical-grade dopaminergic neuron progenitor cells (or mature neurons) under controlled, standardized protocols, which improves safety, reproducibility, and quality control compared to earlier fetal-tissue transplantation (Cha et al, 2023).

11 DISADVANTAGES OF STEM CELL APPROACHES FOR PARKINSON'S DISEASE

1. Significant heterogeneity exists among studies with respect to cell sources (e.g., MSCs, NSCs, and pluripotent stem cells), differentiation strategies, and modes of delivery. Such variablity hampers meaningful comparison, undermines reproducibility, and diminishes the extent to which results can be reliably generalized to diverse patient groups. Because many studies remain preclinical (animal or in vitro), with only a few early-phase human trials, their findings may not translate to real-world clinical settings (Cueva et al, 2025).
2. One of the major challenges is the inability to have a good survival of the transplanted dopaminergic (DA) neurons. It has been shown that more than 90 percent of transplanted neurons degenerate regardless of whether the cells used are autologous, allogeneic, or xenogeneic which highly limits the therapeutic benefit attainable (Kim, 2026). The surviving cells even are not properly integrated into the neuronal circuits of the host brain (i.e. the correct connections between the synaptic functions, proper functional integration) with a lot of efficiency. Unless integration is done correctly, transplant cells may fail to restore functions of the lost neurons (Zeng & Qin, 2022).
3. Pluripotent stem cells include ESCs and iPSCs, which have an intrinsic risk of tumorigenicity and genomic instabilization. Such concerns, therefore, remain among the most salient and incumbent safety concerns in the development of such cells to clinical use (Sancho-Bielsa, 2022). With differentiation protocols in place, the possibility still exists of uncontrolled differentiation or the production of undesired cell types, which may not result in functional neurons, but instead tissue growth in the wrong place (ectopic tissue growth). (Marei, 2025).
4. Host immune activates can be developed by transplanted cells, most notably, allogeneic cells. Although there is relative immune privilege of the brain, the grafts cannot be assured to survive in the long term without immune mediated rejection. Immunosuppressive drugs might be necessary to avoid rejection, but it is still unclear which type of immunosuppression is appropriate, what dosage is needed, and how long should immunosuppression continue in case of stem-cell grafts.

This complicates long-term safety and feasibility (Zeng & Qin, 2022).

5. For certain stem-cell types (e.g., MSCs), although they have shown neuroprotective or modulatory effects in animal models, their capacity to restore full brain function (e.g., restoration of lost DA neurons and circuitry) in humans remains limited and unproven (Hwang et al, 2018).

6. The use of certain stem cell sources, particularly embryonic stem cells, raises ethical concerns, which can limit acceptability and regulatory approval (Dong et al, 2024).

12 THE FUTURE PERSPECTIVE OF STEM CELL TREATMENT OF PARKINSON'S DISEASE IN UNDER- RESOURCED SETTINGS

With the growing burden of NCDs in low- and middle-income regions, there is increasing need for therapies that do more than relieve symptoms. Stem-cell therapy (SCT) offers a regenerative strategy that targets the neuronal loss at the root of Parkinson's disease. (Atewologun et al, 2024).

Therapies using mesenchymal stem cells (MSCs) or induced pluripotent stem cells (iPSCs) can ease the ethical and supply issues associated with donor tissue. IPSC-based strategies are now central to international research initiatives (Morizane, 2023).

Current PD treatments (e.g., dopamine replacement) mainly relieve symptoms without halting neuronal loss. As argued in recent reviews, stem-cell–based regenerative therapies may eventually restore dopaminergic function at the cellular and circuit levels, offering the possibility of more durable disease-modifying effects (Kim, 2026).

13 CHALLENGES

1. A major barrier is the limited availability of trained scientists, clinicians, and lab infrastructure in many Low- and Middle-Income Countries (LMICs). As documented for African countries, "brain drain" (loss of skilled professionals) and weak innovation ecosystems hamper the establishment of robust cell-therapy programs (Atewologun et al, 2024).
2. Stem-cell therapies, especially personalized or iPSC-based options, are expensive to produce and deliver. In many LMICs, reliance on out-of-pocket payments and weak health insurance systems makes these treatments accessible only to wealthier patients.
3. Many LMICs lack comprehensive regulatory frameworks for advanced therapies such as SCT. In the absence of guidelines, oversight, and quality standards, unregulated, unsafe, or unfair deployment may cause harm to patients or lead to a loss of trust in the society (Atewologun et al, 2024).

4. Other challenges include the inability to achieve good survival of transplanted dopaminergic (DA) neurons, cell population heterogeneity, variability in differentiation protocols, and the possibility of undesirable cell types or immune response even with well-resourced settings (Kim, 2026).
5. Research done in Africa and other limited resources is scarce. In the absence of local generated information (safety, efficacy, long-term results in various genetic and environmental conditions), it is not easy to extrapolate global results to local conditions (Atewologun et al, 2024).

14 RECOMMENDATION

Based on the challenges faced by the LMIC, the following recommendations have been made:

1. To overcome cost barriers, LMICs could explore decentralized production manufacturing stem-cell products locally or regionally to reduce import costs and reliance on foreign labs. This could involve public-private partnerships and support from international agencies. Indeed, some propose "place-of-care bio-manufacturing" as a pathway forward (Atewologun et al, 2024).
2. Building human capital is vital: training neurologists, neuroscientists, translational-medicine specialists, lab technicians and regulatory experts in LMICs. Regional or continental collaborations (e.g., among African universities and research centers) can help share expertise and resources (Atewologun et al, 2024).
3. It is critical to conduct clinical trials in under-resourced settings, to assess efficacy, safety, cost-effectiveness, and long-term outcomes in populations that may differ genetically, environmentally, or in comorbid conditions from those in high-income countries (Atewologun et al, 2024).

15 CONCLUSION

In conclusion, stem cell therapy could be explored in the treatment of PD because it is a promising and emerging field in PD drug discovery; however, appropriate conditions should be put in place to overcome its challenges to a great extent.

REFERENCES

Aarsland, D., Brønnick, K., Larsen, J. P., & Alves, G. (2021). Parkinson disease-associated cognitive impairment. *Nature Reviews. Disease Primers*, *7*, 61.

Abbaszadeh, H., Ghorbani, F., Derakhshani, M., Movassaghpour, A., & Yousefi, M. (2020). Human umbilical cord mesenchymal stem cell-derived extracellular vesicles: A novel therapeutic paradigm. *Journal of Cellular Physiology*, *235*(2), 706–717. PMID: 31254289

Arya, R., Haque, A. A., Shakya, H., Billah, M. M., Parvin, A., Rahman, M. M., Sakib, K. M., Faruquee, H. M., Kumar, V., & Kim, J. J. (2024). Parkinson's disease: Biomarkers for diagnosis and disease progression. *International Journal of Molecular Sciences*, *25*(22), 12379. PMID: 39596444

Atewologun, F. A., Okesanya, O. J., Okon, I. I., Kayode, H. H., Ukoaka, B. M., Olaleke, N. O., Ogaya, J. B., Okikiola, L. A., Manirambona, E., & Lucero-Prisno, D. E.III. (2024). Examining the potentials of stem cell therapy in reducing the burden of selected non-communicable diseases in Africa. *Stem Cell Research & Therapy*, *15*(1), 253. PMID: 39135088

Balzanelli, M. G., Distratis, P., Lazzaro, R., Pham, V. H., Tran, T. C., Dipalma, G., Inchingolo, F., Serlenga, E. M., Aityan, S. K., Ballini, A., Nguyen, K. C. D., & Isacco, C. G. (2023). The Anti-Viral Activity of Stem Cells: A Rational Explanation for their Use in Clinical Application. *Endocrine, Metabolic & Immune Disorders Drug Targets*, *23*(6), 739–747. PMID: 37254275

Barker, R. A., Björklund, A., & Parmar, M. (2024). The history and status of dopamine cell therapies for Parkinson's disease. *BioEssays*, *46*(12), 2400118. PMID: 39058892

Barker, R. A., Carpenter, M. K., Forbes, S., Goldman, S. A., Jamieson, C., Murry, C. E., & Weir, G. (2018). The challenges of first-in-human stem cell clinical trials: What does this mean for ethics and institutional review boards? *Stem Cell Reports*, *10*(5), 1429–1431. PMID: 29742388

Barker, R. A., & Parmar, M. (2025). Stem cell-derived dopamine cell therapies for Parkinson's disease: What have the first trials shown? *Brain*, *148*(10), 3428–3430. PMID: 40898774

Bátiz, L. F., Castro, M. A., Burgos, P. V., Velásquez, Z. D., Muñoz, R. I., Lafourcade, C. A., Troncoso-Escudero, P., & Wyneken, U. (2016). Exosomes as Novel Regulators of Adult Neurogenic Niches. *Frontiers in Cellular Neuroscience*, *9*, 501. PMID: 26834560

Ben-Shlomo, Y., Darweesh, S., Llibre-Guerra, J., Marras, C., San Luciano, M., & Tanner, C. (2024). The epidemiology of Parkinson's disease. *Lancet*, *403*(10423), 283–292. PMID: 38245248

Bloem, B. R., Okun, M. S., & Klein, C. (2021). Parkinson's disease. *Lancet*, *397*(10291), 2284–2303. PMID: 33848468

Brummer, T., Zipp, F., & Bittner, S. (2022). T cell–neuron interaction in inflammatory and progressive multiple sclerosis biology. *Current Opinion in Neurobiology*, *75*, 102588. PMID: 35732103

Cerneckis, J., Cai, H., & Shi, Y. (2024). Induced pluripotent stem cells (iPSCs): Molecular mechanisms of induction and applications. *Signal Transduction and Targeted Therapy*, *9*(1), 112. PMID: 38670977

Cha, Y., Park, T. Y., Leblanc, P., & Kim, K. S. (2023). Current Status and Future Perspectives on Stem Cell-Based Therapies for Parkinson's Disease. *Journal of Movement Disorders*, *16*(1), 22–41. PMID: 36628428

Cueva, E., Wiesheu, A., Sordo, Z., González, J., Falconi, S., Rodas, J. A., & Leon-Rojas, J. E. (2025). Tissue Stem Cell-Based Therapies in Parkinson's Disease: A Scoping Review of Therapeutic Mechanisms and Translational Outcomes. *Cells*, *14*(11), 822. PMID: 40497998

Das, S., & Ramteke, H. (2024). A comprehensive review of the role of biomarkers in early diagnosis of Parkinson's disease. *Cureus*, *16*(2). PMID: 38500934

Dong, W., Liu, S., Li, S., & Wang, Z. (2024). Cell reprogramming therapy for Parkinson's disease. *Neural Regeneration Research*, *19*(11), 2444–2455. PMID: 38526281

Fan, Y., Winanto, & Ng, S. Y. (2020). Replacing what's lost: A new era of stem cell therapy for Parkinson's disease. *Translational Neurodegeneration*, *9*(1), 2. PMID: 31911835

Gage, F. H. (2000). Mammalian neural stem cells. *Science*, *287*(5457), 1433–1438. PMID: 10688783

Geranmayeh, M. H., Nourazarian, A., Avci, Ç. B., Rahbarghazi, R., & Farhoudi, M. (2017). Stem cells as a promising tool for the restoration of brain neurovascular unit and angiogenic orientation. *Molecular Neurobiology*, *54*, 7689–7705. PMID: 27844280

Gilbert, E. A. B., Lakshman, N., Lau, K. S. K., & Morshead, C. M. (2022). Regulating Endogenous Neural Stem Cell Activation to Promote Spinal Cord Injury Repair. *Cells*, *11*(5), 846. PMID: 35269466

Golchin, A., Chatziparasidou, A., Ranjbarvan, P., Niknam, Z., & Ardeshirylajimi, A. (2021). Embryonic Stem Cells in Clinical Trials: Current Overview of Developments and Challenges. *Advances in Experimental Medicine and Biology, 1312*, 19–37. PMID: 33159303

Gugliandolo, A., Bramanti, P., & Mazzon, E. (2019). Mesenchymal Stem Cells: A Potential Therapeutic Approach for Amyotrophic Lateral Sclerosis? *Stem Cells International, 2019*, 3675627. PMID: 30956667

Han, Y., Yang, J., Fang, J., Zhou, Y., Candi, E., Wang, J., Hua, D., Shao, C., & Shi, Y. (2022). The secretion profile of mesenchymal stem cells and potential applications in treating human diseases. *Signal Transduction and Targeted Therapy*, *7*(1), 92. PMID: 35314676

Heris, R. M., Shirvaliloo, M., Abbaspour-Aghdam, S., Hazrati, A., Shariati, A., Youshanlouei, H. R., Niaragh, F. J., Valizadeh, H., & Ahmadi, M. (2022). The potential use of mesenchymal stem cells and their exosomes in Parkinson's disease treatment. *Stem Cell Research & Therapy*, *13*(1), 371. PMID: 35902981

Hess, D. C., Wechsler, L. R., & Clark, W. M.. (2017). Safety and efficacy of multipotent adult progenitor cells in acute ischaemic stroke (MASTERS): A randomised, double-blind, placebo-controlled, phase 2 trial. *Lancet Neurology*, *16*(5), 360–368. PMID: 28320635

Hussen, B. M., Taheri, M., Yashooa, R. K., Abdullah, G. H., Abdullah, S. R., Kheder, R. K., & Mustafa, S. A. (2024). Revolutionizing medicine: Recent developments and future prospects in stem-cell therapy. *International Journal of Surgery*, *110*(12), 8002–8024. PMID: 39497543

Huynh, P. D., Tran, Q. X., Nguyen, S. T., Nguyen, V. Q., & Vu, N. B. (2022). Mesenchymal stem cell therapy for wound healing: An update to 2022. *Biomedical Research and Therapy*, *9*(12), 5437–5449.

Hwang, S., Gill, S., Pathak, S., & Subramanian, S. (2018). A Comparison of Stem Cell Therapies for Parkinson Disease. *Georgetown Medical Review, 2*(1).

Kim, T. W. (2026). Human stem cell–based cell replacement therapy for Parkinson's disease: Enhancing the survival of postmitotic dopamine neuron grafts. *Neural Regeneration Research*, *21*(2), 689–690. PMID: 40326986

Kirkeby, A., Main, H., & Carpenter, M. (2025). Pluripotent stem-cell-derived therapies in clinical trial: A 2025 update. *Cell Stem Cell*, *32*(1), 10–37. PMID: 39753110

Li, M., Jiang, Y., Hou, Q., Zhao, Y., Zhong, L., & Fu, X. (2022). Potential pre-activation strategies for improving therapeutic efficacy of mesenchymal stem cells: Current status and future prospects. *Stem Cell Research & Therapy*, *13*(1), 146. PMID: 35379361

Liang, X., Ding, Y., Zhang, Y., Tse, H. F., & Lian, Q. (2014). Paracrine mechanisms of mesenchymal stem cell-based therapy: Current status and perspectives. *Cell Transplantation*, *23*(9), 1045–1059. PMID: 23676629

Lindvall, O., & Kokaia, Z. (2011). Stem cell research in stroke: How far from the clinic? *Stroke*, *42*(8), 2369–2375. PMID: 21757669

Liu, Z., & Cheung, H. H. (2020). Stem cell-based therapies for Parkinson disease. *International Journal of Molecular Sciences*, *21*(21), 8060. PMID: 33137927

Lund University. (2024, May 6). *Update on STEM-PD clinical trial* - stem cell based transplant for parkinson's disease. Lund University; Accessed on November, 2025.

Mao, A. S., Özkale, B., Shah, N. J., Vining, K. H., Descombes, T., Zhang, L., Tringides, C. M., Wong, S. W., Shin, J. W., Scadden, D. T., Weitz, D. A., & Mooney, D. J. (2019). Programmable microencapsulation for enhanced mesenchymal stem cell persistence and immunomodulation. *Proceedings of the National Academy of Sciences of the United States of America*, *116*(31), 15392–15397. PMID: 31311862

Marei, H. E. (2025). Stem cell therapy: A revolutionary cure or a pandora's box. *Stem Cell Research & Therapy*, *16*(1), 255. PMID: 40405306

Mass General Brigham. (2025, March 6). Clinical trial tests novel stem-cell treatment for parkinson's disease; Accessed on November, 2025. http://www.massgeneralbrigham.org/en/about/newsroom/press-releases/clinical-trial-novel-stem-cell-treatment-for-parkinson's

Mokhtari, Y. G., Varnava, I., Kyrgiannis, K., Ampatsidou, V., & Giakoumettis, D. (2025). Stem cell therapy for Parkinson's disease: A new hope for neural regeneration. *World Journal of Biological Chemistry*, *16*(2), 106850. PMID: 40476258

Morizane, A. (2023). Cell therapy for Parkinson's disease with induced pluripotent stem cells. *Inflammation and Regeneration*, *43*(1), 16. PMID: 36843101

Mousaei Ghasroldasht, M., Seok, J., Park, H. S., Liakath Ali, F. B., & Al-Hendy, A. (2022). Stem cell therapy: From idea to clinical practice. *International Journal of Molecular Sciences*, *23*(5), 2850. PMID: 35269990

Osborn, T. M., Hallett, P. J., Schumacher, J. M., & Isacson, O. (2020). Advantages and recent developments of autologous cell therapy for Parkinson's disease patients. *Frontiers in Cellular Neuroscience, 14*, 58. PMID: 32317934

Park, S., Park, C. W., Eom, J. H., Jo, M. Y., Hur, H. J., Choi, S. K., Lee, J. S., Nam, S. T., Jo, K. S., Oh, Y. W., & Kim, D. W. (2024). Preclinical and dose-ranging assessment of hESC-derived dopaminergic progenitors for a clinical trial on Parkinson's disease. *Cell Stem Cell, 31*(1), 25–38. PMID: 38086390

Roda, A. R., Serra-Mir, G., Montoliu-Gaya, L., Tiessler, L., & Villegas, S. (2022). Amyloid-beta peptide and tau protein crosstalk in Alzheimer's disease. *Neural Regeneration Research, 17*(8), 1666–1674. PMID: 35017413

Rodríguez-Pallares, J., García-Garrote, M., Parga, J. A., & Labandeira-García, J. L. (2023). Combined cell-based therapy strategies for the treatment of Parkinson's disease: Focus on mesenchymal stromal cells. *Neural Regeneration Research, 18*(3), 478–484. PMID: 36018150

Sancho-Bielsa, F. J. (2022). Parkinson's disease: Present and future of cell therapy. *Neurology Perspectives, 2*(1), 58–68.

Sawamoto, N., Doi, D., Nakanishi, E., Sawamura, M., Kikuchi, T., Yamakado, H., Taruno, Y., Shima, A., Fushimi, Y., Okada, T., & Takahashi, J. (2025). Phase I/II trial of iPS-cell-derived dopaminergic cells for Parkinson's disease. *Nature*, •••, 1–7. PMID: 40240591

Schweitzer, J. S., Song, B., Herrington, T. M., Park, T. Y., Lee, N., Ko, S., Jeon, J., Cha, Y., & Kim, K. S. (2020). Personalized iPSC-derived dopamine progenitor cells for Parkinson's disease. *The New England Journal of Medicine, 382*(20), 1926–1932. PMID: 32402162

Shi, Y., Inoue, H., Wu, J. C., & Yamanaka, S. (2017). Induced pluripotent stem cell technology: A decade of progress. *Nature Reviews. Drug Discovery, 16*(2), 115–130. PMID: 27980341

Sivandzade, F., & Cucullo, L. (2021). Regenerative stem cell therapy for neurodegenerative diseases: An overview. *International Journal of Molecular Sciences, 22*(4), 2153. PMID: 33671500

Sonntag, K. C., Song, B., Lee, N., Jung, J. H., Cha, Y., Leblanc, P., Neff, C., Kong, S. W., Carter, B. S., Schweitzer, J., & Kim, K. S. (2018). Pluripotent stem cell-based therapy for Parkinson's disease: Current status and future prospects. *Progress in Neurobiology, 168*, 1–20. PMID: 29653250

Sosero, Y. L., & Gan-Or, Z. (2023). LRRK2 and Parkinson's disease: From genetics to targeted therapy. *Annals of Clinical and Translational Neurology*, *10*(6), 850–864. PMID: 37021623

Tabar, V., Sarva, H., Lozano, A. M., Fasano, A., Kalia, S. K., Yu, K. K. H., & Henchcliffe, C. (2025). Phase I trial of hES cell-derived dopaminergic neurons for Parkinson's disease. *Nature*, •••, 1–6. PMID: 40240592

Takahashi, K., Tanabe, K., Ohnuki, M., Narita, M., Ichisaka, T., Tomoda, K., & Yamanaka, S. (2007). Induction of pluripotent stem cells from adult human fibroblasts by defined factors. *Cell*, *131*(5), 861–872. PMID: 18035408

Thomson, J. A., Itskovitz-Eldor, J., Shapiro, S. S., Waknitz, M. A., Swiergiel, J. J., Marshall, V. S., & Jones, J. M. (1998). Embryonic stem cell lines derived from human blastocysts. *science, 282*(5391), 1145-1147.

Uccelli, A., Moretta, L., & Pistoia, V. (2008). Mesenchymal stem cells in health and disease. *Nature Reviews. Immunology*, *8*(9), 726–736. PMID: 19172693

Wang, F., Sun, Z., Peng, D., Gianchandani, S., Le, W., Boltze, J., & Li, S. (2023). Cell-therapy for Parkinson's disease: A systematic review and meta-analysis. *Journal of Translational Medicine*, *21*(1), 601. PMID: 37679754

Wu, H., Fan, Y., & Zhang, M. (2023). Advanced Progress in the Role of Adipose-Derived Mesenchymal Stromal/Stem Cells in the Application of Central Nervous System Disorders. *Pharmaceutics*, *15*(11), 2637. PMID: 38004615

Xie, B., Chen, M., Hu, R., Han, W., & Ding, S. (2020). Therapeutic Evidence of Human Mesenchymal Stem Cell Transplantation for Cerebral Palsy: A Meta-Analysis of Randomized Controlled Trials. *Stem Cells International*, *2020*(1), 5701920. PMID: 32765613

Xiong, Y., Mahmood, A., & Chopp, M. (2017). Emerging potential of exosomes for treatment of traumatic brain injury. *Neural Regeneration Research*, *12*(1), 19–22. PMID: 28250732

Yamashita, K. Y., Bhoopatiraju, S., Silverglate, B. D., & Grossberg, G. T. (2023). Biomarkers in Parkinson's disease: A state of the art review. *Biomarkers in Neuropsychiatry*, *9*, 100074.

Zeng, X., & Qin, H. (2022). Stem cell transplantation for Parkinson's disease: Current challenges and perspectives. *Aging and Disease*, *13*(6), 1652. PMID: 36465172

Zhang, W., Xiao, D., Mao, Q., & Xia, H. (2023). Role of neuroinflammation in neurodegeneration development. *Signal Transduction and Targeted Therapy*, *8*(1), 267. PMID: 37433768

Zhang, Y., Chopp, M., Meng, Y., Katakowski, M., Xin, H., Mahmood, A., & Xiong, Y. (2015). Effect of exosomes derived from multipluripotent mesenchymal stromal cells on functional recovery and neurovascular plasticity in rats after traumatic brain injury. *Journal of Neurosurgery*, *122*(4), 856–867. PMID: 25594326

Zhidu, S., Ying, T., Rui, J., & Chao, Z. (2024). Translational potential of mesenchymal stem cells in regenerative therapies for human diseases: Challenges and opportunities. *Stem Cell Research & Therapy*, *15*(1), 266. PMID: 39183341

Chapter 6
Immunotherapy and Targeted Molecular Therapies for Parkinson's Disease in Under-Resourced Settings

K. Gayathri
http://orcid.org/0009-0007-3786-2009
Department of Microbiology, Sacred Heart College, Tirupattur, India

S. Kavi Karunya
http://orcid.org/0009-0003-4667-4393
Marudhar Kesari Jain College for Women, Vaniyambadi, India

P. Saranraj
http://orcid.org/0000-0002-5052-6532
Department of Microbiology, Sacred Heart College, Tirupattur, India

Mukesh Kumar Dharmalingam Jothinathan
Saveetha Medical College and Hospital, Saveetha Institute of Medical and Technical Sciences, Saveetha University, Chennai, India

J. Arish
Department of Microbiology, Sacred Heart College, Tirupattur, India

Alexander Machado Cardoso
Rio de Janeiro State University, Brazil

ABSTRACT

Parkinson's disease presents a growing global health challenge, particularly in under-resourced settings where access to specialized care and advanced therapies remains limited. This book explores the evolution and innovation of Parkinson's disease therapies, examining historical developments, current treatment standards, and emerging strategies adapted for resource-constrained environments. Emphasis is placed on cost-effective pharmacological approaches, technological innovations,

DOI: 10.4018/979-8-3373-7437-6.ch006

community-based interventions, and sustainable care models. By highlighting challenges, opportunities, and future directions, the book aims to promote equitable access to effective Parkinson's disease management and support the development of inclusive, patient-centered healthcare systems worldwide.

INTRODUCTION

The second most frequent neurodegenerative disorder is Parkinson's disease (PD), which is becoming one of the primary health issues in low- and middle-income countries (LMICs) at an extremely high rate. PD is characterized by progressive degradation of dopaminergic neurons in the substantia nigra as well as consequential deposition of misfolded α-synuclein protein that causes motor symptoms including tremor, rigidity and bradykinesia, and non-motor symptoms including cognitive impairment and sleep disturbances. In high-income countries, development of healthcare has enhanced the process of diagnosis and management; however, in low-resource settings, access to the services of neurologists, diagnostic imaging, and long-term treatment remains low (Asuku et al., 2025). With a growing life expectancy worldwide, the PD burden in these areas in the future is likely to increase greatly, which explains the necessity of disease-modifying therapies accessible, scalable, and affordable (Dekker et al., 2020).

The existing methods of PD treatment are mostly symptomatic and rely mainly on the dopamine replacement therapy, especially levodopa (Ajagun et al., 2024). These therapies are effective in enhancing quality of life, nevertheless, they neither decelerate nor prevent the development of the disease, and after long-term use, complications may arise in the form of motor fluctuations, dyskinesia (Abdel et al., 2021). This weakness has necessitated a paradigm shift in studies to curements that focus on the molecular and cellular pathways of neurodegeneration. Immunotherapy and targeted molecular therapies are among the most promising methods that can alter the course of a disease by addressing causes of neuronal damage instead of relieving the symptoms (Tannenbaum et al., 2019).

The use of immunotherapy has been of particular interest to the advancement considering that increasing evidence has shown that misfolded alpha-synuclein is a central key to PD development and propagation between neurons in a prion-like fashion. Active immunization techniques aim to induce the immune system of the body to form antibodies against 2 pathological 2 forms of 2 synuclein, whereas passive immunotherapy entails the administration of monoclonal antibodies that directly bind and clear up the toxic aggregates of protein (Bhidayasiri et al., 2021). Furthermore, immunomodulatory therapies also work to minimize neuroinflammation which is also a major cause of neuronal damage in PD. These strategies have the possibility to bring about long-term disease alteration, though its application in under-resourced environments is exasperated by a high cost, cold-chain storage demands, and scarce clinical resources (Palmer et al., 2019).

The specific molecular therapies are used to supplement immunotherapy but target the genetic and biochemical pathways of PD. Recent discoveries in the field of molecular neuroscience have revealed mitochondrial dysfunction, oxidative stress, disrupted autophagy, and genetic mutations (including LRRK2 and GBA) as the most important mechanisms in the development of the disease (Yu et al., 2023). New forms of therapy are gene suppression therapies, neuroprotective drugs that can result in better mitochondrial activity, and therapies that can stimulate ways to clear waste out of cells. Such precision-medicine strategies will potentially make neurodegeneration slower and, importantly, it may be possible to prevent the development of the disease in people with genetic vulnerabilities, which will switch the focus to the personalized approach to treatment (Bello et al., 2016).

Although they have shown promise, translating these advanced therapies into under-resourced environments is a challenging endeavor, with such barriers as insufficient healthcare infrastructure, late diagnosis, prohibitive cost of treatment, and a lack of awareness (Valencia et al. 2021). However, such areas also have innovation opportunities especially in the development of low-cost vaccine-based immunotherapies, formulations of long-acting drugs, and easy-to-use diagnostic tools. Immunotherapy and targeted molecular therapies can also change the way the world manages Parkinson with regards to affordability, scalability and collaboration with other countries worldwide, to decrease the increasing inequality in neurological care (Adelson et al., 2003).

HISTORICAL EVOLUTION OF PARKINSON'S DISEASE THERAPIES

The clinical observation, neurobiology, pharmacology, and health systems organization have seen remarkable developments in the past two centuries that led to the therapeutic management of Parkinson's disease (PD). It is of special significance to under-resourced environments to comprehend this historical path since most of the initial principles of therapeutic approaches, including symptom-related management, the use of relatively inexpensive medications, and the use of non-pharmacological methods, are still very topical in under-resourced settings where there is no access to the latest technologies (Okunoye et al., 2023).

Early Descriptions and Symptomatic Management

Symptomatic management entails managing the symptoms of an illness or condition, and is often employed before the acquisition of treatment or preventive measures aimed at curing or preventing the disease. Early descriptions Early symptomatic treatments consist of the management of the symptoms of an illness or condition without the acquisition of treatment or preventive interventions with the aim of curing or preventing the disease. It was James Parkinson in 1817 who described Parkinson's disease in a systematic fashion placing him in a seminal position as he outlined the cardinal motor characteristics of tremor, rigidity, postural instability, and gait disorder in his work titled An Essay on the Shaking Palsy (Walker et al., 2023). Therapeutic choices during this era and until early in the 20th century were mostly empirical and symptomatic and were not based on an appreciation of underlying pathophysiology. They were treated using herbal treatments, blood-letting, purgatives, and eventually, plant-based anticholinergic agents, including Atropa belladonna. Massage, exercise and rest were frequently used as physical interventions to relieve the stiffness and mobility restrictions. Though these interventions had a low level of benefit but beneficence, they made a very early acknowledgment of the necessity of multidisciplinary and supportive care- a theme that still has merit in low resource settings where there is no curative or disease-modifying treatment (Bianco et al., 2024).

Discovery of Dopamine Deficiency and Levodopa Era

The management of Parkinson disease came in the mid-20th century when the cause of the condition was discovered through dopamine deficiency in the basal ganglia. Oleh Hornykiewicz and others showed a significant decrease in dopamine concentration in the striatum of people with PD, which proved a neurochemical basis of PD. The discovery resulted in the introduction of the dopamine precursor levodopa that is able to cross the blood-brain barrier and thus changed the management of PD. Levodopa was first administered to patients in the late 1960s and yielded significant and impressive improvements in motor symptoms and quality of life, turning PD into a condition that could be managed successfully over many years (Helmer et al., 2024). Although long-term effects of PD were only identified much later, levodopa has always been the gold standard of PD treatment. Its relative low cost, strong effectiveness, and status as a World Health Organization Model List of Essential Medicines makes it specifically important in under-resourced settings, where it can universally be the foundation, and in other cases the sole, pharmacological treatment option (Contini et al., 2024).

Development of Adjunct Pharmacotherapies

The limitations of the long-term levodopa treatment becoming apparent, the focus was on the development of the adjunct pharmacological therapies that would improve the dopaminergic function of the brain and diminish the occurrence of motor complications. Dopamine agonists, monoamine oxidase-B (MAO-B) inhibitors, catechol-O-methyltransferase (COMT) inhibitors, amantadine, and anticholinergic medications were introduced to the therapeutic portfolio, and thus more specific and flexible treatment options became possible. These agents allowed reduction of dosage of levodopa, retarded onset of motor complications and enhanced the treatment of certain symptoms like tremor or dyskinesia. Most of these drugs are however costlier, more complicated to side-effects or need close monitoring, which restricts their application in low-resource locations. However, access has been enhanced tremendously by generic formulations and easier dosing schedules in certain areas, which demonstrates how small changes in pharmacology may be modified to resource-limited health care systems (Bhidayasiri, 2024).

Evolution of Non-Pharmacological Interventions

In line with the gains made in the field of pharmacology, non-pharmacological interventions have become a significant part of the management of the disease of Parkinson. The early understanding of the advantages of exercise transformed into formal physiotherapy efforts to address the abilities of gait, balance and strength. Speech and language therapy came up to counter dysarthria and dysphagia whereas occupational therapy aimed at sustaining independence in daily lives. Exercise interventions including dance, tai chi, yoga and group-based movement programs have also been found to have beneficial effects on motor function, balance, and psychosocial well-being more recently. These interventions are especially useful in under-resourced environments when it comes to their affordability, flexibility, and possible community-based implementation. A good example of how non-pharmacological treatments can be scaled when workforce is limited is the use of task-shifting models which train community health workers or caregivers to provide basic rehabilitative support (Sharma et al., 2024).

IMMUNOTHERAPY APPROACHES IN PARKINSON'S DISEASE

Principles of Immunotherapy in Neurodegenerative Disorders

Immunotherapy is the newly developed paradigm in the treatment of neurodegenerative disorders such as Parkinson's disease (PD) by targeting disease pathophysiology as opposed to merely treating the symptoms. The general idea is to utilize the body immune system to identify, eliminate, block the presence of pathological proteins or inflammatory cytokines that cause neuronal degeneration (Hajzer et al., 2025).. Misfolded α-synuclein aggregates build up in the neurons and spread across neuronal networks in PD causing neuroinflammation and progressive dopaminergic neuron loss. Immunotherapy is focused on disrupting these pathological processes by means of specific immune response and increasing protein clearance and decreasing inflammatory damage. In contrast to traditional pharmacotherapy, which mainly manages the lack of dopamine, immunotherapy is directed against its upstream disease determinants, which promises to be able to change the disease meaningfully in the long term. Nevertheless, it is unique to develop effective immunotherapies of the brain because of immune privilege, blood-brain barriers, and the necessity to prevent autoimmune reactions against normal neural tissue (Dias et al., 2024).

Active Immunization Strategies

Active immunization is where the immune system of the patient is made to generate antibodies against disease related proteins like alpha-synuclein. The structure of vaccines is usually created based on some peptide fragments or modified protein structures that induce an immune response but not the development of harmful inflammation. When given, the effect of these vaccines is the stimulation of long-term antibodies which are capable of binding extracellular aggregates and triggering the clearance of these aggregates by immune-mediated clearance processes. Such vaccines have shown the capability to induce long lasting antibody response with reasonable safety profiles through early clinical trials. The fact that active immunization can result in therapies of long-term effects with fewer doses than those of passive antibody therapy is one of the benefits. Nevertheless, the immune responses may be quite different in different people, particularly the elderly or those individuals whose immunity is weakened. Under-resourced environments, malnutrition, chronic infections, and lack of access to follow-up care are the factors that under-vaccinated individuals and vaccine safety monitoring might be affected by, so a cautious choice of patients and the education of the community is needed (Hassan et al., 2024).

Passive Immunotherapy (Monoclonal Antibodies)

Passive immunotherapy could be used whereby monoclonal antibodies are generated externally and used to bind pathologically formed forms of α-synuclein. These antibodies facilitate neutralization of toxic aggregates, blockage of their movement among neurons and facilitate their clearance by microglial phagocytosis. Passive therapies, in comparison to vaccines, offer immediate therapeutic activity and give the clinicians the ability to regulate dosage and duration of treatment. Multiple monoclonal antibodies have also gone through clinical and have shown engagement of the target and biological activity, with mixed clinical results. Difficulties are the high cost of production, repeated intravenous infusion procedures, and the possibility of a side effect like infusion reaction or immune mediated complications. Under-resourced health systems could have logistical limitations, like the number of infusion centers, cold-chain storage facilities, and insufficient monitoring systems, which could limit widespread use. However, passive immunotherapy is among the most developed immunological treatment options being investigated on PD.

α-Synuclein Targeted Immunotherapies

PD immunotherapy is also targeting α-synuclein because it takes up a central location in the pathology of the disease. The goal of both active and passive methods is to decrease the load of the extracellular aggregates, which increase neuronal toxicity and disease progression. Immunity response through antibodies or the inoculation of vaccines specifically targets misfolded alpha-synuclein but not normal physiological proteins. These therapies will reduce the rate of disease progression and maintenance of neural functions by inhibiting aggregates between neurons. Clinical studies have indicated that early intervention can be essential in delivering significant clinical outcome because disease at advanced stages could have caused permanent damage to neurons. Biomarkers include neuroimaging markers and cerebral levels of α-synuclein in cerebral fluid and are becoming more popular to assess therapeutic response. Further studies are required to optimize the efficacy of antibodies by improving their specificity, dose regimens, and patient selection strategies (Rashid et al., 2025).

Anti-Inflammatory Immunomodulation

One of the main causes of PD development is neuroinflammation, which is caused by the activation of microglia that secrete pro-inflammatory cytokines and reactive oxygen species, which further increases neuronal damage. Immunomodulatory treatments are used in order to decrease destructive inflammation but maintain protective immunities. Cytokine-targeting biologic, small molecules, which regulate immune signaling pathways, and those that facilitate regulatory immune activity are some of the strategies. The point is to normalize the immunity of the central nervous system, minimize the chronic inflammation of the neurons. Nevertheless, immunosuppression can cause over immunosuppression, which can make one more susceptible to infections, especially in a resource-limited setting where there are frequent infections. Consequently, attentive observation and personalized dosage regimens are necessary to attain beneficial treatment effects without imposing any harm on patients (Padma, 2024).

Cell-Based Immunotherapies

Cell-based immunotherapies involve using engineered immune cells or stem cell-derived products to modulate neuroinflammation and support neuronal survival. These approaches are still largely experimental but hold promise for delivering targeted immunoregulatory effects directly within affected brain regions. For example, regulatory immune cells may be designed to suppress excessive inflammation, while stem cell-derived products may release neurotrophic factors that promote neuronal repair. Although these therapies offer potential long-lasting effects, they face significant challenges including high costs, complex manufacturing requirements, and regulatory hurdles. Implementing such advanced therapies in under-resourced settings will require substantial investment in infrastructure and training, as well as simplified treatment protocols to ensure safety and accessibility (Lee et al., 2024).

Mechanisms of Action

Immunotherapies act in several different ways such as neutralization of toxic proteins using antibodies, complementation of immune-mediated clearance, prevention of protein aggregation, and influencing of inflammatory signaling pathways. Antibodies can be used to bind extracellular aggregates and facilitate their absorption by immune cells, whereas vaccines elicit long-term adaptive immune responses. Immunomodulators change the cytokine pattern to suppress neurotoxic inflammation and cell-based therapies can offer localized immunosuppression. These mechanisms are important in understanding how to maximize treatment combinations and those patients who will most likely respond. Development of biomarkers can also be facilitated by mechanistic studies, as it allows the clinicians to track the treatment effects and adjust treatment plans (Serrano et al., 2024).

The Figure 1: provides a immunotherapy approaches in Parkinson's disease, highlighting how targeted immune-based strategies aim to reduce toxic α-synuclein aggregation, a key pathological hallmark of the disorder. It contrasts active immunization (vaccines stimulating the body's own immune response) with passive immunotherapy (monoclonal antibodies), summarizes evidence from clinical trials, and illustrates the practical challenges of implementing these therapies in low-resource settings, including cost, infrastructure, and cold-chain requirements.

Figure 1. Immunotherapy Approaches in Parkinson's Diseases

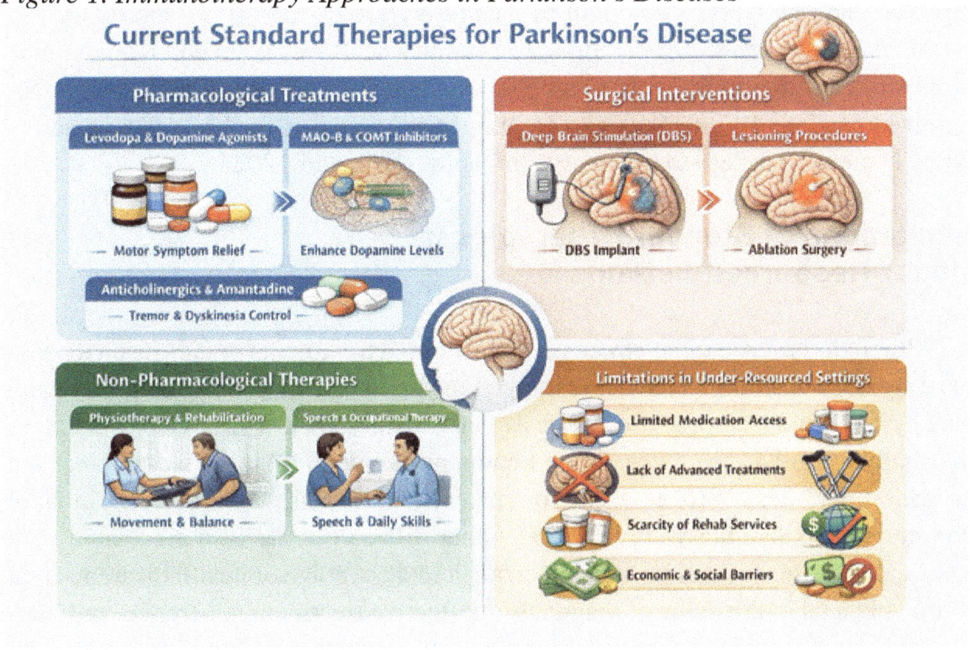

Efficacy and Safety Profiles

Evaluating efficacy requires long-term follow-up to determine whether immunotherapy slows disease progression or improves quality of life. Safety considerations include the risk of autoimmune reactions, infusion-related events, and unintended immune suppression (Su et al., 2025). Vaccine design focuses on minimizing pro-inflammatory responses, while monoclonal antibodies are engineered for high specificity to reduce off-target effects. Monitoring systems must track adverse events and ensure early detection of complications. In under-resourced settings, limited laboratory capacity and specialist availability may hinder comprehensive monitoring, emphasizing the need for simplified safety protocols and accessible reporting mechanisms (Liu et al., 2024).

Adverse Effects and Risk Management

Potential adverse effects of immunotherapy include local injection reactions, systemic immune responses, neuroinflammation, and rare autoimmune complications. Risk management strategies involve careful patient selection, gradual dose escalation, and ongoing monitoring of immune markers. Education of healthcare providers and patients is essential to ensure early recognition of side effects. In resource-limited healthcare systems, community health workers and telemedicine platforms can support follow-up and pharmacovigilance efforts. Establishing standardized treatment guidelines and training programs can further enhance safety while expanding access to innovative therapies (Bril et al., 2024).

Limitations of Standard Therapies in Under-Resourced Settings

Although these are quite effective, conventional treatments of Parkinson disease have serious constraints in under resourced locations like money, inadequate health care systems and lack of skilled professionals. Availability of necessary medicines is usually irregular, more developed treatment like deep brain stimulation are not as widespread, and there is a lack of rehabilitation facilities, especially in rural communities (Chaudhary et al., 2025). Other difficulties are also associated with low health literacy, social stigma, and insufficient coverage of health insurance that ultimately lead to the delay of diagnosis, ineffective treatment adherence, and optimal disease outcomes. To manage these barriers, systemic policy change, capacity building and new low cost care models are needed to ensure equitable management of Parkinson's disease (Sande et al., 2001).

The Figure 2: gives a succinct representation of the existing range of standard therapies of the Parkinson disease, grouping the approaches to treatment into pharmacological, surgical, and non-pharmacological treatment options, and also outlining major drawbacks of under-resourced environments. It shows how the initial severe treatments as levodopa and enzyme inhibitors are used as the baseline of symptom management, how advanced treatment approaches, including deep brain stimulation and lesioning, are used to treat refractory motor symptoms, and how rehabilitation treatments address mobility, speech, and daily functioning. Other issues that are highlighted in the image include access to drugs, complex treatment, and rehabilitation whereby the global differences in the management of Parkinsonism diseases are highlighted.

Figure 2. Current Standard Therapies for Parkinson's Disease

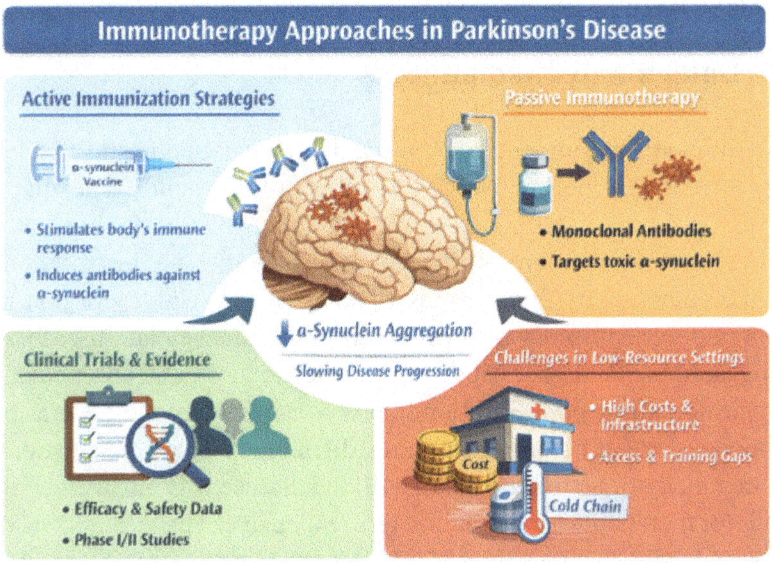

CHALLENGES IN PARKINSON'S DISEASE MANAGEMENT IN UNDER-RESOURCED SETTINGS

Limited Access to Neurological Care

Limited access to specialist neurological services remains one of the major obstacles in caring for people with Parkinson's disease in low-resource settings. Neurologists tend to be over-represented in urban and tertiary care settings, resulting in reduced or no access to specialist review for rural and remote patients. In many low- and middle-income countries the number of neurologists is very small compared to the population with Parkinson's disease, which often receive care from general practitioners or non-specialist clinicians with probably limited education in movement disorders. This lack of expertise results in late diagnosis, suboptimal treatment strategies and poor management of disease progression and complications. Referral networks are often weak or broken, and long travel distances, expenses related to transportation and loss of income also hinder patients from consulting specialist care. Consequently, an even greater number of people with Parkinson's disease go undetected or undertreated for extended periods, causing unnecessary disability and poor quality of life (Bloem et al., 2020).

Diagnostic Delays and Misdiagnosis

In resource-limited environments, diagnostic delays and diagnostic misclassification are frequent and influence disease outcomes in Parkinson's. The diagnosis of PD is largely a clinical one, dependent on meticulous history taking and close bedside neurological examination – competencies which may not be well honed in generalist health practitioners. Initial signs of bradykinesia, rigidity or non-motor features are commonly confused with normal aging, musculoskeletal disease, stroke or psychiatric disorders. Poor accessibility to diagnostic tools, and absence of standardized diagnostic pathways, in addition to low awareness among general public as well as clinicians further contribute to these difficulties. Hence, the patients are given wrong treatment, or no treatment at all till the disease is in an advanced stage and the options for therapeutic intervention less responsive. The lack of confidence in the diagnosis also undermines the confidence/ adherence to treatment, creating a vicious cycle exacerbating delay and poor outcomes (Baguet et al., 2023).

Infrastructure and Workforce Constraints

An inherent structural barrier to optimal care of Parkinson's disease in under-resourced areas is the lack of infrastructure and trained manpower. There are few resources for diagnostics, laboratory services with minimal quality control and space for long-term ambulatory care. Overall, MD services are rarely or poor in importance for a comprehensive management of PD (i.e., physiotherapy; speech therapy; occupational therapy; and psychosocial support). Alzheimer's and Related Dementias clinicians shortages are seen not only with neurologists, but also include other care providers such as allied health workers, nurses, and rehabilitation therapists trained in neurodegenerative diseases. Already weak health systems are further stretched as high workloads, limited opportunities for training and poor retention of expert staff conspire. Such restrictions inhibit the ability to provide seamless and coordinated care and favor patients with advanced stage disease who need complex, multidisciplinary interventions (Kirmani & Afaq, 2024).

Sociocultural Beliefs, Stigma, and Health Literacy

Sociocultural attitudes and stigma toward neurologic disease have pronounced effects on how Parkinson's is managed in low-resource settings. The symptoms, tremor, slowness and speech disturbance are interpreted as those of normal aging, possession by spirits or related to madness that results in delayed help-seeking and social exclusion. Stigma may prevent patients and their families from reporting symptoms or seeking care from the formal healthcare system, and those who do seek care regularly delay diagnosis by consulting traditional or faith healers. Additionally, patients who have low health literacy have even greater difficulty understanding the disease process, treatment choices as well as the necessity of long-term adherence. Caregivers — often family members — may lack the skills and resources to offer effective help; this can lead to economic and emotional stress. Overcoming these social and cultural obstacles is key to enhancing early detection, adherence into care, and quality of care (Makanjuola et al., 2021).

The following table 1 summarizes the key challenges in the management of Parkinson's disease in under-resourced settings. It highlights structural, clinical, sociocultural, and policy-related barriers that impede timely diagnosis, optimal treatment, and comprehensive care. Each challenge is described in terms of its impact on patients and care delivery, with specific implications for resource-limited environments, providing a concise overview of the multifactorial obstacles to effective Parkinson's disease management.

Table 1. Challenges in Parkinson's Disease Management in Under-Resourced Settings

Challenge Area	Description	Impact on Patients and Care Delivery	Implications for Under-Resourced Settings
Limited Access to Neurological Care	Severe shortage and unequal distribution of neurologists and movement disorder specialists, often concentrated in urban tertiary centers	Delayed diagnosis, suboptimal treatment plans, inadequate management of disease progression and complications	Necessitates reliance on general practitioners and non-specialists; highlights need for task-shifting, tele-neurology, and capacity building
Diagnostic Delays and Misdiagnosis	Clinical diagnosis requires expertise often lacking; early symptoms misattributed to aging, stroke, or psychiatric illness	Late-stage presentation, reduced treatment effectiveness, patient mistrust, and inappropriate therapies	Emphasizes need for simplified diagnostic algorithms, training of primary care providers, and awareness programs
Medication Availability, Cost, and Supply Chain Issues	Frequent stock-outs of essential drugs (e.g., levodopa), high out-of-pocket costs, weak procurement and distribution systems	Treatment interruptions, poor symptom control, non-adherence, increased disability and caregiver burden	Calls for inclusion of PD drugs in essential medicines lists, improved supply chains, and generic drug production
Infrastructure and Workforce Constraints	Inadequate healthcare facilities, lack of diagnostic equipment, and shortage of allied health professionals	Absence of multidisciplinary care, poor follow-up, limited rehabilitation services	Supports development of community-based care models and integration of PD services into primary healthcare

continued on following page

Table 1. Continued

Challenge Area	Description	Impact on Patients and Care Delivery	Implications for Under-Resourced Settings
Sociocultural Beliefs, Stigma, and Health Literacy	Misconceptions about PD, stigma, reliance on traditional healers, low disease awareness	Delayed care-seeking, social isolation, poor adherence to treatment	Highlights importance of culturally sensitive education, caregiver training, and community engagement
Policy, Financing, and Health System Barriers	Low prioritization of neurological disorders, limited insurance coverage, weak health information systems	Financial hardship, fragmented care, lack of long-term planning	Demonstrates need for policy inclusion of PD, sustainable financing, and integration into national NCD strategies

TARGETED MOLECULAR THERAPIES FOR PARKINSON'S DISEASE

Specific molecular therapies of PD are a new form of therapy that does not aim at the global alleviation of symptoms but addresses specific molecular events leading to neurodegeneration. The goals of these therapies are to disrupt cellular and genetic pathways of loss of dopaminergic neurons, protein aggregation, mitochondrial dysfunction, and neuroinflammation. In contrast to the conventional pharmacological interventions, which mainly adjust the dopamine deficiency, specific molecular therapies are intended to alter the progression of the disease by using specific biological pathways, including kinase signaling, regulation of gene expression, response to oxidative stress, and intracellular protein transport systems. These therapies are usually classified as gene therapies, RNA-based therapies, small molecule inhibitors, neuroprotective agents, growth factor therapies and advanced delivery technologies. All classes are aimed at different aspects of PD pathology, which allows making interventions more personal and, possibly, disease-modifying. Molecular biology, genomics and bioinformatics have increased the rate at which therapeutic targets such as LRRK2 mutations, mitochondrial pathways, and alpha synuclein processing are identified and employed. Such a focused strategy is also in line with the larger trend of precision medicine, in which interventions are adapted to fit specific molecular phenotypes and subtypes of disease (Pereira et al., 2024).

Gene Therapy Approaches

The goal of gene therapy is to implant, alter or silence certain genes that are involved in the pathogenesis of PD to re-establish normal cellular activity or to increase neuroprotection. Some of the strategies involve the delivery of genes that encode enzymes to boost the production of dopamine, introduction of neurotrophic factors that help to preserve the survival of neurons, and correction of genetic defects that cause PD in families. The therapeutic genes are most frequently delivered to specific brain regions by the use of viral vectors like adeno-associated viruses. As a case in point, the aromatic L-amino acid decarboxylase activity can be increased with the help of gene therapies to boost dopamine production or a copy of genes can be inserted that controls the behaviour of the mitochondrion and mitochondria oxidative stress reactions. These interventions are potentially effective in terms of long-term therapeutic impact after one administration, that is, it does not have to be dosed frequently. The difficulties in doing so, however, involve the need to particularly target, the risk of immune response to viral vectors, and the question of ethical issues of genetic modification. In a resource strained environment, the complexity and high cost of gene therapy infrastructure can constrain its wide adoption and the accessibility rates of the technology are likely to increase with future studies into simplified delivery systems and scalable methods of manufacturing.

RNA-Based Therapies (siRNA, Antisense Oligonucleotides)

The objective of the gene therapy is to implant, modify or suppress some of the genes that are implicated in the pathogenesis of PD to re- normalize the cellular functioning or enhance neuro protection. These are some of the approaches that include transfer of genes that encode enzymes to accelerate the formation of dopamine, transfer of neurotrophic factors that enhance the survival of neurons, and repair genetic defects that lead to PD in families. The viral vectors such as adeno-associated viruses are mostly used to deliver the therapeutic genes to particular areas of the brain. The aromatic L-amino acid decarboxylase activity, as an example, could be enhanced through gene therapies to promote the amount of dopamine or a duplicate of genes could be placed in it that regulates the behaviour of the mitochondrion and the mitochondria oxidative stress responses. Such interventions may be potentially useful in respect of long-term therapeutic effectiveness following a single administration i.e. it does not have to be administered with any frequency. The challenges in doing so however include the fact that one is specifically required to do so, the danger of immune reaction to viral vectors, and the issue of ethical problems of genetic modification. The complexity and expensive nature of gene therapy infrastructure in a resource constrained environment may limit its large scale implementation and the rate of technology accessibility is likely to improve as future researchers seek to work on simplified delivery systems and scalable ways of producing the technology.

Small Molecule Inhibitors

Small molecule inhibitors are engineered to manipulate particular biochemical processes that contribute to PD development, which are protein aggregation, mitochondrial dysfunction, and inflammatory signaling. These drugs are normally orally taken and can reach the blood-brain barrier with relative ease compared to large biologics. Small molecules can also regulate cellular functions by affecting enzymes, receptors, or intracellular signaling pathways and include oxidative stress regulation, lysosomes, or synaptic transmission. Other types of inhibitors focus on lowering the process of α-synuclein aggregation, and others increase autophagy processes, which clear damaged proteins. Small molecules especially are of interest in under-resourced healthcare as they are relatively affordable and easy to administer. Nevertheless, it is difficult to reach a high level of specificity and reduce the off-target effects. The safety and efficacy studies should be done on a long-term basis to make sure that chronic manipulation of cellular pathways does not interfere with normal physiological functions.

LRRK2 Inhibitors and Kinase Modulators

One of the most common genetic causes of PD is the mutation of the leucine-rich repeat kinase 2 (LRRK2) gene, so it is of interest as a molecular therapeutic target. LRRK2 inhibitors are expected to suppress abnormal detection of kinase relevant to neuronal poisonousness and defective cellular signaling. These therapies attempt to normalize cellular homeostasis and decrease the neurodegenerative mechanisms by adjusting the kinase pathways. Preclinical results of LRRK2 inhibitors have displayed potential clinical results regarding neuroinflammation and survival of neurons. Nevertheless, the involvement of kinase signaling pathways in many physiological processes has raised the concern over the possibility of side effects on the entire system. Researchers are coming up with very specific inhibitors in order to reduce non-specific interactions with other kinases. Individualized methods to detect patients with particular genetic mutations could enhance treatment effects and lessen the unneeded exposure of individuals to a particular therapy (Marino et al., 2021).

Mitochondrial Protective Agents

One of the pathological features of PD is mitochondrial dysfunction that leads to energy deficits, oxidative stress, and neuronal susceptibility (Asuku et al, 2024). Specific molecular therapeutic agents designed to preserve or repair the activity of the mitochondrion are intended to increase the cellular resistance and inhibit neuronal apoptosis. These can be antioxidants, mitochondrial membrane stabilizers and energy metabolism stabilizers. Others are therapies that act via pathways of mitochondrial biogenesis and quality control, which facilitates the elimination of damaged organelles requiring mitophagy. These interventions would help to slow down disease progression and enhance neuronal survival by maintaining mitochondrial integrity. Most of the mitochondrial protective agents are yet to be implemented in practice, but their relatively simple administration and reduced cost of manufacture could render them appropriate to be used more widely, even in under-resourced environments (McFall et al., 2000).

Neurotrophic Factors and Growth Factor Therapies

Neurotrophic factors are proteins which help in the growth, survival and maintenance of the neurons. During PD, there is a decrease in the neurotrophic support which leads to the degeneration of dopaminergic neurons. Growth factor therapies, including glial cell line-derived neurotrophic factor, are in place to strengthen neuronal resistance and stimulate restoration procedures. The delivery strategies involve direct infusion into the parts of the brain, the expression systems using gene therapy, and the engineered biomaterials that leak growth factors. There have proved to be varied outcomes in clinical trials in part because of the difficulty in obtaining sufficient distribution in the brain and consistent therapeutic levels. Improvements in technologies of delivery and molecular engineering can enhance efficacy. The growth factor therapy can be used to supplement other specific therapies by offering favorable conditions to neuronal recovery (Li et al., 2025).

Stem Cell-Derived Molecular Interventions

The molecular interventions which can be derived using stem cell include the cell engineered to generate therapeutic molecules like neurotrophic factors, anti-inflammatory mediators or enzymes which help in stimulating the production of dopamine. Instead of substituting neurons as such, these approaches aim at providing molecular assistance that alters disease pathways. The exosomes and secreted factors produced by stem cells have the ability to modify the immune response, decrease inflammatory processes, and stimulate neuronal regeneration. These methods are highly promising, but still fairly experimental and have difficulties on safety, scalability, and regulatory approval. The uniformity of quality and the avoidance of the occurrence of tumors are important issues. The complexity and cost of cell-based manufacturing can pose a challenge in resource-limited setting, but further progress in standardized production could eventually change the situation (Poplawska et al., 2024).

Precision Medicine and Biomarker-Based Therapies

Precision medicine is a form of medicine that consists of the design of targeted molecular therapy using individual genetic, molecular, and clinical attributes. Biomarkers, including genetic mutations, levels of protein expression, and neuroimaging, are useful in determining which subgroups of the patient are the most likely to respond to particular interventions. As an example, patients with LRRK2 defects might be sensitive to kinase inhibitors, and patients with indicators of mitochondrial dysfunction may also be treated with targeted protective therapy. The development of genomic sequencing and bioinformatics allows more precise classification of diseases and choice of therapy. End-of-life biomarker-based strategies also make it easy to diagnose and track treatment response early on, which enhances clinical outcome and lowers unwarranted interventions. Nevertheless, in most under-resourced contexts, the use of highly sensitive diagnostic tools is an unattainable option, which underscores the necessity to develop cost-efficient biomarker-based technologies and streamlined testing procedures (Sampaio et al., 2022).

Nanotechnology-Based Drug Delivery Systems

Nanotechnology-delivery systems provide new avenues of overcoming the barriers that have been presented on the way of derived molecular therapies especially the barrier of blood brain barrier. Nanoparticles may be designed to ferry drugs, genes, or RNA molecules directly to regions of the brain that may be affected and be much more effective in treatment and preventing systemic side effects (Ajibare et al., 2026; Asuku et al., 2026; Ayoola et al., 2026). Such delivery methods can be lipid nanoparticles, polymer-based delivery, and targeted nanovesicles that target particular neuronal receptors. Controlled-release delivery enables prolonged drug effect and lower dosage rate. Nanotechnology is also an effective way of employing combination therapies because various agents can be administered at the same time. Still in development, the systems can revolutionize the PD treatment process by enhancing the bioavailability and accuracy of the drug. Among the obstacles, there are long-term safety, prevention of immune responses, and the development of scalable production methods that can be adopted by various healthcare facilities (Rashidi et al., 2021).

TECHNOLOGICAL INNOVATIONS AND ADAPTATIONS

Telemedicine and Remote Neurology Consultations

Telemedicine has become a game changer in making neurological care accessible where resources are limited and unaffordable for patients with Parkinson's disease who have financial, geographical and mobility challenges to access specialist neurological care. By facilitating remote consultations with neurologists and movement disorders specialists, telemedicine overcomes the obstacles found in city-driven systems of care and decreases long-distance travel expenses (Fezeu et al., 2018). Video telemedicine, tele-assessment of symptoms by patients at home and video follow-up visits now enable clinicians to titrate medications, monitor disease evolution and counsel on non-pharmacological management. Additionally, telemedicine enables the training and support of front-line health workers by connecting them with specialists to discuss cases and receive decision-making support. In resource-limited settings, scaleable telehealth solutions (such as low-bandwidth telemedicine as applied to mobile devices) can enhance continuity of care, patient follow-up, and prompt management of complications despite infrequent in-person visits (Faruqui et al., 2021).

Mobile Health (mHealth) Applications for Monitoring and Adherence

mHealth applications promise novel methods for the monitoring of PD symptoms, adherence to medication as well patient reported outcomes where resources are scarce. Apps installed on a smartphone also are available for monitoring tremor, bradykinesia, dyskinesia, sleep disturbance and medication schedules in real time to help physicians make treatment choices. They can also disseminate reminders, educational materials and motivational interventions to enhance adherence and independence in patient self-management. In resource-poor settings where specialist follow-up is often patchy, such mHealth technologies provide a cost-effective means of disease surveillance at a distance and without the reliance on caregivers or healthcare infrastructure. In addition, collection of the aggregated anonymized data could be used for population surveillance and tracking disease outcomes as well as to inform health policy. High penetration of mobile phones in many low- and middle-income countries makes mHealth a practical and scalable intervention even in resource poor areas (Wolff et al., 2023).

Wearable Technologies and Low-Cost Diagnostic Tools

Wearable technologies and inexpensive diagnosis tools By imposing a low-cost approach, wearable technologies also seem to be another interesting innovation for Parkinson's disease care in resource-limited setting. Accelerometers, gyroscopes and smartwatches can measure motor signs like tremor, gait abnormalities and bradykinesia objectively and continuously which supplement conventional clinical assessments (Stocchi et al., 2024). Low-cost portable diagnostic devices such as smartphone-based gait analysis systems or simplified finger-tapping tests could enable community health workers or primary care physicians to conduct initial screenings, track progress and triage patients for specialist referral. Such technologies minimize reliance on costly equipment and highly trained personnel, facilitating accessibility of an objective measurement approach in remote or resource-limited settings. Additionally, wearables can enable early detection of complications and inform therapeutic adjustments; and they can power trials by building large datasets with no need for expensive infrastructure (Watabe et al., 2025).

Artificial Intelligence and Decision-Support Systems

The application of artificial intelligence (AI) and clinical decision-support systems has significant potential to support Parkinson's disease care in regions with limited specialist resources. By leveraging AI algorithms to process patient information in electronic health records, mHealth apps, and wearable devices, disease patterns can be recognized; motor fluctuations may be forecasted; and personalized treatment adjustments might be suggested. Decision-support systems can help non-neurologist healthcare workers with diagnostic, titration of therapy and referral decisions- thus enhancing the neurologists' reach to underserved areas (Dorsey et al., 2018). In resource limited settings, AI-enhanced tools can help minimize misdiagnosis, standardize care and promote evidence-based clinical decisions when there is an inadequate healthcare workforce. Moreover, machine learning models can detect patterns in population level data at scale, and inform public health policies and allocation of limited healthcare resources. When applied strategically, AI can help to fill gaps in expertise and access with provisioning of quality patient-centered care (Shlisky et al., 2022).

Barriers to Technology Adoption in Resource-Limited Contexts

Technological advancements can offer much hope, a number of challenges prevent their implementation in resource-poor settings. Cost and limited infrastructure – including poor internet connectivity – are barriers to telemedicine platforms, mHealth apps and wearables. Patients, caregivers and health professionals often lack digital literacy which hampers an optimal use of technology-based interventions. Cultural acceptability, concerns about privacy and clinical workflow resistance to change may also inhibit uptake. Also, regulatory and policy for digital health is often nascent leaving questions about safety, data security and reimbursement. Another challenge includes sustainability – technology solutions need maintaining, updating and technical support, which may not be achievable within resource-limited health systems. Overcoming these barriers will require locally-contextualized implementation strategies, user-centered design principles, capacity building efforts and enabling policies to ensure that technological advances in Parkinson's disease yield concrete benefits (Chaudhuri et al., 2024).

NON-PHARMACOLOGICAL AND COMMUNITY-BASED INNOVATIONS

Task-Shifting and Community Health Worker Models

Task-shifting, the rational redistribution of tasks among health workforce teams and its decentralization of service delivery through utilisation of trained non-specialist health personnel is a pragmatic approach to provide care for Parkinson's disease in resource-limited environments lacking specialists and allied professionals. (2016) CHWs can be trained to recognize early motor and non-motor sign/symptoms, deliver layperson information (e.g., medication adherence), follow treatment response, support end-referral osmosis to a third level of care facilities also when indicated (Emilio et al., 2024). Using existing human resources from the community, task-shifting improves access to care, decreases the load on busy facilities and allows structured follow-up without multiple specialist visits. Success of service delivery relies on uniform training, ongoing tele-supervision and integration within the health care system to maintain quality, standardization and safety for patients. Evidence emerging from low- and middle-income countries suggests that CHW-led interventions could result in disease awareness, early identification, and continuity of care, whilst also being scalable for the management of Parkinson's disease (Khalid et al., 2025).

Integration of Traditional and Complementary Medicine Practices

From low-and middle-income countries, Traditional and Complementary Medicine practices are still relevant culturally and have been an approach frequently sought by people with Parkinson's disease. Incorporating evidence-informed elements from traditional approaches to care, including herbal preparations, acupuncture or mindfulness activities, into community-based models of delivery may improve acceptability and facilitate engagement with patients. This collaboration between modern health labour force and traditional practitioners may enable safe concurrence usage of these interventions in complementing standard pharmacologic and rehabilitative agents. Certain complementary approaches have some promise for symptom management, stress relief, and quality of life based on research but require rigorous study and continued oversight to establish safety and effectiveness. Adopting a sustainable culturally competent approach in PD care enhances trust, promotes utilization of health care services and maximizes existing community resources which are valuable for patient-centered care in resource-limited settings (Deb et al., 2020).

FUTURE DIRECTIONS AND EMERGING OPPORTUNITIES

The landscape of PD care is expected to change dramatically over the next few decades, influenced by genomics, therapeutics, digital health and systems-based approaches. New opportunities include pharmacological discovery, technological fusion, community-focused interventions and health system strengthening that have the potential to overcome these discrepancies in access and quality. Because cutting-edge treatments and personalized interventions have historically been focused on high-income countries, there is emerging awareness of the importance of tailoring and scaling these innovations for low- and middle-income countries to bring progress in PD treatment to populations worldwide. The discussion that follows covers a number of critical avenues defining the future of Parkinson's disease care including translational approaches to new opportunities and serves as an approach to articulating those efforts toward sustainable equitable therapy (Fagiani et al., 2022).

Personalized medicine is one of the most exciting opportunities to change outcomes for people with Parkinson's. When correlations among these data and clinical information are incorporated, personalized strategies help selectively model therapies based on disease characteristics of individual patients to maximize efficacy and to minimize undesired toxicities. In high-resource countries, biomarker discovery, genomic sequencing and imaging are showing promise for predicting progression of disease, identifying patient subgroups responsive to particular pharmacologic or surgical interventions and informing approaches to early intervention (Zhou et al., 2024). Translating personalized medicine for low-resource settings will necessitate thinking about creative solutions, such as simplified versions of biomarker assays and algorithm-driven support for decision making, as well as population-level clinical risk stratification. Even in resource-poor environments, it is possible to improvise a structured approach to prescription based on demographic characteristics and clinical symptoms which could allow individualized drug treatment, optimize its titration as well as monitoring of the progression of the diseases. Personalized medicine in these settings could lead not only to better patient outcomes but also to more efficient use of limited healthcare resources by focussing interventions where they are most likely to be beneficial (Wang et al., 2024).

Gene- and cell-based treatments, such as transplantation of dopaminergic neurons, stem cells-derived neural replacement therapy as well gene editing provide a hope of modifying or even reversing neurodegeneration in Parkinson's disease. Such therapies are designed to repair neuronal function, preserve surviving neurons or intervene in the pathological pathways leading to loss of dopaminergic cells. As promising as they are scientifically, these interventions are deeply fraught from an economic, logistical and infrastructure standpoint. In high-resource settings, such treatments in being tested in clinical trials and specialized centres, but in low-resource areas the access is very aspirational (Gonçalves et al., 2024). International cooperation, technology transfer and regional centers of excellence, innovative financing mechanisms ought to be employed with greater levels of international collaboration and in order that equity is addressed globally in advanced therapeutics including through the mitigation of cost barriers. In addition, attention to ethical issues, regulatory alignment and culturally-specific patient inclusion are key to ensuring that new treatments reach and are acceptable to a wide range of populations. Failure to address these equity challenges through intentional strategies could create the next generation of PD therapies that risks adding new insult to global injury rather than addressing it (Bray et al., 2024).

Sustainable models of innovation are also a key area for further growth especially in low resource settings. These models focus on cost, scale and context relevance by converging pharmacological, technological and community-based interventions in to comprehensive care structures. For drug development, this encompasses use of generics, repurposed low-cost compounds and pared down treatment algorithms for non-specialist providers. Technical integration may include telemedicine, mHealth apps, wearables monitoring tools, and decision-support systems driven by AI designed for low-bandwidth environments and low-literacy users (Kumar et al., 2024). Community-based interventions such as home-based rehabilitation, task-shifting to community health workers and caregiver support programs are complementary strategies addressing workforce limitations and continuity of care. Sustainable innovation also needs to match with national health priorities, local capacity-building and research investment, and culturally sensitive intervention. Incorporation of considerations around sustainability, equity and contextual tailoring create an approach to future models of care with the potential to deliver the greatest clinical benefit within financial and operational constraints (García et al., 2025).

A comprehensive vision for global Parkinson's disease care equity incorporates emerging technology, therapeutics, and community-based interventions framed by systemic fortification and policy backing. Health care equity requires universal access to essential medicines, including affordable, generic and locally manufactured medicines, non-pharmacologic interventions and rehabilitation integrated into primary health care. Specialists beyond brick-and-mortar centers can be accessed from remote, supported by telemedicine, follow up with the mother on how to return home with her baby, as well transfer knowledge and skill through utilization of digital tools. Policy roadmaps should emphasize chronic neurologic diseases as a public health priority, address sustainable funding, and create paths for oversight of new treatments (Al-Jaber et al., 2025). International research collaboration and sharing of knowledge between countries are likely to facilitate the uptake and implementation of new interventions. In the end, the new face of Parkinson's disease care will rely on a coordinated and multi-tiered method whereby technological and therapeutic breakthroughs are available, culturally relevant, and sustainable to create a worldwide environment where health equality is achieved independent of societal status or geographic circumstance (Peng et al., 2025).

CONCLUSION

Parkinson disease (PD) is another complicated and progressive neurodegenerative disease, and the available treatment is mostly symptomatic and fails to arrest the disease progression. In that regard, immunotherapy and targeted molecular treatment are the promising directions where the focus is on the pathogenic mechanisms of the disease as opposed to the symptomatic relief of the motor ones. There is growing evidence of implicating α-synuclein aggregation, neuroinflammation, dysfunction in mitochondria, and genetic mutations in the genesis and pathogenesis of PD including LRRK2 and GBA. Targeted therapeutic approaches that activate these pathways in particular have thus become of great interest. The immunotherapeutic interventions, such as the active and passive immunization against α-synuclein, aim at decreasing the toxic protein buildup and prevent its proliferation in the brain. These means provide potential neuroprotective benefits by oscillating the immune response and microglial activity and treating the pathology of the disease at an early stage. Equally, specific molecular therapies, including, but not limited to, small-molecule inhibitors, antisense oligonucleotides, and gene-based interventions, seek to correct particular molecular abnormalities, to reregulate cellular homeostasis, and to increase neuronal survival. Recent progress in drug delivery mechanisms and penetration of the blood brain barrier indicate additionally the promise of these therapies in a translational approach. Although promising preclinical and early clinical results have been noted, there are still major challenges such as long-term safety, individual response variability and methodology of identifying valid biomarkers to be used in individualized treatment. However, with further advances in molecular neuroscience, immunology, and precision medicine, these methods will be likely to be refined and produce better clinical outcomes. Altogether, immunotherapy and targeted molecule therapies have a great potential as disease-modifying approaches to Parkinson disease that bring an opportunity to more effective and tailor-made intervention in future.

REFERENCES

Abdel-Bari, S. H., Amer, H., Ayoub, B. M., & Kamel, R. (2021). Surgical management of Parkinson's disease: The role of lesioning procedures in developing countries in the modern era. *Open Access Macedonian Journal of Medical Sciences, 9*, 1241. DOI: 10.3889/oamjms.2021.6649

Adelson, P. D., Bratton, S. L., Carney, N., Chesnut, R. M., du Coudray, H. E. M., & Goldstein, B.. (2003). Chapter 1: Introduction. *Pediatric Critical Care Medicine, 4*. Advance online publication. DOI: 10.1097/01.ccm.0000066600.71233.01 PMID: 12847337

Ajagun, E. J., Asuku, A. O., Ayinla, M. T., Abdulsalam, T. A., Ajibare, A. J., Olajide, T. S., Hamza, Y. O., & Ganiyu, K. O. (2024). Pharmacotherapy of Parkinson's Disease and their Limitations. In: Zebrafish as a Model for Parkinson's Disease. Taylor and Francis, CRC, https://doi.org/DOI: 10.1201/9781003402893-17

Ajibare, A. J., Akintoye, O. O., Aransi-Ola, K. T., Adejumo, M. O., Folarin, E. O. A., & Asuku, A. O. (2026). Nanoformulations of Plant Compounds for Metabolic Syndrome: A Multitarget Approach. In Gosh, V., Bhardwaj, A. K., & Maddela, N. R. (Eds.), *Applications of Plant Bioactive Compounds-Based Nanoformulations. Nanotechnology in the Life Sciences*. Springer., DOI: 10.1007/978-3-032-13086-0_17

Al-Jaber, H., Biswas, K. H., & Al-Mansoori, L. (2025). Advancing targeted therapy for colorectal cancer: Harnessing ligand-directed enzyme prodrug therapy for highly specific interventions. *Frontiers in Oncology, 15*. Advance online publication. DOI: 10.3389/fonc.2025.1570712 PMID: 40510154

Asuku, A. O., Adebayo, P. O., Ajibare, A. J., & Ayoola, S. A. (2026). Application of Plant Based Nanomaterials for Treating Dementia. In Gosh, V., Bhardwaj, A. K., & Maddela, N. R. (Eds.), *Applications of Plant Bioactive Compounds-Based Nanoformulations. Nanotechnology in the Life Sciences* (pp. 263–280). Springer., DOI: 10.1007/978-3-032-13086-0_8

Asuku, A. O., Ayinla, M. T., Olajide, T. S., Oyerinde, T. O., Yusuf, J. A., Bayo-Olugbami, A. A., & Fajemidagba, G. A. (2024). Coffee and Parkinson's disease. In. Progress in Brain Research: Vol. 289. *Neuroscience of Coffee*. Elsevier., DOI: 10.1016/bs.pbr.2024.06.001

Asuku, A. O., Ogungbangbe, G. O., & Fajemidagba, G. A. (2025). Gene therapy for Parkinson's disease: A new frontier in neurodegenerative diseases. *Exploration of Neuroprotective Therapy, 5*, 1004119. DOI: 10.37349/ent.2025.1004119

Ayoola, S. A., Ajijolakewu, A. K., Ajadi, A. A., Asuku, A. O., & Adamu, S. B. (2026). Controlled Release of Antimicrobial Biomolecules by Plant-Based Nanomaterials. In Gosh, V., Bhardwaj, A. K., & Maddela, N. R. (Eds.), *Applications of Plant Bioactive Compounds-Based Nanoformulations. Nanotechnology in the Life Sciences* (pp. 263–280). Springer., DOI: 10.1007/978-3-032-13086-0_11

Baguet, C., Larghero, J., & Mebarki, M. (2023). Early predictive factors of failure in autologous CAR T-cell manufacturing and/or efficacy in hematologic malignancies. *Blood Advances*, *8*, 337. DOI: 10.1182/bloodadvances.2023011992 PMID: 38052048

Bello-Mojeed, M. A., Ani, C., Lagunju, I., & Omigbodun, O. (2016). Feasibility of parent-mediated behavioural intervention for behavioural problems in children with autism spectrum disorder in Nigeria: A pilot study. *Child and Adolescent Psychiatry and Mental Health*, *10*. Advance online publication. DOI: 10.1186/s13034-016-0117-4 PMID: 27594900

Bhidayasiri, R. (2024). Old problems, new solutions: Harnessing technology and innovation in Parkinson's disease—Evidence and experiences from Thailand. *Journal of Neural Transmission (Vienna, Austria)*, *131*, 721. DOI: 10.1007/s00702-023-02727-1 PMID: 38189972

Bhidayasiri, R., Virameteekul, S., Sukoandari, B., Tran, T. N., & Lim, T. T. (2021). Challenges of Parkinson's disease care in Southeast Asia. https://doi.org/DOI: 10.1007/978-3-319-56015-1_442-1

Bianco, L., Linardi, A., & Stilhano, R. S. (2024). Effect of the anti-inflammatory action of β-carbolines on SH-SY5Y cell line (human neuroblastoma) and modulation of TMPRSS11 and Furin receptors. *Arquivos de Neuro-Psiquiatria*, *1*. Advance online publication. DOI: 10.5327/cbn240003

Bloem, B. R., Henderson, E. J., Dorsey, E. R., Okun, M. S., Okubadejo, N., & Chan, P.. (2020). Integrated and patient-centred management of Parkinson's disease: A network model for reshaping chronic neurological care. *Lancet Neurology*, *19*, 623. DOI: 10.1016/S1474-4422(20)30064-8 PMID: 32464101

Bray, F., Laversanne, M., Sung, H., Ferlay, J., Siegel, R. L., & Soerjomataram, I.. (2024). Global cancer statistics 2022: GLOBOCAN estimates of incidence and mortality worldwide for 36 cancers in 185 countries. *CA: a Cancer Journal for Clinicians*, *74*, 229. DOI: 10.3322/caac.21834 PMID: 38572751

Bril, E., Fedorova, N. D., Кулуа, T. K., & Zimnyakova, O. S. (2024). Treatment of the early stages of Parkinson's disease. Differences in approaches to the choice of therapy in different countries. *Neurology Neuropsychiatry Psychosomatics*, *16*, 130–135. DOI: 10.14412/2074-2711-2024-3-130-135

Chaudhary, S., Chaudhary, S., & Rawat, S. (2025). Understanding Parkinson's disease: Current trends and its multifaceted complications. *Frontiers in Aging Neuroscience, 17*. Advance online publication. DOI: 10.3389/fnagi.2025.1617106 PMID: 41049533

Chaudhuri, K. R., Azulay, J., Odin, P., Lindvall, S., Domingos, J., & Alobaidi, A.. (2024). Economic burden of Parkinson's disease: A multinational, real-world, cost-of-illness study. *Drugs - Real World Outcomes, 11*, 1. DOI: 10.1007/s40801-023-00410-1 PMID: 38193999

Contini, N., Martins, W. A., & Schilling, L. P. (2024). Unsteadiness of gait in terminal renal failure: Miller Fisher syndrome triggered by haemodialysis. *Arquivos de Neuro-Psiquiatria, 481*. Advance online publication. DOI: 10.5327/cbn241718

Deb, S., Retzer, A., Roy, M., Acharya, R., Limbu, B., & Roy, A. (2020). The effectiveness of parent training for children with autism spectrum disorder: A systematic review and meta-analyses. *BMC Psychiatry, 20*. Advance online publication. DOI: 10.1186/s12888-020-02973-7 PMID: 33287762

Dekker, M. C. J., Coulibaly, T., Bardien, S., Ross, O. A., Carr, J., & Komolafe, M. (2020). Parkinson's disease research on the African continent: Obstacles and opportunities. *Frontiers in Neurology, 11*. Advance online publication. DOI: 10.3389/fneur.2020.00512 PMID: 32636796

Dias, J., García, J., Agliardi, G., & Roddie, C. (2024). CAR-T cell manufacturing landscape—Lessons from the past decade and considerations for early clinical development. *Molecular Therapy. Methods & Clinical Development, 32*, 101250. DOI: 10.1016/j.omtm.2024.101250 PMID: 38737799

Dorsey, E. R., Elbaz, A., Nichols, E., Abbasi, N., Abd-Allah, F., & Abdelalim, A.. (2018). Global, regional, and national burden of Parkinson's disease, 1990–2016: A systematic analysis for the Global Burden of Disease Study 2016. *Lancet Neurology, 17*, 939. DOI: 10.1016/S1474-4422(18)30295-3 PMID: 30287051

Emilio, A. R., & Portes, J. R. M. (2024). Modelo híbrido de entrenamiento parental para madres de niños en edad preescolar con trastorno del espectro autista basado en el análisis de comportamiento aplicado para reducir el estrés parental. *Ciencias Psicológicas (Montevideo), 18*. Advance online publication. DOI: 10.22235/cp.v18i2.3285

Fagiani, F., Marino, D. D., Romagnoli, A., Travelli, C., Voltan, D., & Mannelli, L. D. C.. (2022). Molecular regulations of circadian rhythm and implications for physiology and diseases. *Signal Transduction and Targeted Therapy, 7*, 41. DOI: 10.1038/s41392-022-00899-y PMID: 35136018

Faruqui, N., Yousuf, M. A., Whaiduzzaman, M., Azad, A., Barros, A., & Moni, M. A. (2021). LungNet: A hybrid deep-CNN model for lung cancer diagnosis using CT and wearable sensor-based medical IoT data. *Computers in Biology and Medicine, 139*, 104961. DOI: 10.1016/j.compbiomed.2021.104961 PMID: 34741906

Fezeu, F., Ramesh, A., Melmer, P. D., Moosa, S., Larson, P., & Henderson, F. (2018). Challenges and solutions for functional neurosurgery in developing countries. *Cureus*. Advance online publication. DOI: 10.7759/cureus.3314 PMID: 30473947

García, S. F. R., Morón-Duarte, L. S., Arango, G., López, C. L. M., & González, N. Y. (2025). Generadores de pulso implantable recargables y no recargables para la estimulación cerebral profunda en pacientes con enfermedad de Parkinson. *Acta Neurologica Colombiana, 41*. Advance online publication. DOI: 10.22379/anc.v41i1.1861

Gonçalves, J., & Caliceti, P. (2024). Optimizing pharmacological and immunological properties of therapeutic proteins through PEGylation: Investigating key parameters and their impact. *Drug Design, Development and Therapy, 5041*. Advance online publication. DOI: 10.2147/DDDT.S481420 PMID: 39529843

Hajzer, Z. E., Alibrahem, W., Helu, N. K., Oláh, C., & Prokisch, J. (2025). Functional foods in clinical trials and future research directions. *Foods, 14*, 2675. DOI: 10.3390/foods14152675 PMID: 40807611

Hassan, A., Khan, H., Ali, A., Din, I. U., Sajid, A., & Husain, M.. (2024). An enhanced lung cancer identification and classification based on advanced deep learning and convolutional neural network. *Bulletin of Business and Economics, 13*, 136. DOI: 10.61506/01.00308

Helmer, R. S., Merscher, M. N., Lobo, C. C., de Souza, V. M., de Jesus, M. A., & Ganho, T.. (2024). A rare case of hemichorea secondary to giant perivascular space: A case report. *Arquivos de Neuro-Psiquiatria, 13*. Advance online publication. DOI: 10.5327/cbn240046

Khalid, T., Malik, A., Rasool, N., Kanwal, A., Nawaz, H., & Almas, I. (2025). Cracking the code: The clinical and molecular impact of aminopyridines; A review (2019–2024). *RSC Advances, 15*, 688. DOI: 10.1039/D4RA07438F PMID: 39781020

Kirmani, M. A., & Afaq, Y. (2024). Developments in deep learning approaches for apple leaf Alternaria disease identification: A review. *Computers and Electronics in Agriculture, 227*, 109593. DOI: 10.1016/j.compag.2024.109593

Kumar, L., Malhotra, M., Sharma, A., & Singh, A. P. (2024). A holistic approach to Parkinson's disease: Integrating advances in pathophysiology, diagnosis, and therapy. *Journal of Drug Delivery and Therapeutics, 14*, 141. DOI: 10.22270/jddt.v14i5.6558

Lee, J., Lim, J., Kang, S., Kim, S., Jung, S. Y., & Kim, S.. (2024). Mobile app–assisted parent training intervention for behavioral problems in children with autism spectrum disorder: Pilot randomized controlled trial. *JMIR Human Factors, 11*. Advance online publication. DOI: 10.2196/52295 PMID: 39466295

Li, Y., Lv, Z., Dai, Y., Yu, L., Zhang, L., & Wang, K.. (2025). The global, regional, and national burden of Parkinson's disease in 204 countries and territories, 1990–2021: A systematic analysis for the Global Burden of Disease Study 2021. *BMC Public Health,* Liu, B., Zhou, H., Tan, L., Siu, K. T. H., & Guan, X. (2024). Exploring treatment options in cancer: Tumor treatment strategies. *Signal Transduction and Targeted Therapy, 9*, 175. DOI: 10.1038/s41392-024-01856-7

Makanjuola, A., Taiwo, F., Yaria, J., Akinyemi, R., & Ogunniyi, A. (2021). Parkinson's disease – A review of pathogenesis, recent advances in management, and challenges of care in sub-Saharan Africa. *Journal of Global Medicine*. https://doi .org/DOI: 10.51496/jogm.v1.35

Marino, F., Failla, C., Chilà, P., Minutoli, R., Puglisi, A., & Arnao, A. A.. (2021). The effect of acceptance and commitment therapy for improving psychological well-being in parents of individuals with autism spectrum disorders: A randomized controlled trial. *Brain Sciences, 11*, 880. DOI: 10.3390/brainsci11070880 PMID: 34209171

McFall, S. L., Yerkes, A. M., & Cowan, L. D. (2000). Outcomes of a small group educational intervention for urinary incontinence. *Journal of Aging and Health, 12*, 301. DOI: 10.1177/089826430001200302 PMID: 11067699

Okunoye, O., Zewde, Y. Z., Azar, J., Ayele, B. A., Dindayal, S., & Moustafa, A.. (2023). The state of play of Parkinson's disease in Africa: A systematic review and point of view. *bioRxiv*. https://doi.org/DOI: 10.1101/2023.07.07.23292392

Padma, V. V. (2024). An overview of targeted cancer therapy. *Biomedicine (Taipei), 5*. Advance online publication. DOI: 10.37796/2211-8039.1512 PMID: 26613930

Palmer, M., Tarver, J., Perez, J. P., Cawthorne, T., Romeo, R., & Stringer, D.. (2019). A novel group parenting intervention to reduce emotional and behavioural difficulties in young autistic children: Protocol for the Autism Spectrum Treatment and Resilience pilot randomised controlled trial. *BMJ Open, 9*. Advance online publication. DOI: 10.1136/bmjopen-2019-029959 PMID: 31248932

Peng, S., Liu, P., Wang, X., & Li, K. (2025). Global, regional and national burden of Parkinson's disease in people over 55 years of age: A systematic analysis of the Global Burden of Disease Study, 1991–2021. *BMC Neurology, 25*, 178. DOI: 10.1186/s12883-025-04191-8 PMID: 40269818

Pereira, G. M., dos Santos, D. T., Soares, N. M., Marconi, G. A., Friedrich, D. C., & Awad, P. S.. (2024). A systematic review and meta-analysis of the prevalence of Parkinson's disease in lower- to upper-middle-income countries. *npj. Parkinson's Disease, 10*. Advance online publication. DOI: 10.1038/s41531-024-00779-y PMID: 39349513

Rashid, M. R. A., Korim, M. A. E., Hasan, M., Ali, M. S., Islam, M. M., & Jabid, T.. (2025). An ensemble learning framework with explainable AI for interpretable leaf disease detection. *Array (New York, N.Y.), 26*, 100386. DOI: 10.1016/j.array.2025.100386

Rashidi Fakari, F., Hajian, S., Darvish, S., & Alavi Majd, H. (2021). Explaining factors affecting help-seeking behaviors in women with urinary incontinence: A qualitative study. *BMC Health Services Research, 21*, 60. DOI: 10.1186/s12913-020-06047-y PMID: 33435931

Sampaio, F., Nystrand, C., Feldman, I., & Mihalopoulos, C. (2022). Evidence for investing in parenting interventions aiming to improve child health: A systematic review of economic evaluations. *European Child & Adolescent Psychiatry, 33*, 323. DOI: 10.1007/s00787-022-01969-w PMID: 35304645

Serrano, M., Elías, M., Llorens, M., Bolasell, M., Vall-Roqué, H., & Villalta, L. (2024). Early treatment for children with mental health problems and genetic conditions through a parenting intervention (The GAP): Study protocol for a pragmatic randomized controlled trial. *Trials, 25*. Advance online publication. DOI: 10.1186/s13063-024-08278-4 PMID: 39033111

Sharma, A., Verwilst, P., Li, M., Ma, D., Singh, N., & Yoo, J.. (2024). Theranostic fluorescent probes. *Chemical Reviews, 124*, 2699. DOI: 10.1021/acs.chemrev.3c00778 PMID: 38422393

Shlisky, J., Mandlik, R., Askari, S., Abrams, S. A., Belizán, J. M., & Bourassa, M. W.. (2022). Calcium deficiency worldwide: Prevalence of inadequate intakes and associated health outcomes. *Annals of the New York Academy of Sciences, 1512*, 10. DOI: 10.1111/nyas.14758 PMID: 35247225

Stocchi, F., Bravi, D., Emmi, A., & Antonini, A. (2024). Parkinson disease therapy: Current strategies and future research priorities. *Nature Reviews. Neurology, 20*, 695. DOI: 10.1038/s41582-024-01034-x PMID: 39496848

Su, D., Cui, Y., He, C., Yin, P., Bai, R., & Zhu, J.. (2025). Projections for prevalence of Parkinson's disease and its driving factors in 195 countries and territories to 2050: Modelling study of Global Burden of Disease Study 2021. *BMJ (Clinical Research Ed.), 388*. Advance online publication. DOI: 10.1136/bmj-2024-080952 PMID: 40044233

Tannenbaum, C., Fritel, X., Halme, A., Van Den Heuvel, E., Jutai, J., & Wagg, A. (2019). Long-term effect of community-based continence promotion on urinary symptoms, falls and healthy active life expectancy among older women: Cluster randomised trial. *Age and Ageing*, *48*, 526. DOI: 10.1093/ageing/afz038 PMID: 31220200

Valencia-Agudo, F., Urbiola, E., Romero-González, M., Navas, I., Elías, M., & Garriz, A.. (2021). Protocol for a randomized pilot study (FIRST STEPS): Implementation of the Incredible Years-ASLD® program in Spanish children with autism and preterm children with communication and/or socialization difficulties. *Trials*, *22*. Advance online publication. DOI: 10.1186/s13063-021-05229-1 PMID: 33879224

van der Sande, M. A. B., Walraven, G., Milligan, P., Banya, W., Ceesay, S. M., & Nyan, O.. (2001).. . *Bulletin of the World Health Organization*, *79*, 321. PMID: 11357211

Walker, R., Fothergill-Misbah, N., Kariuki, S., Ojo, O. O., Cilia, R., & Dekker, M.. (2023). Transforming Parkinson's care in Africa (TraPCAf): Protocol for a multimethodology National Institute for Health and Care Research Global Health Research Group project. *BMC Neurology*, *23*, 373. DOI: 10.1186/s12883-023-03414-0 PMID: 37858118

Wang, J., Zhang, S., Yuan, L., Tang, H., She, W., Zou, Y., ... (2024). Global, regional, and national burden of Parkinson's disease 1990–2021: A systematic analysis of the Global Burden of Disease Study 2021. SSRN *Electronic Journal*. https://doi .org/DOI: 10.2139/ssrn.5058486

Watabe, T., Hirata, K., Iima, M., Yanagawa, M., Saida, T., & Sakata, A.. (2025). Recent advances in theranostics and oncology PET: Emerging radionuclides and targets. *Annals of Nuclear Medicine*, *39*, 909. DOI: 10.1007/s12149-025-02090-z PMID: 40717183

Wolff, A., Schumacher, N. U., Pürner, D., Machetanz, G., Demleitner, A. F., & Feneberg, E.. (2023). Parkinson's disease therapy: What lies ahead? *Journal of Neural Transmission (Vienna, Austria)*, *130*, 793. DOI: 10.1007/s00702-023-02641-6 PMID: 37147404

Yu, T., & Li, X. (2023). Development of ZD2767P–carboxypeptidase G2–ultrasound therapy against cisplatin-resistant cancer. *Frontiers in Oncology*, *13*, 1151613. DOI: 10.3389/fonc.2023.1151613 PMID: 37274240

Zhou, L., Wang, Q., Gao, H., Tan, Y. X., Xu, Q., & Zhang, J.. (2024). Trends in the global burden of Parkinson's disease 1990–2021. *Findings from the Global Burden of Disease Study, 2021*. Advance online publication. DOI: 10.2139/ssrn.4950652

Chapter 7
Deep Brain Stimulation and Neuromodulation Advances for Parkinson's Disease

Olaniyan Tope Olugbemi
http://orcid.org/0009-0006-0351-4666
Kwara State University, Malete, Nigeria & Korea University, Seoul, South Korea

Abraham Olufemi Asuku
http://orcid.org/0000-0003-0071-0531
National Biotechnology Research and Development Agency, Nigeria

ABSTRACT

Recent studies have indicated that the incidence of Parkinson's disease has been on the increase as a neurodegenerative disease globally. While treatment using drugs like levodopa has offered much assistance, many are limited due to increased side effects. Several research on the role of neuromodulation and deep brain stimulation in Parkinson's disease have revealed much more beneficial properties. Neuromodulation and deep brain stimulation is an innovative and safe therapeutic approach in neurodegenerative diseases that can effectively improve neuroimaging, structure and functions of the brain to enhance movement functions. The approach can enhance electrophysiological markers as feedback signals mechanism within the brain highlighting the potential of integrating and making an informed decision on selecting non-invasive and invasive neuromodulation techniques for the condition. This book chapter is to give an overview on the recent advances in the novel application of deep brain stimulation and neuromodulation technology in the therapeutic treatment of Parkinson's disease.

DOI: 10.4018/979-8-3373-7437-6.ch007

INTRODUCTION

Foote et al. (2025) reported that the death of dopamine generating neurons result into neurodegenerative condition called Parkinson's disease. This condition causes dysfunctional motor cortex with movement disorders like tremor, difficulty in swallowing and speaking. The conventional medical treatment using surgery or medications have been reported to have several limitations, thus the search for alternative approach in the management of Parkinson's disease. Deep brain neurostimulation technology is gaining more attention as a result of inventions in hardware, targeting techniques and software. Martinez-Nunez et al. (2024) reported the underlying physiological symptoms of Parkinson's disease such as bradykinesia, tremor, rigidity and postural instability. These symptoms are as a result of defective non-motor and motor contributions from the basal ganglia pathways involve in the neuromodulation network. Furthermore, magnetic or electrical field neuromodulation therapy can be utilized as deep brain neurostimulation for the management of Parkinson's disease. Advancement in science and technological development has resulted into more sophisticated approach of deep brain neurostimulation like imaging-guided planning, closed-loop neurostimulation, brain leads with sensing capabilities and segmented leads coupled with guiding navigation. More less invasive approaches have been introduced for disease-specific networks applications like transcranial magnetic neurostimulation, electroconvulsive therapy and transcranial direct electrical neurostimulation. Other advanced laboratory methods have been developed such as temporal interference stimulation, magnetoelectric stimulation and low-frequency focused ultrasound.

Davidsona et al. (2024) reported that deep brain neurostimulation is an important therapeutic approach in Parkinson's disease management. This technique is widely utilized for several neuropsychiatric conditions owing to the intricate mechanism of action yet to be established. The authors revealed that the mechanism of action of deep brain neurostimulation is linked to stimulation of myelinated axons, the surrounding microenvironment and neurotransmitter release. The deep brain circuitry stimulation stimulates the neuronal activity within the basal ganglia resulting into neurobiological effects, epigenetic modification, neuroprotective role and changes in dopamine production in Parkinson's disease. Fang & Tolleson, (2017) demonstrated that damage of neuronal dopamine generation in the brain across the motor cortex result into Parkinson's disease. Over the years, oral administration of medications to augment the dopamine level of the brain has yielded little results with several side effects such as continuous delivery of drugs as disease progresses, thus, the need for more effective and efficient approach. Deep brain stimulation is reported to effectively assist patients suffering from pharmacotherapy complications ameliorate the disease condition. Deep brain stimulation offers more novel hardware options like leads, several software options enhancing the ability for better effectiveness and lower adverse effects.

Burns et al. (2021) revealed that deep brain neurostimulation is a very reliable, effective and innovation approach for neuromodulation therapy in Parkinson's disease. The authors demonstrated that further research in the area of neuroimaging, biomedical technology, neurophysiology and neuroanatomy will establish the mechanism of action of deep brain neurostimulation. Recently, deep brain neurostimulation has emerged as an alternative method to the conventional traditional neurosurgical lesioning treatments due to lower side effect and improved safety. The authors demonstrated that deep brain stimulation exerts dampening effects (local neuronal suppression) on the overactive neurons across the basal ganglia in the brain. Furthermore, other hypothesis has also suggested that deep brain neurostimulation performs an important function in disrupting normal communication system of the basal ganglia. Subsequently, deep brain neurostimulation may also cause alteration in the real-time dynamics of neurotransmitter movement resulting into synaptic suppression across brain network. Umemura, (2023) revealed that over the years, surgery has been utilized for the treatment of Parkinsons's disease. Due to the complications and side effects of surgery, other approaches are beginning to emerge such as the deep brain neurostimulation. Deep brain neurostimulation is a reversible and adjustable management for refractory Parkinson's disease. This can be done using implanted medical device to deliver excellent amount of electrical current to the brain to the specific target site. The modulatory impact of deep brain neurostimulation particularly for patients suffering from dopaminergic complications is effective. The author suggested that the combination of deep brain neurostimulation and medical management protocol will provide a long-term relief for patients. This book chapter provides an overview on the recent advances in the novel use of deep brain neurostimulation and neuromodulation technology in the therapeutic management of Parkinson's disease.

DEEP BRAIN NEUROSTIMULATION AND NEUROMODULATION ADVANCES FOR PARKINSON'S DISEASE

Umemura, (2023) reported that deep brain stimulation involves implanting medical device to deliver electric current precisely to the brain. This will alter the functionality of the target area of the brain resulting into activation of the neuronal system network. Deep brain stimulation involves three major components such as the lead with 4-8 contacts, the implantable pulse generator and the extension wire. Furthermore, deep brain neurostimulation is reversible and adjustable management regime for adjusting the functionality of nerves across the basal ganglia. Sandoval-

Pistorius et al. (2023) reported that deep brain neurostimulation is an effective therapeutic approach for the management and treatment of Parkinson's disease. The process involves the implantation of medical device using electrode into the target brain region and delivery of electric current to stimulate the area. The authors noted that despite the advancement in safety and efficacy of deep brain neurostimulation, the utilization remains very poor. John-Stuart & Hayriye (2018) revealed that deep brain neurostimulation is a recent trend in the electrical stimulation of the brain for therapeutic treatment of disease conditions through neuromodulation particularly in Parkinson's disease. The transcranial direct electrical neurostimulation can positively impact the basal ganglia motor activity.

Koirala et al. (2025) reported that the crucial component of today's strategies for the management of Parkinson's disease are the neuromodulation techniques. These techniques offer a valuable approach to complement the conventional pharmacotherapy. With deep brain neurostimulation, the intervention is well established as a noninvasive and invasive methods using ultra sound neurostimulation, transcranial direct electrical neurostimulation and transcranial magnetic neurostimulation. Furthermore, the application of electrophysiology markers in the brain are clinical correlated to motor symptoms severity (Olaniyan et al., 2022a; 2022b; 2022c; 2022d; 2022e; 2022f; 2022g). Shah et al. (2022) reported that neuronal degeneration is the cardinal feature of Parkinson's disease-causing dopamine depletion and motor dysfunction. Among the management options available today, deep brain neurostimulation remains a reliable management protocol for Parkinson's disease. Deep brain stimulation is cost effective, has less side effects and very effective.

Wang et al. (2024) revealed that recently more progress has been achieved across the field of neuro-modulation for the management of Parkinson's disease. The advancement in the production and generation of medical innovations, neuroscience and technological driven products has massively led to novel approaches in the management of patients with motor dysfunctions. For instance, deep brain modulation is a noninvasive approach with evolving promising solution in the management of Parkinson's disease (Olaniyan et al., 2022a; 2022b; 2022c; 2022d; 2022e; 2022f; 2022g). Mondal et al. (2024) further revealed that noninvasive neurostimulation of the brain like deep brain neurostimulation is an established protocol for therapeutic treatment of Parkinson's disease. The authors demonstrated that deep brain neurostimulation is effective and reliable in the management of staggering gait and other motor dysfunction in Parkinson's disease. Little et al. (2013) revealed that pathological brain signal can be interacted with using computer brain interfaces to ameliorate or intervene in the disease progression. The authors revealed that in Parkinson's disease, deep brain neurostimulation can deliver efficient and effective therapeutic neuromodulation.

Wójcik, et al. (2025) reported that deep brain stimulation target motor symptoms that are not responsive to pharmacotherapy in Parkinson's disease. Moreso, several target site in the brain can be stimulation for motor activity such as dentatorubrothalamic tract, subthalamic nucleus, pedunculopontine nucleus, nucleus basalis of Meynert globus pallidus internus, and zona incerta. These sites in the brain are potential areas for cognitive and axial symptoms. The authors recognized the paradigm shift as the combination of multimodal imaging with electrophysiological biomarkers therapeutic approach to direct neuromodulation in Parkinson's disease treatment. Moshayedi, et al. (2025) revealed that Parkinson's disease can be managed with brain activation techniques such as invasive and noninvasive methods like transcranial magnetic neurostimulation, transcutaneous vagus nerve stimulation, transcranial focused ultrasound neurostimulation, and transcranial electrical neurostimulation. These techniques can reduce the effects of motor impairments like bradykinesia, rigidity, cognitive decline, impulse control disorders and depression. Noninvasive approach is effective and safe in the management of Parkinson's disease. More research in this field of neuromodulation will illuminate more therapeutic potential and tools in the management of Parkinson's disease (Olaniyan et al., 2022a; 2022b; 2022c; 2022d; 2022e; 2022f; 2022g).

Malek, (2019) reported that deep brain neurostimulation is an established therapeutic approach for treatment patients with Parkinson's disease. The author noted that in addition to the efficacy and reliable, deep brain neurostimulation also enhances the quality of life of the patients by ameliorating the motor symptoms and improving clinical outcomes. Carina et al. (2022) revealed that over the years, deep brain neurostimulation has been utilized for the management of Parkinson's disease. Though, still underutilized as a result of lack of awareness and information on the clinical outcomes and safety. Groiss et al. (2009) revealed that deep brain neurostimulation has been utilized for more 15 years and established as a highly effective therapeutic approach in treating Parkinson's disease.

Schnitzler et al. (2022) reported that deep brain neurostimulation directional range for amplitudes to achieve symptoms relief with low side effects yielded a wider therapeutic window as compared with omnidirectional stimulation. Lavano et al. (2016) reported that innovations across the field of deep brain neurostimulation are emerging solutions to the management of Parkinson's disease. Moscovich et al. (2024) noted that in the past few years the field of neuromodulation has emerged meaningfully through the development of innovations in hardware, stimulation techniques, electrode placement and software for therapeutic interventions. The deep brain stimulation releases electrical signals to specific region of the brain to restore physiological balance. Wang et al. (2024) showed that in recent years important attention has been witnessed in the field of neuromodulation in the management of Parkinson's disease. The authors noted that deep brain neurostimulation is a non-invasive approach that is rapidly evolving with promising solution for improving quality of life and reducing motor defects.

Ramirez-Zamora et al. (2018) revealed that deep brain neurostimulation provides opportunity multidisciplinary ensemble in neuromodulation for the management of Parkinson's disease. The recent advances in the technology have brought about deep brain stimulation electrodes, neuronal signal processing, improved sensors, uses of responsive deep brain stimulation and advancements in development applications in practice and research. Hartmann et al. (2019) reported that in the past few decades deep brain neurostimulation has appeared as standard clinical protocol that is highly effective for the management of Parkinson's disease. The advancement in the development of hardware allows for more individualized, focused and optimal brain neurostimulation in Parkinson's disease. The noninvasive and invasive techniques alter the brain function through the utilization of electric, radio wave, magnetic, electric current to targeted areas to improve neurochemical regulation, gene expression, functional brain activity, cognitive or sensorimotor function, and affective processes as shown in figure 1.

Paff et al. (2020) revealed that deep brain neurostimulation is gaining a dominant focus in the management of Parkinson's disease. There has been tremendous improvement in the development of advanced deep brain neurostimulation tools such as implantable pulse generation and deep brain stimulation lead improve the potentials of therapeutic management of Parkinson's disease. Jost et al. (2024) reported that deep brain neurostimulation can enhance the quality of life among patients with Parkinson's disease. The authors investigated the long-term impact of subthalamic nucleus deep brain neurostimulation and compare with standard drug. In their study, it was revealed that deep brain neurostimulation improved outcomes and quality of life in long term assessment among patients with Parkinson's disease. Deep brain stimulation has been described as a neurostimulator consisting of surgical implant for the generation of electrical impulse using electrode to a precise area of the brain to modulate physiological functions. Many of these devices are referred to as brain pacemakers often utilized where patients show resistance to oral medications. Most often, deep brain stimulation is combined with medication for improvement of clinical outcomes among patients.

Franzoi et al. (2018) showed that motor fluctuation is a key characteristic of Parkinson's disease such as dyskinesia. The authors noted that the technique is safe, reversible and with advantage of low side effects. The mechanism of action involved in deep brain neurostimulation has been suggested to be blockade of sodium channels, stimulation of local inhibitory neurons in the target nucleus, release of GABA neurotransmitter, cortical activation and blockade of synaptic depolarization. Suarez-Cedeno et al. (2017) reported that neuromodulation of the subcortical region of the brain are utilized as therapeutic approach in Parkinson's disease. The

FDA approved the utilization of deep brain neurostimulation in the year 2002 as an effective neuromodulation approach in the management of Parkinson's disease due to the effectiveness and safety. Picillo et al. (2016) showed that deep brain neurostimulation has been established for the management of Parkinson's disease. The authors investigate the optimal stimulation parameters using extensive programming sessions by relying on the physician's experience. This approach made the patient to be subjected to inefficient and inconsistent stimulation changes and visit. From their results, it was discovered that four different algorithms assist in the management of symptoms through individualized approach.

Pycroft et al. (2018) reported that deep brain neurostimulation has transformed the clinical approach in the treatment of Parkinson's disease. The authors noted that deep brain neurostimulation is safe and effective and there are several emerging advanced techniques like cybersecurity risk, optogenetics, implantation timing, impediments to undertaking high-quality research that needs further investigation to establish the effectiveness of these tools. Parastarfeizabadi & Kouzani, (2017) reported that deep brain neurostimulation is a medical based remedy utilized for the management of Parkinson's disease with lower side effects. The authors demonstrated that advancement in closed loop deep brain neurostimulation offers a brighter future for patients with Parkinson's disease. Bange et al. (2025) reported that non-invasive deep brain stimulation is clinically utilized for the management of Parkinson's disease. Many of these non-invasive deep brain neurostimulation like Transcranial magnetic neurostimulation, transcranial electric neurostimulation, and ultrasound neuromodulation as shown in figure 1. Busch et al. (2025) showed that the stimulation amplitude in deep brain neurostimulation is evaluated by the level of feedback of neurophysiological motor fluctuations. The authors setup a programming strategy to determine the potential clinical benefits of deep brain neurostimulation in Parkinson's disease. The findings from the study revealed that three step programming is an important strategy to guide the implementation of deep brain neurostimulation in the clinical settings. There are many factors that contribute to the positive results of deep brain neurostimulation in Parkinson's patients such as lead placement, effective programming and careful patient selection.

Lozano et al. (2019) reported that the medical application of deep brain neurostimulation is one of the most significant advances in clinical neurosciences over the last few decades. Furthermore, deep brain neurostimulation is an invasive intervention that potentially measures the brain pathophysiological activity to deliver timely reversible electrical impulses for therapeutic purposes. Martinez-Ramirez et al. (2015) showed that deep brain neurostimulation is a safe invasive procedure utilized for the management of Parkinson's disease. In the last few decades, it has provided huge therapeutic advantage over the conventional approaches like medication use. Deep brain neurostimulation improves motor function particularly across the subthalamic nucleus, zona incerta, ventralis intermedius and globus pallidus pars interna and enhance quality of life.

Figure 1. Deep Brain Stimulation and Neuromodulation Advances for Parkinson's Disease

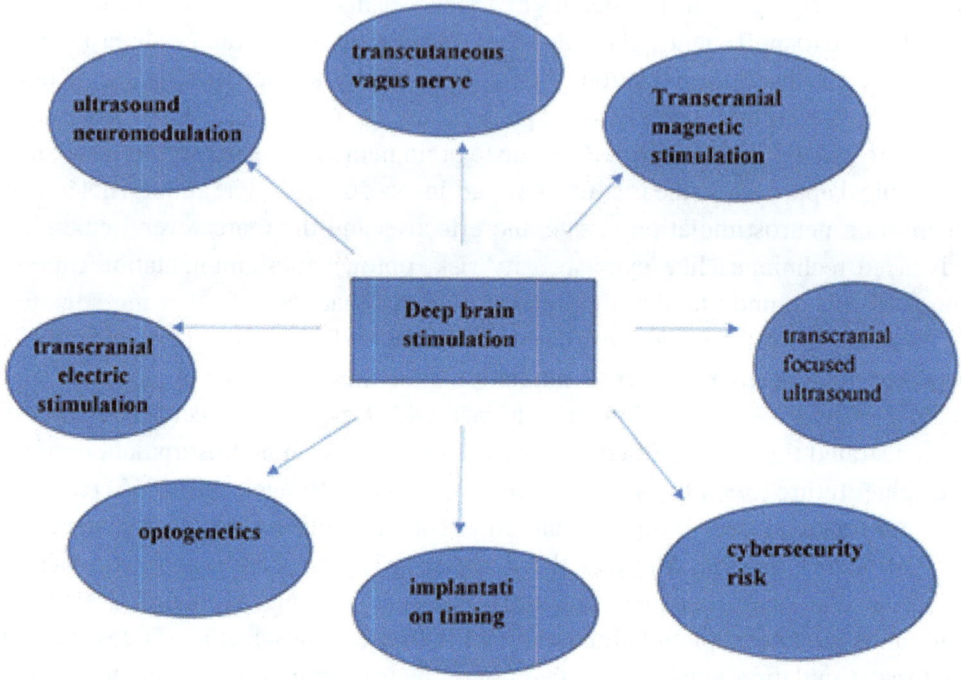

CHALLENGES, LIMITATIONS AND FUTURE PERSPECTIVES

Advancement in technology and understanding in the management, treatment and monitoring of neurological disorders using neurostimulation and acquisition of advance signal in brain neurophysiology has increased the growing interest. The utilization of microelectrode has been shown to increase the risk of intracranial hemorrhage. Furthermore, more patients with depression, suicide, long hospital stay and infection are noticed with neurostimulation compared to normal group. Deep brain neurostimulation has been revealed to possess serious complications such as perioperative, medium and long-term. Many of the adverse effects include intracerebral hemorrhage, scalp infections, infarction, foreign body intolerance, transient postoperative mental status changes and pain. Others include increased electrode impedance, lead displacement, lead fracture, lead migration, battery drain, device failure and skin erosion. Therapy linked complications are hemiballismus, dyskinesia, dysarthria, diplopia, paraesthesia, mild impairments in verbal fluency, executive function and learning.

Further research will continue to shape our understanding in neuromodulation in neurological disorders. Future collaboration and research in the areas of controlled trials, long term safety, persistent efficacy and ethical guidelines and principles will be important. In ameliorating the signs, symptoms and complications of Parkinson's disease, future perspective and research should be focused on therapeutic intervention for both genotypic and phenotypic expression through individualized treatment targeting specific symptoms and circuits. More multidisciplinary approach should be utilized for evaluation and decision making. More study on the next-generation of electrical neuromodulation techniques for more physiological and anatomical specificity is required. In addition, emerging wearable technologies development should improve sensors memory, rechargeable batteries, external signals and increase lead electrodes to enhance recording capacities and stimulation.

CONCLUSION

This book chapter provides an overview on the recent advances in the novel utilization of deep brain neurostimulation and neuromodulation technology in the therapeutic management of Parkinson's disease. Deep brain neurostimulation has been described as a surgical technique which is well accommodated and its complications rate is very minimal. Advancement in technology has resulted into more sophisticated approach of deep brain stimulation such as imaging-guided planning, closed-loop neurostimulation, segmented leads with guiding navigation and brain leads with sensing capabilities. More less invasive approaches have been introduced for disease-specific networks applications like transcranial magnetic neurostimulation, electroconvulsive therapy and transcranial direct electric current neurostimulation. Other advanced laboratory methods have been developed such as temporal interference stimulation, magnetoelectric stimulation and low-frequency focused ultrasound.

REFERENCES

Bange, M., Rick, C.G.H, Aparna, A. W. S, Günther, D. & Muthuraman, M. (2025). Non-invasive brain stimulation to modulate neural activity in Parkinson's disease. npj | parkinson's disease. (2025) 11:68. https://doi.org/.DOI: 10.1038/s41531-025-00908-1

Burns, M. R., Shannon, Y. C., Bhavana, P., Sotiris, G. M., Joshua, K. W., & Ramirez-Zamora, A. (2021). Advances and Future Directions of Neuromodulation in Neurologic Disorders. *Neurologic Clinics*, *39*, 71–85. DOI: 10.1016/j.ncl.2020.09.004 PMID: 33223090

Busch, J.L., Jonathan, K, Jennifer, K.B, Victoria, S.W, Luisa, D, Jeroen, G.V.H & Andrea, A.K. (2025). Chronic adaptive deep brain stimulation for Parkinson's disease: clinical outcomes and programming strategies. (2025) 11:264.

Carina, F., Rafael, B. C., Juliete, M. D., Renato, P. M., & Rubens, G. C. (2022). Deep brain stimulation in Parkinson's disease: State of the art and future perspectives. DBS in Parkinson's disease. *Arquivos de Neuro-Psiquiatria*, *80*(5, Suppl. 1), 105–115. DOI: 10.1590/0004-282X-ANP-2022-S133 PMID: 35976323

Davidsona, B., Luka, M., Laura, K., Lorraine, V. K., & Suneil, K. K. (2024). Neuroscience fundamentals relevant to neuromodulation: Neurobiology of deep brain stimulation in Parkinson's disease. *Neurotherapeutics; the Journal of the American Society for Experimental NeuroTherapeutics*, *21*, e00348. PMID: 38579455

Franzoi, A. E. A., Bonchoski, A. B., & Koerbel, A. (2018). The advances of Deep Brain Stimulation (DBS) for treatment of Parkinson's Disease (PD). *Clinical & Biomedical Research*, *38*(4).

Fang, J. Y., & Tolleson, C. (2017). The role of deep brain stimulation in Parkinson's disease: An overview and update on new developments. *Neuropsychiatric Disease and Treatment*, *2017*(13), 723–732. PMID: 28331322

Foote, A., de Waal, E., Caiado, F., Samman, A., & Ukolov, A. (2025). A comprehensive review of deep brain stimulation for Parkinson's disease: The history, current state of the art and future possibilities. *Medicine in Novel Technology and Devices*, *26*, 100362.

Groiss, S.J.L., Wojtecki, M., Su¨dmeyer, & Schnitzler, A. (2009). Deep brain stimulation in Parkinson's disease. Ther Adv Neurol Disord (2009) 2(6) 379 391 DOI: .DOI: 10.1177/ 1756285609339382

Hartmann, C.J., Sabine, F., Stefan, J.G, Lars, W. & Alfons, S. (2019). An update on best practice of deep brain stimulation in Parkinson's disease. Therapeutic Advances in Neurological Disorders. 2019, Vol. 12: 1–20 https://doi.org/ https://doi.org/.DOI: 10.1177/1756286419838096

John-Stuart, B., & Hayriye, C. (2018). Recent Trends in the Use of Electrical Neuromodulation in Parkinson's Disease. *Current Behavioral Neuroscience Reports, 2018*(5), 170–178. DOI: 10.1007/s40473-018-0154-9 PMID: 29862163

Jost, S. T., Salima, A., Julian, E., Keyoumars, A., Anna, S., Alexandra, R., Jan, N. P. S., Alexandra, G., & Gereon, R. F. V. (2024). Visser-Vandewalle, Angelo, A., Monty, S., Lars, T.P., Martinez-Martin, K. R., Chaudhuri, Haidar, S., & Dafsari, M. (2024). Neurostimulation for Advanced Parkinson Disease and Quality of Life at 5 Years A Non-Randomized Controlled Trial. *JAMA Network Open*, *7*(1), e2352177. DOI: 10.1001/jamanetworkopen.2023.52177 PMID: 38236600

Koirala, N., Manuel, B., Aparna, W.S. & Muthuraman, M. (2025). Advancements in invasive and non-invasive neuromodulation for Parkinson's disease: current findings and future directions. | (2025) 11:221. https://doi.org/.DOI: 10.1038/s41531-025-01071-3

Lavano, A., Attilio, D.T. & Giusy, G. (2016). Directional Deep Brain Stimulation. Brain Disord The 2016, 5:3. 1000220. DOI: .DOI: 10.4172/2168-975X.1000220

Little, S., Alex, P., Spencer, N., Baltazar, Z., Ludvic, Z., Marwan, H., Thomas, F., Patricia, L., Keyoumars, A., James, F., Alexander, L. G., Tipu, Z. A., & Peter, B. (2013). Adaptive Deep Brain Stimulation in Advanced Parkinson Disease. *Annals of Neurology*, *74*, 449–457. PMID: 23852650

Lozano, A. M., Lipsman, N., Bergman, H., Brown, P., Chabardes, S., Chang, J. W., Matthews, K., McIntyre, C. C., Schlaepfer, T. E., Schulder, M., Temel, Y., Volkmann, J., & Krauss, J. K. (2019). Deep brain stimulation: Current challenges and future directions. *Nature Reviews. Neurology*, *15*(3), 148–160. DOI: 10.1038/s41582-018-0128-2 PMID: 30683913

Malek, N. (2019). Deep Brain Stimulation in Parkinson's Disease. *Neurology India*, *67*, 968–978. PMID: 31512617

Martinez-Nunez, A. E., Maria, B. J., Michael, S. O., & Alfonso, F. (2024). Emerging therapies for neuromodulation in Parkinson's disease. *Neurotherapeutics; the Journal of the American Society for Experimental NeuroTherapeutics*, *21*, e00310.

Martinez-Ramirez, D., Wei, H., Alberto, R. B., Michael, S. O., & Aparna, W. S. (2015). Update on deep brain stimulation in Parkinson's disease. *Translational Neurodegeneration, 2015*(4), 12. DOI: 10.1186/s40035-015-0034-0 PMID: 26257895

Mondal, B., Choudhury, S., Banerjee, R., Roy, A., Chatterjee, K., Basu, P., Singh, R., Halder, S., Shubham, S., Baker, S. N., Baker, M. R., & Kumar, H. (2024). Effects of non-invasive vagus nerve stimulation on clinical symptoms and molecular biomarkers in Parkinson's disease. *Frontiers in Aging Neuroscience, 15*, 1331575. DOI: 10.3389/fnagi.2023.1331575 PMID: 38384731

Moscovich, M., Camila, H. de A., Murilo, M. M., Lorena, B. B., André, C. F., Matthew, H., Clement, H., Henrique, B. F., & Munhoz, R. P. (2024). Fundamentals of deep brain stimulation for Parkinson's disease in clinical practice: part2. *Arquivos de Neuro-Psiquiatria, 82*(4), s00441786037. PMID: 38653486

Moshayedi, A.J., & Mokhtari, T., & Emadi, Andani, M. (2025). Brain Stimulation Techniques in Research and Clinical Practice: A Comprehensive Review of Applications and Therapeutic Potential in Parkinson's Disease. *Brain Sciences, 2025*(15), 20. DOI: 10.3390/brainsci15010020 PMID: 39851388

Olaniyan, O., Adetunji, C. O., Adeyomoye, O., Dare, A., Adeniyi, M. J., & Enoch, A. (2022g). *Computational methods for translational brain-behavior analysis. In book: ARTIFICIAL INTELLIGENCE FOR NEUROLOGICAL DISORDERS. Publisher*. Elsevier., DOI: 10.1016/B978-0-323-90277-9.00025-0

Olaniyan, O. T., Adetunji, C. O., Adeyomoye, O., Dare, A., Adeniyi, M. J., & Alex, E. (2022e). *Cognitive therapy for brain diseases using deep learning models. In book: ARTIFICIAL INTELLIGENCE FOR NEUROLOGICAL DISORDERS. Publisher*. Elsevier., DOI: 10.106/B978-0-323-90277-9.00017-1

Olaniyan, O. T., Adetunji, C. O., Adeyomoye, O., Dare, A., Adeniyi, M. J., & Alex, E. (2022f). *Clinical applications of deep learning in neurology and its enhancements with future directions. In book: ARTIFICIAL INTELLIGENCE FOR NEUROLOGICAL DISORDERS. Publisher*. Elsevier., DOI: 10.1016/B978-0-323-90277-9.00026-2

Olaniyan, O.T., Adetunji, C.O., Dare, A., Adeyomoye, O., Adeniyi, M.J., & Alex, E. (2022a). Clinical applications of deep learning in neurology and its enhancements with future predictions. In book: ARTIFICIAL INTELLIGENCE FOR NEUROLOGICAL DISORDERS. Publisher: Elsevier. September 2022. DOI: .DOI: 10.1016/B978-0-323-90277-9.00016-X

Olaniyan, O. T., Adetunji, C. O., Dare, A., Adeyomoye, O., Adeniyi, M. J., & Alex, E. (2022b). *Cognitive therapy for brain diseases using artificial intelligence models. In book: ARTIFICIAL INTELLIGENCE FOR NEUROLOGICAL DISORDERS. Publisher*. Elsevier., DOI: 10.1016/B978-0-323-90277-9.00013-4

Olaniyan, O. T., Adetunji, C. O., Dare, A., Adeyomoye, O., Adeniyi, M. J., & Alex, E. (2022c). *Artificial intelligence-based early detection of neurological disease using noninvasive method based on speech analysis. In book: ARTIFICIAL INTELLIGENCE FOR NEUROLOGICAL DISORDERS. Publisher*. Elsevier., DOI: 10.1016/B978-0-323-90277-9.00008-0

Olaniyan, O. T., Adetunji, C. O., Dare, A., Adeyomoye, O., Adeniyi, M. J., & Alex, E. (2022d). *Prevention and diagnosis of neurodegenerative diseases using machine learning models. In book: ARTIFICIAL INTELLIGENCE FOR NEUROLOGICAL DISORDERS. Publisher*. Elsevier., DOI: 10.1016/B978-0-323-90277-9.00009-2

Paff, M., Aaron, L., Can, S., Andres, M. L., & Alfonso, F. (2020). Update on Current Technologies for Deep Brain Stimulation in Parkinson's Disease. *Journal of Movement Disorders*, *13*(3), 185–198. DOI: 10.14802/jmd.20052 PMID: 32854482

Parastarfeizabadi, M., & Kouzani, A. Z. (2017). Advances in closed-loop deep brain stimulation devices. *Journal of Neuroengineering and Rehabilitation*, *2017*(14), 79. DOI: 10.1186/s12984-017-0295-1 PMID: 28800738

Picillo, M., Andres, M. L., Nancy, K., Renato, P. M., & Alfonso, F. (2016). Programming Deep Brain Stimulation for Parkinson's Disease: The Toronto Western Hospital Algorithms. *Brain Stimulation*, *9*, 425–437. PMID: 26968806

Pycroft, L., John, S., & Tipu, A. (2018). Deep brain stimulation: An overview of history, methods, and future developments. *Brain and Neuroscience Advances*, *2*, 1–6. DOI: 10.1177/2398212818816017 PMID: 32166163

Ramirez-Zamora, A., Giordano, J. J., Gunduz, A., Brown, P., Sanchez, J. C., Foote, K. D., Almeida, L., Starr, P. A., Bronte-Stewart, H. M., Hu, W., McIntyre, C., Goodman, W., Kumsa, D., Grill, W. M., Walker, H. C., Johnson, M. D., Vitek, J. L., Greene, D., Rizzuto, D. S., & Deeb, M. S. (2018). Evolving Applications, Technological Challenges and Future Opportunities in Neuromodulation: Proceedings of the Fifth Annual Deep Brain Stimulation Think Tank. *Frontiers in Neuroscience*, *11*, 734. DOI: 10.3389/fnins.2017.00734 PMID: 29416498

Sandoval-Pistorius, S.S., Nicole, R., Provenza, Coralie, de H., Mallory, L., Hacker, Allison, C.W., Kara, A.J., Jing, W., Melanie, A.M., & Stephanie, C. (2023). Advances in Deep Brain Stimulation: From Mechanisms to Applications. The Journal of Neuroscience, November 8, 2023. 43(45):7575–7586. 7575.

Schnitzler, A., Pablo, M., Matthew, A. B., Leonard, V., Sergiu, G., Andrew, E., Ramiro, A., Marta, B., Julie, G. P., & Sean, N. M. (2022). Pötter-Nerger, Winona, T., Leonardo, A., Jimenez-Shahed, J., Nestor, T., Witold, L., Fatima, C., Christian, J.H., Stefan, J.G., Martin, G., Florence, D., Edward, K., Binith, C., & Jan, V., (2022). Directional Deep Brain Stimulation for Parkinson's Disease: Results of an International Crossover Study With Randomized, Double-Blind Primary End-point. Neuromodulation: Technology at the Neural Interface. *Neuromodulation*, *25*, 817–828. DOI: 10.1111/ner.13407 PMID: 34047410

Shah, H., Omer, U., Habib, U. R., Sharan, J., Chaithanya, A., Kamran, H., Hamza, I., & Sailesh, I. S. K. (2022). Deep Brain Stimulation in the Treatment of Parkinson's Disease. *Cureus*, *14*(9), e28760. DOI: 10.7759/cureus.28760 PMID: 36211107

Suarez-Cedeno, G., Jessika, S., & Mya, C. S. (2017). Earlier Intervention with Deep Brain Stimulation for Parkinson's Disease. Hindawi Parkinson's Disease Volume. 2017, Article ID 9358153, 9 pages https://doi.org/DOI: 10.1155/2017/9358153

Umemura, A. (2023). Deep Brain Stimulation for Parkinson's Disease. *Juntendo Medical Journal*, *69*(1), 21–29. PMID: 38854848

Wang, K., Meng, F., Zhang, Y., Ramirez-Zamora, A., & Chen, S.-Y. (Eds.). (2024). *Advances in neuromodulation treatment of Parkinson's disease and aging-related movement disorders*. Frontiers Media SA., DOI: 10.3389/978-2-8325-4818-9

Wang, K. L., Meng, F., Chen, S., Ramirez-Zamora, A., & Zhang, Y. Q. (2024). Editorial: Advances in neuromodulation treatment of Parkinson's disease and aging related movement disorders. *Frontiers in Aging Neuroscience*, *16*, 1407216. DOI: 10.3389/fnag.2024.1407216 PMID: 38659703

Wójcik, R., Debska, A., Zaczkowski, K., Szmyd, B., Podstawka, M., Bobeff, E. J., Piotrowski, M., Ratajczyk, P., Jaskólski, D. J., & Wisniewski, K. (2025). Deep Brain Stimulation for Parkinson's Disease—ANarrativeReview. *Biomedicines*, *2025*(13), 2430. DOI: 10.3390/ biomedicines13102430 PMID: 41153713

Chapter 8
Digital and Wearable Technology in Therapeutic Monitoring of Parkinson's Disease in Under-Resourced Settings

Olaniyan Tope Olugbemi
http://orcid.org/0009-0006-0351-4666
Kwara State University, Malete, Nigeria & Korea University, Seoul, South Korea

Duyilemi Chris Ajonijebu
University of Johannesburg, Doornfontein, South Africa

Danwahab O. Ambali
Kwara State University, Malete, Nigeria

ABSTRACT

Parkinson's disease has been described as a neurodegenerative disease characterized by non-motor and motor symptoms that impact negatively on individual's lifestyle. Due to the nature of this condition, it requires constant monitoring to evaluate the progress of treatment, clinical assessment and therapeutic interventions. Consequently, wearable and digital technologies are emerging advances in artificial intelligence that are now recently being mobilized to provide real-time, promising solutions, personalized intervention and objective data collection for neurodegenerative diseases. These technologies are very specific and highly sensitive in tracking

DOI: 10.4018/979-8-3373-7437-6.ch008

non-motor and motor variations, tremors and gait abnormalities. Furthermore, many of these devices are able to provide feedback mechanisms, cognitive impairment, sleep/autonomic and gastrointestinal comorbidities. The aim of the book chapter is to give an overview on the recent advances in the novel application of digital and wearable technology in the therapeutic monitoring of Parkinson's disease.

INTRODUCTION

According to Paccoud et al. (2024), it is estimated that Parkinson's disease affects about 8.5 million people globally and this figure is estimated to increase to about 12 million by the year 2040. The authors further revealed that Parkinson's disease has both nonmotor and motor fluctuating symptoms which demands constant medical attention. For accurate and adequate monitoring of this condition, the use of advanced digital medical devices such as AI wearable tools has been suggested, although the success of these technologies is largely determined by the willingness of the patients to wear these devices for healthcare purposes. Thus, the authors carried out research to understand the perspective of the patients with Parkinson's disease on the use of digital medical devices across Europe. From their study, it was revealed that patient's perspective is important in considering the deployment of digital technologies for more advanced disease stage. Sigchaa et al. (2023) reported that Parkinson's disease is a neurodegenerative disease that affects the quality of life. The authors noted that wearable devices utilization combined with machine learning algorithm can provide continuous monitoring and objective methods for data analysis among Parkinson's disease patients. More supportive use of artificial intelligence particularly deep learning has provided platforms for data analysis and new approaches in prognosis, diagnosis, and monitoring of Parkinson's disease among patients (Adetunji et al., 2022 a, b). The authors equally noted several challenges associated with the use of wearable devices among patients such as implementation conditions (a large amount of computational processing or data), the transparency of the algorithms and imbalance in the type of symptoms analyzed. Laar et al. (2023) reported that the prevalence of Parkinson's disease is on the increase with attending consequences such as nonmotor and motor symptoms. Several non-pharmacological and pharmacological interventions have been utilized to alleviate the symptoms of Parkinson's disease. The authors noted that technology is currently being use to improve the accessibility, efficiency and feasibility of these diagnosis and treatments outcomes. Olaniyan et al. (2022 a, b, c, d, e, f, g) reported that there is ongoing increasing attention on the use of wearable technology in addressing the issues linked to Parkinson's disease. The authors noted that these technologies can be utilized for monitoring or diagnosis of Parkinson's disease symptoms, alleviating and management. Parkinson's disease symptoms that can be addressed using advanced technology include gait, limb movements, Electromyography abnormalities, freezing of gait, tremor, activities of daily living, bradykinesia, dyskinesia, posture, balance, nocturnal hypokinesia, handwriting, swallowing, speech, heart rate, Electroencephalogram abnormalities, cognitive activities, depression, dementia, emotions, fatigue, blinking, facial expression, breath, cortical activity and saccades. Channa et al. (2020) reported that the use of wearable devices for transforming the management of neurocognitive diseases in mental health is gaining more attention. Wearable technology is being utilized for the rehabilitation, diagnosis, monitoring and assessment of Parkinson's disease among patients. The authors noted that sensor based wearable devices have more positive impact in advancing the tracking of numerous exercise activities, monitoring and early diagnosis of Parkinson's disease among patients, thus improving the quality of life in such patient. Recent advances in the development of information technology and artificial intelligence in wearable medical devices have significantly gained serious attention for the treatment and diagnosis of Parkinson's disease. These devices use sensors and real time approaches which is an intelligent portable device utilized for data collection from human body (Olaniyan et al., 2022a; 2022b; 2022c; 2022d; 2022e; 2022f; 2022g; Yuexuan, 2024). These approaches can be described as computer human interaction for various services such as exercise measurement, health management, social entertainment. Polvorinos-Fernández et al. (2024) showed that Parkinson's disease contributes significantly to the reduction in the quality of life among affected subjects globally. The authors noted that computing resources possess great potential in ameliorating the effects of the symptoms through early diagnosis, monitoring and prognosis. Little has been done in the study of digital biomarkers in Parkinson's disease, but the authors demonstrated that more studies should be done in this regard. Terry & Vazquez, (2025) reported that prompt and effective treatment of symptoms requires timely intervention and continuous monitoring which are often not provided by the traditional clinical evaluation. Using wearable devices, there can be real time data assessment, evaluation and prompt intervention towards improving clinical outcomes. Many wearable devices are very sensitive and specific for evaluating and tracking motor activity, tremor, gait abnormalities. It will also provide feedback mechanism towards improving medication intervention and adherence. The authors also noted several challenges in utilization of wearable devices such as user-friendly nature, device adherence, data integration into clinical workflows and device widespread-adoption. Ultimately, wearable devices are important tools in the management and enhanced treatment of Parkinson's disease for personalized interventions. The aim of the book chapter is to give an overview on Digital and Wearable Technology in Therapeutic Monitoring of Parkinson's Disease.

DIGITAL AND WEARABLE TECHNOLOGY IN THERAPEUTIC MONITORING OF PARKINSON'S DISEASE

Toshiki et al. (2024) reported that the understanding of the purpose and pattern of istradefylline adherence to treatment is important in Parkinson's disease target intervention. There are different factors associated with the adherence to istradefylline treatment in Parkinson's disease. The authors characterized each factor utilizing univariable multinomial logistic regression models. In their study, it was revealed that declining adherence group got lower MAO-B inhibitors and amantadine treatment resulting into a higher prevalence of dementia/ mild cognitive impairment while the declining and then recovering adherence group had a higher prevalence of mood/ anxiety disorders. Kehnemouyi et al. (2024) showed that Parkinson's disease is linked to gastrointestinal dysfunction, sleep/autonomic disturbances and cognitive impairment. In their study, they revealed that constant monitoring is important for fluctuating symptoms. To achieve this, wearable devices must be adopted to evaluate and track objective measures of Parkinson's disease comorbidities. These devices can monitor real-time pathological function and physiological responses in Parkinson's disease for optimized treatment protocol.

Bruno et al. (2019) demonstrated that the state of art of wearable technologies for monitoring of patients with Parkinson's disease have a very rich field of application but more research is essential in this regard for adequate reliability and effectiveness. The authors noted that wearable medical devices are an evolving area in medicine for medical assistance providing more precise and effective treatment and diagnostic approach. These technologies use sensors for data collection, analysis and processing to enable healthcare providers take informed decision, assess progress, monitoring, remote management of Parkinson's disease. The authors concluded that the utilization of wearable devices improves medical care, intervention and research data collection. Ymeri et al. (2023) reported that the assessment of Parkinson' disease often have reliability issues but these can be overcome using smart devices such as smartwatches and smartphones. The signal obtain by these devices can be processed using machine learning algorithms. The authors conducted a study to investigate the compliance, user experience of actively and passively analysis of symptoms from home environments and the feasibility using data obtained from sensors incorporated in a wrist- wearable device and smartphones. In their study, it was observed that user aspects and Compliance will support the long- term feasibility of the wearable devices. Signal processing and machine learning approaches will support the analyses of the data collected from the GENEActiv, Mobistudy app and correlate them with the MDS- UPDRS using sleep disorders from Parkinson's patients.

Terry & Alvarez-Vazquez, (2017) showed that effective management of Parkinson's disease symptoms requires constant timely intervention and continuous monitoring. This is so because the traditional clinical management and assessment often fail to provide timely intervention and monitoring. The authors revealed that wearable devices are an emerging technology with promising effective solutions for the real time data collection, analyses, monitoring and personalized intervention among Parkinson's disease patients. From the study conducted by the authors, it was demonstrated that wearable devices possess high specificity and sensitivity in tracking gait abnormalities, tremors and motor fluctuations. Wearable-based technological interventions, like feedback mechanisms and cueing, have provided opportunity in enhancing reduced bradykinesia, motor control, improved medication adherence and data support. The challenges of using wearable devices include user friendliness, data integration into clinical workflows, and device adherence. The authors concluded that wearable technology is a valuable tool for improving Parkinson's disease management via continuous personalized interventions and monitoring.

Channa, et al. (2024) revealed that wearable Internet of Things devices are an emerging field in medicine for the timely intervention, detection, analysis and diagnosis of Parkinson's disease. The authors demonstrated that computational algorithms and inertial sensors can support these devices in providing accurate, sensitive and specific results in Parkinson's disease management. In their study, it was revealed that wearable technology gave about 90.0% accuracy in tremor detection among Parkinson's disease patients. Advancement in computing resources and wearable technologies have greatly enhanced the potential application of technology in the diagnosis, detection, prognosis, monitoring, analysis and timely intervention of Parkinson's disease. Hirczy et al. (2024) revealed that Parkinson's diseases monitoring using wearable devices has gain tremendous attention due to the compelling supportive therapeutic advantage and diagnosis even though there are some limitations. The authors demonstrated that larger percentage of respondents agree to have interest in emerging technologies such as wearable devices for Parkinson's disease detection, monitoring and analysis.

Rodríguez-Martín et al. (2022) showed that wearable medical devices are important for clinical practice, research, and clinical trials in the field of Parkinson's disease in order to save time, improve data collection, and timely intervention. Kenny et al. (2022) reported that wearable devices can monitor, diagnose and track neurological disorders like Parkinson's disease. The authors conducted a study on the needs of people and to understand their views with regards to Parkinson disease using wearable devices for disease diagnosis and monitoring. Using a mixed method parallel design, the authors demonstrated that wearable devices are seen by the participants to mainly provide data for health care professionals rather than supporting feedback for their timely interventions. They concluded that wearable devices are important for remote assessment and monitoring of patients with Parkinson's disease. Bacanoiu et al. (2025) reported that Parkinson's disease symptoms include abnormal posture, falls, instability, gait variability, executive dysfunction, neuropsychiatric symptoms and Parkinson's disease dementia. These symptoms affect the quality of life among patients. To manage this condition, the use of mobile platforms, digital health technologies, and sensory cues has been revealed to effective monitor and diagnose these symptoms. The authors revealed that developing efficient strategies in Parkinson's disease management involves remote monitoring solutions, using home-based digital health assessments, semi-structured activities are reported to offer unique advantages in recent times. In addition, it was noted that clinical rating scales, digital biomarkers and wearable inertial sensors, enhance the ability to monitor and characterize motor symptoms among Parkinson's disease patients. The authors concluded that accurate detection of motor alterations and support for clinical evaluations in Parkinson's disease requires the use of digital health technologies which are scalable, specific and sensitive for improving the clinical management of Parkinson's disease.

Bougea, (2025) revealed that wearable sensors are emerging technologies in the management of neurodegenerative diseases like Parkinson's disease. The technology through the sensor offers continuous real time monitoring of Parkinson's disease symptoms such as gait, bradykinesia, dyskinesia and tremor for early intervention and detection. The author concluded that wearable technology plays a significant role in Parkinson's disease management. Ruirui et al. (2020) suggested that the incidence of Parkinson's disease is a growing concern estimated to increase due to increasing aging population. The use of wearable devices is reported to revolutionize the monitoring and early diagnosis of Parkinson's disease symptoms such as tremor, bradykinesia, myotonia and gait by clinicians. Bagrodia et al. (2022) suggested that lack of awareness of Parkinson's disease among patients may increase the prevalence of the disease. The use of digital healthcare platforms embedded with technologies has been suggested to assist in reducing the burden of the disease. Wearable sensors and smartphones are noninvasive approach for effective monitoring of Parkinson's disease symptoms among patients, though some limitations have been suggested such as limited technological capabilities, lack of awareness of wearables devices and cost of digital devices. The approach is noted to promote efficient remote monitoring of symptoms in real time through the support of cost-effective, simple and inconspicuous wearable device.

Mughal et al. (2022) reported that wearable technology is an essential part of mobile health for rehabilitation, treatment, and diagnosis, of several neurodegenerative diseases like Parkinson's disease. The authors suggested that till date, there is no reported standard cure for the diseases, but early intervention, detection and treatment through assistive care can ameliorate the disease. The authors noted that Sensor devices are gaining attention due to the accuracy and low cost for monitoring, detection and management of Parkinson's disease. Reid et al. (2024) noted that digital devices provide huge opportunity in the clinical settings to promptly monitor and detect symptoms associated with Parkinson's disease. These devices can help to gather information for research support and clinical care for the delivery and development of validated measures. de Graaf et al. (2024) showed that the quality of life and functionality is measured by physical activity and capacity. In Parkinson's disease patients, this physical activity is grossly reduced affecting the quality of life of the patients. Thus, wearable sensor technology may provide a solution to enable clinicians monitor, assess and detect changes in physical activity of their patients towards improving personalized treatment strategy.

Polvorinos-Fernández et al. (2025) noted that the monitoring of Parkinson's disease symptoms may be a difficult challenge due to fluctuation, complex nature of disease condition, and the progression of symptoms. Recently, wearable devices with sensors have gained significant attention owing to the ability to accurately and objectively measure parameters in real time across clinical settings among Parkinson's disease patients. Generally, Parkinson's is characterized by complex intrinsic condition with diverse range of nonmotor and motor symptoms. Smart devices and wearable gadgets with sensors like accelerometers, GPS, electromyography, temperature sensors, electrocardiography, magnetometers, and gyroscopes are able to accurately detect, diagnose and monitor physical activity level among Parkinson's patients (Mirelmoan et al. 2022). Yanjie et al. (2025) reported that Parkinson's disease affects over 8.5 million individuals globally impacting negatively on the quality of life. The current method of management using levodopa and brain stimulation are limited and often require constant adjustment. thus, there is need for alternative solution. The use of wearable devices offers real time monitoring to enhance personalized care. Challenges in the use of wearable devices such as comfort, patient adherence and usability blocks widespread adoption of the technology. The authors noted that individuals with Parkinson's disease often witness discomfort, interface difficulties, emotional distress, and low long-term adherence. The author in their study demonstrated that wearable devices assist in managing Parkinson's disease, improve patient's care and support and prevent diseases.

Reichmann et al. (2023) reported that the increasing population of individuals affected by Parkinson's disease is on the rise. These individuals suffer from difficulties in traveling long distances to seek medical attention while some lack adequate care due to insufficient specialist. Thus, newer approaches and options are being suggested such as wearable devices for the management of Parkinson's disease. The development of wearable technology with sensors promotes continuous monitoring and detection of symptoms. The authors noted that smartphone app can detect bradykinesia, voice abnormalities, changes in facial expression and tremor among patients with Parkinson's disease. Silva-Batista et al. (2023) reported that Parkinson's disease may lead to balance impairments leading to fall of the patient.

The authors suggested that telerehabilitation is an emerging area using wearable sensor devices as home based balanced telemedicine and virtual assistance for the monitoring of Parkinson's disease remotely. Moreau et al. (2023) reported that the prevalence of Parkinson's disease is on the rise globally with corresponding decrease in the number of expert neurologists for care. This thus, requires emergency solution in order to ameliorate this situation. The authors noted that the use of innovative tools and wearable sensor-based technology is becoming acceptable measure to combat the complexity of this condition. The advanced technology can provide real time monitoring and detection of symptoms like motor fluctuations, tremor, dyskinesia, bradykinesia, gait disturbances and freezing of gait among Parkinson's disease patients.

Thankathuraipandian et al. (2024) reported that digital health devices are emerging ways to solve the challenges associated with the diagnosis, monitoring and treatment of Parkinson's disease among patients. The authors demonstrated that the conventional approach such as the use of deep brain stimulation may be difficult to maintain, limited accessibility, and discrete assessments. Thus, mobile health platforms and Wearable technology may provide alternative solutions to the current challenges in Parkinson's management. Furthermore, remote monitoring, digital biomarkers can be utilized for real-time virtual programming, data collection, identify the symptoms, onset, side-effects, and medication-linked fluctuations. Yue-meng et al. (2024) reported that among Parkinson's disease patients, 60% of them suffer from dopaminergic neuron damage with irreversible features. Thus, early diagnosis and timely intervention is needed to ameliorate the condition. The authors suggested that the advancement in the development of digital health technology has enhanced the impact of digital biomarkers in early detection, treatment evaluation and monitoring of Parkinson's disease. van Uem et al. (2016) noted that wearable devices could be utilized for the measurement of health-related quality of life among Parkinson's disease patients. Rapidly evolving new technologies like wearable devices have been reported to facilitate patient-driven management changes, enhancing likelihood of improvements in wellbeing, enabling greater control by Parkinson's disease patients and health-related quality of life (Olaniyan et al., 2022a; 2022b; 2022c; 2022d; 2022e; 2022f; 2022g). Xu et al. (2025) reported that great progress has been made in assessing motor dysfunction using wearable technology, little focus has been seen in the bulbar challenge such as swallowing difficulty in Parkinson's disease. The authors suggested that digital health solution can leverage upon advanced acousto-mechanic sensors for the evaluation of bulbar and motor dysfunction via artificial intelligence-enhanced haptic bio-feedback to improve swallowing rate in Parkinson's disease.

Digital and Wearable Technology

Apple Watch

The Apple Watch Parkinson Disease symptom device utilizes inbuilt motion senso to monitor and process symptoms like tremors, gaits and dyskinesia. The device can track several events such as adverse effects, medication use, patient-reported outcomes like mood, and overall physiological health parameters like sleep, fall detection, mobility, heart rate variation and blood pressure.

Garmin Vívomove

The Garmin Vívomove is described as a smartwatch device that is able to track different sleep, fall, stress and movement patterns to support the management resources.

Fitbit Sense

The Fitbit Sense is described as a smartwatch device for the tracking of day-to-day activity, stress levels, fall and sleep pattern among patients.

Amazfit GTS 2

The Amazfit GTS 2 is described as a smartwatch tool that can track and monitor daily events such as sleep, stress and fall movement among patients.

Parkinson's Kinetigraph

This is a wearable device and mobile app combine together for tracking movement patterns among patients with Parkinson's disease. This app provides a range of tools for monitoring and tracking medications use, symptoms, support and accessing educational resources. There are different wearable technologies for monitoring and detecting Parkinson’s disease such as PKG, STAT- ON, Kinesia360 and KinesiaU, PDMonitor, Cala Trio, MotiMove, Tremelo, Gondola, Bravo, SKYWALK, Dyna Port7, Feet-me, MATRIX, mobility Lab and CUE1 as shown in figure 10.1. These technologies are specific, sensitive and accurate in generating information regarding Parkinson’s disease.

Figure 1. Digital and Wearable Technology in Therapeutic Monitoring of Parkinson's Disease

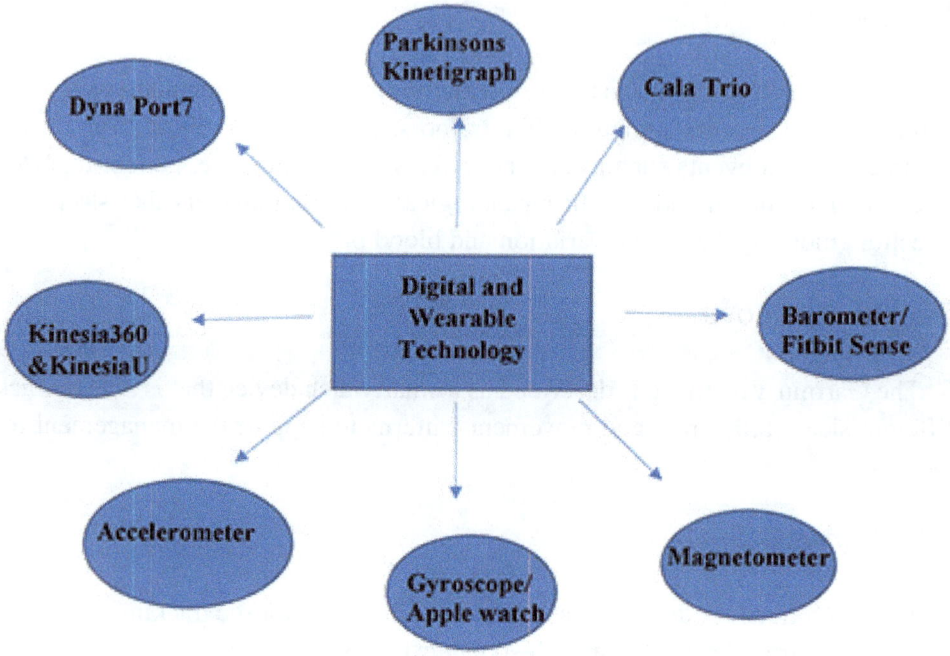

CHALLENGES, LIMITATIONS AND FUTURE PERSPECTIVES

There are increasing effort to encourage patients with Parkinson's disease to utilize wearable digital technology for the management of the condition. These devices provide simple solution to complex problems like associated symptoms linked to the disease. Some of the limitations encounter with the use of wearable and digital devices for the monitoring and measurement of symptoms is that many devices cannot successfully quantify the main feature of Parkinson's disease such as gait, tremor, and Parkinson's kinetograph. In addition, there is general lack of consensus on the main feature of Parkinson's disease for monitoring and diagnosis. Furthermore, lack of empirical data on non-motor symptoms monitoring and diagnosis using wearable digital technology is missing. It is suggested that wearable digital technologies are only designed to monitor physical parameters rather than cognitive aspects. As promising as the topic is, there is currently lack of commercially available wearable digital devices for the monitoring and diagnosis of Parkinson's disease in clinical settings even though many has been approved. The necessary platforms or algorithm to support these wearable devices for compatibility are lacking. More of the available wearable digital technologies are not compatible with each other. In general, wearable digital technology have been reported to reshape and significantly contribute to the landscape of healthcare system globally among people living with Parkinson's disease, the realization of the full potential has not been achieved. To fully achieve this, there must be consensus guidelines on sone important aspect of monitoring, diagnosis and treatment in the treatment of Parkinson's disease.

Most often, research around wearable digital devices is centered on technologically advanced countries thus excluding lower resource based socioeconomic communities. Targeted research for inclusivity of these poor communities will strengthen advancing the utilization of wearable digital technology for the monitoring of Parkinson's disease. For broader perspective, infusing the experiences of caregivers, patient's perspectives and health care professional will provide more valuable information on the acceptability of these technologies. In the algorithm domain, some of the results generated by wearable digital devices are difficult to interpret like statistical interpretability and explainability of model prediction mechanisms. This further reduce the implementation of the technology in clinical settings. Many of the studies reported in this review focused on monitoring parameters such as tremor and gait while leaving other aspects such as postural instability, dyskinesia, and rigidity. Most of the studies evaluated in this review showed significant heterogeneity in intervention types, design, outcome measures and target symptoms affecting the generalization of efficient outcomes and sizes. Future research should focus more in providing model performance comparison between study. Research focus on reliability and accuracy in symptom measurement by devices should be reduced but more of assessment in terms of potential for actively reducing symptoms by delivery of therapeutic effects, neurostimulation, feedback mechanism, and therapeutic exercise. More studies should be focused on ideally randomized controlled trials, clinical trial designs, and evaluating the effectiveness of wearable technologies in alleviating symptoms.

CONCLUSION

This chapter gives an overview on the role of digital and wearable technology in therapeutic monitoring of Parkinson's disease. Many of these wearable devices are able to provide feedback mechanisms, cognitive impairment, sleep/autonomic and gastrointestinal comorbidities using real-time physiological and pathological indices with embedded sensors that help track various signals. The various signals that are picked up by sensors are sleep, cerebral oxygenation, heart rate variability, metabolites, and waves that are linked to Parkinson's disease. Rapidly evolving new technologies like wearable devices have been reported to facilitate patient-driven management changes, enhancing likelihood of improvements in wellbeing, enabling greater control by Parkinson's disease patients and health-related quality of life.

REFERENCES

Adetunji, C. O., Olaniyan, O. T., Adeyomoye, O., Dare, A., Adeniyi, M. J., & Alex, E. (2022a). *Classification of neurodegenerative disorders using machine learning techniques. In book: ARTIFICIAL INTELLIGENCE FOR NEUROLOGICAL DISORDERS. Publisher*. Elsevier., DOI: 10.1016/B978-0-323-90277-9.00028-6

Adetunji, C. O., Olaniyan, O. T., Adeyomoye, O., Dare, A., Adeniyi, M. J., & Alex, E. (2022b). *An intelligent diagnostic approach for epileptic seizure detection and classification using machine learning. In book: ARTIFICIAL INTELLIGENCE FOR NEUROLOGICAL DISORDERS. Publisher*. Elsevier., DOI: 10.1016/B978-0-323-90277-9.00011-0

Bacanoiu, M. V., Rusu, L., Marin, M. I., Piele, D., Rusu, M. R., Danoiu, R., & Danoiu, M. (2025). Digital Health in Parkinson's Disease and Atypical Parkinsonism—New Frontiers in Motor Function and Physical Activity Assessment [Review]. *Journal of Clinical Medicine*, *2025*(14), 4140. DOI: 10.3390/jcm14124140 PMID: 40565895

Bagrodia, V., Vikram, V.H., Nitish, L.K., Pramod, K.P., & Ravi, Y. (2022). Parkinson's Disease and Wearable Technology: An Indian Perspective. Annals of Indian Academy of Neurology | Published by Wolters Kluwer – Medknow. Vol 25(5). 817-820. DOI: .DOI: 10.4103/aian.aian_653_22

Bougea, A. (2025). Application of Wearable Sensors in Parkinson's Disease: State of the Art. *J. Sens. Actuator Netw.*, *2025*(14), 23. DOI: 10.3390/jsan14020023

Bruno, B. G., Gabriel, D. A., Daniel, G. Q., Vanessa, M. H., Thiago, J., & Marcelo, B. T. (2019). Parkinson's disease and wearable devices, new perspectives for a public health issue: An integrative literature review. *Revista da Associação Médica Brasileira*, *65*(11), 1413–1420. DOI: 10.1590/1806-9282.65.11.1413 PMID: 31800906

Channa, A., Nirvana, P., & Vlad, C. (2020). Wearable Solutions for Patients with Parkinson's Disease and Neurocognitive Disorder: A Systematic Review. *Sensors (Basel)*, *2020*(20), 2713. DOI: 10.3390/s20092713 PMID: 32397516

Channa, A., Ruggeri, G., Ifrim, R. C., Mammone, N., Iera, A., & Popescu, N. (2024). Cloud-Connected Bracelet for Continuous Monitoring of Parkinson's Disease Patients: Integrating Continuous Wavelet Transform and AlexNet Network. *Electronics (Basel)*, *2024*(13), 1002. DOI: 10.3390/electronics13061002 de Graaf, D., de Vries, N. M., van de Zande, T., Schimmel, J. J. P., Shin, S., Kowahl, N., Barman, P., Kapur, R., Marks, W. J., Jr., van 't Hul, A., & Bloem, B. R. (2024). Measuring Physical Functioning Using Wearable Sensors in Parkinson Disease and Chronic Obstructive Pulmonary Disease (the Accuracy of Digital Assessment of Performance Trial Study): Protocol for a Prospective Observational Study JMIR Res Protoc 2024; 13: e55452 URL: https://www.researchprotocols.org/2024/1/e55452 doi: DOI: 10.2196/55452

Hirczy, S., Zabetian, C., & Lin, Y. H. (2024). The current state of wearable device uses in Parkinson's disease: A survey of individuals with Parkinson's. *Frontiers in Digital Health, 6*, 1472691. DOI: 10.3389/fdgth.2024.1472691 PMID: 39764207

Kehnemouyi, Y. M., Coleman, T. P., & Tass, P. A. (2024). Emerging wearable technologies for multisystem monitoring and treatment of Parkinson's disease: A narrative review. *Frontiers in Network Physiology, 4*, 1354211. DOI: 10.3389/fnetp.2024.1354211 PMID: 38414636

Kenny, L., Moore, K., O' Riordan, C., Fox, S., Barton, J., Tedesco, S., Sica, M., Crowe, C., Alamäki, A., Condell, J., Nordström, A., & Timmons, S. (2022). The Views and Needs of People with Parkinson Disease Regarding Wearable Devices for Disease Monitoring: Mixed Methods Exploration. *JMIR Formative Research, 6*(1), e27418. https://formative.jmir.org/2022/1/e27418. DOI: 10.2196/27418 PMID: 34989693

Laar, A., Silva de Lima, A. L., Maas, B. R., Bloem, B. R., & de Vries, N. M. (2023). Successful implementation of technology in the management of Parkinson's disease: Barriers and facilitators. *Clinical Parkinsonism & Related Disorders*.

Moreau, C., Tiphaine, R., David, G., Isabelle, B., Philippe, R., Ana-Raquel, M. S. D., Louise-Laure, M., Emmanuel, R., David, D., Gwendoline, D. M. B., & Margherita, F. (2023). Overview on wearable sensors for the management of Parkinson's disease. npj. *Parkinson's Disease, 2023*(9), 153. DOI: 10.1038/s41531-023-00585-y PMID: 37919332

Mughal, H., Abdul, R. J., Muhammad, R., Ahmads, A., & Natalia, K. (2022). *Parkinson's Disease Management via Wearable Sensors: A Systematic Review. IEEE Access. VOLUME 10, 35219- 35237.* Digital Object Identifier., DOI: 10.1109/ACCESS.2022.3162844

Olaniyan, O., Adetunji, C. O., Adeyomoye, O., Dare, A., Adeniyi, M. J., & Enoch, A. (2022g). *Computational methods for translational brain-behavior analysis. In book: ARTIFICIAL INTELLIGENCE FOR NEUROLOGICAL DISORDERS. Publisher.* Elsevier., DOI: 10.1016/B978-0-323-90277-9.00025-0

Olaniyan, O. T., Adetunji, C. O., Adeyomoye, O., Dare, A., Adeniyi, M. J., & Alex, E. (2022a). *Ensemble sparse intelligent mining techniques for cognitive disease. In book: ARTIFICIAL INTELLIGENCE FOR NEUROLOGICAL DISORDERS. Publisher*. Elsevier., DOI: 10.1016/B978-0-323-90277- 9.00027-4

Olaniyan, O. T., Adetunji, C. O., Adeyomoye, O., Dare, A., Adeniyi, M. J., & Alex, E. (2022e). *Cognitive therapy for brain diseases using deep learning models. In book: ARTIFICIAL INTELLIGENCE FOR NEUROLOGICAL DISORDERS. Publisher*. Elsevier., DOI: 10.106/B978-0-323-90277-9.00017-1

Olaniyan, O. T., Adetunji, C. O., Adeyomoye, O., Dare, A., Adeniyi, M. J., & Alex, E. (2022f). *Clinical applications of deep learning in neurology and its enhancements with future directions. In book: ARTIFICIAL INTELLIGENCE FOR NEUROLOGICAL DISORDERS. Publisher*. Elsevier., DOI: 10.1016/B978-0-323-90277-9.00026-2

Olaniyan, O. T., Adetunji, C. O., Dare, A., Adeyomoye, O., Adeniyi, M. J., & Alex, E. (2022b). *Neural signaling and communication using machine learning. In book: ARTIFICIAL INTELLIGENCE FOR NEUROLOGICAL DISORDERS. Publisher*. Elsevier., DOI: 10.1016/B978-0-323-90277-9.00010-9

Olaniyan, O. T., Adetunji, C. O., Dare, A., Adeyomoye, O., Adeniyi, M. J., & Alex, E. (2022c). *New trends in deep learning for neuroimaging analysis and disease prediction. In book: ARTIFICIAL INTELLIGENCE FOR NEUROLOGICAL DISORDERS. Publisher*. Elsevier., DOI: 10.1016/B978-0-323-90277-9.00012-2

Olaniyan, O. T., Adetunji, C. O., Dare, A., Adeyomoye, O., Adeniyi, M. J., & Alex, E. (2022d). *Cognitive therapy for brain diseases using deep learning models. In book: ARTIFICIAL INTELLIGENCE FOR NEUROLOGICAL DISORDERS. Publisher*. Elsevier., DOI: 10.1016/B978-0-323-90277-9.00017-1

Paccoud, I., Valero, M. M., Marín, L. C., Bontridder, N., Ibrahim, A., Winkler, J., Fomo, M., Sapienza, S., Khoury, F., Corvol, J. C., Fröhlich, H., & Klucken, J. (2024). Patient perspectives on the use of digital medical devices and health data for AI-driven personalised medicine in Parkinson's Disease. *Frontiers in Neurology*, *15*, 1453243. DOI: 10.3389/fneur.2024.1453243 PMID: 39697442

Polvorinos-Fernández, C., Sigcha, L., Borzì, L., Olmo, G., Asensio, C., López, J. M., de Arcas, G., & Pavón, I. (2024). Evaluating Motor Symptoms in Parkinson's Disease Through Wearable Sensors: A Systematic Review of Digital Biomarkers. *Applied Sciences (Basel, Switzerland)*, *2024*(14), 10189. DOI: 10.3390/app142210189

Polvorinos-Fernández, C., Sigcha, L., Centeno-Cerrato, M., de Arcas, G., Grande, M., Marín, M., Pareés, I., Martínez-Castrillo, J. C., & Pavón, I. (2025). Evaluation of Free-Living Motor Symptoms in Patients With Parkinson Disease Through Smartwatches: Protocol for Defining Digital Biomarkers JMIR Res Protoc 2025;14: e72820 URL: https://www.researchprotocols.org/2025/1/e72820 doi: DOI: 10.2196/72820

Reichmann, H., Lisa, K., & Jonas, B. (2023). The use of wearables for the diagnosis and treatment of Parkinson's disease. *Journal of Neural Transmission (Vienna, Austria), 2023*(130), 783–791. DOI: 10.1007/s00702-022-02575-5 PMID: 36609737

Reid, K., Emily, B., Johnny, T., Alexander, S., Dawn, L., Judy, N., David, P., Jonathan, N., Siddharthan, C., & Suvankar, P. (2024). Perceptions of digital technology use for monitoring health in people living with neurological disorders. JournaloftheNeurologicalSciences462(2024)123072.

Rodríguez-Martín, D., Cabestany, J., Pérez-López, C., Pie, M., Calvet, J., Samà, A., Capra, C., Català, A., & Rodríguez-Molinero, A. (2022). A New Paradigm in Parkinson's Disease Evaluation With Wearable Medical Devices: A Review of STAT-ONTM. *Frontiers in Neurology, 13*, 912343. DOI: 10.3389/fneur.2022.912343 PMID: 35720090

Ruirui, L., Yan, X., Xiaohui, L., Yongli, F., Weiqi, Z., Yang, T., Kang, R., Wenwu, C., & Xuebing, C. (2020). Evaluation of Wearable Sensor Devices in Parkinson's Disease: A Review of Current Status and Future Prospects. Hindawi Parkinson's Disease Volume 2020, Article ID 4693019, 8 pages https://doi.org/DOI: 10.1155/2020/4693019

Sigchaa, L., Luigi, B., Federica, A., Irene, R., Ramos-Romero, C., Andrés, C., Luis, G., & Gabriella, O. (2023). Deep learning and wearable sensors for the diagnosis and monitoring of Parkinson's disease: A systematic review. *Expert Systems with Applications, 229*, 120541.

Silva-Batista, C., Jennifer, L. W., Kathleen, T. S., Margaret, S., Carlson-Kuhta, P., Siting, C., William, L., Tomas, N. G de la H., Fay, B. H., Martina, M., & Laurie, A. K. (2023). Balance telerehabilitation and wearable technology for people with Parkinson's disease (TelePD trial). *BMC Neurology, 3*, 33. DOI: 10.1186/s12883-023-03403-3 PMID: 37833645

Terry, M.A., & Alvarez-Vazquez, E. (2017). Efficacy of Wearable Devices in Monitoring and Treating Parkinson's Disease Symptoms: A Systematic Review and Meta Analyses. Preparation of Papers for IEEE Access. 1-9. DOI DOI: 10.1109/ACCESS.2025.3569056

Terry, M. A., & Vazquez, E. (2025). *Efficacy of Wearable Devices in Monitoring and Treating Parkinson's Disease Symptoms: A Systematic Review and Meta Analyses. IEEE. 13. 84240-84258.* Digital Object Identifier., DOI: 10.1109/ACCESS.2025.3569056

Thankathuraipandian, S., Walter, G., Anahita, K., Tucker, T., Binesh, B., Erika, R., & Yagna, P. (2024). Development of a remote therapeutic monitoring platform: applications for movement disorders. Scientific Reports | (2024) 14:29837 | https://doi.org/.DOI: 10.1038/s41598-024-80567-z

Toshiki, T., Etsuro, N., Hiroo, S., Katsumi, S., Satoru, I., Shinji, A., Satomi, Y., Tanaka-Mizuno, S., Kayoko, M., Ryosuke, T., & Koji, K. (2024). Adherence to istradefylline in patients with Parkinson's disease: A group-based trajectory analysis. JournaloftheNeurologicalSciences462(2024)123092.

van Uem, J. M. T., Tom, I., Alan, L., Eros, B., Dina, S., Alberto, J. E., Helen, M., & Walter, M. (2016). AViewpoint on Wearable Technology-Enabled Measurement of Wellbeing and Health-Related Quality of Life in Parkinson's Disease. [IOS Press.]. *Journal of Parkinson's Disease*, *6*, 279–287. DOI: 10.3233/JPD-150740 PMID: 27003779

Xu, S., Cagla, K., Keum, S.C., Rabab, R., Dylan, R., Abigail, N., Keum, S.C., Dylan, R., Albert-Smet, I., Matthew, K., Hope, C., Joy, H., Shiv, P., Jacqueline, T., Albert, Y., Aejin, S., Jessica, W., Sarah, C., Hyoyoung, J., Jong, Y.L., & Martin-Harris, B., (2025). Digital health technology for Parkinson's disease with comprehensive monitoring and artificial intelligence-enabled haptic biofeedback for bulbar dysfunction. Journal of Parkinson's Disease 2025, Vol. 15(3) 630–645 © The Author(s) 2025 Article reuse guidelines: sagepub.com/journals-permissions DOI: .DOI: 10.1177/1877718X251329354

Yanjie, M., Yifan, Z., Rui, L., Wenlin, C., & Fang, W. (2025). The experience and perception of wearable devices in Parkinson's disease patients: A systematic review and meta-synthesis of qualitative studies. *Journal of Neurology*, *2025*(272), 350. DOI: 10.1007/s00415-025-13085-1 PMID: 40252116

Ymeri, G., Salvi, D., Olsson, C. M., Wassenburg, M. V., Tsanas, A., & Svenningsson, P. (2023). Quantifying Parkinson's disease severity using mobile wearable devices and machine learning: The ParkApp pilot study protocol. *BMJ Open*, *13*, e077766. DOI: 10.1136/ bmjopen-2023-077766 PMID: 38154904

Yue-meng, S., Zhi-yun, W., Yuan-yuan, L., Chen-wei, H., & Chang-heShi, (2024). Digital biomarkers for precision diagnosis and monitoring in Parkinson's disease. npj | digital medicine. 7:218. https://doi.org/.DOI: 10.1038/s41746-024-01217-2

Yuexuan, L. (2024). *Development of Wearable Medical Devices in Parkin son's Disease. In2024InternationalConferenceonSmartHealthcareandWear able Intelligent Devices (SHWID2024), October18–20, 2024, Guangzhou, China*. ACM., DOI: 10.1145/3703847.3703874

Chapter 9

Transcranial Magnetic Stimulation as a Novel Therapeutic Strategy for Parkinson's Disease in Under-Resourced Settings

Alexander Zakharov
http://orcid.org/0000-0003-1709-6195
Samara State Medical University, Russia

Yuliya Komarova
http://orcid.org/0000-0003-3435-1477
Samara State Medical University, Russia

Mariya Sergeeva
http://orcid.org/0000-0002-0926-8551
Samara State Medical University, Russia

Igor Shirolapov
http://orcid.org/0000-0002-7670-6566
Samara State Medical University, Russia

Elena Khivintseva
http://orcid.org/0000-0002-1878-7951
Samara State Medical University, Russia

Vladimir Kalinin
http://orcid.org/0009-0004-0440-2928
Samara State Medical University, Russia

Natalia Romanchuk
Samara State Medical University, Russia

DOI: 10.4018/979-8-3373-7437-6.ch009

ABSTRACT

Parkinson's disease (PD) is a progressive neurodegenerative disorder characterized not only by motor deficits but also by cognitive impairment and network-level dysfunction. This chapter explores the therapeutic potential of Transcranial Magnetic Stimulation (TMS), a non-invasive neuromodulation technique. We posit that TMS can directly target maladaptive cortico-subcortical dynamics—such as pathological beta oscillations—and induce beneficial neuroplasticity, thereby addressing both motor and cognitive symptoms. The rationale for network-level intervention is supported by empirical data linking functional connectivity patterns, measured via EEG and source localization, to working memory performance. By reviewing physiological mechanisms, clinical protocols, and methodological integration, we argue that TMS represents a paradigm shift towards personalized, circuit-based remediation in PD, offering a promising adjunct to standard therapies for treatment-resistant symptoms.

INTRODUCTION

Parkinson's disease (PD) is one of the most common neurodegenerative diseases in the world and poses a serious challenge to the global health system. The epidemiological feature of PD is that its prevalence and morbidity continue to grow, surpassing the rate of population aging. According to the 2019 Global Burden of Disease Report, from 1990 to 2021, the number of people with Parkinson's disease increased by hundreds of %, and the global prevalence of the disease is approximately 1.51 cases per 1,000 people of all ages. This trend persists even after statistical adjustments are made to take into account the age structure of the population, indicating the influence of factors unrelated to life expectancy (Yang et al., 2026). A recent meta-analysis confirmed these findings and showed that the prevalence of the disease increased significantly after the age of 60 and was close to 1% in the elderly (Pringsheim et al., 2014). This growth cannot be explained only by the aging of the population. Important factors leading to the spread of the disease are considered to be the evolution of diagnostic criteria, increased access to medical care, more frequent detection of preclinical stages, and possible changes in the environment and lifestyle (Zhu et al., 2024). These data highlight the emergence of a persistent global trend that positions PD as an increasingly relevant medical and social issue, requiring interdisciplinary research and clinical attention.

The clinical manifestations of PD are very diverse and are not limited to the main motor symptoms. PD has traditionally been classified as a movement disorder based on three characteristics: tremor at rest, muscle stiffness, and slow movement (Postuma & Berg, 2016). However, studies have shown that clinical phenotypes include a wide range of low-dynamic manifestations, such as cognitive impairment, neuropsychiatric symptoms (such as depression, apathy), sensitivity problems, and autonomic nervous dysfunction (Asuku et al., 2024; Asuku et al., 2025). It is important to note that many of these non-motor symptoms may appear in the early stages of the disease, years or even decades before the onset of traditional motor symptoms (Poewe, 2008). Scientists are increasingly concluding that Parkinson's disease is not one disease, but multiple diseases, and treatments should take this into account. Patients can be very different from each other. Some people may have tremors, others may have stiffness and slow movement, and others may have balance and gait problems. In addition, there are forms of disease in which non-motor symptoms play a significant role, such as changes in mood, sleep, or smell. More and more evidence shows that genetics is one of the main factors that determine the course of Parkinson's disease in a particular population. In the future, personalized medical methods such as transcranial magnetic stimulation (TMS) are likely to be tailored according to the patient's genetic characteristics, affecting the selection of target areas and stimulating neuroplasticity (Kalinderi et al., 2019).

When using clustering methods to analyze data, it is clear that different types of diseases represent more than just clinical differences. They reflect significant differences in the underlying process, rate of progress, and treatment effect (Deng et al., 2025). This study confirms the need to shift from considering PD as a single nosological condition to studying its spectrum as a heterogeneous neurodegenerative syndrome. Pathological changes caused by α-synuclein The accumulation of α-synuclein is related to neurodegeneration and impaired protein excretion, especially in the glandular system, where aquaporin-4 plays an important role (I. Shirolapov et al., 2023).

Cognitive impairment, especially working memory defects, is a distinctive feature of this diverse phenotype, and it is also a good prognostic factor that determines the degree of disability and quality of life. Working memory is one of the most fragile cognitive functions in neurodegenerative diseases. Working memory disorders are observed in 40-60% of patients with PD, and are usually associated with broader executive dysfunction due to weakening of the anterior striatum connection (Komarova et al., 2025; Owen, 2004). These violations are manifested as a decrease in the amount of information, a slowdown in data processing speed, an increase in the number of errors during psychological operations, and the difficulty of retaining task-related information in memory. This symptom is used as a sensitive marker for progressive deterioration of the condition, and is increasingly becoming the subject of diagnosis and treatment research. The various manifestations of the phenotype of Parkinson's disease affect motor activity, cognitive function, and mental state, which emphasizes the systemic nature of the disease. Neuromorphological studies have shown that pathological alpha-synuclein (lewy body) is widely present in the brainstem, limbic structures, cerebral cortex, and the nuclei of the peripheral autonomic and enteric nervous systems (Halliday & Murphy, 2010). This multifocal disease is accompanied by the progressive appearance of precursor symptoms, such as hypoglycemia, (Rapid Eye Movement) REM sleep behavior disorders, and autonomic dysfunction of the gastrointestinal tract (Mahlknecht et al., 2015). Systematically identify people at risk through large-scale prospective studies such as «PPMI» and «PROSPECT». In vivo biomarkers, such as skin biopsy for detecting phosphorylated alpha-synuclein and amplification in cerebrospinal fluid, are revolutionizing the field of early and accurate diagnosis, and may even allow the use of neuroprotective therapy before the onset of dyskinesia (Gibbons et al., 2024).

Among non-motor symptoms, some autonomic nervous disorders, such as orthostatic hypotension and severe constipation, are increasingly seen as clear signs of accelerated disease development and cognitive impairment. Their severity is usually reflected in the first part of the Parkinson's Disease Severity Scale (MDS-UPDRS), which provides useful prognostic information that can be used to stratify patients during clinical trials and treatment plans.

Levodopa, a precursor of dopamine, continues to form the basis of drug treatment for Parkinson's disease. It still does not have the equal ability to reduce key movement disorders, especially slow movement and muscle stiffness. This is why it can be regarded as the "gold standard" of treatment. However, with long-term use of levodopa, its limitations and risks become clearer, which clearly highlights the purely symptomatic nature of the drug and its impact on the disease process. One of the most common and difficult-to-control complications is drug-induced dyskinesia, which develops a few years after treatment begins. They are based on obvious striatal denervation and related non-physiological pulse stimulation of dopamine receptors, which significantly limits the possibility of purely pharmacological correction (Bezard et al., 2001). In addition, the progress of PD is accompanied by systemic diseases, especially dysfunction of the glandular system, which may contribute to the accumulation of toxic proteins and accelerate neurodegeneration (Shirolapov et al., 2023). Amantadine is considered an effective remedy to reduce the severity of dyskinesia, but its use is usually limited by side effects, and it remains an exception among the few successful alternatives (Oertel & Schulz, 2016). Melatonin is considered an additional treatment method because of its neuroprotective properties and its ability to improve sleep patterns in PD patients (Zakharov et al., 2017).

In addition to dyskinesia, the treatment window of levodopa narrows over time, which leads to movement fluctuations-debilitating phenomena of "dose depletion" and "on-off" fluctuations that seriously impair the quality of life. Further dose increases often lead to poor tolerance: psychotic episodes, impulse control disorders, orthostatic hypotension and sleep disorders often force doctors to stop, forcing doctors to choose between symptom control and the risk of side effects. It is worth noting that many disabled manifestations show significant resistance to dopaminergic therapy. Axial dyskinesia-unstable posture, stiffness when walking, dysphonia poor correction of levodopa, has become the main cause of falls and loss of independence (Gao et al., 2020).

When the possibility of drug treatment is exhausted, invasive surgical methods appear, mainly deep stimulation of the inferior ocular nucleus or the inner segment of the globus pallidus. In carefully selected patients, Deep Brain Stimulation (DBS) provided significant improvements: it reduced the duration of tremors, "shutdowns" and movement disorders, increased motor activity and quality of life (Deuschl et al., 2006). But this method is not universal either. Its use is limited by strict selection criteria: significant cognitive impairment, mental impairment or old age as contraindications. Surgery carries the risk of bleeding, infection, and complications associated with the implant, and requires complex, long-term programming of the stimulator. Most importantly, like levodopa, DBS is ineffective in the symptoms of levodopa resistance and many non-motor manifestations. A newer technique, focused ultrasound under magnetic resonance imaging (MRI) control, provides a less invasive way to unilaterally destroy the thalamus or globus pallidus. However, the evidence base for a wide range of PD symptoms, especially gait and balance disorders, is still not as good as traditional methods, and long-term results and safety profiles require further research (Helmers et al., 2025).

A common and fundamental disadvantage of all these methods is that their focus is mainly on regulating the effector link of a single node of the dopamine nigra striatum system or the basal-thalamic-cortical motor circuit. At the same time, the actual pathological reorganization of the neural network that is the basis of PD still exceeds the direct impact. As mentioned earlier, PD is increasingly considered to be a disorder of distributed neural networks today, characterized by pathological synchronization (mainly excessive β activity on electroencephalogram), impaired interregional interactions, and loss of adaptive plasticity of cortical-subcortical connections (Jahanshahi et al., 1995). Exercise deficiency is not just the result of dopamine deficiency, but the result of unbalanced network frequency patterns and ineffective participation of compensatory cortical resources. Cognitive impairment, especially working memory impairment, is related to dysfunction of the frontal lobe and frontal lobe network. Although its activity depends on the level of dopamine, it is far from restricted by it.

Therefore, there is still an urgent need for methods that can directly affect the pathokinetics of neural networks. The ideal method can not only reduce symptoms, but also change the nature of the connections between nerves, enhance the compensatory process, and promote adaptive plasticity. In this field of treatment of defects, non-invasive brain stimulation methods, mainly rhythmic transcranial magnetic stimulation, are of particular interest. By affecting cortical regions from the outside, rhythmic transcranial magnetic stimulation (rTMS) enables the regulation of neuronal excitability, affects oscillatory activity, and rebuilds functional connections in pathologically changed networks.

In order to more clearly identify the treatment niche and justify the use of TMS in PD, it should be compared with other key treatment methods. Table 1 shows the comparative characteristics of the main methods-rhythmic TMS, deep brain stimulation, transcranial direct current stimulation and standard dopaminergic therapy. The comparison is based on key parameters: aggressiveness, level of action and mechanism, main advantages and limitations, usage instructions and safety profile. As can be seen from the table, TMS occupies a unique position: it is a noninvasive method that allows targeted action on the cortical nodes of a distributed network. This is the ability that systemic drug therapy lacks and is not obvious in other noninvasive stimulation methods.

Table 1. Comparison of Neuromodulation Techniques and Pharmacotherapy in Parkinson's Disease

Parameter	TMS (rTMS / TBS)	Deep Brain Stimulation (DBS)	Transcranial Direct Current Stimulation (tDCS)	Standard Pharmacotherapy (Levodopa)
Invasiveness	Non-invasive (external)	Invasive (neurosurgical)	Non-invasive (external)	Non-invasive (systemic)
Level of Action	Cerebral cortex (superficial)	Deep nuclei (subthalamic nucleus, globus pallidus internus)	Cerebral cortex (superficial)	Systemic, with predominant action on the nigrostriatal pathway
Mechanism	Electromagnetic induction; modulation of cortical excitability and network connectivity	High-frequency electrical stimulation; suppression of pathological nuclei activity	Weak direct current; modulation of neuronal membrane potential	Dopamine precursor; replenishment of neurotransmitter deficit
Key Advantages	Focality, favorable safety profile, potential for network targeting, non-invasiveness	Powerful and sustained effect on core motor symptoms, correction of dyskinesias	Low cost, portability, potential for home-based use	"Gold standard," powerful and rapid effect on hypokinesia and rigidity, wide availability

continued on following page

Table 1. Continued

Parameter	TMS (rTMS / TBS)	Deep Brain Stimulation (DBS)	Transcranial Direct Current Stimulation (tDCS)	Standard Pharmacotherapy (Levodopa)
Key Limitations	Moderate effect size, short-lived aftereffects, protocol heterogeneity, high equipment cost	Surgical risks (hemorrhage, infection), strict selection criteria, limited efficacy for axial and cognitive symptoms	Low focality and penetration depth, weak evidence base in PD, variable individual response	Side effects (dyskinesias, psychosis), development of motor fluctuations, resistance of axial and many non-motor symptoms
Indications (in PD)	Adjunctive therapy for motor fluctuations, mild cognitive impairment, postural instability (investigational/adjuvant status)	Severe motor fluctuations and medication-induced dyskinesias, refractory tremor in carefully selected patients	Investigational method, studied for depression, fatigue, cognitive impairment (primarily within clinical trials)	First-line therapy for core motor symptoms at all disease stages
Safety Profile	Excellent; rare transient headaches, scalp discomfort; very low seizure risk with protocol adherence	Substantial; surgical and hardware-related complications, risks of neuropsychiatric changes	Excellent; mild tingling or burning under electrodes	Satisfactory; high risk of long-term motor and neuropsychiatric complications

Rationale for Non-Invasive Neuromodulation

The mature "Substantia nigra striatum model" of PD directly leads to the depletion of striatum dopamine reserves, and provides an extremely important but still incomplete picture of the disease. Understanding this model is not enough to capture the full complexity of PD, nor is it enough to develop a truly comprehensive treatment. The degeneration of dopaminergic neurons in the compact part of the substantia nigra is still the pathological anatomical basis of diagnosis-it is indisputable. However, modern research has no doubt that PD is a multisystem neurodegenerative disease. The pathological staging scheme shows how alpha-synuclein aggregates spread from bottom to top, capturing the trunk (blue area, dorsal nucleus of vagus nerve), limbic structures (amygdala, hippocampus), basal ganglia, and ultimately the cerebral cortex. This process begins long before the first motor symptoms appear (Takahashi & Wakabayashi, 2001). It is precisely because of this extensive pathological matrix that the precursor period is related to its non-motor performance. Therefore, the inevitable conclusion is: the clinical manifestations of PD include the failure of several large-scale neural network operations and the interruption of their interactions.

Therefore, modern thinking on the pathogenesis of Parkinson's disease has changed from a model where everything is explained by the lack of a neurotransmitter to a model that focuses on the dysfunction of distributed neural networks. We are talking about the pathological synchronization of activities (especially in the β range), the weakening of the connection between regions and plasticity disorders. In this context, TMS seems to be not just another symptom remedy, but a fundamentally different approach: by non-intrusively and specifically affecting the cortical nodes of the affected network, it allows you to directly.

This has led to several interrelated treatment hypotheses, which are well integrated into the network model:

1. Normalization of pathological oscillatory activity. High-frequency rhythmic TMS (≥5Hz) targeting the primary motor cortex or additional motor areas can inhibit excessive β synchronization in the cortical-basal-thalamic-cortical ring. This releases the motor system from the pathological "frozen" state and promotes the beginning of exercise (Li et al., 2020).
2. Strengthen compensation procedures. Stimulation of the premotor cortex or dorsolateral prefrontal cortex can stimulate the activity of alternative, less dopamine-dependent pathways. In fact, it supports those compensatory mechanisms that the patient's body has tried to use to avoid striatal dysfunction. The result is improved exercise planning, exercise preparation, and cognitive motor control.
3. Change the function connection. Under the influence of TMS, not only the intensity changes, but the connection pattern between the stimulated area and the remote area also changes. For example, DLPFC stimulation can normalize the damaged frontal chamber connection responsible for controlling function. And exposure to additional exercise areas can strengthen its connection to M1, which directly affects gait .
4. Restoration of cortical plasticity. In PD, the long-term enhancement mechanism of synapses is affected. Protocols such as intermittent theta flashes, which mimic natural theta rhythm and cause long-term potentiation (LTP) - like changes, can partially reverse this deficit. There is reason to believe that the effect here may be more lasting (Suppa et al., 2017).

Therefore, TMS should not be regarded as another way to eliminate symptoms. This is a targeted strategy aimed at restoring network operation. Using the natural pathway of signal transmission in the brain, she tried to directly correct the pathological dynamics of motor and non-motor symptoms. In this sense, it is closer to a modern, networked understanding of PD.

PHYSIOLOGICAL FOUNDATIONS AND MECHANISMS OF TMS ACTION IN PD

Basic Principles and Biophysics of TMS

Transcranial magnetic stimulation refers to a non-invasive method in which an electric current coil placed on the scalp generates an electric field in the brain tissue, capable of transferring the membrane potential of neurons to depolarization or hyperpolarization (Guerra et al., 2021).

However, when repeated pulses—the rTMS applied, the key neuromodulatory effects of this method are revealed. The direction of cortical excitability changes depends on the protocol parameters and persists from a few minutes to a few hours after the stimulation ends, indicating the induction of synaptic plasticity. According to the classic, although somewhat simplified scheme, high-frequency rTMS (from 5Hz and above) enhances cortical excitability, while low-frequency rTMS (1Hz and below) has an inhibitory effect (Lefaucheur et al., 2020). The nature of these sequelae is usually considered to be related to a mechanism similar to the long-term enhancement and inhibition of synaptic transmission, which involves the N-methyl-D-aspartate (NMDA) receptor pathway (Huang et al., 2005).

With the introduction of theta flash stimulation, the development of this method has taken a qualitative leap. This is a patterned protocol that reproduces the natural theta rhythm of the hippocampus. Intermittent theta-burst stimulation (iTBS), in which the two-second burst of three pulses at 50Hz is repeated every 10 seconds, gives a major activation effect, while continuous theta-burst stimulation (cTBS), lasts for 40 seconds without pause, resulting in activity suppression. The theta-burst stimulation (TBS) is not as good as classic rTMS in terms of total pulse count and session duration, but tends to surpass it in terms of modulation severity and duration, which makes them more convenient in clinical practice (Suppa et al., 2017).

Today, the joint registration of TMS and EEG is actively used to analyze the rearrangement of neural network levels. The TMS-EEG method can directly evaluate the cortical response to magnetic stimulation with millisecond accuracy, and obtain data on the local excitability and effective connectivity of the cortical area-and there is no need to refer to motor behavior or conscious informational indicators are the amplitude and spatial distribution of the evoked potential, its oscillation component, and the signal complexity index (Formaggio et al., 2023). As pointed out in modern reviews, this combination of techniques makes it possible to non-intrusively assess the neuronal excitability and functional connectivity of the area of interest, which is important for basic research and the diagnosis of pathological conditions.

Use TMS to Regulate of the Cortical-Subcortical Network in PD

It is important to understand that strictly dividing effects into "stimulation" and "inhibition" is a significant simplification. The final result of stimulation depends on many variables: the initial functional state of the cortex in the affected area, the type of activated neurons and insertion circuits, the structural and functional connections of the stimulated area, and the oscillatory activity of the brain when a pulse is applied (Duecker & Sack, 2015). This ambiguity is particularly obvious in the neurodynamics of pathological changes in patients with PD, in which the basal excitability of the cortex, inhibitory processes (for example, short-delayed intracortical inhibition) and network synchronization are impaired.

According to one of the key hypotheses, high-frequency rTMS in the primary motor cortex inhibits the pathological β activity characteristics of PD. There is evidence that this stimulation reduces the power of β oscillations in local and related cortical regions, contributes to the "smooth flow" of the motor system and restores its dynamic flexibility (Li et al., 2020).

The impact of TMS depends on the selected target, which makes it possible to target specific symptoms. Stimulation of the supplementary motor area (SMA), which is responsible for the initiation and sequence of movement, as well as internal cues, has shown its effectiveness in axial disorders, especially in the case of stiff gait. PD is characterized by the dysfunction of SMA and its weakened connection to M1. High-frequency rTMS or iTBS targeting SMA increased its excitability and restored functional interaction with the motor cortex, which was accompanied by improved gait and reduced freezing episodes (Kim et al., 2019). Studies combining TMS and functional magnetic resonance imaging have confirmed that SMA stimulation not only causes changes in blood oxygenation level dependent (BOLD) signals in the cortex, but also causes changes in BOLD signals in subcortical structures (such as the subcranial nucleus, thalamus, and shell), indicating that the effect.

Stimulating the dorsolateral prefrontal cortex (DLPFC) is a classic method of treating depression. By affecting the networks related to cognitive and emotional processes, it also has a positive impact on PD. Exposure to DLPFC can correct damaged frontal striatum interactions and improve working memory and control functions.

Moreover, it can influence motor network dynamics indirectly; for example, by reducing excessive inhibitory connectivity from the DLPFC to the SMA, it may facilitate motor circuit activity. This underscores the interconnectedness of motor and non-motor networks in PD and highlights how a "cognitive" target can yield motor benefits.

Figure 1. Correlations between brain functional connectivity and accuracy in the 2-back task before TMS.

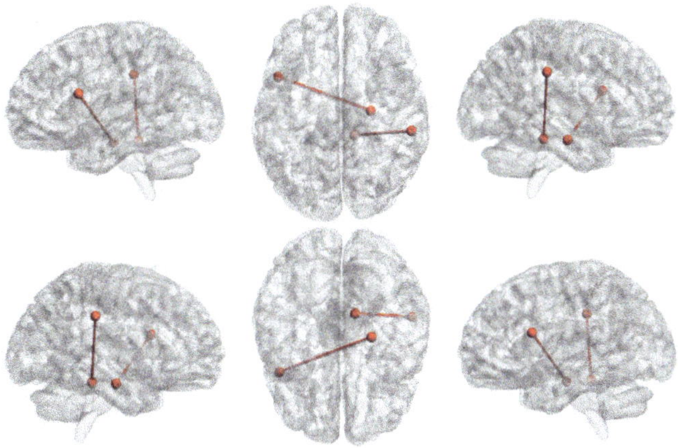

The figure 1 illustrates significant positive correlations between the strength of functional connections in specific brain regions and accuracy on a working memory task (2-back). Notably, a significant association was found between accuracy and the connectivity of the left inferior frontal gyrus (Left Inferior Frontal Gyrus, Opercular Part) with the right parahippocampal gyrus (Right Parahippocampal Gyrus), as well as between the right supramarginal gyrus and the right cerebellar lobule III. These findings indicate the involvement of fronto-limbic and parietal-cerebellar networks in successful working memory performance in the studied group prior to therapeutic intervention.

These correlational maps identify specific connections that are behaviorally relevant. A therapeutic TMS protocol that successfully modulates the strength of these identified pathways, for example, by stimulating a frontal node to enhance its connection to the hippocampus or cerebellum, would provide direct evidence for a network-mediated cognitive improvement.

Activation and Registration of Neuroplasticity

The ability of transcranial magnetic stimulation to provide stable therapeutic transformations in Parkinson's disease directly depends on its impact on neuroplasticity, the nature of nerve tissue reconstruction of synaptic connection strength and recombination under the influence of external factors. A key link in the pathogenesis of PD is the violation of synaptic plasticity, which depends on the activity of neurons, especially in the cortex and striatum. This is obvious. Clinically, this is manifested as a response to weakening or qualitative changes in TMS protocols designed to assess plasticity, such as paired associative stimulation or theta flashes, which indicate a failure of a mechanism similar tlong-term potentiation (Morgante et al., 2006). Such a "plastic deficit" is not only considered to be the reason why motor skills are difficult to form, but also considered to be a factor in the rigidity of motor and cognitive stereotypes, limiting the possibility of compensatory adjustments. Therefore, the key task of the therapeutic use of TMS is to overcome this defect and stimulate the plasticity of adaptive forms.

It is generally believed that the standard rhythmic TMS pattern involves synaptic mechanisms similar to long-term potentiation and long-term depression. As mentioned earlier, high-frequency stimulation (for example, 10 or 20 Hz) and intermittent theta burst protocols usually have aactivating n effect, which increases the excitability of the cortex due to an effect similar to TBS. Conversely, low-frequency TMS (1 Hz) and continuous theta stimulation can lead to inhibition of neuronal activity (Huang et al., 2005). However, the response of the changed Parkinson's brain depends to a large extent on its current functional state. Therefore, the ability of iTBS to trigger plastic rearrangement was significantly reduced during the "shutdown" of dopaminergic therapy, and partially restored after taking levodopa, which emphasizes dopamine as a necessary condition for effectively enhancing synaptic transmission (Suppa et al., 2017). This situation determines the need to carefully monitor drug intake during treatment and shows that TMS can bring the greatest benefits in the context of activating the dopamine link.

To objectify plastic displacement, it is necessary to go beyond biomarkers that record the evoked potential of the motor. In this regard, the combination of TMS and EEG is considered to be one of the most informative methods. This method makes it possible to directly evaluate cortical reactivity and effective connectivity in the stimulated area with a time resolution of up to milliseconds. Among the key EEG markers of TMS-induced plasticity, one can distinguish:

The amplitude and morphology of the TMS evoked potential. Changes in the severity and spatial distribution of response components in the early (up to 100 ms) and late (over 100 ms) stages reflect the rearrangement of cortical local excitability and the response of neural networks to plasticizing effects (Formaggio et al., 2023).

- Oscillating activity: The power and frequency characteristics of the vibration triggered by the magnetic pulse (for example, in the range of α, β, or γ) give the concept of the functional state of the cortical ensemble and its synchronization tendency. In the context of the activation protocol, the weakening of β activity associated with the stimulation moment may be a sign of overcoming the pathological stability of the oscillation pattern.

- An indicator of disturbance complexity: This indicator evaluates the spatial and temporal expansion of the brain's response to a single stimulus, and characterizes the ability of neural networks to integrate information. The increase in this index is seen as a sign of the transition from a rigid, over-synchronized state to a more flexible and adaptive network configuration.

In addition, as described in detail in the review of EEG analysis methods, the use of advanced computational methods, especially graph theory related to resting or cognitive load data, makes it possible to quantify neural network reorganization at the macro level. Indicators such as global efficiency, clustering coefficient, and the severity of the "small world" architecture make it possible to track whether the TMS curriculum brings the topology of the brain network closer to the optimal balance of integration and isolation, and overcomes pathological extremes (excessive disconnection or conversely, chaotic connections).

TMS PROTOCOL AND ITS EFFECT ON PD MOTOR SYMPTOMS

Effect on the Symptoms of Parkinson's Disease

The effect on the primary motor cortex (M1) is the most studied and traditional field of rTMS in PD, because of the key role of this field in achieving exercise and the possibility of objective neurophysiological assessment of the changes caused. The main therapeutic hypothesis is that high-frequency (≥5 Hz) rTMS exceeding M1 increases the excitability of the cortical space tract and modulates pathology to weaken the thalamocortical drive, thereby weakening this basic manifestation as motor slowness and rigidity.

According to the systematic evaluation and meta-analysis of randomized controlled trials, high-frequency M1 stimulation has a moderate but statistically significant positive effect on motor symptoms, as described in Part III of the UPDRS (Lefaucheur et al., 2020). The induced changes are related to the trigger of ltp-like plasticity in the stimulated cortical protrusions, which leads to increased cortical drive. This is also confirmed by promoting an increase in neurophysiological recording of the amplitude of motor evoked potential (MVP) after M1 stimulation, which indicates an increase in cortical spinal cord excitability.

In addition to affecting the efferent pathway, TMS evaluation of the intracortical contour revealed more subtle changes. The pathophysiology of PD is characterized by the imbalance between inhibition and promotion of intracortical mechanisms. Therefore, γ-Aminobutyric acid sub-type A receptors (GABAA) receptor mediated short-delayed intracortical inhibition (SICI) is often reduced, while intracortical remission can vary in different directions. The high-frequency rTMS on M1 can partially normalize these parameters, enhance SICI and shift intracortical remission to more physiological balance.

Modern protocols have enriched pattern patterns, especially intermittent theta burst stimulation (iTBS), with a focus on M1. This protocol achieves a mitigating effect in a physiologically related mode in a short period of time, and compared with the classic rTMS, it exhibits considerable or even higher efficiency in improving motor performance (Suppa et al., 2017). At the same time, the effects of iTBS are characterized by a clear dependence on the disorder: more stable ltp-like changes are recorded in the context of dopaminergic therapy, which emphasizes exogenous neuromodulation and endogenous neurochemistry.

Influence on the Secondary Motor Area

The primary motor cortex (M1) serves as the ultimate executor of commands. However, it is the higher — order regions — SMA and the dorsal premotor cortex (PMd) - that play a key role in the movement disorders of Parkinson's disease. Perhaps the most fragile of these structures provides motor planning, sequence organization, internal initiation and integration of sensory information. In PD, these processes are mainly affected, manifested as akinesia, slow movement and freezing (fog) episodes. This is why stimulating secondary motor areas with TMS is becoming an increasingly popular strategy aimed at correcting complex symptoms of dopamine resistance.

SMA plays a central role in initiating movement "from the inside" without relying on external signals. In PD, the activity of this area is reduced and the connection to the basal ganglia is destroyed, which is directly related to the development and hardening of akinesia (Kim et al., 2019).

In clinical trials, the use of high-frequency rhythmic TMS (10Hz) or intermittent theta flash stimulation (iTBS) on SMA produced promising outcomes. These treatments are intended to promote cortical excitability and cause long-term heightened forms of plastic changes. According to meta-analysis, SMA stimulation can improve walking parameters—stride length, speed, turning-and reduce the frequency of freezing episodes (Kim et al., 2019). The mechanism of action is most likely twofold: on the one hand, the downward flow of signals from the SMA to the motor structure increases, while the abnormal oscillation activity normalizes. High-frequency stimulation of SMA has been shown to inhibit excessive β synchronization in the sensorimotor cortex, and this effect is associated with clinical improvement (Li et al., 2020).

Addressing the Therapeutic Gap: TMS for Axial Symptoms, Gait, and Freezing

Axial symptoms such as unstable posture, gait disorders, and stiffness episodes are one of the most crippling and difficult to treat manifestations of the advanced stage of PD. The weak response to dopaminergic drugs and deep brain stimulation indicates the special pathogenesis of these diseases associated with the participation of the non-dopamine system: the motor center of the brainstem (peduncle nucleus), the cerebellum-thalamus-cortical pathway and the medial frontal cortex (Iansek & Danoudis, 2017).

Axial damage, and, more crucially, fog, are caused by a failure to integrate motor, cognitive, and affective inputs at the super-spine motor network. The major goal here is to support the motor cortex (internal initiation), prefrontal cortex (executive control, conflict resolution), and primary motor cortex (motor realization). The breakdown of the connection between these areas and the subcortical center results in the fact that automatic stereotyped movements-especially when turning, multitasking, or in restricted spaces-are no longer properly produced. (Kelly et al., 2012).

The TMS method makes it possible to influence these mechanisms at the cortical level. As mentioned earlier, SMA is becoming the main target. The high-frequency rhythmic TMS or iTBS in this area is designed to compensate for its dysfunction and enhance the descending path of internal steps to initiate and activate the spine pattern generator. According to clinical studies, this stimulation can objectively improve walking parameters (stride length, pace, variability) and subjectively reduce freezing frequency. Although the controlled studies produced optimistic results, there is still significant heterogeneity among the results. Differences in target placement (pre-SMA and SMA suitable), stimulation parameters, the initial severity of axial damage, and evaluation methods (diary and instrument analysis) account for the majority of data alterations. The effect is usually moderate, necessitating repeated or supporting meetings. This reminds us that TMS is not a radical therapy strategy, but rather a modulation tool that can temporarily move the network's state to a more functioning channel, thereby expanding the treatment window for subsequent rehabilitation.

A promising direction is the combined use of TMS and exercise therapy. We are talking about the concept of activation: stimulation immediately before walking training will temporarily increase the plasticity of the cortex, creating conditions for more effective consolidation of correct motor skills (Benninger et al., 2010).

The Preservation of the Effect, the Time of Extinction and the Maintenance of Treatment Issues

Although the meta-analysis persuasively shows the short-term effects of TMS in PD, what happens to patients after three, six, or nine months is still vague. Data on long-term results are decentralized and are usually collected as auxiliary tasks for different design studies, so clear answers are rarely provided. In fact, the key issue in translating this method into actual clinical practice today is not so much the proof of its immediate effect as the lack of a general understanding of how long it can last in the context of progressive neurodegenerative processes. In the absence of sufficient external support, the plastic changes triggered by the final process of rhythmic stimulation are gradually erased. As a result, the improvement in gait, speech, or motor function gradually disappeared, and performance returned to baseline.

The changes that affect the duration and the general uncertainty of this issue are composed of several factors. First of all, the starting protocol varies greatly in the duration of the course, the total number of pulses, and the selected impact area-this sets a completely different "depth" of intervention. In addition, the stage of the disease and its main phenotypes are important.: In patients with emphysema tremor and patients with dominant walking disorders and unstable posture, the benefits of the same surgery may last for different times. Background treatment with dopaminergic drugs is still an important distorting factor, and its dose and regimen often change during follow-up, which makes it difficult to identify the contribution of TMS. Finally, when the main effects have subsided, the measuring scale itself is not always sensitive to small but clinically significant changes.

Overcoming these limitations requires reviewing the research design. Protocols whose follow-up period is extended to one year or more should be the focus of attention. But most importantly, it is necessary to develop a strategy to maintain the results achieved. We are talking about so-called "booster" or support meetings, which follow intensive courses and have been held at long intervals-monthly or quarterly. However, it has not been determined which parameters of stimulation should be optimal (target, frequency, duration) in this case. Perhaps the solution lies not in the technical configuration of the equipment, but in the combination of stimulation and exercise or cognitive training. If you set up a TMS session as a trigger to prepare your brain for the next lesson, then the consolidation of new skills will be more active and the structural adjustment will be more stable. Without the formalization of these plans and the introduction of evidence-based support protocols, TMS may become a tool for intermittent rather than long-term management of patients with PD.

TMS FOR THE DETERMINATION OF COGNITIVE AND NEUROBEHAVIORAL DYSFUNCTION IN PD

The Continuum of Cognitive Impairment in PD

Cognitive decline is a common and often debilitating non-motor manifestation of Parkinson's disease. It can manifest in the early stages of the clinical process and develop into obvious dementia in a significant proportion of patients. Although many cognitive areas may be impaired, defects in executive function and working memory are usually particularly obvious, with the most serious consequences for daily function and overall quality of life (Owen, 2004). Sleep disorders, usually associated with PD, can further exacerbate these cognitive disorders. One of the proposed mechanisms is related to impaired lymphatic metabolism, which leads to the accumulation of metabolic waste and accelerated neurodegeneration (Shirolapov et al., 2024). Working memory refers to the cognitive system responsible for temporarily storing information and actively manipulating it. It plays a key role in high-level processes such as reasoning, planning, and problem solving. In Parkinson's disease, working memory dysfunction is usually manifested as decreased memory capacity, slower information processing speed, increased distraction, and difficulty in updating task-related information.

Mechanically, the shortage of working memory in PD can be expressed as a failure of large-scale network integration. Data from functional neuroimaging and electrophysiology show that the distributed network includes impaired activation and reduced connectivity of the dorsolateral prefrontal cortex, anterior cingulate gyrus, posterior parietal lobe region and striatum. These deviations are accompanied by changes in oscillatory activity, especially in the theta and gamma frequency ranges, which play an important role in the time coordination of neural ensembles when performing memory tasks. The empirical evidence of this study supports these explanations at the network level. During the 1.5-month follow-up period, working memory indicators showed a significant positive correlation with the strength of functional connections in several specific areas. They include the right lingual gyrus and the right globular pallidum, the connection between the right lingual gyrus and the right thalamus, and the right pedicle of the right fusiform gyrus and cerebellum I. These data show that the visual-limbic and visual-cerebellar circuits can contribute to the process of postoperative cognitive function recovery (see fig. 2).

Figure 2. Correlations between functional connectivity and 2-back task accuracy at 1.5 months post-TMS

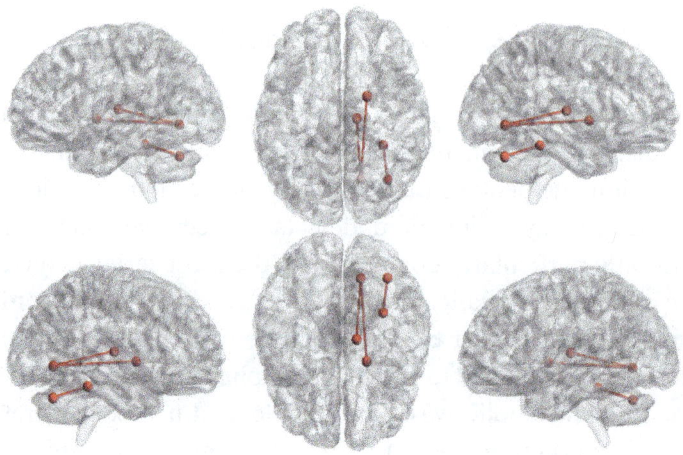

These results show that effective working memory depends on a widely distributed network, including coordinated activities of cortical, subcortical, and cerebellar structures. In addition, the integrity of certain relationships in this architecture directly depends on individual differences in task performance.

Looking at working memory through the lens of this network, we believe that it is not only a symptom to be evaluated, but also the real goal of neuromodulatory intervention. Although dopaminergic drugs provide inconsistent and usually limited relief from the cognitive symptoms of Parkinson's disease, TMS provides a direct impact on the cortical nodes involved in these circuits. The basic premise is simple: regulating the excitability of key centers by applying repetitive or patterned stimuli—especially in the dorsolateral prefrontal cortex (DLPFC)-can change the functional dynamics of the broader network embedded in these centers.

Effect on Anterior Striatum and Anterior Parietal Lobe Circuits

DLPFC has become a leading cortical center for noninvasive neuromodulation aimed at eliminating the cognitive and emotional symptoms of Parkinson's disease. Its prominent position stems from its role as an important node in the anterior striatum and anterior parietal lobe systems, which support executive functions such as updating working memory, switching attention, and managing competitive responses. These functions are often destroyed by PD. DLPFC does not work in isolation, but plays a regulatory role through the dense mutual projection of the striatum (especially the caudate), medial thalamus, and posterior parietal lobe regions. These integrated circuits are heavily dependent on dopaminergic and noradrenergic signaling, and their destruction in PD destroys the precise time and coordination required to effectively perform control.

The repeated application of TMS to DLPFC is based on the idea that changes in excitability in this central node can lead to a broader functional reorganization of the connection circuit. Excitatory protocols-whether it is conventional high-frequency (e.g. 10Hz) stimulation or template examples such as intermittent theta pulse stimulation (iTBS)-are usually used to provide long-term plasticity similar to local and transsynaptic enhancement (Lefaucheur et al., 2020). The expected effect is twofold. First, stimulation can directly counteract local low activity or inefficient processing in DLPFC. Secondly, and perhaps more importantly, it can regulate effective communication between DLPFC and other areas involved in cognitive control. For example, studies have shown that stimulation of the left DLPFC changes its connections to the anterior cingulate gyrus, caudate nucleus, and posterior parietal cortex, areas related to performance control, cognitive flexibility, and spatial working memory, respectively. (Fox et al., 2013).

Behavioral evidence supports the functional significance of these effects. Several studies have reported that high-frequency RTMS through the left DLPFC improves the performance of working memory tasks (for example, n-back), as well as indicators of fluency and cognitive flexibility, and may reduce apathy, which is a common neuropsychiatric feature associated with damaged prefrontal cortex in PD (Fregni et al., 2006). It is worth noting that these cognitive advances are accompanied by significant changes in network-level activities. The relevant results shown in Figure 3 provide a physiological basis for these behavioral changes (see fig. 3). Six months after the intervention, the improvement in working memory performance was related to a widely improved functional connection between multiple circuits. Among them, the strongest correlation is the correlation related to the frontal lobe pathway (for example, the left orbitofrontal cortex and the right paratemporal gyrus; the right orbitofrontal cortex and the left amygdala), the trans-modal visual integration pathway (for example, the right dorsomedial prefrontal cortex and bilateral mid-occipital gyri) and the cortex-cerebellum loop (for example, the left posterior cingulate gyrus and the right lobule of cerebellum VIIb). The results of these studies show that the continuous cognitive improvement reflects the continuous reorganization of the distributed network connecting the prefrontal, limbic, parietal, occipital, and cerebellar regions.

Figure 3. Significant correlations between functional connectivity and 2-back task accuracy at 6 months post-TMS

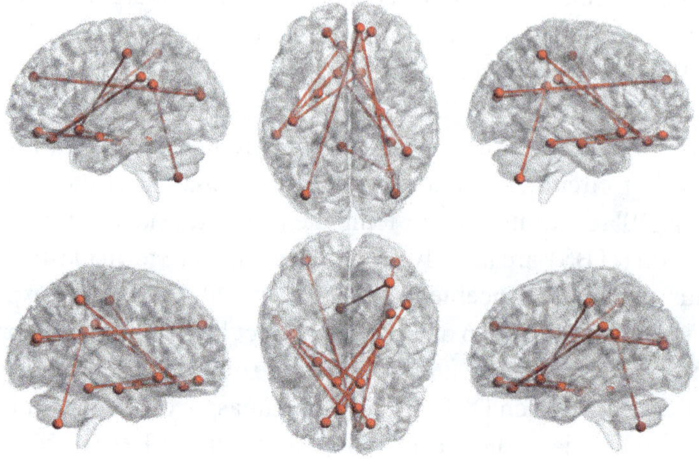

Therefore, an effective DLPFC-TMS protocol should influence not only the local excitability of the cerebral cortex, but also the functional significance of remote pathways related to behavior. This observation is consistent with the idea of a network reboot, in which targeted stimuli trigger a distributed cascade of effects, and eventually the pathological network is rebuilt into a more adaptive configuration.

Clinically convincing and theoretically sound results indicate the effect of DLPFC stimulation on athletic performance. Although this area is traditionally regarded as cognitive, its activation can lead to improved motor function, especially in conditions of high performance requirements, such as walking with two tasks. This interdisciplinary effect reflects the deep anatomical intertwining of cognitive and motor circuits. For example, in older people, compensatory mechanisms involving perceptual integration may become particularly evident during the performance of cognitively complex tasks — this is an important consideration in the development of personalized neuromodulation protocols (Frolov et al., 2023). Anatomically, DLPFC supports the direct projection of the premotor region and the additional motor cortex of the brain

Empirical Evidence and Changes at the Network Level

The claim that TMS mainly improves cognitive abilities in PD by regulating large-scale networks rather than isolated cortical points should be supported by direct measurements of functional connections related to behavior. The results of electrophysiological studies and neuroimaging confirm this network approach, and task-based behavioral indicators provide a link between changes in connections and observed cognitive gains.

The combination of high-density EEG techniques and source reconstruction provides a non-invasive window for rapidly changing network configuration during task execution. As discussed in the Methods section, modern analysis methods, including artifact suppression, virtual reality modeling (for example, the boundary element model associated with the Automated Anatomical Labeling (AAL) atlas), and time-varying connectivity estimation, allow researchers to quantify cognitive abilities after constructing a functional connectivity matrix, as well as statistical structures such Network-Based Statistic (NBS) can identify individual changes in the subnet related to disease status or intervention effects.

At the most basic level, relevant data linking brain connections to behavior provides an essential foundation. A detailed description of such relationships is shown in the figure 4, for example, the relationship between the regional connection configuration file and the execution of the n—back task.

Figure 4. Network correlates of reaction time in the 2-back task before TMS

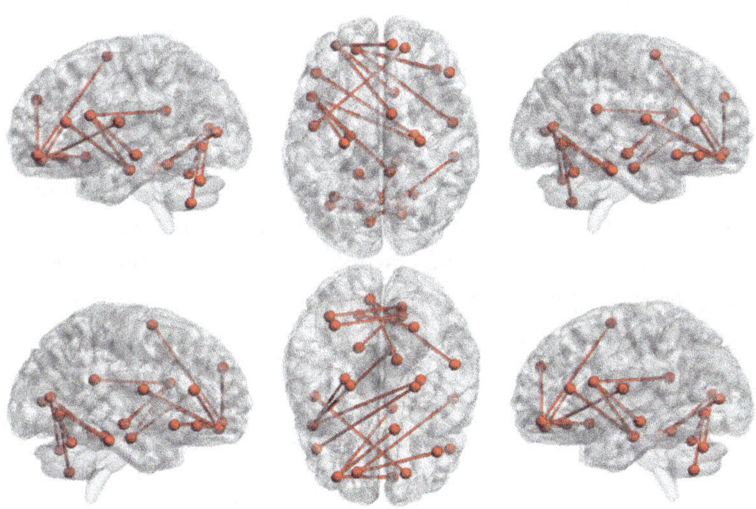

The main conclusions of the study are:

The connection between the frontotemporal area and the hippocampus. Positive correlation between the activity of the frontal region (in particular, the operating part of the inferior frontal gyrus) and the medial temporal structures (hippocampus, parahippocampus) and the 2nd gyrus test showed that effective working memory requires the execution of control systems and situational memory.

- Fronto-striato-thalamus pathway. The revealed connections between the dorsolateral prefrontal cortex (the triangular part of the inferior frontal gyrus), the orbitofrontal cortex, the thalamus, and the globus pallidus emphasize the importance of the cortical-striatal-thalamus cycle for switching cognitive attitudes and updating working memory content.\
- The interaction of the cortex, visual area and cerebellum. The connections found between the occipital bones (lingual sulcus, lingual gyrus), temporal and cerebellar regions associated with task success confirm that the cerebellum is not only involved in motor synchronization, but also in the precise time organization of cognitive processes. This function is particularly affected by Parkinson's disease.

These data are obtained at the initial level and can describe the network structure of cognitive defects-their unique "phenotypes". From this, it is concluded that effective neuromodulation should aim to change the strength of these behavioral significant connections. Many studies using combined TMS and EEG techniques before and after the intervention have confirmed this hypothesis.

The analysis of the dynamics of network changes presented in the material contains a clear illustrative example. Using the NBS method to compare the connection matrix between the groups (healthy controls and patients with Parkinson's disease, or experimental and control groups of patients at different time intervals), it is possible to identify subnets that have undergone significant changes (see Figure 5). Therefore, in one of the identified subnets, the connection between the frontal pole, amygdala, and temporal regions—nodes involved in the integration of executive control, emotional meaning, and memory information retrieval processes-appeared in the intergroup comparison.

Figure 5. Longitudinal Changes in Functional Connectivity Associated with 3-back

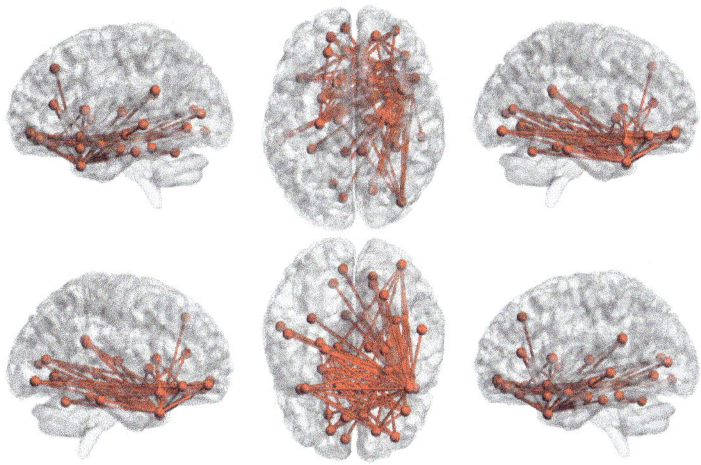

Performance in the Experimental Group: Pre-TMS vs. 6-Month Follow-up

In addition, accurate analysis of how neural network characteristics change over time (for example, before stimulation, one and a half months later, and six months later) makes it possible to separate short-term changes in excitability from long-term, uncertain network reorganization. If the functionally favorable connection pattern lasts for several months, this indicates the formation of stable neuroplasticity, which is a key task of therapeutic neuromodulation.

Empirical research strongly confirms that the cognitive impairment of PD is directly related to the state of certain macroscopic neural networks. The correlation diagram obtained during the execution of cognitive tasks outlines the target area for directional modulation.

Comprehensive Method: Use EEG and Source Positioning for TMS Navigation

The key task on this path is to solve the inverse problem: to determine the location of the neurogenesis that produces the potential recorded on the scalp. It is solved by localizing the source. First, build a direct model, which requires a geometric model of the head that describes the electrical conductivity of the scalp, skull, and brain. As shown in the method, the boundary unit model based on the MNI template is usually used to assign appropriate conductivity values to each type of organization. This model, combined with the coordinates of the electrodes, allows us to mathematically describe how current from any part of the earth's crust is projected onto the sensor. Then the inverse solution calculates the most likely distribution of cortical activity and interprets the obtained data. In order to solve this misstatement problem, methods such as dynamic statistical parameter mapping (dSPM) or standardized low-resolution electromagnetic tomography (sLORETA) are used. Anatomical antecedents and dipole orientation constraints are used to increase accuracy. Modern methods of classifying EEG patterns make it possible to more accurately identify neurophysiological markers and distinguish the functional state of the cortex (Agapov et al., 2017).

Based on the time series of regional activities, estimate functional connectivity-the statistical relationship between signals in different regions, reflecting their functional interactions. Common indicators include Pearson correlation, phase indicators (such as phase delay index (antibody conduction artifacts), and envelope correlation). Calculating the pairwise connectivity between all selected areas generates a symmetrical connectivity matrix for each subject and each condition. As shown in the attached network analysis, these individual matrices can be averaged to build a population network or statistically compared to identify differences between groups (patients and controls) or conditions (before and after TMS).

Key metrics for the network's global and local topology:

- Global efficiency-convenience of information exchange between networks;
- Clustering coefficient-the degree of local interconnection and separation;
- The characteristic path length is the average shortest distance between any two nodes.

The final and most important stage is the use of TMS to target the resulting network model. The identified dysfunctional subnets-for example, the hyperconnection between the supplementary motor area and the shell of patients with walking stiffness or the anterior thalamus-the hyperconnection in the cerebellar circuit of patients with tremor-become therapeutic targets.

LIMITATIONS OF CURRENT METHODS, CONCLUSIONS AND FURTHER RESEARCH DIRECTIONS

Transcranial magnetic stimulation confidently occupies a place in the noninvasive treatment of PD, at the junction of neurophysiology, neural network methods and clinical neurology. Her treatment logic comes from the modern concept of PD, as a disorder of large-scale neural network dynamics with pathological rhythm (excessive synchronization in the β range), weakened connections, and impaired neuroplasticity. A series of magnetic impulses applied to certain cortical areas—the motor cortex (M1) in motor delay, additional motor areas in gait disorders and stiffness, and the dorsolateral prefrontal cortex in cognitive difficulties—can not only come from clinical trials, neurophysiological experiments, and generalized data from our own correlation analysis results show in the work that TMS can lead to statistically significant in the motor and cognitive fields, although to a moderate extent this is particularly valuable in the context of symptoms resistant to dopaminergic therapy. In fact, we are facing a paradigm shift: from pure pharmacological supplementation to targeted correction of neural networks.

The further development of this method is inextricably linked to overcoming existing limitations and introducing technical solutions that can transfer TMS to personalized and precise intervention categories.

1. Closed loop and brain-dependent stimulation. The logical next step is to move from a hard-coded protocol to an adaptive system controlled by feedback signals. EEG or other physiological indicators can determine the moment when stimulation is applied in real time: for example, the pulse is synchronized with the β oscillation stage that needs to be suppressed, or conversely, with the peak activity in the gamma range to enhance cognition. The implementation of this method requires advanced signal processing methods and compact equipment, but it opens up opportunities for fundamentally different time accuracy.
2. A well-thought-out combination with other types of treatment. The greatest effect is likely to be achieved through synergy. Combining TMS with behavioral interventions is promising: stimulating SMA immediately before physical therapy, promoting motor learning, or activating DLPFC paired with cognitive training to enhance neuroplasticity in memory and executive dysfunction. It is also important to establish a reasonable plan for drug treatment (for example, to set the stimulation time as the optimal "oh" period), and to study how TMS interacts with deep brain stimulation, especially in the case of persistent, resistant sym.
3. Personalized and digital phenotypes based on biomarkers. The future of TMS can be seen in the individual choices of goals. We are talking about using in-

dividual resting function MRI maps or EEG data to identify the cortical nodes with the most obvious abnormalities in the connection within the symptomatic network (for example, the task of weak stimulation of the caudate nucleus in the prefrontal cortex and patients with performance difficulties is to normalize this unique "network portrait" of a particular person. In this context, interpretable artificial intelligence can play a special role. Its multidimensional array based on TMS-EEG data will help identify complex predictors of responses and identify previously unknown electrophysiological markers.

4. Special attention should be paid to the development of methods aimed at improving the functionality of the glymphatic system. This direction can slow down the progress of the disease and improve cognitive function (I. V. Shirolapov, et al., 2023)

REFERENCES

Agapov, S. N., Bulanov, V. A., Zakharov, A. V., & Sergeeva, M. S. (2017). Comparison of classifiers in the tasks of the single-trial vep classification. *Zhurnal Vysshei Nervnoi Deyatelnosti Imeni IP Pavlova, 67*(4), Article 4.

Asuku, A. O., Ayinla, M. T., Olajide, T. S., Oyerinde, T. O., Yusuf, J. A., Bayo-Olugbami, A. A., & Fajemidagba, G. A. (2024). Coffee and Parkinson's disease. In. Progress in Brain Research: Vol. 289. *Neuroscience of Coffee*. Elsevier., DOI: 10.1016/bs.pbr.2024.06.001

Asuku, A. O., Ogungbangbe, G. O., & Fajemidagba, G. A. (2025). Gene therapy for Parkinson's disease: A new frontier in neurodegenerative diseases. *Exploration of Neuroprotective Therapy*, *5*, 1004119. DOI: 10.37349/ent.2025.1004119

Benninger, D. H., Lomarev, M., Lopez, G., Wassermann, E. M., Li, X., Considine, E., & Hallett, M. (2010). Transcranial direct current stimulation for the treatment of Parkinson's disease. *Journal of Neurology, Neurosurgery, and Psychiatry*, *81*(10), 1105–1111. DOI: 10.1136/jnnp.2009.202556 PMID: 20870863

Bezard, E., Brotchie, J. M., & Gross, C. E. (2001). Pathophysiology of levodopa-induced dyskinesia: Potential for new therapies. *Nature Reviews. Neuroscience*, *2*(8), 577–588. DOI: 10.1038/35086062 PMID: 11484001

Deuschl, G., Schade-Brittinger, C., Krack, P., Volkmann, J., Schäfer, H., Bötzel, K., Daniels, C., Deutschländer, A., Dillmann, U., Eisner, W., Gruber, D., Hamel, W., Herzog, J., Hilker, R., Klebe, S., Kloß, M., Koy, J., Krause, M., Kupsch, A., & Voges, J. (2006). A Randomized Trial of Deep-Brain Stimulation for Parkinson's Disease. *The New England Journal of Medicine*, *355*(9), 896–908. DOI: 10.1056/NEJMoa060281 PMID: 16943402

Duecker, F., & Sack, A. T. (2015). Rethinking the role of sham TMS. *Frontiers in Psychology*, *6*. Advance online publication. DOI: 10.3389/fpsyg.2015.00210 PMID: 25767458

Formaggio, E., Tonellato, M., Antonini, A., Castiglia, L., Gallo, L., Manganotti, P., Masiero, S., & Del Felice, A. (2023). Oscillatory EEG-TMS Reactivity in Parkinson Disease. *Journal of Clinical Neurophysiology*, *40*(3), 263–268. DOI: 10.1097/WNP.0000000000000881 PMID: 34280941

Fox, M. D., Liu, H., & Pascual-Leone, A. (2013). Identification of reproducible individualized targets for treatment of depression with TMS based on intrinsic connectivity. *NeuroImage*, *66*, 151–160. DOI: 10.1016/j.neuroimage.2012.10.082 PMID: 23142067

Fregni, F., Boggio, P. S., Nitsche, M. A., Marcolin, M. A., Rigonatti, S. P., & Pascual-Leone, A. (2006). Treatment of major depression with transcranial direct current stimulation. *Bipolar Disorders, 8*(2), 203–204. DOI: 10.1111/j.1399-5618.2006.00291.x PMID: 16542193

Frolov, N., Pitsik, E., Grubov, V., Badarin, A., Maksimenko, V., Zakharov, A., Kurkin, S., & Hramov, A. (2023). Perceptual Integration Compensates for Attention Deficit in Elderly during Repetitive Auditory-Based Sensorimotor Task. *Sensors, 23*(14). *Scopus*. Advance online publication. DOI: 10.3390/s23146420 PMID: 37514714

Gao, C., Liu, J., Tan, Y., & Chen, S. (2020). Freezing of gait in Parkinson's disease: Pathophysiology, risk factors and treatments. *Translational Neurodegeneration, 9*(1), 12. DOI: 10.1186/s40035-020-00191-5 PMID: 32322387

Gibbons, C. H., Levine, T., Adler, C., Bellaire, B., Wang, N., Stohl, J., Agarwal, P., Aldridge, G. M., Barboi, A., Evidente, V. G. H., Galasko, D., Geschwind, M. D., Gonzalez-Duarte, A., Gil, R., Gudesblatt, M., Isaacson, S. H., Kaufmann, H., Khemani, P., Kumar, R., & Freeman, R. (2024). Skin Biopsy Detection of Phosphorylated α-Synuclein in Patients With Synucleinopathies. *Journal of the American Medical Association, 331*(15), 1298. DOI: 10.1001/jama.2024.0792 PMID: 38506839

Guerra, A., Rocchi, L., Grego, A., Berardi, F., Luisi, C., & Ferreri, F. (2021). Contribution of TMS and TMS-EEG to the Understanding of Mechanisms Underlying Physiological Brain Aging. *Brain Sciences, 11*(3), 405. DOI: 10.3390/brainsci11030405 PMID: 33810206

Helmers, A.-K., Stieglitz, L. H., & Werner, B. (2025). Focused Ultrasound in Parkinson's Disease. In E. Ch. Wolters & C. R. Baumann (Eds.), *International Compendium of Movement Disorders* (pp. 328–338). Cambridge University Press. Cambridge Core. https://doi.org/DOI: 10.1017/9781108989855.029

Huang, Y.-Z., Edwards, M. J., Rounis, E., Bhatia, K. P., & Rothwell, J. C. (2005). Theta Burst Stimulation of the Human Motor Cortex. *Neuron, 45*(2), 201–206. DOI: 10.1016/j.neuron.2004.12.033 PMID: 15664172

Iansek, R., & Danoudis, M. (2017). Freezing of Gait in Parkinson's Disease: Its Pathophysiology and Pragmatic Approaches to Management. *Movement Disorders Clinical Practice, 4*(3), 290–297. DOI: 10.1002/mdc3.12463 PMID: 30868095

Jahanshahi, M., Jenkins, I. H., Brown, R. G., Marsden, C. D., Passingham, R. E., & Brooks, D. J. (1995). Self-initiated versus externally triggered movements. I. An investigation using measurement of regional cerebral blood flow with PET and movement-related potentials in normal and Parkinson's disease subjects. *Brain, 118*(Pt 4), 913–933. DOI: 10.1093/brain/118.4.913 PMID: 7655888

Kalinderi, K., Papaliagkas, V., & Fidani, L. (2019). Pharmacogenetics and levodopa induced motor complications. *The International Journal of Neuroscience, 129*(4), 384–392. DOI: 10.1080/00207454.2018.1538993 PMID: 30359152

Kelly, V. E., Eusterbrock, A. J., & Shumway-Cook, A. (2012). The Effects of Instructions on Dual-Task Walking and Cognitive Task Performance in People with Parkinson's Disease. *Parkinson's Disease, 2012*, 1–9. DOI: 10.1155/2012/671261 PMID: 23326758

Kim, Y. W., Shin, I.-S., Moon, H. I., Lee, S. C., & Yoon, S. Y. (2019). Effects of non-invasive brain stimulation on freezing of gait in parkinsonism: A systematic review with meta-analysis. *Parkinsonism & Related Disorders, 64*, 82–89. DOI: 10.1016/j.parkreldis.2019.02.029 PMID: 30902526

Komarova, Y., Zakharov, A., Sergeeva, M., Romanchuk, N., Vladimirova, T., & Shirolapov, I. (2025). Modeling Working Memory in Neurodegeneration: A Focus on EEG Methods. *Diagnostics (Basel), 15*(23), 2992. DOI: 10.3390/diagnostics15232992 PMID: 41374372

Lefaucheur, J.-P., Aleman, A., Baeken, C., Benninger, D. H., Brunelin, J., Di Lazzaro, V., Filipović, S. R., Grefkes, C., Hasan, A., Hummel, F. C., Jääskeläinen, S. K., Langguth, B., Leocani, L., Londero, A., Nardone, R., Nguyen, J.-P., Nyffeler, T., Oliveira-Maia, A. J., Oliviero, A., & Ziemann, U. (2020). Evidence-based guidelines on the therapeutic use of repetitive transcranial magnetic stimulation (rTMS): An update (2014–2018). *Clinical Neurophysiology, 131*(2), 474–528. DOI: 10.1016/j.clinph.2019.11.002 PMID: 31901449

Li, J., Mi, T.-M., Zhu, B., Ma, J.-H., Han, C., Li, Y., Yang, W.-M., & Chan, P. (2020). High-frequency repetitive transcranial magnetic stimulation over the primary motor cortex relieves musculoskeletal pain in patients with Parkinson's disease: A randomized controlled trial. *Parkinsonism & Related Disorders, 80*, 113–119. DOI: 10.1016/j.parkreldis.2020.07.006 PMID: 32980772

Mahlknecht, P., Seppi, K., & Poewe, W. (2015). The Concept of Prodromal Parkinson's Disease. *Journal of Parkinson's Disease, 5*(4), 681–697. DOI: 10.3233/JPD-150685 PMID: 26485429

Morgante, F., Espay, A. J., Gunraj, C., Lang, A. E., & Chen, R. (2006). Motor cortex plasticity in Parkinson's disease and levodopa-induced dyskinesias. *Brain, 129*(4), 1059–1069. DOI: 10.1093/brain/awl031 PMID: 16476674

Oertel, W., & Schulz, J. B. (2016). Current and experimental treatments of Parkinson disease: A guide for neuroscientists. *Journal of Neurochemistry, 139*(Suppl 1), 325–337. DOI: 10.1111/jnc.13750 PMID: 27577098

Owen, A. M. (2004). Cognitive Dysfunction in Parkinson's Disease: The Role of Frontostriatal Circuitry. *The Neuroscientist, 10*(6), 525–537. DOI: 10.1177/1073858404266776 PMID: 15534038

Poewe, W. (2008). Non-motor symptoms in Parkinson's disease. *European Journal of Neurology, 15*(s1), 14–20. DOI: 10.1111/j.1468-1331.2008.02056.x PMID: 18353132

Postuma, R. B., & Berg, D. (2016). Advances in markers of prodromal Parkinson disease. *Nature Reviews. Neurology, 12*(11), 622–634. DOI: 10.1038/nrneurol.2016.152 PMID: 27786242

Pringsheim, T., Jette, N., Frolkis, A., & Steeves, T. D. L. (2014). The prevalence of Parkinson's disease: A systematic review and meta-analysis. *Movement Disorders, 29*(13), 1583–1590. DOI: 10.1002/mds.25945 PMID: 24976103

Shirolapov, I., Zakharov, A., Gochhait, S., Pyatin, V., Sergeeva, M., Romanchuk, N., Komarova, Y., Kalinin, V., Pavlova, O., & Khivintseva, E. (2023). Aquaporin-4 as the Main Element of the Glymphatic System for Clearance of Abnormal Proteins and Prevention of Neurodegeneration: A Review. *WSEAS TRANSACTIONS ON BIOLOGY AND BIOMEDICINE, 20*, 110–118. DOI: 10.37394/23208.2023.20.11

Shirolapov, Igor V., Zakharov, A. V., Bulgakova, S. V., Khivintseva, E. V., Sergeeva, M. S., Romanchuk, N. P., Pavlova, O. N., & Kazantsev, V. B. (2023). Glymphatic dysfunction in the pathogenesis of neurodegenerative diseases and pathological aging. *Genes to Cells, 18*(4), 309–322. DOI: 10.23868/gc546022

Shirolapov, I. V., Gribkova, O. V., Kovalev, A. M., Shafigullina, L. R., Ulivanova, V. A., Kozlov, A. V., Ereshchenko, A. A., Lyamin, A. V., & Zakharov, A. V. (2024). The Role of Interactions along the Brain–Gut–Microbiome Axis in the Regulation of Circadian Rhythms, Sleep Mechanisms, and Their Disorders. *Neuroscience and Behavioral Physiology, 54*(8), 1177–1183. DOI: 10.1007/s11055-024-01712-9

Shirolapov, I. V., Zakharov, A. V., Smirnova, D. A., Lyamin, A. V., & Gayduk, A. Ya. (2023). The significance of the glymphatic pathway in the relationship between the sleep—Wake cycle and neurodegenerative diseases. *Zhurnal Nevrologii i Psikhiatrii Imeni S. S. Korsakova, 123*(9), 9. Advance online publication. DOI: 10.17116/jnevro202312309131 PMID: 37796065

Suppa, A., Quartarone, A., Siebner, H., Chen, R., Di Lazzaro, V., Del Giudice, P., Paulus, W., Rothwell, J. C., Ziemann, U., & Classen, J. (2017). The associative brain at work: Evidence from paired associative stimulation studies in humans. *Clinical Neurophysiology, 128*(11), 2140–2164. DOI: 10.1016/j.clinph.2017.08.003 PMID: 28938144

Takahashi, H., & Wakabayashi, K. (2001). The cellular pathology of Parkinson's disease. *Neuropathology, 21*(4), 315–322. DOI: 10.1046/j.1440-1789.2001.00403.x PMID: 11837539

Yang, R., Sun, M., Chen, W., Feng, H., Chen, B., Liu, Y., He, Q., Wang, L., Zou, C., Luo, X., Li, Z., Fu, A., Qiao, F., Tang, H., Yang, J., & Ren, H. (2026). Global, regional and national burden of Parkinson's disease, 1990–2021: Update from the GBD 2021 study. *Journal of the Neurological Sciences, 480*, 125703. DOI: 10.1016/j.jns.2025.125703 PMID: 41435482

Zakharov, A. V., Khivintseva, E. V., Pytin, V. F., Sergeeva, M. S., & Antipov, O. I. (2017). Melatonin—Known problems and perspectives of clinical usage. *Zhurnal Nevrologii i Psikhiatrii Im. S.S. Korsakova, 117*(4. Vyp. 2), 74. https://doi.org/DOI: 10.17116/jnevro20171174274-78

Zhu, J., Cui, Y., Zhang, J., Yan, R., Su, D., Zhao, D., Wang, A., & Feng, T. (2024). Temporal trends in the prevalence of Parkinson's disease from 1980 to 2023: A systematic review and meta-analysis. *The Lancet. Healthy Longevity, 5*(7), e464–e479. DOI: 10.1016/S2666-7568(24)00094-1 PMID: 38945129

Chapter 10
Surgical Intervention for Parkinson's Disease in Under-Resourced Settings

Christopher Oloruntoba Akintayo
http://orcid.org/0009-0008-3446-466X
Obafemi Awolowo University Teaching Hospital Complex, Ile-Ife, Nigeria

Samuel Obiosa Onyekweli
http://orcid.org/0000-0002-4715-7932
Lagos University Teaching Hospital, Idi-Araba, Nigeria

Gloria Osayamen Omoruyi
Obafemi Awolowo University Teaching Hospital Complex, Ile-Ife, Nigeria

Joseph Oluwatomi Akintayo
University of Ibadan, Nigeria

Tobi Opeyemi Olaleye
http://orcid.org/0009-0001-3655-2259
Achievers University, Nigeria

ABSTRACT

The advancements and challenges of surgical interventions for Parkinson's disease (PD), a neurodegenerative disorder characterized by the progressive loss of dopaminergic neurons. We provided a comprehensive overview of the limitations of pharmacological treatments and emphasize the necessity for surgical options in advanced cases. By critically analyzing various surgical techniques such as Deep

DOI: 10.4018/979-8-3373-7437-6.ch010

Brain Stimulation (DBS), ablative procedures like pallidotomy and thalamotomy, and emerging methods such as focused ultrasound and gene therapy, we reviewed and evaluated their efficacy, risks, and impact on patients' quality of life. Furthermore, we also focused on the ethical considerations and complications associated with these interventions, while also examining future directions for surgical innovation aimed at overcoming current limitations. This review article underscores the significance of a multifaceted approach in treating PD, combining surgical, pharmacological, and rehabilitative therapies to enhance patient outcomes.

INTRODUCTION

Parkinson's disease is a progressive neurological disorder that affects millions of people across the world. PD is in fact one of the most severe health consequences that patients, their caregivers and the healthcare system experience, and includes symptoms of motor symptoms, including tremors, rigidity, bradykinesia, postural instability, as well as cognitive decline, mood disorders and sleep disorders (Ajagun et al., 2024; Asuku et al., 2024). Recently, these numbers were introduced to indicate that PD is present in over 100 countries and that there are about 10 million people worldwide with PD (Etukudoh & Ejinaka, 2024). This decline is not only related to improving diagnoses and ageing populations but also to the need for effective treatment of this terrifying disease. Despite the dramatic change in the use of pharmacological drugs in the highly comorbid cases of PD, the limitations to treatment for advanced PD are beginning to emerge. PD is characterized by drugs that have been shown to reduce symptoms in many patients, including levodopa and dopamine agonists. But they're easy to break and can cause dyskinesia and off periods in the motor. Second, there is not sufficient clinical data to support the neurodegenerative processes associated with PD, and therefore, pharmacological interventions are very ineffective (Kotyal et al. 2024). These issues highlight the need to explore other treatment options, including surgical treatments, which are effective in controlling higher-grade PD symptoms and improving patient quality of life. PD also affects the individual for some patients. It is viewed by families and caregivers as particularly burdened by a lack of access to assistive devices, rehabilitation services and social services. But the economic and psychological effects of diseases are also amplified by poor productivity, long-term care costs and social stigma. The burden is growing, but many in those areas still have no access to modern treatments such as surgery. This lack also creates a global disconnect in the delivery of health care and must be addressed in this context. But because they are sick, the problem is there is no standard form of treatment for Parkinson's disease, including surgery, and if so, how safe is that? This is particularly true because the recent developments in neuroscience and medicine have put therapies such as DBS, targeted ultrasound, and gene therapy among the most lauded, of which is brain stimulation. The quality, safety, and ethical nature of these interventions and their potential impact on PD treatment practice must be considered. The problem is that even surgical treatments like DBS and new techniques are problematic. This study represents an important one that provides information about the potential threat of these procedures, ethical concerns regarding patient consent, and the nature and extent of these practices' outcomes. This study is important in order to improve the treatment of PD and guide future research and medicine in an effort to improve patient outcomes. Parkinson's disease is a neurodegenerative condition caused by the loss of dopaminergic neurons in the substantia nigra, the area of the brain that controls motion. Dopamine subsequently disrupts the basal ganglia circuit and causes the motor symptoms of PD. Neuronal conditions that cause nonmotor symptoms are even worse: depression, anxiety, autonomic dysfunction and cognitive impairment (Alassaf, 2024). People need to be able to participate in everyday activities, function, and socially normalise due to the disease. PD has also had emotional and financial consequences, illustrating the devastating nature of this disease.

The PD burden is particularly high among the older population, who are around 60 years of age on average. But this PD, or early onset PD, is also a genetic disease. It is a public health crisis, and by 2040, the number of cases would double, Weerarathna et al. 2024 wrote. This poses huge challenges for hospitals and emphasizes the need for appropriate approaches to manage motor and nonmotor processes. PD drugs must be able to refuel dopamine or behave like dopamine in the brain. Levodopa is a common medication that helps reduce symptoms but is converted into dopamine in the brain to help relieve symptoms. It is, but its associated complications, including dyskinesias and motor dystrophy, can impact patients' lives. Alternatives include dopamine agonists and MAO-B inhibitors, although in some cases not as effective, and can cause hallucinations, impulse control and stomach problems (Ezike et al., 2023). It is a nonsymptomatic palliative measure that targets illness rather than symptoms. Other things include that patients take more medications simultaneously to control symptoms since they become sick and are therefore at greater risk of side effects and complications. This lack of efficacy of drugs combined with increased need for more effective alternative therapies to help patients address long-term relief and the underlying mechanism of disease suggests that alternatives to drugs, such as surgery, may be needed in addition to those prescribed by the drugs used in advanced PD to better address long-term relief and maybe even lessen symptoms. Today surgery is the focus of PD treatment, especially in patients who exhibit serious motor symptoms with appropriate medical attention but have significant motor problems after effective pharmacological treatment. These programs target specific areas of the brain that trigger abnormal neuronal activity that affects motor function, to avoid tremors, rigidity and dyskinesia symptoms. The gold standard PD treatment, DBS, is the most widely used PD treatment. DBS is the electrode placement of a pulse generator in the chest, in the target brain region, such as STN or GPi. It is electrically activated so that it changes neuronal activity and restores balance in circuits of deficient basal ganglia. In clinical trials of DBS, this approach has been shown to work well against motor symptoms, to reduce the occurrence of prescriptions longer and to improve patient life expectancy (Zhou et al., 2021). It is dangerous, but it's dangerous surgery and complications of DBS, and it has neuropsychiatric consequences.

Other procedures, such as ablative surgery, such as thalamotomy and pallidotomy, and new procedures, such as focused ultrasound and gene therapy, are being discussed. These interventions may also be useful for patients who do not qualify for DBS and are willing to take less aggressive medications. All of these means are risky, inflexible, morally motivated, and should be tested for potential profit. Since then, PD has been very difficult to detect and treat using neuroscience and medicine. Recent technological innovations that have simplified and enhanced surgery include imaging, neuromodulation and molecular biology. For example, closed-loop DBS systems that real-time alter stimulus parameters based on neuronal activity have better outcomes with fewer side effects (Tushar et al., 2021). The same is true of gene therapy and stem cell research. Changes in this process can even prevent or reverse the neurodegenerative process.

But there are many problems. Infection, bleeding, or cognitive or psychiatric complications can accompany surgical procedures. The reason for that is also that they are not inexpensive and are even less readily available in low-resource environments. These include informed consent, patient selection, and experimental procedures to ensure appropriate use responsibly and justly (Hanson et al. 2025). Lastly, while surgery, such as DBS and new treatments, have made positive changes in the landscape of Parkinson's disease, these treatments remain controversial. These procedures are legal, ethical, and dangerous in that they need to be considered thoroughly for proper implementation and safety. In an era where innovation will always lead to innovation, these interventions have to balance the benefits of these new therapies with risks and problems. Low-sourced environments present two problems: 1) the population aging with more Parkinson's disease; and 2) the lack of neurosurgical expertise needed to treat patients on time. A similar question, about surgery in these situations, is whether treatments are clinically necessary and whether treatment is sustainable and fair. This problem of addressing these problems in low income or middle income countries or eras could help to make PD better, more effective and fairer so that it becomes easier to get effective and fair treatment, improving the lives of patients and their families. But DBS in general is becoming more complex and expensive. The modern surgeries reach some poor patients, not entire populations of patients that would have been excluded from the health care system.

TECHNIQUES OF SURGICAL TREATMENT FOR PARKINSON'S DISEASE

Historical Development of Surgical Treatments

Parkinson's disease treatment options range from invasive treatments to therapies that promise to combat symptoms of motor dysfunction by disabling basal ganglia circuits. These kinds of interventions are scientifically relevant in each case, but they vary in intensity and frequency with resources. The surgical option is likely to be appropriate to the sub-sourced environment because of its efficacy, cost, durability and model maintenance and follow-up. Over the last few decades PD has transformed from a deficient and primitive model to one that is more efficient. This is a signal of an increased awareness of the pathology and medical innovations that helped to create this disease. PD operation can be grouped into steps with ablative surgery at the pre-surgery point and up to the DBS. This chapter outlines the evolution from ablative to DBS surgery in the case of PD and the role that historians and some of the best men in the field played in shaping progress and evidence associated with it. In the early twentieth century, babies had the same kinds of surgeries. For the moment, though, ablative surgery was the preferred strategy because ablative surgery became the preferred treatment for PD, due to the lack of drugs available. Thalamotomy, and pallidotomy were most commonly utilized to treat the painful motor symptoms of the disease such as tremors, rigidity, and bradykinesia. Thalamotomy is a tumor of the thalamus, which controls motor behavior. The first development of this method was in response to doctors' advice that patients suffering accidental thalamic injuries have a slightly less tremor than those suffering from traumatic trauma. On top of that, pallidotomy targets the globus pallidus in the basal ganglia, which is the motorcircuitry of PD in PD. These methods were designed to interfere with the abnormal neural processes that induced motor symptoms. Chilvery et al. (2020) found that early surgery can collaterally damage surrounding tissues and have worse effects, such as speech problems and weakness, such as tissue destruction. The most powerful effects of such procedures were tremor anddyskinesia. Usually treatment helped to relieve symptoms; decreasing mobility or reducing medication can help to relieve symptoms. But ablative surgeries can also be risky. They often required very little imaging or surgical precision, but often resulted in complications such as hemorrhage, infection and cognitive decline. These problems, but, also position inablative surgery as a promising move. It was the first step in the progression from destructive to neuromodulating treatment history of PD. To date, the damage to the brain tissue has been removed through neuromodulation, such asablative surgeries. Rather, they use electrical stimulation to alter abnormal neuronal activity. But it also brought with it new discoveries in neuroscience and technology, and new insight into the complex neural circuits of PD. DBS was another method that brought it into the late twentieth century. In the 1960s, elective stimulation was first proposed to control the brain activity but was accepted into medical schools in the 1980s and 1990s. DBS was also linked to a resurgence of instereotactic surgery targeting specific areas of the brain including STN and GPi.

Tufail et al. (2023) argue that technology is playing a role in modern surgical techniques, such as DBS, and speculate on how machine learning and computational models could be employed to improve surgical outcomes. DBS is performed by inserting electrodes into areas of the brain which are connected to a pulse generator in the chest. This electrical generator inhibits PD symptoms, and electrical signals that inhibit PD symptoms may be of use to relieve PD symptoms. Early studies found that DBS may improve motor symptoms among patients who did not respond well to medications and especially among patients who did not respond well to treatment. It can be adjusted and stimulated in reverse, something that would be helpful for ablative surgery. But, as BB Sinha and R Dhanalakshmi (1922) show, DBS failure is a product of patient selection, surgical skill and electrode placement, but an evolving surgical process. Some of these researchers, physicians and pioneers have led to surgical treatments for PD. One of the first physicians to offer pallidotomy in the 1950s was Dr Irving Cooper. Cooper finds that ablative therapies may help alleviate symptoms of PD but are risky nonetheless. He was involved in another study of surgery as well. It was designed by French neurosurgeon and researcher Dr Alim-Louis Benabid. Benabid found that high-frequency electric stimulation of the thalamus could be interpreted as similar to ablative surgery but would not cause permanent damage. This was the beginning of functional neurosurgery, and Benabid refused to give up on international fame. Kotyal et al. (2024) stress that there must be "deep collaboration and innovation in the pursuit of excellence in medical practice" and have also drawn attention to some of the leaders in surgical procedures, such as Benabid. Some important studies were helpful in determining the safety and efficacy of surgical treatment of PD. Early findings from DBS's early trials in the 1990s were of a more compelling nature to look for in easing motor symptoms and boosting quality of life. These data also reflected the importance of long-run follow-up and carefully selected patients to ensure the best results. Failures such as those described by Etukudoh & Ejinaka, (2024) will push doctors to conduct intensive clinical research to assess the safety and efficacy of new medical technologies.

PD surgery was new but limited. They were also extremely irreparably damaging, because they could cause brain damage. But, not all of this required the best imaging and surgery skills, and the lack of modern imaging technology and high complications augmented this risk. Further, nonmotor symptoms such as cognitive decline and mood disorders were rare in achieving full relief of PD symptoms. DBS filled many of these voids, since it was safer and more flexible than ablative procedures. DBS is more problematic than it may seem, though. It is quite complex and requires a good deal of surgical experience and a great deal of preoperative testing prior to hiring a candidate. DBS can also cause infection, hardware, and neuropsychiatric complications, such as neuropsychiatric side effects. As R Rajagopalan et al. (2020) address, further studies on such problems and improvement in DBS safety and efficacy are warranted. Research and neuroscience, and medicine have long supported the use of surgery for Parkinson's disease. From ablative treatments such as thalamotomy and pallidotomy to Deep Brain Stimulation and from the early years of ablative treatments such as thalamotomy and pallidotomy, new knowledge and innovations have emerged. Historical figures and well-known papers have shaped the modern discourse on PD therapy. Summation, Kumar and Sathiya (1921) indicate that "the continuing evolution in surgical practice given the technological developments and the collaboration" suggests that future management of PD is highly conjectured. These advances are slow and unhelpful, but they can provide a fertile space for development that can have a lasting impact on those affected by this devastating disease. The rise of ablative treatments for Parkinson's disease has fueled modern neuromodulation. Researchers and physicians have come out on top in Parkinson's disease research, and technology has changed treatments for patients and families. As Pulgar (2019) shows, surgical innovation is still not in progress and there may be new data to inform future surgical strategies to better navigate the demanding and difficult world of this complicated and complicated disease. The construction of a history of history and the breaking of the deadlock will allow the medical community to continue to push the boundaries of possible treatment for Parkinson's disease. Many of the challenges facing low and middle-income families include: hardware costs; additional imaging and intraoperative neurophysiology; short-term follow-up, programming and replacement batteries; and technical support. But these were overcome, and DBS programs have benefited low-resource centres through international collaboration, patient selection, and rechargeable devices to maintain cost in check.

Figure 1.

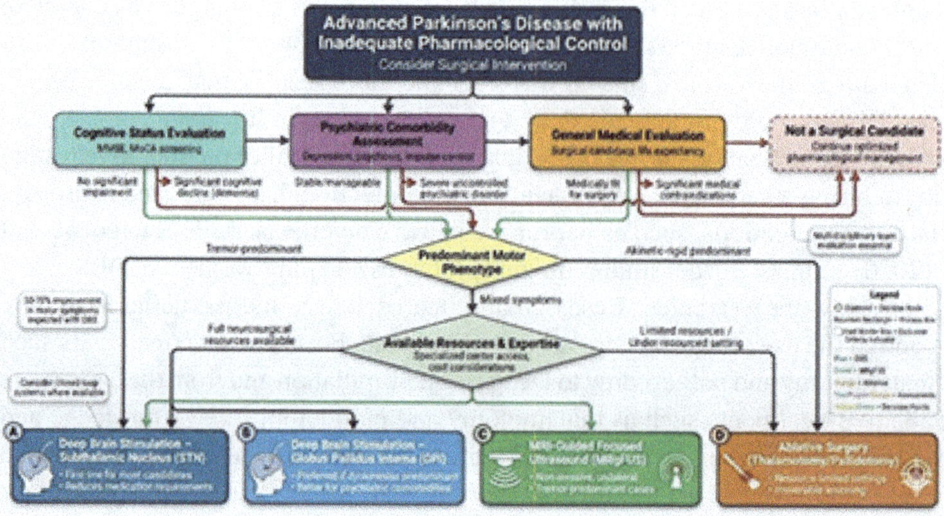

THE PATHOPHYSIOLOGY OF PARKINSON'S DISEASE IN UNDER-RESOURCED SETTINGS

Parkinson's disease is a progressive neurodegenerative disease that produces symptoms such as motor symptoms such as bradykinesia, resting tremor, rigidity and postural instability, and a host of other nonmotor symptoms such as mood disorders, sleep disorders and autonomic dystrophy. In addition, dopaminergic neurons become degenerated in the SNpc, in which both basal ganglia circuits and striatal dopamine depletion are dysregulated in PD pathophysiology (Obeso et al., 2017). It is rare that the neuropathology and mechanisms can be directly identified to the extent they are similar across contexts, but there is concern among low-income populations who encounter particular barriers to disease development, detection, management, and outcome. These include delayed diagnosis, limited neuroimaging and specialist care, economic barriers to long-term therapy, and underrepresented studies. Chapters were also provided on factors involved in the pathophysiology of PD and other concerns facing the under-sourced community that included: Dopaminergic neurodegeneration, Lewy bodies and alpha-synuclein pathology, mitochondrial dysfunction and oxidative stress, neuroinflammation, genetics and environmental interaction, clinical expression and delay in diagnosis.

Dopaminergic Neurodegeneration

PD is the most common pathological condition; if dopaminergic neurons accumulate in the SNpc, then dopamine accumulates in the striatum and most putamen. This control of motor coordination involves dopamine via the direct and indirect basal ganglia pathways. By contrast, dopamine loss disrupts the communication between these pathways, causing the inner portion of GPi and SNr to increase ion output, which inhibits thalamocortical receptors and affects cardinal motor symptoms of PD (Obeso et al., 2017). Patients who may have recovered from heavy limb loss may also become infected earlier in the progression of the disease.

Lewy Bodies and Alpha-Synuclein Pathology

Unsurprisingly, PD has very detailed microscopic features such as Lewy bodies, which are intracellular molecules made primarily of misfolded alpha-synuclein protein. But, it remains to be determined whether this is the cause or a consequence of other pathologies (Spillantini & Goedert, 2018). Instead, analysis of alpha-synuclein pathology reveals peripheral tissues, such as the enteric nervous system or olfactory bulb, but can be diffused centrally through synaptic networks in the Braak staging hypothesis (Braak et al., 2003). These underfunded populations are particularly vulnerable in that Lewy pathology cannot be definitively assessed at follow-mortem by the neuropathology services, making these populations particularly impacted in cases where the infection is less endemic and has an elevated risk for under- or misdiagnosing Parkinsonian syndrome.

Parkinson's disease is a progressive neurodegenerative disorder that causes motor symptoms, including bradykinesia, resting tremor, rigidity and postural instability, and other nonmotor symptoms, including mood disorders, sleep disorders, and motor dysfunction. Also, the dysregulation of the striatal dopamine depletion and basal ganglia circuits in PD pathophysiology also suggests the loss of dopaminergic neurons in the substantia nigra pars compacta (Obeso et al., 2017). The prevalence of neuropathology and mechanisms in other contexts is perhaps less important here at this point, but there is one problem specific to those living in low-resource areas who have particular difficulties addressing disease development, detection, management, and outcome. These include late diagnosis, low neuroimaging and specialist care, long-term treatment costs and low research representation. Other underlying mechanisms of pathophysiology of PD and other major problems of the subsourced population included: Dopaminergic neurodegeneration, Lewy bodies and alpha-synuclein pathology, mitochondrial dysfunction and oxidative stress, neuroinflammation, genetics and environmental interaction, clinical expression and tardiness of diagnosis.

Dopaminergic Neurodegeneration

Pathology is the main cause of PD; when dopaminergic neurons are lost in the SNpc, dopamine is lost in the striatum and most putamen. One part of this function is provided by dopamine, which controls motor coordination in the direct and indirect basal ganglia. Also, dopamine loss does alter the chemistry of these pathways, and results in lower-than-optimal output from the inner portion of GPi and SNr, limiting the expression of thalamocortical receptors, leading to cardinal motor symptoms of PD (Obeso et al., 2017). In small spaces, such as those for dopaminergic impairment diagnostic testing for positron emission tomography where there is usually limited space, patients may be in the early stages of illness and later infected, thus early detection is critical for patients with significant limb loss.

Lewy Bodies and Alpha-Synuclein Pathology

This is not surprising, considering that PD possesses extremely detailed microscopic features, such as Lewy bodies and intracellular molecules containing the dominant disseminated alpha-synuclein protein. This is not understood or is a response to other pathologies and is associated with neuronal dysfunction and death (Spillantini & Goedert, 2018). Instead, the mechanism of pathology for alpha-synuclein is hypothesized to be centrally diffused by synaptic networks in peripheral tissues such as the enteric nervous system or the olfactory bulb, as in the Braak staging hypothesis (Braak et al., 2003). These low-income populations **are at risk in that neuropathology** services cannot definitively rule out Lewy pathology at post-mortem, which is particularly problematic in areas where Lewy is less commonly detected, because it may be a factor in the failure or inability to exclude or misdiagnose Parkinsonian syndromes.

Impact of Nutritional and Comorbid Conditions

Poor areas are more likely to be malnourished and to contract HIV, tuberculosis, and parasitic diseases. Vitamins C and E, along with a poor diet, may contribute to oxidative stress in prey neurons (Mythri & Bharath, 2012). Also, systemic infections and immune reactions may further increase neuroinflammatory processes and even induce neurodegeneration. The accumulation of chronic disease also poses a challenge for PD management since polypharmacy and interaction with antiparkinsonian drugs increase the risk of adverse outcomes and therapy failure.

Treatment Barriers and Pathophysiological Consequences

Among prescription medications, most commonly prescribed for PD, are those designed to repair or modulate the downstream effect of dopamine, but levodopa is the most effective symptomatic therapy for PD (Olanow et al., 2009). But levodopa and dopamine agonists are scarce, poorly available and inconsistent. Without physiotherapy, speech therapy, or occupational therapy, the onset of functional outcomes can be delayed. PD also causes falls, aspiration pneumonia, depression and cognitive decline more severe than those of the central motor (Schrag et al., 2000).

Research Gaps and Global Health Implications

The low and middle-income subrepresentation in PD research raises serious questions about disease epidemiology, environmental risk factors, gene variation and drug response. Most of these studies have taken place in populations within developing countries and are potentially relevant to the pathophysiology and care models. Increased funding for research, international cooperation and capacity building in poor countries are important step towards a more just understanding and management of PD (Dorsey et al., 2018).

VARIOUS SURGICAL INTERVENTIONS IN PARKINSON'S DISEASE

Deep Brain Stimulation (DBS)

The country's poor history has largely limited the treatment of the PD. This is useful, but not representative of the situation for clinicians and patients with inadequate sources. The risk-benefit equation of surgery is undermined by the lack of imaging technology, inexperienced staff and high health care costs. If policy-makers and government are willing to respond to the problem, Deep Brain Stimulation would be an excellent idea for improving the surgical response to PD in the context of under-source. Now, this is a step forward that could even be even more revolutionary in the treatment of symptoms of PD, Parkinson's disease. This type of neurosurgery involves electrodes that are positioned on the brain for years, and has been studied and used in the past in the hope of advanced patients with PD who cannot talk because of severe motor symptoms. I will then return to explaining in detail the nature of DBS, its application to clinical practice, how it might work, the side effects and risks of using it, and what is being done. With data from recent developments and research we will explore how DBS functions in our modern world in more ways than ever. DBS sends electrical signals to areas of the brain such as STN and globus pallidus interna, but also uses electrical energy to send impulses to the subthalamic nucleus and interglobus pallidus. These are the circuits of the basal ganglia for motor control. Because there are no dopaminergic neurons in the substantia nigra of Parkinson's disease, these circuits also have no dopaminergic neurons and cause abnormal firing and motor symptoms such as tremors, rigidity and bradykinesia. DBS's electrical stimulation does not induce re-regulation of dopamine levels but stimulates abnormal neuronal activity in these targets. Chilvery et al. (2020) hypothesize that such modulation occurs by manipulating the pathological neural oscillations and synchrony in the basal ganglia-thalamocortical loop in order to induce a more normalized pattern of activity. Electrophysiological studies support this hypothesis; some experimental evidence supports the hypothesis that pathological beta-band oscillations were exclusionary during DBS in the STN (Tufail et al. 2023). But how precisely does this type of modulation actually happen? While some authors have speculated that DBS promotes neuroplasticity over time, others seem to be implicated. DBS is reversible and flexible, an approach often applied in other ablative procedures such as pallidotomy or thalamotomy. This allows the clinician to adjust the stimulation parameters to ensure an optimal response to symptom control and minimal side effects. But, as Sinha and Dhanalakshmi (1922) describe, DBS systems like directional leads and closed loop systems were technically improved to improve targeting and responsive stimulation. DBS has been proven in many studies and is particularly effective in reducing motor symptoms, off-time and quality of life among appropriate patients.

This can extend over years if the device is programmed continuously and periodically monitored. BDS is indicated for patients with advanced Parkinson's disease who have not responded well to appropriate pharmacological treatments, and/or severe motor problems such as dyskinesia and motor fluctuation. One of the factors, as discussed in Kotyal et al. (2024), may be the good candidates for DBS. To be considered for surgery, one must undergo neurological testing, neuroimaging, and neuropsychological testing. For example, most patients are admitted if they have symptoms related to levodopa responsive motor. DBS may be helpful in patients who have severe motor impairment after levodopa. In addition, serious cognitive impairment or psychopathology is necessary because the condition may become more severe if there are no underlying conditions or if they do occur (Etukudoh & Ejinaka, 2024). But, age may have been associated with two other factors influencing patient selection, although recent studies suggest that age should not be considered a contraindication since older patients may benefit from age because they are much more able to cope with quality-of-life problems. Clinical studies have shown that DBS helps reduce motor symptoms. Rajagopalan et al. (2020) reported significant reductions in tremor, rigidity and bradykinesia in this meta-analysis of randomized controlled trials with STN-DBS. In sub-sourced settings, the results were slightly different, but in well-prepared centers with well trained staff, these might be similar to those in high income countries. Yet, in the long run, poor postoperative planning, inconsistent follow-up or device problems can be costly as well. There are also studies that suggest DBS prevents sleep disorders and mood disorders, but the extent of those benefits is a bit different among individuals. Short-term periosteal studies have found that motor function persists for 10 years following the operation and suggest DBS treatment may be warranted (Kumar & Sathiya, 2021).

DBS is great, but not a king. Electrodes and hardware for the pulse generator may also be infected, hemorrhaged, and hardware complications as they are surgically installed. But, Pulgar has demonstrated intracranial hemorrhage is a risk factor for 1–22% of DBS surgery and may result in stroke or death. Other complications of the device. Some are lead migration, fracture or malfunction; they can require revision surgery. The pulse generator is currently on but patients have to replace batteries and that is simple and expensive (Younas et al. 2016). In nature, the rechargeable batteries would help combat this issue, extending the life of the battery and minimizing device replacement costs. DBS is also one of the most problematic neuropsychiatric side effects. But some patients may experience post-operation mood disorders such as depression, anxiety or mania. Cognitive consequences in particular with STN-DBS are also associated with cognitive side effects, such as poor verbal fluency and low executive function (Ezike et al. 2023). These side effects are not confirmed but appear to be the result of stimulation of non-motor pathways in the basal ganglia circuit. DBS is also used in people of sensitivity, such as elderly or to manage chronic symptoms, to avoid discrimination. Access to this new treatment option is a tough question, though: how high the cost and healthcare gaps can make access to this new treatment strategy difficult? One of the possible explanations for this is that, among the many new technologies, such as closed-loop DBS systems being developed in the testing phase of studies, ethics is sensitive to patient consent and potentially false proven interventions (Chilvery et al., 2020). Deep Brain Stimulation is, of course, a revolutionary new surgery for Parkinson's disease. It has been substantially improved in motor and nonmotor advanced PD patients by modulating abnormal neuronal activity in target areas of the brain. But, surgery can also be problematic because of the risks of surgery, device complications, and neuropsychiatric side effects. These problems are being addressed with research and technology to improve the safety, effectiveness and access of DBS. Because the mechanism for DBS is still poorly understood, the potential benefit of this intervention is not known, but has implications in terms of quality of life that may be improved through continued treatment of Parkinson's patients.

Figure 2.

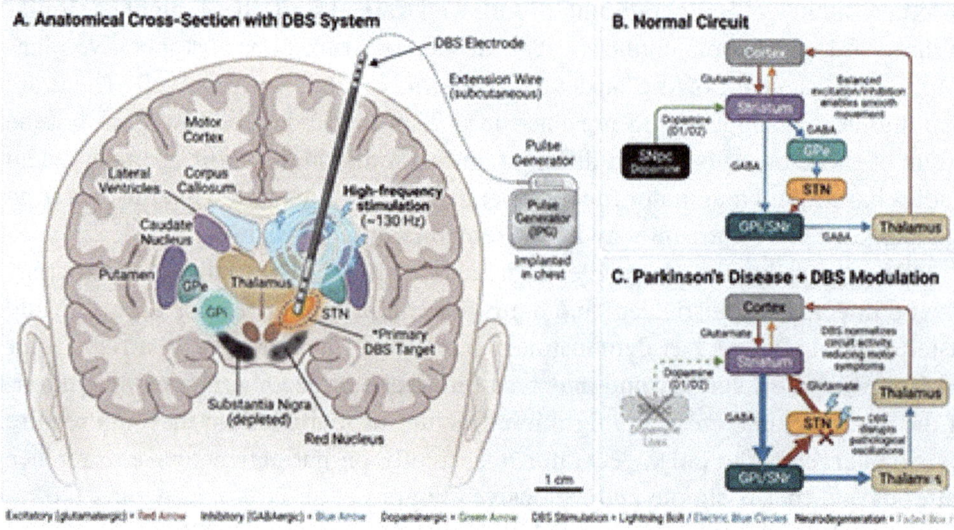

Ablative Procedures: Pallidotomy and Thalamotomy

Over the decades, relative procedures have become a major part of the pallidotomy andthalamotomy surgical approach toParkinson's disease. These were some of the first steroids to relieve crippling motor symptoms of PD, such as tremors, rigidity and bradykinesia. While such procedures have been relatively marginalized by new techniques like DBS, they are indeed unique, and what constitutes their action, its benefits, and challenges gives us information about how neurosurgical approaches to PD have evolved.

By the mid-19th century, a surgeon performed both pallidotomy and thalamotomy to treat the severe motor symptoms associated with PD under the supervision of an endocrinologist. During the most successful efforts to prevent advanced PD, most patients responded to the most effective treatments available, such as levodopa, but surgery was among the few interventions that improved quality of life. During this time period, somelesions were found to decrease the tremors and rigidity of the disease and eventually to initiate individualized ablative treatments.

Pallidotomy is the name given to a tumour of theglobus pallidus interna that controls the movements of objects in the brain. It was first developed in the 1950s and widely used for tremors and dyskinesia. Similarly, thalamotomy targets the VIM of thethalamus that transmits motor signals. This treatment became especially popular among tremor-like antidepressants.

They became less popular after the advent of levodopa during the 1960s, when it was common, and drugs seemed to be effective in halting motor symptoms. But as the symptoms of prolonged levodopa use, including motor impairment and dyskinesia, recede, ablative procedures become increasingly popular in older patients with high levels of PD. The resumption of interest in pallidotomy and thalamotomy during the 1990s set the stage for surgical treatment of PD and later, the development of DBS (Chilvery et al., 2020).

To understand the role of pallidotomy and thalamotomy on motor symptoms, we need to look at the basal ganglia circuitry, or brain regions that control motor behaviour. Because PD causes progressive loss of dopaminergic neurons in the substantia nigra, there is animbalance in this circuitry which overexerts some areas such as GPi and STN. During this time, the motor symptoms increase.

Pallidotomy targets the GPi, one of the principal basal ganglial output structures, which affects motor control by impairing the concentration of thalamocortical activity. Pallidotomy induces the GPi, which is hypersensitive and depresses the recruitment of basalganglia to the motor cortex. This reduces symptoms of bradykinesia, rigidity and tremors. Pallidotomy has been found to improve motor function and reduce prescribing among advanced PD patients (Tufail et al., 2023). On the other hand, Thalamotomy, the relay centre of motor signals, is the heart of the VIM of thethalamus. PD is affected by an abnormal neuronal activation of the VIM. This is the area where thlamotomy causes a lesion which stops aberrantsignal transmission, and reduces the intensity of tremors. This procedure is especially helpful in patients with tremor-dominant PD that are not responsive to pharmacological agents. But pallidotomy and thalamotomy have shown some promising results in specific motor symptoms, although each treatment containing both is unique. It is determined based on the symptoms, health history, and response to treatment. Neuroimaging and surgery, of course, have improved the accuracy and safety of these procedures, so that more precise interventions are made and outcomes are better.

Pallidotomy and thalamotomy are both of historical relevance, clinical benefits and risks and risks. One of the problems with these procedures is that they are irreversible. Unlike DBS in which neurons can be controlled and redirected, ablative procedures are permanent cures of brain tissue. This irreversibility can also be a source of longer-term complications, which makes it less flexible to change with the changes in patient's condition over time (Sinha & Dhanalakshmi, 2022).

Pallidotomy and thalamotomy are both potentially fatal procedures on an operative and neurologic level. All invasive procedures are potentially deadly, including infection, hemorrhage and anaesthesia complications. The other type of neurological risk is cognitive, speech and balance problems. These are especially alarming because tissue loss in an ablative procedure is permanent (Kotyal et al., 2024). Pallidotomy and thalamotomy have not been shown to be effective in treating non-motor PD symptoms such as cognitive decline, mood disorders and autonomic dysfunction. These adverse symptoms can persist even after effective treatment of motor symptoms and are harmful to the quality of life. This leads to the generalization of treatment for PD in relation to motor PD and nonmotor PD (Etukudoh & Ejinaka, 2024). Another problem with pallidotomy and thalamotomy is patient selection. Identify appropriate patients for these procedures based on symptom patterns, patient progression, and health. Complications and worse outcomes can be caused by high age, complications and cognitive impairment. This calls attention to individualized response to treatment that is based on the needs and preferences of the individual patient (Rajagopalan et al., 2020). In recent years, some of the complications of pallidotomy and thalamotomy have been surgically and neuroimaging treated. Intraoperative imaging and neurophysiological monitoring have facilitated better placement of the lesion, resulting in minimal brain injury. In addition, more minimally invasive procedures, such as focused ultrasound are emerging as viable alternatives to ablative procedures and are in high demand in the market (Kumar & Sathiya, 2021). Although pallidotomy and thalamotomy are often used with DBS as therapies for PD, research has been conducted to understand the efficacy of this treatment and how it might help. One concern is that ablative procedures should be combined with other therapeutics, such as pharmacology and rehabilitation, to provide a holistic approach to the treatment of symptoms. Plus, the use of neuroimaging and computational modelling can be used in the patient selection process as well as in improving the surgery outcome (Pulgar, 2019). On the other side of this promising road are therapies that can modulate PD development not only in terms of symptoms. Gene therapy and stem cell therapy, for example, are designed to restore dopaminergic function and reduce the likelihood of disease. These drugs are still under investigation, but may combine with surgical interventions to produce the most novel of new therapies for PD (Younas et al., 2016).

Finally, pallidotomy and thalamotomy are important developments in Parkinson's disease treatments. In some cases, this type of ablative therapy has significantly decreased symptoms of motor function in advanced PD amongst patients not responding well to pharmacological treatment. But because of their irreversibility and risk, adoption has decreased, especially with less intrusive, more flexible forms such as DBS. With the evolving nature of neuroscience, I think it is highly unlikely that pallidotomy and thalamotomy will be used to inform new and improved treatments for PD. Researchers and clinicians must put into place the tools to overcome the limitations of current surgical intervention and find new avenues to make PD much less burdensome, so that patients are better off. The case of pallidotomy and thalamotomy is also part of a narrative of attempts to combat this incurable disease, and in terms of further research and improvements in these areas (Ezike et al., 2023). The ablative procedure procedures (lesioning) also offer some advantages to poor and middle-income countries because they require no implanted hardware, are economical, hence less expensive, and need very little time to acquire technology. Some risks vary; irreversible risk, permanent neurological deficits, particularly bilateral lesions, moderate progression and nonmotor symptoms. Unilateral prelesioning would be an attractive alternative to DBS in cases with tremor-dominant PD where local expertise is useful. The non-invasive therapies, such as focused ultrasound thalamotomy, are promising but require substantial infrastructure and capital investment and are not available in low-income communities.

Emerging Techniques: Focused Ultrasound and Gene Therapy

More recently, FUS, as well as gene therapy, have expanded the surgical treatment of PD. These new approaches are welcome additions to the existing approaches, but can also be used to develop new processes and interventions addressing PD mechanisms. In this chapter, we describe how these new technologies work, what they do, their applications, and their problems, as well as briefly describe a few other promising avenues, including stem cell therapy and optogenetics. Focused ultrasound is the most popular non-invasive therapy for Parkinson's. FUS targets and abuts portions of the brain via ultrasonic waves, unlike thalamotomy and pallidotomy, where the incision is small with the risk of infection and complications. This approach has been particularly useful in treating PD motor symptoms such as tremors and rigidity. FUS sends high-frequency sound waves to a targeted brain region, such as the thalamus or globus pallidus. These sound waves produce localized heat that is damaging to the defective neural tissue but not the surrounding tissue (Chilvery et al., 2020). This accuracy also arises from the latest imaging technologies, such as magnetic resonance imaging or computed tomography, in which ultrasound beams are focused on a given location. In PD patients, the efficacy of FUS as a tremor drug has been noted. For example, Sinha & Dhanalakshmi (2022) reported that tremors were better controlled among FUS patients, without side effects. FUS is also non-invasive, requires less recovery time and is less likely to infect or bleed. FUS is therefore approved for essential tremor therapy and is currently being investigated for PD treatment. FUS is no cakewalk, but Reversibility is one of the main constraints. These results are permanent after ablation of the targeted neural tissue, and one should be cautious of the potentially fatal consequences of not mapping the target region (Tufail et al. 2023). In addition, the long-run efficacy and safety of FUS are still being tested. Researchers are currently working on more accurate and effective methods of treating PD. Gene therapy is another new treatment strategy for PD that may be useful in treating the cause of PD rather than in reverse. Gene therapy in PD focuses in the first place on restoring dopamine production, or preventing neurodegeneration that may cause the loss of dopaminergic neurons in the substantia nigra. Gene therapy may also be pursued by smuggling genes which encode dopamine synthesis enzymes like tyrosine hydroxylase and aromatic.

Recent developments in FUS and gene therapy, surgery for PD, and the area of focused ultrasound have created a growing interest. These new techniques are welcome improvements over those from previous generations, but they also allow for more sophisticated processes and measures to address mechanisms of PD. In this section we describe the mechanisms, applications, and challenges of these new approaches as well as briefly describe some other promising directions, including stem cell therapy and optogenetics.

Focused ultrasound is the most recently approved non-invasive method for treating Parkinson's disease. FUS uses ultrasonic waves to target and ablate specific areas of the brain, unlike thalamotomy and pallidotomy, which involve incisions which are extremely prone to infection and complications. This strategy has been particularly useful in treating PD motor symptoms such as tremors and rigidity. FUS sends high-frequency sound waves to one brain target, such as the thalamus or globus pallidus. These sounds produce heat to the defective neural tissue but not to the surrounding tissue (Chilvery et al., 2020). This accuracy is because new imaging methods, such as magnetic resonance imaging and computed tomography, focus the ultrasound beams on a specific area. PD patients have described clinical evidence for FUS as an effective treatment for tremors. Similarly, Sinha & Dhanalakshmi (2022) reported tremor control significantly higher among FUS patients but not without side effects. FUS is also less invasive, requires fewer incisions and therefore requires less recovery time, infection and bleeding. FUS has been accepted to be used in essential tremor therapy and is being investigated in the treatment of PD. FUS is not isolated, but. Reversibility is one of the major limitations. These effects persist after ablation of target neural tissue, and therefore, some caution should be exercised about the potentially damaging effects of not mapping the target area (Tufail et al. 2023). In addition, the long-term efficacy and safety of FUS are also a concern. Researchers are now attempting to make the technology more precise and effective in the treatment of PD. Gene therapy is another new PD treatment option, and it may be a better way to manage PD symptoms rather than treating them. Gene therapy for PD is designed to resuscitate dopamine production or prevent neurodegeneration that leads to the deletion of dopaminergic neurons in the substantia nigra. Another direction that might be explored is by introducing two of the genes involved in the production of dopamine, namely tyrosine hydroxylase and aromatic.

EFFICACY AND RISKS OF SURGICAL INTERVENTIONS IN PARKINSON'S DISEASE

Clinical Outcomes and Success Rates in Parkinson's Disease

At more advanced stages of the disease, surgeries become increasingly popular because pharmacological treatments are ineffective. In addition, PD has been treated successfully with DBS, pallidotomy or thalamotomy, and more effective medications such as targeted ultrasound or gene therapy. Here we discuss the clinical outcomes and results of these surgeries, how they work, and why long-term sustainability is important in the management of Parkinson's disease. DBS is a new treatment strategy for PD and is particularly helpful to address motor symptoms such as tremors, rigidity and bradykinesia. In other clinical trials it has been shown to enhance motor performance and to reduce dopaminergic effects. Chilvery, Palwai and Guggilla (2020) reported that UPDRS scores in DBS patients were much better and tremor frequency and motor dystrophy were substantially reduced. DBS targets both STN and GPi, a process that modulates abnormal PD neuronal activity. DBS does not reverse neurodegeneration by itself or reverse disease progression. Over the last few decades several alternatives to pallidotomy for PD symptoms such as tremors and rigidity have emerged. During these procedures, certain regions of the brain are burned down in order to break through pathological neuronal circuits. Tufail, Riggs and Tariq (2023) reported the reduction of tremors by thalamotomy with 50-90 per cent success rate and about equal to patient and surgical accuracy. Pallidotomy was also shown to treat dyskinesia and motor symptoms, so it is an effective adjunct to DBS treatment for patients who are not eligible. But they can be cognitively and speechly absent and are irreversible preventing effectiveness as well. Current drugs such as targeted ultrasound and gene therapy are promising alternatives to standard PD care. Focused ultrasound is an non-invasive approach that focused high frequency sound waves on a small portion of the brain. The drug has been shown to reduce tremors and improve motor function among PD patients, but with less side effects than surgery, such as by Sinha and Dhanalakshmi (2022). Gene therapy, on the other hand, prevents neurodegeneration and addresses the cause of PD by eliminating dopamine. The initial findings suggested both motor symptoms and quality of life have been successful and have remained successful.

Whether PD patients receive better treatment depends on surgical approach, procedures and surgical training. DBS was shown to reduce symptoms of motor functions for several years and there was evidence that DBS was effective for at least the longest time in 60% – 80% of patients (Kotyal, Nautiyal, Singh, Semwal, 2024). This strategy is particularly successful in young patients with advanced PD who respond well to levodopa but have motor complications. DBS requires, but mostly, precise placement of electrodes, which requires special imaging equipment and a neurosurgeon trained. Only on rare occasions are successful ablative procedures such as pallidotomy or thalamotomy, in light of its irreversible nature and potential complications. These may be useful in reducing tremors and rigidity, but not for other motor symptoms. Etukudoh & Ejinaka, (2024) compare thalamotomy success rate to 50%-75% recovery with the highest success rate for satisfied patients. Focused ultrasound has improved the accuracy and safety of ablative procedures and may become even more useful, and even more available. Many new therapies, such as gene therapy and focused ultrasound, are being investigated, but not fully tested. Some initial results suggest that they can deliver the same, or better, outcomes than conventional surgery. For example, Pulgar (2019) discusses ultrasound in the context of specific lesions that are less toxic to the surrounding tissue and thus less likely to have side effects in clinical trials.

Kumar and Sathiya suggested gene therapy in preclinical studies (2021), and some patients have shown marked improvement in symptoms and slow disease progression. Several factors have been identified that have a bearing on surgical success rates in PD, including number of patients being treated, surgical training, and technology.

Selection is an important predictor of surgery success, since the success of these procedures is almost entirely dependent on the patient's profile. DBS, for example, is the most effective if motor dysfunction occurs even under the best of medical care and in advancedPD. On the other hand, those with a high level of cognitive impairment or psychiatriccomorbidities are less likely to respond to DBS and may experience worse post-surgery symptoms.

Another important outcome problem is surgical knowledge. Such specific surgical procedures and specialized imaging techniques are needed to correctly place electrodes in DBS, or to perform precise lesioning operations in ablative procedures. Rajagopalan, Tang, Jia and Jia (2020) argue that MRI and CT in the high-resolution retina have made surgery less painful, more successful and more predictable.

Technological advances have also played a role in improving the safety and efficacy of surgical treatment for PD. For example, DBSsystems are closed-loop systems that link the stimuli in real time with neuronalactivity, and have been used to improve therapy outcomes and reduce side effects. Further, as Younas, Kong, Bashir and Nadeem (2016) suggest, artificial intelligence and machinelearning can be used to design and execute procedures that produce improved outcomes and better outcomes for patients.

While the potential for short-term effects and effects on progression of PD treatment have been documented, testing for longer-term effects and effects on progression has also been discussed. In addition, DBS is believed to allow patients to maintain their motor symptoms and quality of life for up to 10 years. But nonmotor symptoms like thinking a loss and motor dysfunction can be fatal to the procedure in general. Ezike,

Okpala, Onoja, Nwike and Ezeako (2023) describe long-run treatment strategies for motor and nonmotor symptoms to minimize residual effects of surgery.

On the other hand, relative procedures can have a long-term outcome, namely speech and cognitive impairment, which can also compromise patient health. Such procedures can also be transversal and can't be changed or reverted to meet evolving clinical needs as they can't be changed or reverted to meet changing clinical needs. Newer diagnostic methods, such as focused ultrasound and gene therapy, may be more effective and viable. Ultrasound is a targeted therapy, and it facilitates specific, irreversible therapies, while gene therapy targets the causes of diseases that slow or stop ageing.

Although surgical interventions forPD have excellent efficacy and clinical applications, there are still a few issues to be addressed and several considerations to be considered to maximize efficacy and accessibility. One problem is that these procedures are expensive and not affordable to low-resource patients. High technology costs and long-term follow-up complicate surgical costs. It is also because these drugs are rare to anyone, especially in the subservience, and it poses ethical concerns of equal and just care for all.

Another factor is the potential for complications of PD after surgery. These complications, infections, hemorrhage and hardware all point to care that requires carefully identified patient and surgical planning. Second, a risk and benefit analysis must be done before surgery to avoid cognitive and psychiatric side effects, especially when considering low-risk patients.

But, currently available surgery cannot combat the disease, and therefore, research and innovation in this area must be completed without a cure. As noted by Rajagopalan et al. 2019, "more and more therapies that use the microenvironmental mechanisms of PD, including neuroprotection and neurooregeneration, are needed to prevent long-term pathology and improve patient outcomes."

The literature of clinical and safety studies of surgery for Parkinson's disease presents an extraordinary potential for such procedures to save and improve the lives of patients with regard to motor and non-motor symptoms. The most commonly used method, Deep Brain Stimulation, is successful with high success rates and long-term success among carefully selected patients. The relative procedures can be effective, or in some cases irreversible and dangerous. Current diagnostic techniques, such as focused ultrasound and gene therapy, might improve the specificity, ad-hoc, or at best preventable, disease. And most importantly, it should be best practice to improve effectiveness, safety and accessibility of such interventions.

Similarly, outcome and cost, surgical training and technology, access, and ethics all make up a major issue. But they will need to continue working on research and improvements to address these problems and find the most cost-effective and equitable surgical approach to Parkinson's disease. As the field continues to evolve, the surgical, pharmacological and rehabilitation methods will be able to marry the most advanced surgical, pharmacological and rehabilitation strategies with the most advanced technologies, such as artificial intelligence and machine learning, to treat Parkinson's disease and improve the lives of millions of people worldwide. This pathophysiological argument for surgery is not static, but contextual. But if medicine is scarce and the patient is working, surgery can provide a very short-term means of reducing symptoms. This translates into the threat of a lack of infrastructure and follow-up. This is a two-fold reality and requires a pragmatic, contextual approach to surgical care. That is, surgery is not an "all or nothing" choice; it is part of a local continuum of care.

Complications and Ethical Considerations in Parkinson's Disease

To be sure, DBS and new treatments like focused ultrasound and gene therapy have adapted the surgical treatments used to treat advanced Parkinson's disease. But they are not easy processes. Surgery can help to account for many of the physical and psychological complications that could have taken place, such as infections and haemorrhage, and cognitive and physical problems that may be devastating to the overall health of a patient not being treated because they have not had access to care or current methods. In addition, the ethical issues of patient consent, access to new treatments and new technologies complicate the considerations of these options. Lastly, surgery has socio-economic dimensions, such as accessibility and price-performance, that suggest that PD therapies should be developed openly and in collaboration. Surgical intervention may be useful, but does not alter the neurodegenerative processes that promote the development of Parkinson's disease. It is possible that illness develops and other mental disorders, such as loss of brain function, autonomic dysfunction and mood disorders, can occur or worsen over time. These limitations indicate that informed patient selection and realistic counselling are critical. The second reason is that surgical outcomes are mediated through expertise, perioperative care and follow-up. But, in low-resource contexts, such limitations can make benefits complex or less valuable. These are limitations that are important to keep in mind when considering surgery as part of a more complete management plan. Surgical treatment of PD is also subject to several serious complications and risks that should be controlled immediately. It is a common surgical problem that occurs at the incision site or within the interior of the implanted device. Chilvery et al. (2020) found that surgical implants are contaminated with potentially toxic foreign compounds that inactivate or even disrupt immune functions. Infections can lead to longer hospital stays, more procedures for removing or replacing equipment, and more medical bills for patients and their health. One of the more serious complications is haemorrhage, which can occur either at the time of or after surgery because the brain is so fragile and there are blood vessels in the area that need to be occluded. Tufail et al. (2023) describe the relevance of imaging and machine learning models for surgical accuracy and hemorrhage prevention.

Nevertheless, bleeding continues to be a concern despite technological advancements, primarily in older patients or those at high risk for comorbidities that inhibit clotting or could worsen cardiac disease. The procedure can have psychological and cognitive effects as well. Pulgar (2019), in addition, concludes that "...the complex circuitry of the brain targeted by DBS may unwittingly affect areas of the brain associated with mood, cognition and behaviour". Some DBS patients have reported they are depressed, anxious or having trouble remembering, and an intense pre- and post-operative screening is a necessity. Kumar and Sathiya (2021) also point out that device error or incompatibility can result in symptoms of motor and non-motor symptoms, or be unpredictable. Surgery for PD is ethically responsible as well.

Consent is moral – a patient must make informed decisions. Etukudoh & Ejinaka, (2024) have found that patients should know the benefits, risks and limitations of surgery so that they can make informed decisions about whether or not to have surgery. But because PD is complex and the new technologies are experimental, patient confusion about the curative utility of their treatment may be a barrier to understanding, and informed consent is not an absolute requirement. Access to the most advanced surgical procedures has moral implications, especially in terms of healthcare inequality. As noted by Sinha and Dhanalakshmi (2022), demographic variables such as location and health infrastructure are also potentially important in predicting the chance of patients. For example, poor or rural patients might not need special care, while patients in developed countries may have access to technology and trained surgeons. At this point, policy and action must be taken to make access to highly effective treatments more equitable. More importantly, experimental research on new technologies like gene therapy and ultrasound is problematic. Kotyal et al. (2024) focus on this conflict between innovation and patient safety because the experimental therapy is included as a last resort for patients with advanced severe disease. Patients who receive non-tested, potentially dangerous drugs also face ethical challenges that require aggressive clinical trials, regulatory review and explicit information regarding the experimental nature of these drugs. Actions against PD have social and economic consequences that extend well beyond the patients themselves, their families, the health system, and society. This raises a very serious question about the cost-effectiveness of these procedures since both procedures are costly at the time of initiation and require periodic cleaning and follow-up after the procedure. As Rajagopalan et al. (2020) point out, surgery can be costly, or even far more costly than people can bear. This burden is not always cheap, but it can make it difficult for families to choose between self-treatment and specialist care; first might be cheaper than other treatments, or you may want to skip the surgery altogether. A similar problem is uneven access to surgery. Younas et al. (2016) believe that the developing countries may not have the infrastructure, training or funding to perform high-quality PD surgery. This divide creates a global gap in access to and quality of care which is compounded by patients suffering in poor countries. To overcome these imbalances, collaboration is needed in improving healthcare infrastructure, training doctors, and providing funding for specialized treatments. General social and public health policy and research goals are surgical treatments.

Ezike et al. (2023) emphasise the need for surgical innovations to be embedded in a variety of therapies that are pharmacological and rehabilitation-based. This combined will allow hospitals to deliver the best outcomes for patients and potentially avoid expensive surgeries. Other public health programs should invest in research and clinical testing for new treatments so that as many patients as possible can gain benefits from innovation. The PD surgical interventions, complications and ethical concerns are complex, and many approaches have been tried. First, improved surgical techniques and equipment could produce a physical infection and haemorrhage. High-speed imaging devices, intraoperative monitoring and precision-guided devices can also be used to improve surgical accuracy and prevent complications. In addition to the material choice for surgical implants, further work on the application of machine learning models to surgical planning would be worthwhile if Chilvery et al. 2019 and Tufail et al. 2023 were used. Second, ethical considerations include patient education and consent. Etukudoh & Ejinaka (2024) also write that "standardized guidelines and educational materials for patients and their families can allow them to better understand surgical options and make informed decisions". Patients' participation in decision-making also provides an opportunity for trust and collaboration between patients and health care workers. Third, there needs to be action at multiple scales against access problems that require surgical intervention. Sinha and Dhanalakshmi (2022) urge subsidies, telemedicine consultations, and international collaboration to make health care more accessible for poor people. In addition, Kotyal et al. (2024) stress the value of ethical supervision in developing and using new technologies so that innovation is not considered a threat to patient safety or equity. Third, surgery and holistic therapy can be combined to improve outcomes for patients and reduce PD management costs. Rajagopalan et al. (2020) and Ezike et al. (2023) discuss the potential for surgery in combination with pharmacological and rehabilitation interventions and the potential for artificial intelligence and machine learning in tailoring treatment plans. This could lead to increased surgical availability, safety and cost, as well as strategies for managing PD at acute sites. Parkinson's surgery has also altered the landscape of new therapies available to those who cannot overcome symptoms effectively alone through pharmacological treatments. But the challenges, moral questions and social outcomes of such processes must also be contained and used in all directions and without any exclusion.

The health systems may provide more strategies to address PD by increasing physical risk, awareness and consent, access to new therapies, and surgical innovations in integrated care systems for patient safety, health equity and well-being. The possibilities will continue to be developed through research and collaboration, and we can make the full possibility of surgical intervention in Parkinson's disease a reality.

FUTURE DIRECTIONS IN SURGICAL INNOVATION IN PARKINSON'S DISEASE

This is an example of a first that fits into the context that will be the future of surgical treatment for Parkinson's disease in the poorly-sourced context. I recommend less invasive procedures, cost-effective neuromodulation programs, and local guidelines for clinical care. Low and middle-income research needs to be encouraged to collect locally relevant evidence as opposed to forcing data from high-income countries. In recent years, the quality of PD surgical care has improved dramatically by reducing intrusive procedures and will undergo intensive procedures, which may yield better results. But as this progress continues, there remain challenges to the efficacy, safety and accessibility of existing surgery. This is what has led to ongoing research on these issues and the best ways to improve the quality of life for PD sufferers. The present chapter discusses the directions for surgical innovation, such as better DBS technology, surgical intervention through pharmacological and rehabilitation therapy, and the use of artificial intelligence and machine learning to improve several aspects of treatment.

DBS is one of the most novel surgical interventions for motor symptoms in advancedPD. DBS is widely used and effective, but it has its problems: improper placement of electrodes, side effects and constant adjustment to adjust stimulus settings. To correct this skewed state, new DBS methods have been devised, including closed-loop systems and adaptive stimulation. Closed-loop DBS systems have become increasingly popular because they overcome the disadvantages of closed-loop DBS. Closed-loop DBS is electrically stimulated continuously at a constant frequency regardless of temporal or temporal activity or patient symptom type. This can lead to poor results and worse side effects. Unlike closed-loop systems, stimuli are stimulated via actual brain electrical activity. For example, LFPs in the STN can act as a biomarker of the response to or stimuli from a system (Chilvery et al., 2019). The first empirical evidence supports the hypothesis that closed-loop DBS can be used to reduce stimuli and to better manage symptoms. A second aspect of DBS technology is adaptive stimulation, in which patients control electricstimulation on a person according to their physiological andpathological characteristics. A new class of algorithms that detect symptoms at the start of the exacerbation and prevent the stimulus change is being developed for adaptive DBS systems. This approach also prolongs the device's life and decreases the number of device replacement surgeries (Tufail et al. 2023), in addition to reducing symptoms. For example, researchers have developed adaptive experimental DBS systems that incorporate wearable sensors to detect and treat symptoms of motor actions in real-time. These sensors can detect tremors, bradykinesia, or rigidity and communicate with the DBS device that adjusts output. But, there are still concerns regarding the commercialisation of closed-loop and adaptive DBS technologies. Identifying and validating appropriate biomarkers for livemonitoring remains an important issue. LFPs are promising but difficult to interpret, and some further analysis is needed to determine whether they are particular or sensitive to patients at different stages of disease. These new systems need to be robust, flexible enough to handle many data points at any given moment, and have accessible interfaces for clinicians and patients to implement these new systems in clinical practice.

Parkinson's disease is complex, with motor symptoms and non-motor symptoms, and requires several treatments such as surgery, pharmaceuticals and rehabilitation. But, while DBS and ablative treatments surgically target the physiology of the symptoms of motor control, they may not adequately treat other symptoms of mental disorder, mood disorders, or autonomic dysfunction. There is also a growing debate about whether integrated therapy will better manage symptomatology. Some promising studies have shown that DBS can be matched with drugs that treat non-motor symptoms. For example, some research has combined DBS and cholinesterase inhibitors in the treatment of PD symptoms. Dopamine agonists and serotonergic drugs are also being studied to help us identify an alternative to DBS for the treatment of mood disorders and sleepstörungs (Sinha & Dhanalakshmi, 2022). Such combinational therapies aim to maximize each treatment regimen's efficacy while avoiding side effects. Other treatments that may help to improve the outcome of surgery include physiotherapy, occupational therapy and speech therapy. Some of the newer studies also indicate that individual PD rehabilitation practices actually improve motor and non-motor functioning.

Physical activity is also thought to promote neuroplasticity and motor coordination, which makes it an appropriate complement to DBS (Kotyal et al.,2024). Also, CBT and mindfulness are being examined as a response to anxiety, depression, and other PD related psychological disorders. While a combination of surgery, pharmacological treatment and rehabilitation may be beneficial, there are some barriers to pursuing them before they are considered clinically useful. Another problem is that multimodal treatment protocols are not protocol-specific and result in inconsistent outcomes. This is also because these kinds of coordinated care would be expensive and difficult to enact in a setting with limited resources (Etukudoh & Ejinaka, 2024). Future research should focus on making sound recommendations and finding cost-effective approaches to ensuring that all patients have full access to integrated therapies.

For example, AI and machine learning are changing the landscape of healthcare, and there is a shift in the field of data-based decision-making and predictive analytics. For Parkinson's disease, these devices could have a major impact on surgical planning, patient selection and prediction. But the most important step in a successful PD surgery is to find the right candidates for procedures such as DBS. The growing use of AI systems for big data analyses using neuroimaging, genetics, clinical, and computational models provides the opportunity to identify patients who could benefit from surgery.

Machine learning models, for example, measure brainconnectivity and neural activity to identify biomarkers of successful surgery (Rajagopalan et al., 2020).

Those tools can help patients become more selective and reduce the risk of disappointing outcomes and unnecessary surgery. AI and ML are also being used for better planning and performing surgery and patient selection. High resolution brain maps are produced by using high-quality imaging techniques such as fMRI and diffusion tensor imaging DTI. This allows AI algorithms to work with such images to determine which DBS electrodes should be placed in the appropriate locations in order to avoid complications and enhance therapeutic efficacy. Plus, AI is merging with robotic-assisted surgery to improve the precise placement of electrodes and ensure safety (Kumar & Sathiya, 2021). AI can be used to manage post-surgical care and for long-term outcomes monitoring. In addition, there are machine learning models available for making informed, real-time treatment decisions on wearable devices that can predict the development of future complications or symptoms. For example, AI-based machines are being developed that sense motor symptoms remotely and manipulate DBS settings as needed without having to be brought to the clinic (Pulgar, 2019). These are better outcomes for patients and save the healthcare systems money. The potential applications of AI and ML in PD surgery management have some difficulties. Another problem is the level of quality and heterogeneity in the data used to construct AI algorithms. Depending upon the data collection practices, patient characteristics, and severity of disease, generalizability may be a concern with predictive models. These ethical issues of data privacy, algorithm transparency and decision-making accountability should also be considered (Younas et al., 2016). Researchers, clinicians and policy makers therefore need to jointly work to guide and educate an informed use of AI. Future surgical approaches to Parkinson's disease will present new frontiers in terms of DBS technology, combinatory therapies, and combined AI/ML. DBS coupled with closed loops and adaptive DBS systems enable individualized, dynamic stimulation that will transform the management of symptoms. The patient does not need only PD for one particular individual. PD treatments often involve multiple approaches to surgery, medications, and rehabilitation therapy. Meanwhile, AI and ML will drive surgery, altering patient selection, surgical planning and monitoring in the long run. But there is no easy way to triumph. These new technologies require extensive research, infrastructure and training to develop and apply. Ethics, such as access to the latest treatment, and data privacy issues, should also be addressed. As surgical innovation and hope grow for Parkinson patients, this will be a response to these concerns and a mechanism of collaboration that will increase in its pace. Despite the surgical means available for preventing Parkinson's disease, new technologies must be developed to overcome barriers and to expand reach. Combining these new technologies with multidisciplinary treatments will certainly change the landscape of PD treatment and – last but not least – the lives of millions of patients across the globe. They believe more research and collaboration will make a successful operation for Parkinson's possible.

LIMITATIONS OF CURRENT SURGICAL APPROACHES IN PARKINSON'S DISEASE

Parkinson's disease is a progressive neurodegenerative disease which causes the loss of dopaminergic neurons in the substantia nigra and neurological symptoms. Surgery, particularly DBS or ablation, has been able to reverseParkinson's disease from the underlying cause. But, while they do relieve symptoms, a few limitations mean that these surgeries will not completely resolve the disease complexity. I discuss in this section the range of limitations and arguments to prevent disease progression through existing surgical procedures or the reverse, to patients' choice and to maintain research to improve safety, efficacy and access. One of the greatest missteps today of invasive treatment of Parkinson's disease is that they focus on symptoms rather than on pathology. Some important behavioural interventions, including DBS have been shown to combat motor symptoms like tremor, rigidity and bradykinesia but not to combat the neurodegenerative mechanism of the disease. Given the ineffectiveness of preventing and reversing PD, it is time to shift to intervention at the root of PD. For example, DBS is linked to abnormal neuronal activity in areas of the brain such as the STN or GPi. This promotes motor function but does not induce retention of dopaminergic neurons or pathologic accumulation of alpha-synuclein aggregates (Chilvery et al., 2020). It might, in turn contribute to a progressive worsening of non-motor symptoms more resistant to DBS, such as cognitive impairment, mood disorders and motor dysfunction. This leads to an increasing need for the pathology of PD, or at least neuroprotective orneurorestorative practices, intervention. Another factor is that the accuracy of surgical intervention in managing symptoms can also vary widely from patient to patient. The frequency and/or stage of disease can be explained by symptoms, brain anatomy and physiology. This range is important because the treatment strategies discussed in this chapter fall within this range. One of the most grave problems with current procedures is that nobody knows who should be treated for such surgery. The patient selection process is a complex one involving multiple variables such as the degree and severity of symptoms, the overall health of the patient, and any changes in the patient's previous treatment. Imaging and diagnostics have improved, but it is important to determine which patients will most benefit from surgery. Deep Brain Stimulation, for example, is primarily used in advanced patients with advanced PD who have severe motor symptoms that cannot be controlled effectively by medications. But not all patients with advanced PD qualify for DBS.

In this study, high levels of cognitive impairment, or those with severe psychiatric disorders or other medical conditions, are not eligible for treatment because they are more complicated (Tufail et al.,2023). Plus, even though outcomes are somewhat variable for all eligible patients, this also indicates more stringent criteria for the selection of patients. One new class of Parkinson's biomarkers may be able to combat this problem. Identifiable biomarkers that characterize pathogens or predict drug responses could help determine which types of patients are most likely to benefit from surgery. For example, recent studies have focused on the use of neuroimaging biomarkers such as DAT scans to examine the integrity of dopaminergic neurons and predict DBS targeting (Sinha & Dhanalakshmi, 2022). This can be done in very short amounts of time since there are no common protocols, and they are expensive. The psychosocial is also used along with the biological aspects of patient selection. A procedure is successful for several reasons, including patient expectations, social support, access to health services and health outcomes. For example, patients who did not believe in the DBS outcome may not be as impressed with the initial impression of the result as they were by the technically successful procedure. This requires extensive preoperative counselling and family support for patients and their families so that they are told the benefits and disadvantages of surgery. As current surgical procedures are very limited, studies and developments will need to be conducted in order to ensure the safety, efficacy and availability of these procedures. Other promising directions of research include the use of DBS technology, less invasive surgery and collaboration among surgery and new treatments. One of the concerns is to develop better DBS technology so that the associated therapeutic results and side effects can be mitigated. Recent work also aimed to develop closed-loop DBS systems that dynamically adjust stimulus parameters via real-time neural activity feedback. These two tools can be combined to provide a more precise and personalized treatment with minimal side effects such as dyskinesia or cognitive deficit

(Kotyal et al., 2024). That and improved electrode placement and targeting may have other effects on DBS results as well. Other promising research areas include less invasive surgical techniques like focus ultrasound (FUS). FUS, unlike other procedures, which require cuts and tissue injury, produces specific lesions in the targeted area of the brain via high-frequency sound waves. The non-invasive option has been shown to reduce tremors and other motor symptoms in PD patients, is cheaper, requires less surgery and has shorter recovery times than the other options (Etukudoh & Ejinaka, 2024). In the long run, the safety and efficacy of this strategy must be explored. In addition to medical advancements, invasive procedures and other treatments may dramatically improve PD outcomes. For instance, DBS combined with gene therapy or stem cell therapy could reverse the pathology and severity of the disease. Preclinical studies have shown that gene therapy that stimulates dopamine production may be useful in restoring or preventing degeneration of dopaminergic neurons (Rajagopalan et al., 2020). Similarly, stem cell therapy may replace lost neurons, allow normal brain functions, and provide a more complete response to PD. The treatments of surgery and opdology are promising, but expensive. The procedure DBS can be expensive and difficult to obtain in specialist surgical centres, especially in low- and middle-income countries. This will require coordinated efforts to reduce the cost of operative procedures, increase the supply of specialized training for health care providers, and make medical treatment affordable and accessible (Kumar & Sathiya, 2021). Ethics also influences the development and administration of surgical treatments for PD. Concerns like informed consent, the use of experimental methods, and the limited use of medical resources must be considered for an equitable distribution of these treatments. Similarly, the use of technology such as gene therapy or neural implants generates complicated ethical questions concerning the balance between benefits and disadvantages as well as long-term consequences for patients and society (Pulgar, 2019).

CONCLUSION

If needed, acute surgical treatment for PD is also available and is effective in low-sourced sources. In addition to deep brain stimulation, a suitable surgical approach is still important, but a less expensive procedure. Plus, the surgery for Parkinson's disease has made some progress in diagnosing this serious disease, but its limitations reflect a growing need for research and innovation. The current DBS and ablative approaches focus on symptomatic management but do not address the mechanisms of neurodegeneration responsible for the disease. These are some of the barriers to optimal and equitable care, including barriers to patient selection, treatment variability and access constraints. Focusing on research and capacity-building in a low-resource setting will lead to better procedures, new treatments, and ethical and economic considerations for these treatments, thus potentially making it easier to access and enhance the efficacy of therapies that really make a difference in the lives of patients with Parkinson's disease in a low-resource setting. It is a long, slow, but ultimately difficult process to overcome those limitations, but with the continued technological advances in neuroscience and medicine, there is hope for a day in which surgery alleviates symptoms and possibly cures this deadly disease.

REFERENCES

Ajagun, E. J., Asuku, A. O., Ayinla, M. T., Abdulsalam, T. A., Ajibare, A. J., Olajide, T. S., Hamza, Y. O., & Ganiyu, K. O. (2024). Pharmacotherapy of Parkinson's disease and their limitations. In *Zebrafish as a model for Parkinson's disease*. CRC Press., DOI: 10.1201/9781003402893-17

Alassaf, Y. (2024). Comprehensive review of the advancements, benefits, challenges, and design integration of energy-efficient materials for sustainable buildings. *Buildings (Basel, Switzerland)*, *14*(9), 2994.

Asuku, A. O., Ayinla, M. T., Olajide, T. S., Ajagun, E. J., Ganiyu, K. O., Hamza, Y. O., Ajibare, A. J., & Abdulsalam, T. A. (2024). Diagnosis and biomarkers of Parkinson's disease. In *Zebrafish as a model for Parkinson's disease*. CRC Press., DOI: 10.1201/9781003402893-15

Braak, H., Del Tredici, K., Rüb, U., de Vos, R. A., Jansen Steur, E. N., & Braak, E. (2003). Staging of brain pathology related to sporadic Parkinson's disease. *Neurobiology of Aging*, *24*(2), 197–211. PMID: 12498954

Chilvery, A., Palwai, S., Guggilla, P., Wren, K., & Edinburgh, D. (2020). Perovskite materials: Recent advancements and challenges. In *Perovskite materials, devices and integration*. IntechOpen., DOI: 10.5772/intechopen.88500

Dorsey, E. R.. (2018). Global, regional, and national burden of Parkinson's disease, 1990–2016. *Lancet Neurology*, *17*(11), 939–953. PMID: 30287051

Etukudoh, N., & Ejinaka, O. (2024). Advancements, challenges, and opportunities in physical systems.

Ezike, T., Okpala, U., Onoja, U., & Nwike, C. (2023). Advances in drug delivery systems: Challenges and future directions. *Heliyon*. PMID: 37416680

Hanson, E., Nwakile, C., & Hammed, V. (2025). Carbon capture, utilization, and storage (CCUS) technologies: Evaluating the effectiveness of advanced CCUS solutions for reducing CO_2 emissions. *Results in Surfaces and Interfaces*.

Kotyal, K., Nautiyal, P., & Singh, M. (2024). Advancements and challenges in artificial intelligence applications: A comprehensive review. *Journal of Scientific Research*.

Kumar, M., & Sathiya, P. (2021). Methods and materials for additive manufacturing: A critical review on advancements and challenges. *Thin-walled Structures*.

Mythri, R. B., & Bharath, M. M. S. (2012). Mitochondrial dysfunction and oxidative stress in Parkinson's disease. *Molecular Neurobiology*, *46*(1), 194–214. PMID: 22821186

Obeso, J. A.. (2017). Past, present, and future of Parkinson's disease. *Movement Disorders*, *32*(9), 1264–1310. PMID: 28887905

Olanow, C. W., Stern, M. B., & Sethi, K. (2009). The scientific and clinical basis for the treatment of Parkinson disease. *Neurology*, *72*(21, Suppl 4), S1–S136. PMID: 19470958

Pulgar, V. (2019). Transcytosis to cross the blood–brain barrier: New advancements and challenges. *Frontiers in Neuroscience*. PMID: 30686985

Rajagopalan, R., Tang, Y., & Ji, X. (2020). Advancements and challenges in potassium ion batteries: A comprehensive review. *Advanced Functional Materials*.

Schrag, A.. (2000). What contributes to quality of life in Parkinson's disease? *Journal of Neurology, Neurosurgery, and Psychiatry*, *69*(3), 308–312. PMID: 10945804

Sinha, B., & Dhanalakshmi, R. (2022). Recent advancements and challenges of Internet of Things in smart agriculture: A survey. *Future Generation Computer Systems*.

Spillantini, M. G., & Goedert, M. (2018). Neurodegeneration and the ordered assembly of alpha-synuclein. *Cell and Tissue Research*, *373*(1), 137–152. PMID: 29119326

Tufail, S., Riggs, H., Tariq, M., & Sarwat, A. (2023). Advancements and challenges in machine learning: A comprehensive review of models, libraries, applications, and algorithms. *Electronics (Basel)*.

Tushar, W., Yuen, C., Saha, T., & Morstyn, T. (2021). Peer-to-peer energy systems for connected communities: A review of recent advances and emerging challenges. *Applied Energy*.

Weerarathna, I. N., Doelakeh, E. S., Kiwanuka, L., Kumar, P., & Arora, S. (2024). Prophylactic and therapeutic vaccine development: Advancements and challenges. *Molecular Biomedicine*, *5*(1), 57. DOI: 10.1186/s43556-024-00222-x PMID: 39527305

Younas, M., Kong, L. L., & Bashir, M. (2016). Recent advancements, fundamental challenges, and opportunities in catalytic methanation of CO_2. *Energy*.

Zhou, T., Yuan, Z., Weng, J., Pei, D., & Du, X. (2021). Challenges and advances in clinical applications of mesenchymal stromal cells. *Journal of Hematology (Brossard, Quebec)*. PMID: 33579329

Chapter 11
Smart Watch-Based Motion and Voice Analysis for Parkinson's Disease in Under-Resourced Settings

R. Jansi
http://orcid.org/0000-0001-9894-0006
Department of Electronics and Communication Engineering, Faculty of Engineering and Technology, SRM Institute of Science and Technology, India

R. Athilakshmi
http://orcid.org/0000-0002-1772-5388
Department of Computational Intelligence, Faculty of Engineering and Technology, SRM Institute of Science and Technology, India

Alvin Ben George
Department of Electronics and Communication Engineering, Faculty of Engineering and Technology, SRM Institute of Science and Technology, India

Daniel Biju Joseph
Department of Electronics and Communication Engineering, Faculty of Engineering and Technology, SRM Institute of Science and Technology, India

Debanshu Roy
Department of Electronics and Communication Engineering, Faculty of Engineering and Technology, SRM Institute of Science and Technology, India

S. Haarish
Department of Electronics and Communication Engineering, Faculty of Engineering and Technology, SRM Institute of Science and Technology, India

DOI: 10.4018/979-8-3373-7437-6.ch011

ABSTRACT

Parkinson's disease (PD) is the second most common neurological disorder in India. Accurate diagnosis of PD is limited due to the unavailability of sufficient resources. In this research, an IoT-based Parkinson's Smart Watch System that combines both the motion and voice analysis models to attain a real-time PD detection is being proposed. This system uses ESP32 microcontroller along with MEMS inertial sensors and microphones to capture and analyze the motor and voice patterns. The acquired voice data was evaluated using tuned K-Nearest Neighbor and Random Forest classifiers to achieve a prediction accuracy of 97.40% and 95%, respectively. The proposed watch also has the capability to detect falls based on the IMU sensor threshold values and gives SOS alerts powered by GSM modules and Twilio messaging systems to achieve immediate response during emergencies. This system also has additional features like individualized medication and meal reminders along with remote monitoring capacity to enhance patient care.

INTRODUCTION

Parkinson's disease (PD) is a long-lasting nervous ailment which includes motor degeneration and affected great numbers of people worldwide. Due to the absence of specific tests, diagnosing the condition is problematic. Medications like Levodopa provide symptomatic relief but may cause motor fluctuations as well as dyskinesia. Clinical assessments such as MDS-UPDRS are subjective and do not always match patients' real motor condition. Wearable motion sensors, specifically IMUs, hold promise for continuously monitoring PD symptoms during normal activities in everyday life (Sica et al., 2021). PD is a neurodegenerative disorder that involves the death of neurons, dopaminergic ones in particular, and this process is usually caused by the interaction between genetic factors and environmental factors (Asuku et al., 2024; Asuku et al., 2025). In familial PD, which makes up 15% of all cases, mutations in such genes as LRRK2 or DJ-1 can lead to the disease (Krokidis et al., 2022).

PD manifests as motor and non-motor symptoms, in about 1% of those above the age of 60, which are mainly managed with Levodopa. Treatment adjustments are marred by motor fluctuations that include "wearing-off" (Ajagun et al., 2024). Clinical examination remains subjective due to symptom fluctuations. For objective assessment, wearable sensors help in symptom monitoring and treatment adjustments. Breakthroughs in sensor technology and AI promote individualized care and distant monitoring. This article will discuss the detection of PD motor fluctuations using sensors as well as machine learning applications to differentiate between on and off states for optimal therapy towards improved patients' quality of life (Barrachina-Fernández et al., 2021).

The diagnosis and treatment of abnormal gait as well as the detection of falls among the elderly population require an analysis of the way people walk. To better understand it, gait cycle which is divided into stance phase and swing phase further goes to break down detailed periods. Stages such as Heel Strike and Toe Off point out these phases (Chatzaki et al., 2021). The prevalence of PD will increase as people grow old with this ailment, the symptoms of which are both motor and non-motor related, worsening significantly one's quality of life especially during the advanced stages. To date, existing assessments are based on patient diaries as well as clinical scales which limit longitudinal follow up surveillance. In this context, wearable gadgets can be utilized for constant monitoring purposes. The data collection for the Levodopa Response Study was carried out both inside a laboratory environment and at home as well (Daneault et al., 2021).

PD exhibits motor swings, and a limited number of tests are done for its accurate tracking. Shimmer sensors were put on the lower back and all four limbs of the hands of nineteen subjects to collect some data related data. Motor tasks and wearables were co-applied to see how it goes. The subjects are staged according to the severity of the disease. Limb specifics, however, measure the degree of symptomality and converge with MDS-UPDRS. The data obtained from sensors and Daphnet also play an important role with focus on motor disorders. When equipment like the upper limb is used in the monitoring of symptoms, they become less dependent on subjective judgment and have the best validation. The information in this dataset will be of help in the development of machine learning algorithms for the monitoring of home patients particularly important in the clinical settings for long-term post-Parkinson's disease treatment (Vergara-Diaz et al., 2021). This disease affects patients with limited access to specialists, rare neurology consultations and unpredictable responses to treatment. Some wearable technologies, especially inertial measurement units (IMUs), may help in this regard if they are well utilized. Despite being a subject of interest among some people, implementing it in clinics has not been feasible. The International Movement Disorder Society acknowledge that wearable sensors have potential but do not provide practical guidance. This compendium focuses on body-worn sensors (BWS) primarily available in Europe for PD management by monitoring its manifestations and adjusting treatments accordingly. This paper provides strength, weaknesses as well as validation processes of these devices so that clinicians, patients' families and other caregivers can benefit from this information (Moreau et al., 2023).

PD was first described as a chronic disorder by James Parkinson in 1817. It is marked by the loss of dopamine-producing neurons that bring about motor and non-motor symptoms, such as shaking, slowed movements, and sadness. In fact, diagnosing PD is difficult especially during its onset stage (Balakrishnan et al., 2022). Clinical diagnosis and management of PD rely heavily on adjustment of L-Dopa therapy and neurological examination because they do not have reliable biomarkers for monitoring its course. The advancement of wearable electrochemical sensing platforms offers exciting perspectives for integrated PD management. Such biosensors are made by depositing organic recognition elements directly on top of transducers for quantitative or semi-quantitative analysis of biological fluids. In this review, we explore the potential of next-generation electrochemical biosensing technologies meant to detect and monitor Parkinson's disease including the role played by their ability to recognize alpha-synuclein and dopamine molecules in such phenomena as early diagnosis and course prognosis of Parkinson's disease (Asci et al., 2022).

Wearable devices such as these can be used for monitoring various human activities daily, making them cost-effective and accessible to everyone. Tri-axial accelerometer data is the most employed method in gait analysis wearable sensors using IMU. But this would need to be balanced against battery life. Recent developments in artificial intelligence including deep neural networks have improved gait analysis from wearable sensor data, thereby enabling continuous long-term monitoring out the clinic settings. To assess continuous at-home monitoring possibilities in clinical populations, this study proposes a single wearable sensor based deep learning pipeline for gait analysis (Peraza et al., 2021). Gait and balance are greatly affected by PD leading to increased chances of falling. Nevertheless, the prevalence and economic burden has not led to the development of more objective methods for assessing falls in PD clinical trials except self-reporting which is prone to subjectivity and inaccuracies. One possible answer comes from wearable sensors that could provide an objective and repetitive estimation of fall risk based on gait analysis. In previous studies conducted among patients with PD, use of sensors during the Timed Up and Go (TUG) test was found promising as a reliable predictor of falls (Greene et al., 2022).

The progression of PD is usually monitored with clinical rating scales that can be subjective and insensitive. On the other hand, using wearable sensors to detect motor symptoms has several advantages; they offer continuous and objective data. Additionally, machine learning models trained in sensor measurements have the potential to tell different stages and phenotypes apart. Therefore, we will use data from wearables recorded every three months for 18 months to model PD progression (Sotirakis et al., 2023). Freezing of gait (FoG), however, is one of the most prevalent and distressing symptoms in PD that is characterized by temporary inability to start or continue walking. Consequently, this can cause falls and affect patients' quality of life negatively. For detecting FoG, wearable sensors, mainly inertial sensors have been studied as they are cheaper and can be used easily. These sensors have an advantage over vision-based systems because they can monitor patients anywhere at any time. Some interventions like Rhythmic Auditory Stimulation (RAS) and visual cues hold promise for managing FoG though their effectiveness still needs to be investigated further. Detecting FoG early enough becomes very important especially in relation to effective management due to lack of proper treatments that are usually applied at later stages. The main goal of improving PD patient care should therefore be focused on developing wearable devices for early detection of FoG (Ren et al., 2022).

Falls and injuries often result from a common symptom called postural instability. To effectively manage the condition, early detection is necessary; however, current clinical methods usually detect instability when symptoms become visible. Nevertheless, wearable sensors could be one solution in detecting such cases earlier on through their provision of objective data (Castelli Gattinara Di Zubiena et al., 2022). The use of these sensors has been mainly in assessment of motor features although studies have largely focused on clinic-based assessments rather than real-life experiences. What we intend to do in our research is examine the prevalence and impact of tremors outside the clinic. By investigating when tremors occur during the day, how much they change in size or frequency, as well as what kind action they relate to, this paper aims at revealing a difference between those two ideas. This variation can be understood by using clock-based visualization based on wearable sensor data (Adams et al., 2021).

Global and Indian Perspective of Parkinson's Disease

Parkinson's disease (PD) is one of the fastest growing neurological diseases (Dorsey et al., 2017) and causes increasing disability worldwide. Although the elderly population is primarily affected by the illness, growing evidence suggests that early-onset Parkinson's disease is being diagnosed more frequently. Due to global increase in life expectancy, urbanization and change in lifestyle, there has been a sharp increase in number of people living with PD. Epidemiological studies show that the load of PD could double in two decades, likely to create crippling pressure on the already resource-constrained healthcare systems.

In terms of India, it appears to be quite serious. India has a large population with a skewed distribution of neurologists and inadequate access to advanced diagnostic facilities that cause delays in diagnosis and long-term management. Patients in rural and semi-urban areas generally seek basic treatment from general physicians rather than movement disorder specialists. This leads to misdiagnosis or under diagnosis. The frequent hospital visits are also not feasible for older patients because of their inability to move, cost factor and dependence on caregivers. The issue calls for developing economical, scalable and tech-driven solutions that enable regular monitoring and early detection of Parkinson's disease outside clinical settings.

One more vital issue is the unavailability of any objective and continuous data for monitoring. Standard evaluations done in hospitals are "one-off" and fail to capture fluctuations in the motor and non-motor symptoms of patients. Given the substantial intra-and inter-day fluctuations in Parkinson's Disease, episodic clinical examinations alone will likely yield less than optimal treatment adjustments. Due to this gap, wearable and IoT based systems are explored to produce real – time and longitudinal patient health insights.

Limitations of Current Parkinson's Disease Evaluation and Monitoring

Parkinson's disease is clinically diagnosed even with neurological and imaging being advanced of achievements. Neurologists place significant reliance upon symptom observation, patient history and validated rating scales, including the Unified Parkinson's Disease Rating Scale (UPDRS) and its revised variant, MDS-UPDRS. While the first and second chairs are widely used scales, they are subjective measures that depend on each examiner's experience and the patient's cooperation.

Another crucial shortcoming of standard diagnosis is the lack of valid biomarkers. Imaging techniques such as DaTscan are costly and not so easily available in many health care settings, particularly in developing countries. Additionally, such methods cannot be used for repeated tracking of disease progression due to costs and logistics, nor can they be used on a repeated basis for continuous monitoring. Patients often document severity of symptoms and response to medicine in diaries but they are affected by recall bias.

Many assessments are done in a short outpatient visit, and it may not truly reflect the patient's motor performance at home. Tremor, freezing of gait, bradykinesia symptoms can significantly differ at different times of day, with the age of medicine, stress or exertion. As a result of this, treatment decisions based on scant clinical observation may be ineffective for patients.

The Part Played by Wearable Technology in Managing Neurodegenerative Disease

Wearable technology is the new hope to connect clinical assessment with real-world symptom measurement. The development of wearable devices that continuously record physiological and behavioural information is made possible by advances in miniaturized sensors, low-power electronics and wireless communication. Wearable sensors measure subtle movement problems that may be missed at the doctor's office in the case of Parkinson's disease.

Wearable systems use inertial measurement units (IMUs) that consist of accelerometers and gyroscopes to enable studying movement patterns, gait characteristics and postural stability. These sensors have demonstrated efficacy for detecting tremors, slowness of movement and balance abnormalities. Unlike camera-based systems, wearable sensors have minimal intrusion on activities, preserve privacy, and support long-term monitoring in the home environment.

Wrist-worn watches are smart wearable devices that are appealing due to their familiarity, ease of use and high patient compliance. A platform designed for smartwatches supports the seamless integration of various sensors such as motion sensors, microphones, etc. The ability to exhibit signals at multiple modalities makes the device quite useful to monitor both motor and speech symptoms of Parkinson's disease quite robustly.

The Importance of Motion Signal Analysis is Highlighted in Parkinson's Disease Detection

Motor impairments are one of the most characteristic and measurable features of Parkinson's disease. Tremor, rigidity, bradykinesia, and postural instability impact the daily activities and quality of life of patients.

Understanding the movement of Parkinsonian patients can be done using gait analysis. Stride length, cadence, variability, symmetry, and other useful parameters can be valuable indicators of disease severity. Wearable IMU sensors can record these parameters during regular walking instead of in specialized gait laboratories. Furthermore, the study of hand tremor and upper limb movement indicate motoric disability.

Integrating threshold-based algorithms with machine learning techniques is a great deal to improve the reliability of motion-based detection systems. By learning individual movement patterns, these models can assist in the differentiation of pathological movements from normal activities to decrease false alarms. The analysis of motion signals also makes it possible to identify early signs of disease, which is important to intervene timely so that it is possible to slow the progress of the disease.

Voice Signal Analysis can be Used as a Diagnostic Modality

Parkinson's disease affects how people are able to speak in addition to causing motor symptoms. It results in a loss of improved control for the respiratory, phonatory, and articulatory muscles. A majority of patients with PD develop voice disorders collectively known as hypokinetic dysarthria in the early disease phase itself. Examples of speech abnormalities are reduced loudness, monotone pitch, and increased pauses.

Detecting Parkinson's disease can be done non-invasively and cost-effectively using a voice signal. Voice recordings can be analyzed using machine learning algorithms to extract various acoustic features, such as jitter, shimmer, fundamental frequency, and spectral features. Voice analysis is less physically strenuous than motor assessments and can be used by people with high levels of motor impairment.

In the wearable device, the integration of microphones enables the acquisition of voice data in real-time without the need for an external recording device. The simultaneous analysis of voice and motion creates a multi-modal diagnostic framework improving the robustness and accuracy of classification. This approach is especially useful for distinguishing Parkinson's disease from other movement disorders that have similar symptoms.

Machine Learning for Intelligent Detection of Parkinson's Disease

One achieved success in creating a safe and effective vaccine for the coronavirus with help of technology. Machine learning algorithms in Parkinson's disease detection can find correlations and features that are challenging to identify manually. Models of supervised learning, like K-Nearest Neighbor and Random Forest classifiers, produce promising outcomes when classifying PD-related features from sensor data.

Machine learning models achieve their best results by optimizing model and feature analysis along with tuning. The processed and normalized wearable sensor data enables us to train robust classifiers with an abundance of information. Random Forest is an ensemble method that offers greater generalization, and KNN is an instance-based method that offers a simple classification model.

It enables real-time inference and decision support through machine learning technologies for wearable IoT systems. The trained models can be deployed on cloud platforms so that the resource- demanding tasks can be offloaded from the wearable device energy-efficiently and scalably. The continuous monitoring and personalized disease management is supported by this architecture.

IoT and Distributed Computing for Real Time Healthcare Monitoring

The Internet of Things is changing everything in our lives, from our homes to businesses to hospitals and much more. Similarly, healthcare IoT has been allocating the right resources at the right place and at the right time. Most importantly, nothing transforms faulty procedures to perfect one through IoT in healthcare. As a result, undesirable behavior and irrelevant data will not disturb the system anymore. Healthcare IoT is an apt way to do it. Similar healthcare RFIDs are also being used nowadays to do the same. End disarray and corruption through IoT in healthcare. Therefore, it is speculated to perform effectively in times to come. Wearable devices, cloud servers, and healthcare professionals exchange information in a framework for monitoring Parkinson's disease with IoT.

Distributed computing is essential for managing large amounts of sensor data streaming. Cloud-based infrastructure enables wearable devices to process, visualize, and store data in real-time without heavy strain. This method can improve scalability, while also allowing remote monitoring of multiple patients.

Healthcare systems with IoT also help to engage the patients as well as the caregivers. Disease management is made more effective with features like remote access to patient data, alerts, and personalized feedback. Furthermore, you may continuously update the model and optimally fine-tune performance on what is being learnt.

Management of Emergencies and Detection of Falls in PD

Patients with Parkinson's disease often injure themselves falling over, which may lead to hospitalization. Freezing of gait and postural instability often increase fall risk late in the course of the disease. If these falls are detected early enough and the emergency response starts immediately, their consequences will be minimized.

Wearable IMU sensors can be used for fall detection because they can capture sudden acceleration and orientation changes. Using threshold-based algorithms with contextual analysis can distinguish falls from everyday activities. An SOS alert will notify caregivers or emergency services immediately if the wearer is in any distress.

Communication modules like the GSM and cloud messaging service provide quick response time even when the patient is alone. Independent living is easier for older adults with this feature. The detection systems for falls enhance safety but also improve feels of reassurance in the patients and caregivers.

Motivation and Objectives of the Present Work

The need for such a solution that is affordable, reliable and scalable to detect and manage Parkinson's disease generated the motivation for this research. Usually, systems are expensive or complex or limited to the laboratory thus preventing real-world usage.

A smartwatch-based (or, smart-watch based) system and its design are made for motion and voice signal analysis by making use of machine learning and IoT technology. Main objective of the proposed solution is to help with real-time monitoring of Parkinson disease symptoms of a patient. Further, it also classifies them using machine learning models. Moreover, it also reliably detects a fall and manages emergency effectively. The system integrates multi-modal sensing and cloud analytics to improve diagnostic accuracy, patient safety and long-term disease management. The present study is a demonstration of a proof-of-concept implementation of a multi-modal wearable monitoring system. Here, the model training and validation were performed based on a publicly available dataset having laboratory quality. The consecutive acquisition of real-time data from the developed smart watch is planned as a future world for the evaluation of real-world performance clinically.

Organisation of the Paper

The rest of this chapter is structured into five sections that provide a systematic presentation of the proposed smartwatch-based approach to detecting and managing Parkinson's disease.

The previous literature relates to Parkinson's disease diagnosis and monitoring using wearables, motion sensors, voice signal analysis, and machine learning techniques (**Section 2**). This section states the limitation and motivation of the currently used method for the proposed system.

The proposed system and its various components are explained in **Section 3** of the chapter. The section talks about architecture, hardware, data collection and signal preprocessing. This section also details the feature extraction techniques for motion and voice signals and the machine learning models employed for classification of Parkinson's disease.

The experimental setup and evaluation of performance of the proposed methodology is outlined. In **Section 4**, datasets, evaluation metrics, and experimental results with comparative analysis are presented to exhibit the efficacy of the proposed method.

In the end, **Section 5** summarizes the paper's contributions and findings respectively. Additionally, it highlights the limitations of the current work and potential avenues for future work such as system improvement and large-scale clinical validation.

LITERATURE SURVEY

Ile an et al. (Ile an et al., 2022) published a forward-thinking study that explored how wearable gadgets might help people with Parkinsons disease (PD). This research introduced a small AI-boosted device that tracks walking, aiming to spot everyday steps that look normal compared with those changed by PD. To do this, the system blends high-precision sensors with deep-learning convolutional networks. Pierleono et al. (Pierleoni et al., 2022) presented a wearable sensor that was placed at the lower back and used a simple algorithm to identify the walking metrics. Similar ideas appear in Tortelli et al. (Tortelli et al., 2021), who linked pocket-sized devices with smart wearables to track Huntingtons disease during daily life. As Tortelli, Rodrigues, and Wild report, that setup gathers data around the clock at much higher resolution than seen on short outpatient checks, capturing both slow trends and sudden symptom spikes.

According to (Vera Anaya & Yuce, 2021), the monitoring of Parkinson's disease has advanced significantly with the development of wearable sensors that facilitate the observation of motor symptoms. In their study, they introduced a stretchable triboelectric sensor designed to measure movements of forearm muscles and finger motions, offering an innovative approach for PD assessment. Rodríguez et al. (Rodríguez-Martín et al., 2022) discussed the benefits of wearable medical devices in the context of Parkinson's disease evaluation. Traditional methods of symptom monitoring in PD patients involve self-reported diaries and retrospective questionnaires that often yield inaccurate evaluations due to their subjective nature. In support of the hardware, Mancini et al. (Mancini et al., 2021) published a key paper titled Measuring freezing of gait during daily life an open-source, wearable-sensors approach. They placed inertial units on the feet, shins, and lower back, then fused the readings into a custom software toolkit that flags freezing episodes.

Han et al. (Han et al., 2023) built a system that pairs off-the-shelf sensors with simple software to monitor how people with Parkinsons disease walk. Because the sensors sit on the body all day without any intrusiveness, doctors easily acquire data, and painless measurements can be turned into tailored rehabilitation plans almost on the spot. Lencioni et al. (Lencioni et al., 2022) tested a small accelerometer attached to the trunk, asking whether it could spot early postural shifts as well as a bulky force plate. They discovered that readings from the lone trunk unit matched the platforms results so closely that the two were practically twins ($r = 0.99$, slope $= 0.97$). That near-perfect overlap hints that a cheap wrist or belt device could guide balance drills at home rather than in a crowded lab.

Gap and Motivation of Research

Many previous studies use assessment tools that are clinical or laboratory based. For instance, imaging systems, specialized motion capture setups, or voice recording systems found in a hospital. Though these methods usually offer high accuracy, they rely on expensive procedures and institutions making them not suitable for on-the-field continuous monitoring. Parkinson's disease is a progressive illness that affects the nervous system. The severity of the symptoms does vary over time. Consequently, strategies necessitating regular hospital visitation are unsuitable for long-term disease management or early disease detection. Moreover, Wearable technologies, despite being advanced and offering good prospects, have not been sufficiently put to test in a practical way for application purposes. A recent review found that most existing wearable-based studies concentrate on single data modality. Numerous works examine motion signals stemming from accelerometers or gyroscopes for tremors, bradykinesia, or gait analysis, while others focus solely on voice signals in the context of speech impairment analysis.

Parkinson's disease has motor and non-motor symptoms including bradykinesia and tremors. Single-modality systems may overlook this complexity, resulting in incomplete or less reliable assessments. Many machine learning approaches described in the literature are evaluated on relatively small datasets or datasets collected under highly controlled experimental conditions. Although studies like these show it is possible to automate the diagnosis of the neurodegenerative disorder, its widespread application is not yet possible. Furthermore, most models focus on classification performance but do not deal adequately with issues of computational efficiency, real-time implementation, and resource constraints which are a vital issue for wearable and embedded systems.

In the present study, a smartwatch-based framework is proposed for the detection of PD. This method performs the analysis of motion and voice signals using machine learning algorithms. Thus, this research proposes a low-cost, user-friendly and scalable technology for PD detection.

PROPOSED PARKINSON'S DISEASE DETECTION SYSTEM

Figure 1 represents the process diagram of the proposed Parkinson's Smart Watch. The process involves a wearable device the comprises of IMU sensors (MPU 6050, accelerometer, gyroscope) and a Microphone (MAX 9814, AGC Enabled) along with an ESP32 microcontroller that is used to capture and transmit motion and voice data to a server. The server then analyses the captured data for the prediction of PD. Also, based on the information from IMU sensors, falls are detected. In cases of emergencies, an SOS message is sent using Twilio or a GSM module when internet is unavailable.

Figure 1. Process diagram of the Parkinson's smart watch

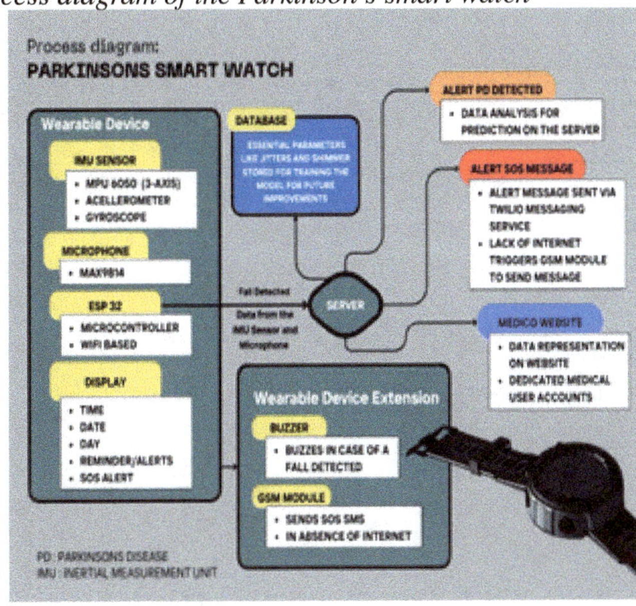

The complete block diagram of the proposed system is shown in Figure 2. It shows the flow of data from the sensors in the smartwatch hardware to the ESP32 microcontroller then to the data processing unit. This unit performs the motion and voice analysis whose output is fed to the machine learning models which are then used for classification and fall detection. This in turn is used for daily monitoring and emergency SOS alerts. Finally, all these are visualized using a clinical dashboard.

Figure 2. Block diagram of the proposed system

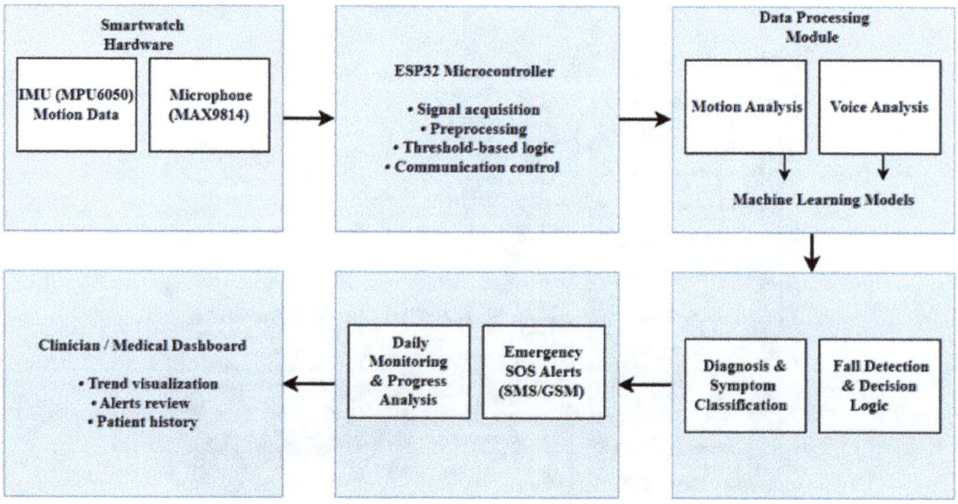

The overall unified decision matrix for the proposed multi-modal clinical support system based on the readings from IMU, Microphone sensors are shown in Table 1.

Table 1. Unified Decision Matrix for Multi-Modal Clinical Decision Support

Sensor Modality	Extracted Parameters	Processing Method	System Function	Clinical Outcome
IMU (MPU6050)	Acceleration (X, Y, Z), Gyroscope (X, Y, Z)	Threshold-based analysis	Fall detection	SOS alert and emergency notification
IMU (MPU6050)	Acceleration and angular velocity patterns	Statistical analysis	Activity and movement monitoring	Daily movement assessment
Microphone (MAX9814)	Jitter, shimmer, pitch-related features	Machine learning (KNN, Random Forest)	Parkinson's disease classification	PD vs non-PD prediction
Integrated outputs	Classification result + fall events	Dashboard visualization	Clinical monitoring support	Longitudinal symptom tracking

Components of the Proposed Parkinson's Smart Watch

ESP32: ESP32 has an integrated Wi-Fi which could be used to communicate with internet such as the backend server. ESP32 acts as the brain of the watch and controls the watch's functionalities and interface. ESP32 receives input from onboard sensors such as the IMU sensor which gives the axis of rotation and gyroscope. This data is processed in ESP32 and is sent to the backend server for further processing and prediction.

IMU Sensor: A device that can measure and report specific gravity and angular rate of an object. Here we use MPU6050 as our IMU sensor. It provides the X, Y, Z data of both rotation and gravitational changes using a gyroscope and accelerometer respectively

Microphone: A device that takes the sound waves as input and converts them into analog signals that the microcontroller can interact with. Here we use MAX 9814 as our microphone that provides the frequency, Pitch, Distortion, Noise and Amplitude of the input sound wave, additionally it has automatic gain control (AGC) feature. The microphone has a sampling rate of 40KHz.

Display: Display module displays vital information such as the time, date, and the day. During specific times of the day, it will display reminders such as breakfast, lunch or dinner and for medicines that the patient has to undertake. When the patient falls, an SOS message is displayed. We used SH110X display module which is a 128 x 64 monochrome OLED display.

SOS Alert: GSM module and an online service (Twilio messaging) was used to send an SMS to the concerned family member, nurse, or a doctor. We also have a buzzer so that anyone around the patient can be aware and take immediate action to the SOS call. The service is fast and can send SMS in less than 1 second after the patient falls. When the patient falls, a trigger is sent to the backend server which quickly contacts the SMS service, and the service sends an SMS to the concerned person. SMS trigger is activated if the person falls. Once the service sends the SMS to the patient's caretakers, it will provide feedback to the backend server. The server then relays the result to ESP32, verifying that the SMS was successfully received by the recipient. If the status response given back by the server was given as false, then ESP32 will try again to ping the server again after 10 seconds to ensure that the message is properly received to the required people. Figure 3 and Figure 4 shows the result of the SOS feature.

Figure 3. SMS alert sent from the online service

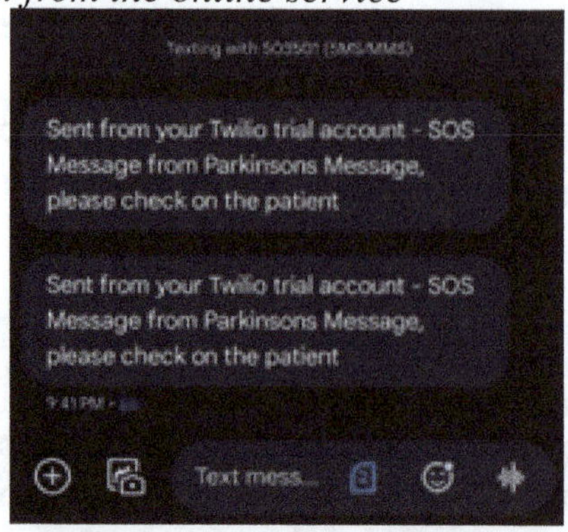

Figure 4. SOS alert after fall detection

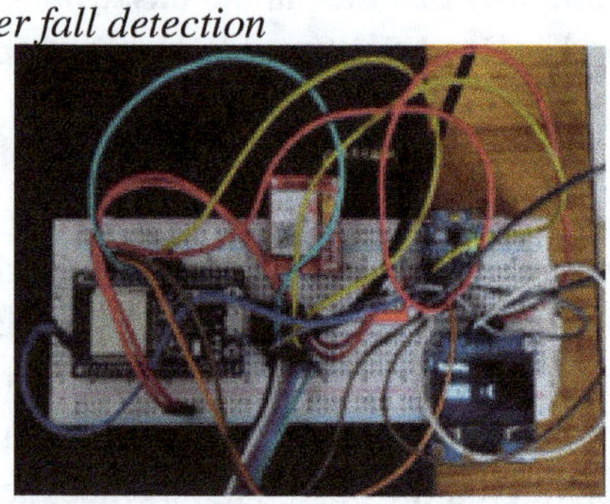

Real time update (Server): The data is obtained from the watch and the data is sent to our server through Wi-Fi (using ESP32). The patient can manually enter his/her vital and essential parameters and clinical conditions to get an accurate prediction. The data includes a JSON containing the X, Y, Z values of Gyroscope data, X, Y, Z values of acceleration and Jitter and shimmer values from the Microphone. The backend server is made in Python to accommodate data analysis and data prediction. REST API, was used that follows constraints of REST. REST Architecture consists of a body, headler and URL, which simplified the work of authentication and data transfer of communication to a minimum. REST architecture consists of 4 main Methods, they are:

GET: To fetch data from the backend server

POST: To add or append data to the backend server

PUT: To modify data which was already added or appended in the previous calls

DELETE: To delete data from the backend server and database

A framework called FastAPI was used to implement the backend server, which increases its speed by 15% when compared to other Python frameworks such as Flask or Django and improves efficiency and modularity while making the project. The deployment could be done in Infrastructure as a Service (IaaS) such as AWS Elastic Computer Cloud (ECC or EC2) instance or Google Computer Engine (GCE) for large scale production and use case, or any Platform as a Service (PaaS) like Heroku. The database used for saving the history of the fall, past readings and the predictions is in a NoSQL Database called MongoDB which is a document-based database developed by Mongo Inc. MongoDB is also trustable, secure, reliable, flexible, and open source which makes it the perfect candidate for data storage and modification.

Medico Website: All the data collected are shown (except for audio) neatly in the front-end using a framework called NextJS, which is an upgraded library of ReactJS and supports server actions which makes data leak to a very minimum. The front end shows all the data such as prediction data, current values of the accelerometer, number of times SOS was called through fall detection, steps walked by the patient and the distance covered on that day. A graph is shown presenting the data of the recent past showing X, Y, Z values of Gyroscope data and X, Y, Z values of Accelerometer. Each of the live data is shown in the screen, including the cholesterol, Age, Blood Pressure and Phone Number of the caretaker or whoever is responsible for the patient's health. The admin can watch as the data varies live, based on the changes made in that instance in the client-side website. Medico Website Interface of the concerned medical authority is shown in Figure 5.

Figure 5. Medico Website Interface of the concerned medical authority

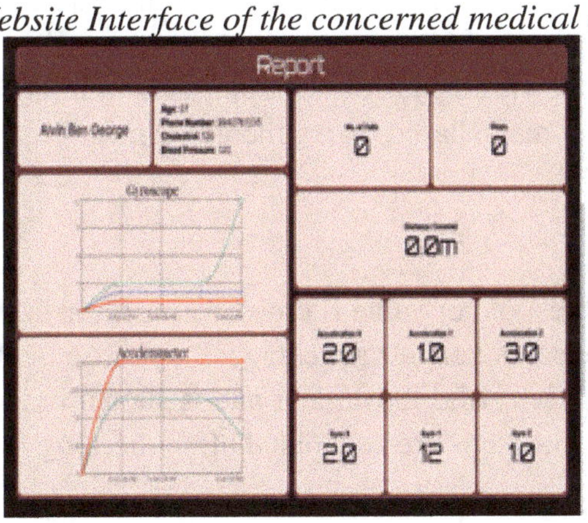

Prediction Based on Real Time Data

With the help of Tuned KNN and Tuned Random Forest Classifier, an accuracy of 97.40% and 95% respectively were attained. We obtain data from the Microphone for the jitter and shimmer. We then process the data received from the sensor to determine if the patient has fallen or has Parkinson disease. The model takes 15 parameters as input, including Fundamental Frequency, Highest Fundamental Frequency, and Lowest Fundamental Frequency. It also considers Jitter, Absolute Jitter, Relative Average Perturbation, and Pitch Perturbation Quotient. Additional parameters are Jitter, Shimmer, Shimmer in dB, Amplitude Perturbation Quotient 3, Amplitude Perturbation Quotient 5, Amplitude Perturbation Quotient, Shimmer, and Noise-to-Harmonics Ratio. Based on the values provided to these parameters, the prediction is made and given to the admin portal. Real-time prediction models for PD detection leverage distributed computing to process and analyze data efficiently. Using cloud-based infrastructure, motion and voice data are streamed and processed in parallel to ensure timely diagnosis.

Fall Detection and Step Counter

Using IMU sensor, the inertial sensor values are acquired. Analysis was done to identify the minimum threshold value to identify the fall threshold so that there is no false fall detection. This is shown in Figure 6. The table presents different threshold values in meters per second squared (m/s^2), ranging from 2 to 10 m/s^2, to detect falls effectively. For each threshold, three aspects are analyzed in this research: successful fall detection, false detection of falls while walking, and missed fall detection during "shimmers". The threshold of 6 m/s^2 was selected as the optimal value as it detected all the falls successfully with any false detections while walking or during shimmers.

Fall Conditions are made based on a general formula:

$$Accl_Z - PreviousAccl_Z > 6 \tag{1}$$

If the minimum threshold of value is crossed according to the IMU sensor data, SOS is called, and the caretaker gets a message. Steps are calculated for the patients to know their daily activity and movement and is shown in the admin portal with the distance walked. The steps are calculated after checking the condition:

$$x_{diff} = (Accl_X - PreviousAccl_X) \tag{2}$$

$$y_{diff} = (Accl_Y - PreviousAccl_Y) \tag{3}$$

$$z_{diff} = (Accl_Z - PreviousAccl_Z) \tag{4}$$

$$\sqrt{x_{diff}^2 + y_{diff}^2 + z_{diff}^2} > 4 \tag{5}$$

Distance and steps are calculated through this condition and when this condition is met, the steps integer is incremented by one. Distance travelled by the patient is calculated through the steps by a factor of 0.74.

Figure 6. Threshold parameters

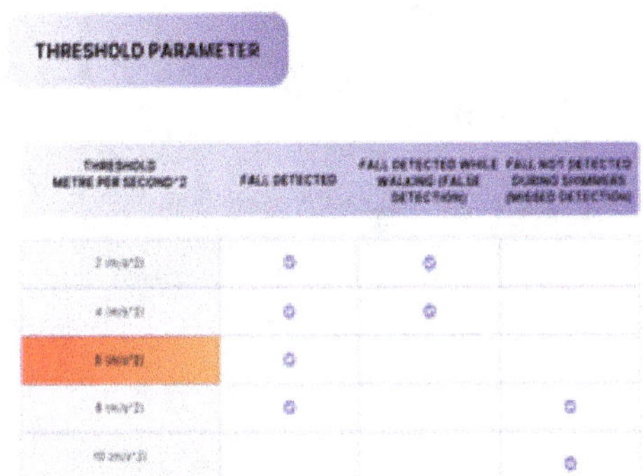
THRESHOLD PARAMETER

THRESHOLD METRE PER SECOND^2	FALL DETECTED	FALL DETECTED WHILE WALKING (FALSE DETECTION)	FALL NOT DETECTED DURING SHIVERING (MISSED DETECTION)
2 (m/s^2)	●	●	
4 (m/s^2)	●	●	
6 (m/s^2)	●		
8 (m/s^2)	●		●
10 (m/s^2)			●

Medicine Indication and Food Indication (Reminders)

Personalized reminders for medication and meals are synchronized using a distributed backend system. Updates to reminders occur every 10 minutes or when the device reconnects to the server, ensuring data consistency across distributed networks. The scalable design accommodates multiple devices and users, enabling efficient coordination in healthcare applications. Using this feature, the user can set personalized reminders with details of medicine and its corresponding timings. Majority of Parkinsons Disease Patients are over the age of 60, hence it is mandatory to have a reminder to vital activities. The administrator, nurse, caretaker or the doctor can manually enter the required medication or food reminder based on the patient's medical situation and health. The frontend admin panel will receive the required data through user input and sends it to the backend for storing in the database. If the watch is offline, the next time it connects, the required data is synced up to update the medication and food reminder in the watch's local storage. If the watch is online throughout, then the update takes place every 10 minutes and if there's a break in the connection between the watch and the backend server, then the next time the watch is online, all the data is synced up. By default, the basic meal timings, such as breakfast, lunch and dinner, are inserted into the watch's local storage. Display showing reminder for Lunch is shown in Figure 7.

Figure 7. Display showing reminder for Lunch

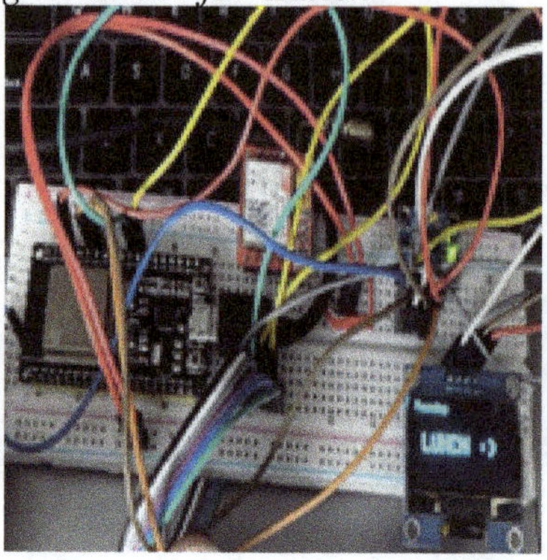

RESULT AND DISCUSSION

Dataset Description

The dataset used in this study (Little et al., 2009) for PD detection was obtained from UCI Machine learning repository (https://archive.ics.uci.edu/dataset/174/parkinsons). This dataset consists of various biomedical voice measurements collected from 31 individuals, 23 of whom have Parkinson's disease. Future extensions to this dataset can support large-scale, distributed studies for training and validating machine learning models in high-performance healthcare systems.

Performance of Tuned Machine Learning Models

The dataset is preprocessed by removing redundant data before training the models. The Random Forest Classifier's hyperparameters are adjusted to find the best combination, and cross-validation is used to evaluate the results. Similarly, the KNN Classifier is tuned by adjusting parameters through cross-validation to achieve the best performance. After fine-tuning, the KNN classifier reached a top accuracy of 97.4% in identifying Parkinsons disease and differentiating it from normal jitters and shimmers. The tuned Random Forest badge followed closely at 95.40%. An untuned KNN fell just behind at 93% yet still proved useful. Together, these figures show that machine-learning tools-can lend real weight to wearables trying to catch Parkinson's early, with the tuned KNN and Random Forest models leading the pack. This system uses k-fold cross validation where k=10 to ensure that the system is robust. The dataset is divided into ten subsets, where nine portions are used for training and remaining for validation. The process is repeated for 10 iterations.

Effectiveness of KNN Classifier and Comparison With Other Models

Table 2 presents the accuracy of Parkinson's disease prediction using the K-Nearest Neighbors (KNN) algorithm for different values of K and two distance metrics: Euclidean and Manhattan.

Table 2. Hyperparameter values for KNN

KNN Value	Distance Metric	Accuracy
1	Euclidean	89.7%
2	Euclidean	92.3%
3	Euclidean	92.3%
4	Euclidean	94.8%
5	Euclidean	94.7%
6	Euclidean	94.8%
7	Euclidean	92.3%
8	Euclidean	92.3%
9	Euclidean	92.3%
1	Manhattan	89.7%
2	Manhattan	89.7%
3	**Manhattan**	**97.4%**
4	Manhattan	96.1%
5	Manhattan	94.8%
6	Manhattan	94.8%
7	Manhattan	94.8%
8	Manhattan	94.8%
9	Manhattan	91.2%

For the Euclidean distance, accuracy increases with higher K values, reaching its peak at around 94.8% for K = 4 and K = 6. However, the Manhattan distance metric produces a higher accuracy, particularly with K = 3, where it reaches an impressive 97.4%. Table 3 shows the tuning of hyperparameters for a Random Forest model so that accuracy can be optimized. From the Table it can be observed that highest accuracy of 95.4% can be achieved with 300 estimators, a maximum depth value of 30, minimum sample split of 10 and sample leaf count of 4.

Table 3. Hyperparameter values for RFC

N Estimator	Max Depth	Minimum Samples Split	Minimum Sample Leaves	Accuracy
3	5	15	5	89.8%
1	1	3	2	87.2%
1	2	5	1	84.8%
40	5	15	5	92.2%
300	30	10	4	95.4%

The confusion matrix for the modified KNN classifier in Figure 8 shows strong performance in predicting Parkinson's disease, with 32 true positives and 6 true negatives. There was only 1 false positive, where the model incorrectly predicted Parkinson's for someone without the disease, and no false negatives, meaning all individuals with Parkinson's were correctly identified.

Figure 8. Confusion Matrix of Tuned KNN

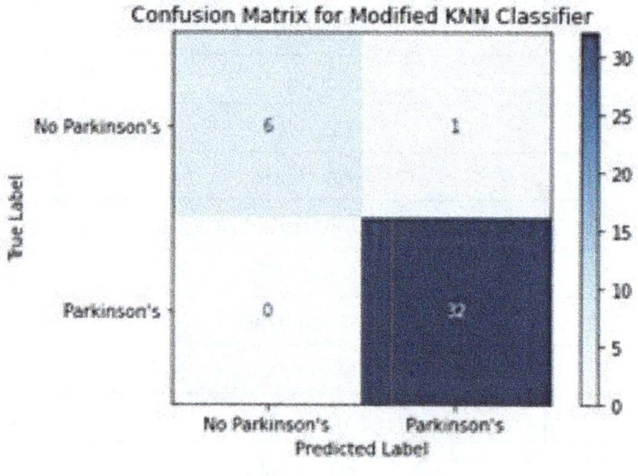

The bar chart in Figure 9 compares the accuracy of different machine learning algorithms for Parkinson's disease detection. The tuned KNN classifier performs best, achieving the highest accuracy of 97.4%, closely followed by the tuned Random Forest (95.4%). Other algorithms like K-Neighbors Classifier, Random Forest Classifier, and SVC show comparable accuracy, while Logistic Regression has the lowest accuracy among the methods tested. This suggests that KNN-based approaches are particularly effective for this task.

Figure 9. Accuracy of various ML algorithms

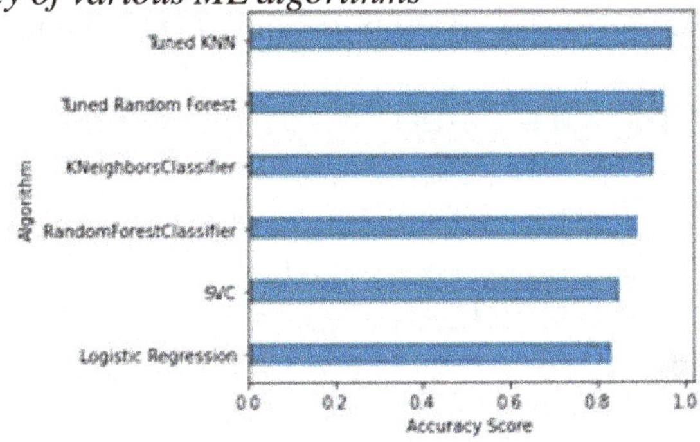

Along with accuracy multiple other metrics were also computed to evaluate the robustness of the proposed system as shown in Table 4. The fall detection module achieved a false alarm rate of **14.29%**, indicating that incorrect fall alerts occurred in a limited number of non-fall events.

Table 4. Performance metrics of the proposed Parkinson's Disease detection model

Metrics	Values
Accuracy	97.4
Sensitivity	100
Specificity	85.71
Positive Predictive Value (PPV)	96.97
Negative Predictive Value (NPV)	100

The 97.4% accuracy obtained is completely based on the publicly available benchmark dataset that were collected under controlled recording conditions. During real-time deployment, its performance may vary due to the presence of environmental noise and also variations in the patient speech captured at everyday setting environments.

ESP32-Based Real-Time Data Monitoring

The ESP32 chip forms the backbone of this IoT-based system, leveraging its Wi-Fi capabilities for real-time data monitoring and transmission to a distributed server for analysis. The device combines the MPU6050 sensor for the collection of acceleration and gyroscope data and the MAX9814 microphone is employed for audio input, both of which are essential for Parkinson's prediction. During situations, when the internet connection gets disrupted, a GSM module is used by the system so that uninterrupted emergency SOS notification is being sent.

Hardware and Software Setup

For hardware implementation a 16GB RAM was used. To implement the machine learning algorithms Jupyter Notebooks, PyTorch, and TensorFlow were used. For implementing the embedded logic in ESP32 Arduino IDE was used. Further, a MacBook Air with M1 chip was used to provide a high speed workflow.

Limitations

The main drawback of this research is that the validation is completely based on the publicly available benchmark dataset that were collected under controlled recording conditions. Thus, this system must be viewed as a proof-of-concept platform for large-scale real-world-validation. As with any emerging technology, voice-enabled interfaces have their advantages and disadvantages. For instance, while the system is accurate in controlled environments, it has only been validated on static datasets and not on live voice or sensor streams. Similarly, the fall detection system is based on fixed thresholds and will likely need customized adjustments for different users. It is clear that clinical validation studies as well as more diverse data inclusion are necessary to evaluate the system's clinical accuracy and reliability comprehensively.

Future Scope

In future, the authors plan to perform a complete pilot study using the developed smart watch so that real-world data could be collected at home environment. This would help in performing end-to-end validation of the system. The proposed method, with continuous refinement and clinical validation can be used as a useful clinical and scalable tool at low-costs for the diagnosis, monitoring and management of Parkinson's disease in real-world healthcare settings.

Clinical Relevance and Deployment Considerations

The smartwatch-based Parkinson's disease detection system has clinical relevance because it offers continuous, objective, and real-time assessments that complement conventional neurological assessments. Routine clinical assessments are performed infrequently and are heavily reliant on observation, which in turn may not capture the true change of symptoms that occur in daily life. The proposed system allows for continuous collection and analysis of motion and voice signals, which could help clinicians in the decision-making process for the patients' future and the treatment plan.

The suggested solution is appropriate for home-based as well as community-level healthcare settings owing to a deployment perspective of using a low-cost wearable platform. The system can especially help earlier-stage patients whose more difficult-to-detect motor and speech issues likely will not be caught in a normal clinic visit. Further, remote monitoring of patients will lessen the burden on the health infrastructure and the need for frequent hospital visits.

Another key deployment consideration is user acceptance and long-term use. In order for a user to keep wearing the device, it must be comfortable, unintrusive, and easy to use. Updating the design based on user feedback in new versions will improve the usability and ensure that the system works well with patients and clinicians. In general, the smartwatch-based system proposed for PD monitoring and management has been presented with a good potential for translation from research prototype to deployment by addressing clinical relevance and deployment challenges.

Pathways to Clinical Implementation

For clinical translation two important aspects must be taken into consideration, namely, daily-life variability and the inter-patient difference aspects. Under such real-world conditions, adaptive learning strategy could be implemented. Future work will involve pilot clinical studies which are conducted along with the neurologist so that the usability, clinical relevance and the reliability of the proposed system can be evaluated. These steps would help to ensure that the proposed system could be effectively used for Parkinson's disease care.

Power Consumption Analysis

Power consumption analysis is a critical step in wearable health system, since continuous monitoring limits the battery capacity. In this proposed system, power consumption analysis is done based on individual components. The ESP32 microcontroller acts as the core processing and communication unit. During Wi-Fi transmission its consumers approximately 160-260 mA and it drops to less than 10 mA while in sleep model. The MPU6050 IMU sensor consumes around 3.9 mA when it performs active sensing. The MAX9814 microphone uses around 3-4 mA when it performs audio acquisition. The OLED modules use around 20-25 mA when it is active and it is switched off during normal monitoring to save power. Thus, the average current consumption is within the range suitable for wearable applications.

CONCLUSION

In this research, a new IoT based system for Parkinson's disease detection is proposed. This system provides real-time monitoring, fall detection and gives emergency indication using SOS alerts especially in environments with limited resources. Machine learning models were used for identification of PD, and it was found that tuned K-NN classifier achieved good accuracy of 97.4% and Random Forest classifier achieved 95.4% accuracy using the UCI dataset. ESP32 module was used to perform real-time data collection in resource constraint environment. Further, this system employes an emergency notification feature at the time of emergency like fall occurrence. The main challenge of this system is that it is trained using a publicly available dataset. In future, this study will be extended to real clinical settings so that the model generalizability is achieved to ensure usability in practical health care applications.

AUTHOR CONTRIBUTIONS

R. Athilakshmi proposed the basic idea behind this research. The work was carried out by the authors Alvin Ben George, Daniel Biju Joseph and Debanshu Roy who were also involved in writing the manuscript. The research was monitored by R. Jansi, who also reviewed the final manuscript.

FUNDING

This research did not receive any specific grant from funding agencies in the public, commercial, or not-for-profit sectors.

DATA AVAILABILITY

The data enabling the findings of this study are available in at UCI Machine learning repository at https://archive.ics.uci.edu/dataset/174/parkinsons

CONFLICT OF INTEREST

The authors declare no competing interests.

ETHICAL APPROVAL AND CONSENT TO PARTICIPATE

This article does not contain any studies with human participants performed by any of the authors.

REFERENCES

Adams, J. L., Dinesh, K., Snyder, C. W., Xiong, M., Tarolli, C. G., Sharma, S., Dorsey, E. R., & Sharma, G. (2021). A real-world study of wearable sensors in Parkinson's disease. *NPJ Parkinson's Disease*, *7*(1). Advance online publication. DOI: 10.1038/s41531-021-00248-w PMID: 34845224

Ajagun, E. J., Asuku, A. O., Ayinla, M. T., Abdulsalam, T. A., Ajibare, A. J., Olajide, T. S., Hamza, Y. O., & Ganiyu, K. O. (2024). Pharmacotherapy of Parkinson's Disease and their Limitations. In: Zebrafish as a Model for Parkinson's Disease. Taylor and Francis, CRC, https://doi.org/DOI: 10.1201/9781003402893-17

Asci, F., Vivacqua, G., Zampogna, A., D'onofrio, V., Mazzeo, A., & Suppa, A. (2022). Wearable Electrochemical Sensors in Parkinson's Disease. *Sensors (Basel)*, *22*(3). Advance online publication. DOI: 10.3390/s22030951 PMID: 35161694

Asuku, A. O., Ayinla, M. T., Olajide, T. S., Ajagun, E. J., Ganiyu, K. O., Hamza, Y. O., Ajibare, A. J., & Abdulsalam, T. A. (2024). Diagnosis and Biomarkers of Parkinson's Disease. In: Zebrafish as a Model for Parkinson's Disease. Taylor and Francis, CRC, https://doi.org/DOI: 10.1201/9781003402893-15

Asuku, A. O., Ogungbangbe, G. O., & Fajemidagba, G. A. (2025). Gene therapy for Parkinson's disease: A new frontier in neurodegenerative diseases. *Exploration of Neuroprotective Therapy*, *5*, 1004119. DOI: 10.37349/ent.2025.1004119

Balakrishnan, A., Medikonda, J., Namboothiri, P. K., & Natarajan, M. (2022). Role of Wearable Sensors with Machine Learning Approaches in Gait Analysis for Parkinson's Disease Assessment: A Review. *Engineering and Science*, *19*, 5–19. DOI: 10.30919/es8e622

Barrachina-Fernández, M., Maitín, A. M., Sánchez-ávila, C., & Romero, J. P. (2021). Wearable technology to detect motor fluctuations in parkinson's disease patients: Current state and challenges. *Sensors (Basel)*, *21*(12). Advance online publication. DOI: 10.3390/s21124188 PMID: 34207198

Castelli Gattinara Di Zubiena, F., Menna, G., Mileti, I., Zampogna, A., Asci, F., Paoloni, M., Suppa, A., Del Prete, Z., & Palermo, E. (2022). Machine Learning and Wearable Sensors for the Early Detection of Balance Disorders in Parkinson's Disease. *Sensors (Basel)*, *22*(24). Advance online publication. DOI: 10.3390/s22249903 PMID: 36560278

Chatzaki, C., Skaramagkas, V., Tachos, N., Christodoulakis, G., Maniadi, E., Kefalopoulou, Z., Fotiadis, D. I., & Tsiknakis, M. (2021). The smart-insole dataset: Gait analysis using wearable sensors with a focus on elderly and parkinson's patients. *Sensors (Basel)*, *21*(8). Advance online publication. DOI: 10.3390/s21082821 PMID: 33923809

Daneault, J. F., Vergara-Diaz, G., Parisi, F., Admati, C., Alfonso, C., Bertoli, M., Bonizzoni, E., Carvalho, G. F., Costante, G., Fabara, E. E., Fixler, N., Golabchi, F. N., Growdon, J., Sapienza, S., Snyder, P., Shpigelman, S., Sudarsky, L., Daeschler, M., Bataille, L., & Bonato, P. (2021). Accelerometer data collected with a minimum set of wearable sensors from subjects with Parkinson's disease. *Scientific Data*, *8*(1). Advance online publication. DOI: 10.1038/s41597-021-00830-0 PMID: 33547309

Dorsey, E. R., Papapetropoulos, S., Xiong, M., & Kieburtz, K. (2017). The first frontier: Digital biomarkers for neurodegenerative disorders. *Digital Biomarkers*, *1*(1), 6–13. DOI: 10.1159/000477383 PMID: 32095743

Greene, B. R., Premoli, I., McManus, K., McGrath, D., & Caulfield, B. (2022). Predicting fall counts using wearable sensors: A novel digital biomarker for parkinson's disease. *Sensors (Basel)*, *22*(1). Advance online publication. DOI: 10.3390/s22010054 PMID: 35009599

Han, Y., Liu, X., Zhang, N., Zhang, X., Zhang, B., Wang, S., Liu, T., & Yi, J. (2023). Automatic Assessments of Parkinsonian Gait with Wearable Sensors for Human Assistive Systems. *Sensors (Basel)*, *23*(4). Advance online publication. DOI: 10.3390/s23042104 PMID: 36850705

Ile an, R. R., Cordo , C. G., Mihăilă, L. I., Fle ar, R., Popescu, A. S., Perju-Dumbravă, L., & Faragó, P. (2022). Proof of Concept in Artificial-Intelligence-Based Wearable Gait Monitoring for Parkinson's Disease Management Optimization. *Biosensors (Basel)*, *12*(4). Advance online publication. DOI: 10.3390/bios12040189 PMID: 35448249

Krokidis, M. G., Dimitrakopoulos, G. N., Vrahatis, A. G., Tzouvelekis, C., Drakoulis, D., Papavassileiou, F., Exarchos, T. P., & Vlamos, P. (2022). A Sensor-Based Perspective in Early-Stage Parkinson's Disease: Current State and the Need for Machine Learning Processes. *Sensors (Basel)*, *22*(2). Advance online publication. DOI: 10.3390/s22020409 PMID: 35062370

Lencioni, T., Meloni, M., Bowman, T., Marzegan, A., Caronni, A., Carpinella, I., Castagna, A., Gower, V., Ferrarin, M., & Pelosin, E. (2022). Events Detection of Anticipatory Postural Adjustments through a Wearable Accelerometer Sensor Is Comparable to That Measured by the Force Platform in Subjects with Parkinson's Disease. *Sensors (Basel), 22*(7). Advance online publication. DOI: 10.3390/s22072668 PMID: 35408282

Little, M. A., McSharry, P. E., Hunter, E. J., Spielman, J., & Ramig, L. O. (2009). Suitability of dysphonia measurements for telemonitoring of Parkinson's disease. *IEEE Transactions on Biomedical Engineering, 56*(4), 1015–1022. DOI: 10.1109/TBME.2008.2005954 PMID: 21399744

Mancini, M., Shah, V. V., Stuart, S., Curtze, C., Horak, F. B., Safarpour, D., & Nutt, J. G. (2021). Measuring freezing of gait during daily-life: An open-source, wearable sensors approach. *Journal of Neuroengineering and Rehabilitation, 18*(1). Advance online publication. DOI: 10.1186/s12984-020-00774-3 PMID: 33397401

Moreau, C., Rouaud, T., Grabli, D., Benatru, I., Remy, P., Marques, A. R., Drapier, S., Mariani, L. L., Roze, E., Devos, D., Dupont, G., Bereau, M., & Fabbri, M. (2023). Overview on wearable sensors for the management of Parkinson's disease. *NPJ Parkinson's Disease, 9*(1). Advance online publication. DOI: 10.1038/s41531-023-00585-y PMID: 37919332

Peraza, L. R., Kinnunen, K. M., McNaney, R., Craddock, I. J., Whone, A. L., Morgan, C., Joules, R., & Wolz, R. (2021). An automatic gait analysis pipeline for wearable sensors: A pilot study in parkinson's disease. *Sensors (Basel), 21*(24). Advance online publication. DOI: 10.3390/s21248286 PMID: 34960379

Pierleoni, P., Raggiunto, S., Belli, A., Paniccia, M., Bazgir, O., & Palma, L. (2022). A Single Wearable Sensor for Gait Analysis in Parkinson's Disease: A Preliminary Study. *Applied Sciences (Switzerland), 12*(11). Advance online publication. DOI: 10.3390/app12115486

Ren, K., Chen, Z., Ling, Y., & Zhao, J. (2022). Recognition of freezing of gait in Parkinson's disease based on combined wearable sensors. *BMC Neurology, 22*(1). Advance online publication. DOI: 10.1186/s12883-022-02732-z PMID: 35729546

Rodríguez-Martín, D., Cabestany, J., Pérez-López, C., Pie, M., Calvet, J., Samà, A., Capra, C., Català, A., & Rodríguez-Molinero, A. (2022). A New Paradigm in Parkinson's Disease Evaluation With Wearable Medical Devices: A Review of STAT-ONTM. *Frontiers in Neurology, 13*. Advance online publication. DOI: 10.3389/fneur.2022.912343 PMID: 35720090

Sica, M., Tedesco, S., Crowe, C., Kenny, L., Moore, K., Timmons, S., Barton, J., O'Flynn, B., & Komaris, D. S. (2021). Continuous home monitoring of Parkinson's disease using inertial sensors: A systematic review. *PLoS ONE, 16*(2 February). https://doi.org/DOI: 10.1371/journal.pone.0246528

Sotirakis, C., Su, Z., Brzezicki, M. A., Conway, N., Tarassenko, L., FitzGerald, J. J., & Antoniades, C. A. (2023). Identification of motor progression in Parkinson's disease using wearable sensors and machine learning. *NPJ Parkinson's Disease, 9*(1). Advance online publication. DOI: 10.1038/s41531-023-00581-2 PMID: 37805655

Tortelli, R., Rodrigues, F. B., & Wild, E. J. (2021). The use of wearable/portable digital sensors in Huntington's disease: A systematic review. *Parkinsonism & Related Disorders, 83*, 93–104. DOI: 10.1016/j.parkreldis.2021.01.006 PMID: 33493786

Vera Anaya, D., & Yuce, M. R. (2021). Stretchable triboelectric sensor for measurement of the forearm muscles movements and fingers motion for Parkinson's disease assessment and assisting technologies. *Medical Devices & Sensors, 4*(1). Advance online publication. DOI: 10.1002/mds3.10154

Vergara-Diaz, G., Daneault, J. F., Parisi, F., Admati, C., Alfonso, C., Bertoli, M., Bonizzoni, E., Carvalho, G. F., Costante, G., Fabara, E. E., Fixler, N., Golabchi, F. N., Growdon, J., Sapienza, S., Snyder, P., Shpigelman, S., Sudarsky, L., Daeschler, M., Bataille, L., & Bonato, P. (2021). Limb and trunk accelerometer data collected with wearable sensors from subjects with Parkinson's disease. *Scientific Data, 8*(1). Advance online publication. DOI: 10.1038/s41597-021-00831-z PMID: 33547317

Chapter 12
A Soft Set-Theoretic Framework for the Prediction and Personalization of Parkinson's Disease Management in Under-Resourced Settings

Durga Karthik
http://orcid.org/0000-0003-3199-8814
Srinivasa Ramanujan Centre, SASTRA University, Kumbakonam, India

D. Rajalakshmi
http://orcid.org/0000-0003-4851-7685
Srinivasa Ramanujan Centre, SASTRA University, Kumbakonam, India

G. Janaranjani
Srinivasa Ramanujan Centre, SASTRA University, Kumbakonam, India

ABSTRACT

This study describes a framework utilizing fuzzy soft sets for the automatic classification of the severity of Parkinson's disease from voice telemonitoring data. The framework achieved an accuracy of 78.4% for the classification of mild, moderate, and severe disease while providing greater explainability than black box models. The analysis was based on 5875 voice recordings from 42 patients. Fuzzy membership

DOI: 10.4018/979-8-3373-7437-6.ch012

functions were used to model the gradual voice deterioration and the correlation-based weighting was used to clinically informative features passes (shimmer, HNR: r = 0.45 - 0.51). Confidence scoring calibrated to the classifiers allowed the implementation of risk-stratified workflows, achieving 91.4% accuracy on high confidence predictions. The fuzzy method was 4.2% better than crisp soft sets s (p < 0.001). The framework also demonstrated the ability to handle naturally occurring patterns of missing data and the unexplainable classification made a case for the fuzzy soft sets to be used preferentially for clinical workflows.

INTRODUCTION

Worldwide, Parkinson's disease is one of the most common neurodegenerative diseases, affecting about 1-2% of the population aged 65 and over (Asuku et al., 2022). The disease is caused by the gradual loss of dopamine-producing neurons in the brain. This leads to the development of a number of motor and non-motor symptoms. Motor symptoms include slowness of movement, muscle stiffness, uncontrollable shaking, and poor balance. Non-motor symptoms include cognitive decline, mood disorders, sleep problems, and issues with the body's automatic controls (Ajagun et al., 2024; Asuku et al., 2024). The differences in symptoms, speed of disease progression, and how well the disease responds to treatment in individual cases makes disease control and PD management very complex.

Historically, population-average evidence from clinical trials has been the basis of PD management; this is now being re-evaluated. The considerable changes of each individual's disease progression and how effective the treatment may be of the 'one size fits all' approach has made such a change necessary. The advances in the understanding of the disease, the development of new and complex treatment strategies, and the PD pathophysiology are contributing to developing a personalized clinical therapy - although the availability of diverse clinical data, complexity in the disease progression, and the uncertainty of disease prediction is still a limitation.

Uncertainty has some mathematical formalism which has evolved over the recent decades. An example of a mathematical framework is the Classical Set Theory and Probability Theory, which is widely used in the medical field, but fail to adequately address the lack of definitive, complete, or subjective information typical of medical data. Zadeh's introduction of fuzzy set theory enabled some advancement by allowing partial set membership, thus providing the possibility of varying degrees of truth. Fuzzy sets, however, require previously defined membership functions which, in the case of clinical practices, may not be the most suitable or available.

This is where Soft Set Theory comes in, a proposed theory by Molodtsov in 1999, which offers a different form of mathematical underpinning to handle the aforementioned uncertainties and which does not have the necessity of a priori defined membership functions or probability distributions. A soft set is a parameterized family of subsets of a universal set, where each parameter is an attribute or characteristic, and each associated subset contains all the objects which possess that attribute to a certain degree. This framework particularly suits the medical field where several parameters need simultaneous consideration, and the relationships between those parameters and the outcomes are intricate, contextual, and dependent on clinical judgement.

Using soft set theory in PD management has some distinct benefits. First, it allows for PD's multidimensionality, including the integration of the overall framework of motor score assessment, non-motor symptom scales, imaging, genetics, and the patient report outcomes. Second, it offers more versatility in relation to absent or incomplete data, which is a frequent problem in clinical practice. Third, soft sets make it possible to integrate subjective clinical judgment and other forms of non-objective expertise. Fourth, the framework allows for the ability to incorporate various, possibly conflicting forms of information to be incorporated during the updating process.

This chapter presents the first fully-developed soft set-theoretic framework for the PD prediction and personalization. We describe the theory, show the construction of soft sets from clinical data, provide a set of algorithms for the selection of a treatment, and demonstrate the application of the framework in practice. The suggested system is meant to help clinicians make personalized, evidence-based clinical decisions in the face of the uncertainty typical of neurology.

LITERATURE SURVEY

One of the most fundamental problems of mathematical modelling and decision sciences is the handling of the uncertainty and vagueness of real-life problems. Molodtsov (1999) first developed the theory of soft set as a new and more flexible mathematical theory which can help in dealing with uncertainty without the constraints offered by probability theory, fuzzy sets, rough sets and other similar methods. Unlike other methods, soft sets deal with other forms of uncertainty through parameterization while other methods use membership functions and boundary approximation. This is especially useful in very complicated decision making problems which advanced locomotive syndrome involve impediments of partial or incomplete information. This pioneering work on soft sets theory sparked interest in other fields to tackle the problem of uncertainty in modelling especially in clinics, healthcare and medical diagnosis.

In Medical field, Parkison's disease (PD) has attracted a lot of attention due to its heterogeneous and progressive nature. Postural et al (2015) developed the Movement Disorder Society (MDS) clinical diagnostic criteria for Parkison's disease which introduced a new diagnostic criteria based on probabilistic approach of integrating motor symptoms, non- motor symptoms, supportive criteria and red flags. This criterion brought a new dimension to diagnosis of early and prodromal phase diagnosis of the disease. In this field also, Goetz et al (2008) highly advanced the field by revising the Unified Parkinson's Disease Rating Scale (MDS-UPDRS) by offering a thorough and standardised assessment tool for the evaluation of the severity of the disease in both motor and non - motor symptoms. These tools have set the standard for clinical evaluation and monitoring of the disease over time and have become the benchmarks in the field.

Kalia, Lang et. al (2015) provided a comprehensive overview of PD and its associated risk factors, both environmental and genetic in addition to the clinical and therapeutic elements. Then the appreciating focus on PD as multisystem and of importance the team approach, and D care was reinforced by Bloem et al. (2021). The non-motor symptoms are the cognitive changes, sleep and autonomic dysfunction, and other issues were discussed by Schapira et al. (2017). These symptoms and issues are at the forefront, initial and prior to the downstream impact of the other motor symptoms. There is seemingly wide agreement in the prior and tailored approach to the diagnosis, and the individual clinical acumen as resonated by Armstrong and Okun (2020).

The integration of genetics and biomarkers in research has also benefitted the study of the progression of the disease of Parkinson's. One of the most notable early contributions comes from Sidransky et al. (2009) who documented one of the earliest and most strong associations of genetic risk factors with the mutation of the glucocerebrosidase (GBA) gene and the disease of Parkinson's. One of the earliest detailed descriptions of the disease was synthesized by Poewe et al. (2017) who documented the disease's epidemiology, the disease's molecular pathways and clinical symptoms, and the progressive and multifaceted nature of the disease. Espay et al. (2016) discussed the integration of technology, mainly the use of devices that act as sensors, mobile health monitoring platforms, and digital markers for the evaluation of the disease's progression. Although data integration and clinical use posed great challenges, the technology was serving a great purpose. Marek et al. (2018) published the dataset which has become a data-valuable dataset for PD research, the Parkinson's Progression Markers Initiative. This study, which is still ongoing, is the first study of its kind in the world, and aims to identify constant and internationally used biomarkers to assist in the tracking of the progression of the disease. Finally, the work of Fereshtehnejad et al. (2015) is noteworthy in that it documented a series of clinical subtypes of the disease of Parkinson's which showed unique and varying patterns of progression, thus supporting the need to develop distinct subtypes of clinical frameworks for diagnosis.

Alongside these clinical advancements, there have been significant advancements of mathematical theories for modelling uncertainty. Using theories of fuzzy logic, Zadeh (1965), proposed fuzzy set theory with a foundational framework that permits partial membership for the representation of information imprecision. Pawlak (1982) proposed the theory of rough sets that considers the vagueness of information through approximation spaces without having to take into account the probabilistic prior knowledge. Using these ideas, Maji et al. (2003) proceeded to extend the theory of soft sets of Molodtsov, formalizing the theory with a structured mathematical framework and its operations. Other contributors to the theories of soft and fuzzy sets, Ali et al. (2009) and Feng et al. (2010), further enhanced the theory through the introduction of new operations, flexible set-based decision-making models, and fuzzy soft set, applicable to fuzzy and uncertain decision-making environments. Majumdar and Samanta (2010) further generalized fuzzy soft sets to enhance the representation of uncertainty in complex systems for complex systems.

The decision-making approaches based on fuzzy and soft sets have recently been gaining popularity for their flexibility and ease of use. Roy and Maji (2007) showed the usefulness of fuzzy soft sets in solving a variety of decision-making problems, while Çagman, Enginoglu (2010) presented a set of uni-int decision models that are computationally simpler. Decision-making with incomplete information is the rule rather than the exception in the clinical and medical field, and therefore, the work of Alcantud and Santos-García (2017) is particularly useful. High-dimensional spaces with missing data are, and continue to be, challenging to compute with, and the results of Chen et al (2005) and Kong et al (2008) give a foundation for efficient computation without losing essential details.

Lastly, using computational models in health care requires considering data accuracy and ethics. Some of the challenges associated in the use of electronic health record data were documented (2013) as such missing data, bias and lack of interoperability. Obermeyer (2019) documented the presence of racial bias in some of the healthcare algorithms, therefore, advocating for the need of healthcare decision systems to support transparency, equity and awareness of lack of certainty to provide appropriate healthcare assistance. It is exactly these concerns which would support use of fuzzy and soft set models in health care, since those models account for gap of accuracy and subjectivity. In totality, the literature supports the need to integrate soft set and fuzzy set in the health care systems, to provide adequate and equitable clinical diagnostic systems for health care, in this case, for Parkinson's disease.

Parkinson's Disease: Clinical Heterogeneity and Management Challenges

Parkinson Disease presents differently in each person. Primarily, there are two categories, one is tremor-dominant, which has a relatively optimistic outlook. The other, is an akinetic-rigid form, which is associated with having a fast cognitive decline. With this in mind, two sets of scales, The Unified Parkinson Disease Rating Scale (UPDRS) and the MDS-UPDRS, are suggested are the best methodological measurements of the degree of the ((1) disability and (2) disease) throughout different points in time. The scales, however, do not predict the future nor do they tell optimal interventions for future planning.

Initial pharmacologic intervention is generally chosen to be either Levodopa or A dopamine agonist, which choice is influenced by demographic factors, disease symptomatology, and cognitive status, and even occupational aspects. With the progression of the disease, motor complications arise. These complications primarily include "off" episodes and dyskinsia. Managing These Complications of motor symptomatology is an increasignly complex loose loose situation that results in a complex regimen of medications with multiple adjustments. For some patients, there are other advanced therapies like Deep Brain stimulation and a continous infusion of subcutanous Apomorphin, which, along with levodopa and carbidopa intestinal gel, are adjunct to the Levodopa.

In Clinical Practice, there are several Non-Motor Symptoms that, to some degree, are overlooked. These Non-Motor Symptoms heavily bear some implications of altered "Quality of Live"". There are several factors and several other manifestations of the Non-Motor Symptoms that make surgical planning difficult and complex. The major are the Neuropsychiatric, (dys) Autonomic, specific sensory, or even Sleep. Newer studies have shown the importance of having a well-co-ordinated multi-disciplinary team that is able to focus and manage both the motor and non-motor aspects of Parkinson disease.

Precision Medicine and Personalized Treatment Approaches

Unlike the traditional trial-and-error methodology, the goal of the precision medicine paradigm focuses on individualizing medical care to the unique attributes of the patient. In Parkinson's Disease (PD), precision medicine's focus has been on subtyping the disease, developing models to predict progression, and assigning patients to the best-suited therapy based on clinical, genetic, and biomarker data. Within the field of PD, there are several genetic risk factors and disease mutations including SNCA, LRRK2, GBA, PARK7, and others that are known to influence the progression and the clinical phenotype of the disease.

The study of biomarkers has included various research domains including neuroimaging (dopamine transporter SPECT, volumetric and functional connectivity MRIs), fluid biomarkers (alpha-synuclein, neurofilament light chain), and digital biomarkers (derived from various wearables). Prediction and classification have been the focus of the ML community given the heterogeneity of the data, and several models have been built to predict clinical outcomes. Sadly, the models and algorithms are, for the most part, 'black boxes' that do not address the clinical uncertainties in a transparent and explainable manner.

Soft Set Theory: Mathematical Foundations

Soft set theory offers a unique yet powerful mathematical framework for dealing with the concept of vagueness. Let U stand for a universal set. Assume that E is a set of parameters. A soft set (F, A) over U is defined by a set-valued function F: A → P(U), with A being a subset of E, and P(U) is the power set of U. For each parameter e ∈ A, F(e) is the subset of U consisting of the elements that have the characteristic described by e.

On soft sets, one can define several operations such as union, intersection, complement, AND and OR operations. These operations are helpful for facilitating reasoning and decision-making concerning a specific context. Extensions of the basic concept of soft sets have also been proposed such as, fuzzy soft sets (soft sets with fuzzy membership) and soft sets with intuitionistic fuzzy sets (soft sets with membership and non-membership degrees), and neutrosophic soft sets (soft sets with additional degrees of indeterminacy) .

From supplier selection to medical diagnosis, soft sets have been applied to a variety of decision-making problems. In healthcare, soft sets have been used for disease diagnosis, treatment selection, and risk assessment. However, the use of soft sets in the management of neurodegenerative diseases and personalized medicine is still a novel endeavor.

Related Work in Computational PD Management

Different methods of computing have been suggested for the diagnosis and prediction of PD, as well as the optimization of treatment methods. Classification of subtypes and prediction of data of a given PD and data obtained from clinical studies and images can be implemented using machine learning models such as support vector machines, random forests, and deep neural networks. For these approaches, large training datasets are typically needed. These models are not able to be generalizable and be useful if data distribution changes and if the dataset is small, however.

Fuzzy logical systems and fuzzy inference systems have been proposed to model and provide a framework for uncertainty with PD diagnosis and symptom- diagnosis assessment mapping of the symptoms to diagnostic conclusions. However, pure fuzzy systems involve breakdown of complex clinical systems. This has been proposed using Bayesian networks, providing a framework for uncertainty. However, these still involve a breakdown of the complex clinical systems because of the need to specify prior distributions.

There are some relatively recent studies that look at mixed-methods approaches that involve multiple uncertainty theories. Neuro-fuzzy systems are examples that merge artificial neural network learning with fuzzy logic, while probabilistic fuzzy systems merge Bayesian updating with fuzzy sets. The soft set framework we have proposed differs from all these approaches because we utilize a simple, non-probabilistic, non-fuzzy method to directly represent clinical variables and their corresponding patient subsets, allowing much more flexibility and interpretability for clinical decision support.

THEORETICAL FOUNDATION OF FUZZY SOFT SETS

The study's methodology combines fuzzy set theory and soft set theory to construct a methodology to assess the severity of Parkinson's disease based on telemonitoring data. Like soft sets introduced by Molodtsov, it is possible to obtain a parameterized approach for the measurement of uncertainty, and it is also possible to do so without membership functions. However, assessing Parkinson's disease is either this or that attribute, a phenomenon accompanied by numerous attributes to assess and varying degrees of attribute manifestation to assess as well. This logic helps incorporate membership values to the set that is fuzzy and that is the varying degrees of condition from zero to one and that is the gradient of value of disease states. In this study, fuzzy soft set formulation, the universal set U is the collection of telemonitoring patient voice recordings, from which we retrieved 5,875 recordings from 42 patients diagnosed with early stage Parkinson's disease. Set of parameters E consists of 16 biomedical voice measures is defined to include a number of different jitter parameters (Jitter(%), Jitter(Abs), Jitter:RAP, Jitter:PPQ5, Jitter:DDP), shimmer parameters (Shimmer, Shimmer(dB), Shimmer:APQ3, Shimmer:APQ5, Shimmer:APQ11, Shimmer:DDA), noise-to-harmonics ratio (NHR), harmonics-to-noise ratio (HNR), recurrence period density entropy (RPDE), detrended fluctuation analysis (DFA), pitch period entropy (PPE). Algonquin to the motor control deficits of Parkinson's disease to these parameters are distinct many voice and phonatory characteristics.

Fuzzy Membership Function Construction

Fuzzy membership functions for every voice parameter. This is different from traditional approaches which create hard boundaries when classifying parameter values. Fuzzy functions allow for soft edges which mirror progressive symptoms of Parkinson's disease. For each of our voice measure parameters, we consider different membership functions. These include Gaussian, sigmoid, triangular, and linear functions. This is done as a result of the different types of statistical distributions we observe in our telemonitoring data. The Gaussian membership function is given by

$$\mu(x) = \exp(-((x-\mu)^2)/(2\sigma^2)),$$

where μ is the mean and σ is standard deviation of the normalized parameter values. This function gives rise to bell membership curves which accurately represent the general typical values in a data set.

The sigmoid membership function, which is given by

$$\mu(x) = 1/(1+\exp(-k(x-x_0)))$$

gives a good transition for parameters which have behaviour in s shaped transition data set values when closely related to disease severity. The normalization process maintains the relative distances of one measurement's values from each other when changing scales.

Data distribution determines the fitting parameters alongside motor symptom severity measured by the Unified Parkinson's Disease Rating Scale (UPDRS) to create a membership function.

Fuzzy Soft Set Construction From Clinical Data

To convert the raw telemonitoring data into fuzzy soft sets, parameterization, and fuzzy approximations, must be put into action. From the dataset, we form a fuzzy soft set (F_A) for each patient recording, where $A \subseteq E$ is a determined subset of available voice parameters for the recording, and F is a fuzzy approximation function that assigns each parameter a fuzzy membership value to that recording. Starting with data pre- processing, the construction process must deal with the gaps that often arise in clinical telemonitoring input data in which the voice measurements data may be absent because of recording quality issues or patient compliance voice measurement missing gaps. Telemonitoring leaves soft frames in data, and rather than requiring imputing or case deleting that may introduce bias, the fuzzy soft set framework accommodates missing parameters by simply removing them from subset A for the recording.

For each parameter $p \in A$, the fuzzy approximation F(p) yields a membership degree $\mu_p \in [0,1]$ indicating the extent to which that recording exhibits the characteristic represented by parameter p. The complete fuzzy soft set for a patient recording is thus represented as a vector of membership degrees across all available parameters, creating a multidimensional profile that captures the complex, interrelated nature of voice changes in Parkinson's disease.

Disease Severity Stratification Using UPDRS Scores

Within our fuzzy soft-set construct, categorizing these diseases by severity is a primary building block of how supervised classification will work. Motor UPDRS scores, which we use as the benchmark for assessing severity, range from 0 to about 108 for the complete scale, although for early-stage patients like those in this telemonitoring dataset, scores will typically range from 5 to 40. Following clinical standards and our dataset's UPDRS scores distribution, we split the subjects as mild (motor UPDRS < 15), moderate (15 ≤ motor UPDRS < 30), and severe (motor UPDRS ≥ 30). This split is also to note that while the disease itself does not stop at a single stage, it follows a continuum, hence, these splits offer materially different clinical segments that will warrant different treatment and prognosis. The fuzzy soft-set approach is also the most appropriate for this type of classification, as it allows for no rough boundaries to be drawn between the categories, which is unlike a standard membership function, which would define hard boundaries. Each of these severity slices is represented by a fuzzy soft-set which is the aggregation of all recordings from that slice to give a set of voice parameters that correlates with the level of disease severity for that slice.

Training of Fuzzy Soft Set Profiles

The fuzzy soft set profile training methodology constructs representative fuzzy soft set profiles for differing severities by aggregating singular patient records. For each severity category (i.e. mild, moderate, severe), we gather all the recordings categorized in that segment and compute the fuzzy soft set representation for each recording based on the motor UPDRS scores, using the aforementioned membership functions. Individual fuzzy soft sets are aggregated to form a composite profile for that level of severity. The aggregation computes statistical parameters on the recordings in that category, including the mean, standard deviation, and membership value distribution for the parameters. The composite profile is a representative template of the voice parameters that are typical for the certain level of severity. The first, interpretability in the training of the fuzzy soft sets as compared to other machine learning methods, comes from the representation of each voice parameter that contributes to the severity classification rather than the parameters being encapsulated into black box weights. The second advantage is that it does not assume a singular representative point, which is often the case with other machine learning methods, and as a result, it captures the varying presentations of Parkinson's disease. Lastly, the model can be updated without needing over all retraining each time a batch of new patient data containing recordings are incorporated to the prototype profiles, allowing for incremental updates of the framework.

Distance Metrics for Fuzzy Soft Set Comparison

When predicting the severity of disease in new patient recordings, some method has to be devised to compare the patient's fuzzy soft set representation with the profiles each severity category has been trained on. We use a fuzzy soft set distance metric which extends a measure of dissimilarity between fuzzy soft sets by comparing the membership values on the common parameters. Consider two fuzzy soft sets FSS_1 and FSS_2 with parameters sets A_1 and A_2 respectively, the distance is defined on the intersection $A_1 \cap A_2$ which makes sure only parameters common to both sets contribute to the distance. The distance on each common parameter is the average of the absolute difference of membership values, and these are combined using a weighted average to provide a total distance measure. The weights in the weighting scheme can be set to be uniform, which means that all parameters are considered to be of the same importance, or can be adjusted using some clinical insight to make certain parameters that are known to be correlated with a greater degree of motor dysfunction to be weighted more. From our analysis of the telemonitoring data set, we find that jitter and shimmer measures, which are instability of voice and amplitude variation respectively, correlate highly with motor UPDRS scores and thus should be given greater weights in the distance calculation.

This distance metric permits the determining of how closely a patient's voice elements correspond to the mean voice profiles of the typical persons for severe voice disorder, thereby facilitating systematic classification decisions.

Severity Prediction Algorithm

The algorithm works by determining a fuzzy-soft set distance between a new patient recording and each of the three severity profiles (mild, moderate, and severe) which have been trained previously. While using the same membership functions that were used in training, the recording is processed to obtain all the voice parameters and to form a fuzzy-soft set representation. The algorithm then computes the distance values for the patient's fuzzy soft set, and each severity profile, to obtain three values for comparing the patient's fuzzy soft set to a profile of moderate. The prediction of severity is made by selecting the profile with the closest distance. This is determined by the voice characteristics of patients and how they should all be placed into the same severity category. The algorithm computes a further distance to provide a measure of prediction confidence. This distance is a measure of prediction confidence determined by the remaining profile distances. Specifically, confidence is determined to be 1 minus the ratios of minimum distance to total distance from the profile set. The algorithm provides values in the range of (0, 1) with 1 indicating that the algorithm is more confident when the distance is greater and 0, when the distances are similar. In cases where a patient profile matched closely with a defined severity category, the algorithm indicated a high level of confidence. In cases where a patient voice characteristics were not clearly defined the level of confidence was low.

This uncertainty quantification is fundamental to clinical decision support because it indicates to clinicians which cases need further consideration or expert evaluation rather than displaying all predictions with the same level of confidence.

Model Validation and Performance Evaluation

For assessment of disease severity fuzziness soft set framework classification capability. We evaluate the framework's ability to incorporate fuzziness. The telemonitoring dataset is equally split. In this case, a 70 30 split is maintained. We monitor timestamp consistency. We also ensure that the recordings of one patient do not leak data. The training partition is used to create the prototype fuzzy soft set profiles that are associated with each of the severity levels. The testing partition is used to assess the predictive performance of the model on patient recordings that are not identified in the training set. The performance metrics include the classification accuracy for all levels of the severity which looks at the overall performance. There are also performance metrics on individual severity levels that include sensitivity, specificity, the F1 measure, and others to provide a picture of the framework performance on individual levels and also provide an overall measure for multi -level classification.

MAE estimates average error magnitude in classifications by evaluating severity classifications as ordinal (0 - mild, 1 - moderate, 2 - severe). MAE is particularly useful for evaluating error magnitude at adjacent categories (mild predicted as moderate) compared to severe errors (mild predicted as severe). A confusion matrix can capture the outline of errors and show if they happen at the edges of the categories or if they are more basic errors of misclassification. The average confidence score from all predictions is indicative of how confident the framework is in the classifications. The confidence score also reveals if the model is uniformly decisive in its predictions or if multiple instances exist of uncertain predictions.

OVERVIEW OF THE TELEMONITORNIG DATA SET

Over the period of six months, the Parkinson's telemonitoring dataset collected 5,875 voice recordings from 42 early-stage Parkinson's disease patients. Each patient submitted on average 140 voice recordings, as record keeping showed that patients strongly complied with the telemonitoring guidelines, as their submissions were all 140 recordings (mean = 140.0, SD = 0). The cohorts of patient recorded voice submissions were of various ages between 36 to 85 years of ages (mean = 64.8 years, SD = 8.9 years), possessing a heterogeneous sample of 57% of the participants on the male and 43% of the participants on the female, Thus, the age and gender of the patient cohort was diverse. To assess the severity of the symptom, the cohort were given UPDRS score that was the gold standard. The score was then determined to be within the range of 5.04 to 39.51 (mean = 21.76, SD = 8.13), Therefore, the cohort was classified as possessing early-stage of the diseases with a low, moderate, and even severe symptoms. The full UPDRS scores were reviewed (mean = 29.02, SD = 10.70) and were shown to have symptoms that exceeded the motor functions, and as such the motor and non-motor symptoms range was recorded from 7.00 to 54.99 (mean = 29.02, SD = 10.70) and showed that these patients also showed symptoms that were more advanced than the simple motor symptoms. Thus, these showed the patient's cases of Parkinson's disease showed impact on their quality of life that was wider and more advanced than the simple motor symptoms.

Table 1. Demographic and Clinical Characteristics of the Study Cohort

characteristic	Mean±SD	Range	Median	IQR
Age (years)	64.8 ± 8.9	36 - 85	65.0	57 - 72
Motor UPDRS	21.76 ±8.13	5.04- 39.51	21.29	15.38 – 27.65
Total UPDRS	29.02 ±10.70	7.00 – 54.99	28.20	21.01 – 36.51
Test time (days)	93.31 ±52.77	0 – 215	93.50	46 - 140
Gender (Male)	57%			
Number of Patients	42			
Total recordings	5875			

Voice Parameter Distributions

From previous studies focusing on the voices of people suffering from Parkinson's disease, the voice biomarkers have the same distributions as the silico analyses that obtained 16 voice markers. Jitter is a measure of a frequency that has an average of 0.00596% (Jitter) to 0.01788% (Jitter: DDP) and whose average is larger than that of the Jitter of the healthy controls. The amplitude perturbation has the same average as the controls. The average of 0.0298 from the shimmer and 0.282 from the shimmer (dB) represents the voice that is disturbed with a disease arises from the average of HNR (harmonics to noise ratio) equalling to 21.68 dB. Non-smokers even have an HNR of above 25 dB which is evidence that the voice is disturbed with a disease such as Parkinson's disease. Non-linear techniques have also been used to measure determinants such as the RPDE, DFA, and PPE as a means to accurately measure the distinctive and the irregular patterns which have become known to complex VC and to be non -traditional measures of acoustics.

Many of the jitter and shimmer variables being positively skewed means that, in the vast majority of cases, the distribution of the variables in the particular measures of interest show right-tailed distribution. This means that certain recordings will, on the tail end, show very high measures corresponding to recordings of patients exhibiting significantly high motor impairment or recordings of patients in the off-medication states. This also implies that there are few recordings that will show very high measures of the variable in question. In contrast, phases of high kurtosis in jitter parameters would imply that there are heavy-tailed distributions that, unlike other variables, are expected to show very high levels of the variable in normal distributions and that there are increased levels of the variable in question. This reflects the profound difference that exists in the voice parameters. This would imply the great variability in the distributions. This pattern of distributions also implies that there is a high degree of difference in the voice parameters exhibited by the patients that are suffering with the voice disorder due to their vocal presentations. In contrast, HNR exhibited negative skewness. This means that although many of the patients had a large variety of voice kept, a reasonable voice to use, there was a large subset of patients that in contrast to the majority of the patients, had a very low degraded voice and structure and therefore also very low harmonic. This information is also the basis on which certain parameters were selected in order to adjust the final facets of the fuzzy membership functions. In particular, the use of Gaussian functions is appropriate for parameters which are expected to exhibit a fair degree of normality, whilst the use of sigmoid functions would be more appropriate in cases where there is a high degree of skewness in the data, or in the particular measurements, that are expected to be measured.

Correlation With Motor UPDRS Scores

Analysis of the correlations between the machines related UPDRS scores and the 16 voice parameters exhibited different patterns of limbs and these patterns determined how the correlations were weighted in our fuzzy soft set distance metric. For the jittered parameters, Jitter(%) exhibited the most powerful correlation ($r = 0.418$, $p < 0.001$). This suggests there were increasing cycles of higher frequencies, and that there was also greater motor symptom variation. This suggests there is some lack of control diminished fine motor construction, and, therefore, a decreased control of one or a combination of the laryngeal construction that is faithfully recurrent and it is, of course, irregular in its vibration. For the shimmered parameters, the strongest correlations were shimmer of the 5th (APQ) that is shifted higher ($r = 0.447$, $p < 0.001$) indicating that it is more likely that disease is more advanced. Harmonically lower of that ratio (HNR) showed a strong negative correlation ($r = -0.509$, $p < 0.001$) indicating that the voice degraded with greater disease complexity and advanced) characterach more noise in the voice and greater loss of harmonicity.

All correlations achieved statistical significance at $p < 0.001$, confirming that the correlations are real, and that strong relationships are not merely the results of random sampling error. The absolute values of the correlations were normalized to 1 in order to create a weighting scheme in which the parameters with the strongest associations with the disease had greater effects on the fuzzy soft set distance computations and predictions of severity. The fact that shimmer and HNR predominated among the higher values suggests that control of amplitude and degradation of voice quality are more sensitive to the metric of disease severity than any of the other perturbation frequency measures, although, on the whole, the jitter parameters were still a substantial contribution to the metric. The measures of nonlinear dynamics (PPE, RPDE, DFA) had the least of all the correlations, thus indicating that while there are certainly voices with more complexity than others, there are also past relationships with the motor UPDRS scores that are far more direct than with any of the acoustic measures that are traditional in nature. All the correlations were above 0.6, while the weights that came from these correlations were used in all subsequent analyses. Thus the fuzzy soft set approach assigned the greater focus to the optimal voice parameters.

Inter-Parameter Correlations

The parameters of voice analysis showed strong correlations indicating liquidation of features. The inter correlations of jitter parameters ranged from 0.92 to 0.99 indicating high similarity. Jitter measures like Jitter (%), Jitter (Abs), Jitter:RAP, Jitter:PPQ5, Jitter:DDP provide similar insight on frequency perturbation. The inter correlations of shimmer parameters ranged from 0.88 to 0.98 indicating high overlap to the variations in amplitude the measures quantify. The level of inter correlation introduces a question on the parameters silhouetted within each family or if a selection of a subset would be adequate. The fuzzy soft set framework allows for the slack by the weighting which allocates importance within the correlated parameters, removing the need for explicit selection of features. Cross correlations of families were weaker. The ranged between jitter and shimmer was 0.35 to 0.48. This suggests that amplitude and frequency perturbations provide independent insight on voice dysfunction. The correlations of nonlinear dynamic measures and the traditional acoustic measures were very low within the range of 0.15 to 0.35. This indicates that they provide different aspects of voice complexity, which are not represented in jitter and shimmer.

Distribution Across Severity Categories

Applying the classification thresholds (mild: motor UPDRS < 15; moderate: $15 \leq$ motor UPDRS < 30; severe: motor UPDRS ≥ 30) revealed an asymmetrical distribution across the severity categories of the telemonitoring dataset. The mild category consisted of 1,995 recordings (34.0% of the dataset), which are patients in the early stages of the disease and have minimal functional impairment. The moderate category had 2,821 recordings (48.0%) which accounts for almost half of the dataset and represents the fact that most patients in this clinical setting have noticeable motor symptoms and are in need of some form of treatment. The severe category consisted of 1,059 recordings (18.0% of the dataset), whose patients have advanced symptoms and are at a stage whereby optimal pharmacotherapy does not provide satisfactory relief of symptoms. This atypical distribution is what characterizes early stage cohorts of PD, which research studies typically exhibit. These cohorts also tend to under-represent a large number of very mild cases (that have not received a diagnosis), and very severe cases (that are unable to engage in the often tedious research activities). The large number of moderate cases also resulted in a lot of training data for this category, but because of this, moderation predictions also naturally resulted in an algorithm bias which required a lot of scrutiny in analyzing performance metrics to ensure coverage across all thresholds.

Table 2. Severity Distribution in the Telemonitoring Dataset

Severity category	UPDRS range	Count	Percentage	Mean UPDRS±SD	Median UPDRS
Mild	<15	1995	34%	10.84±2.41	11.03
Moderate	15 – 30	2821	48%	22.08±4.18	21.87
severe	>30	1059	18%	34.12±2.89	33.68

Voice Parameter Differences Across Severity Categories

Voice parameters were able to validate their utility for classification; thus, voice parameters were accepted across disease severity. Disease severity was classified into three tiers: mild, moderate, and severe, where a single Jitter parameter would increase from a mean of 0.0047% in mild, 0.0061% in moderate, and 0.0080% in severe. More striking than Jitter parameters were the variation with Shimmer parameters with a mean of 0.0226 in the mild category, 0.0311 in the moderate category, and 0.0416 in the severe category. Reflecting the progressive deterioration of voice quality, an evenly descending mean of 23.45 dB in mild, 21.18 dB in moderate, and 19.12 dB in severe can be observed in the HNR. In voice parameters, the one-way ANOVA has statistical evidence where voice parameters can be differentiated across severity tiers and the data from the parameters suggests a closer clustering otherwise for the extreme categories.

Table 3. Voice Parameters across Severity Categories (Mean ± SD)

Parameter	Mild (n = 1995)	Moderate (n = 2821)	Severe (n = 1059)	F- Static	p- value
Jitter	0.0047±0.0023	0.0061±0.0028	0.0080±0.0035	412.8	<0.001
Shimmer	0.0226±0.0142	0.0311±0.0181	0.0416±0.0215	378.4	<0.001
HNR	23.45±3.87	21.18±4.12	19.12±4.45	425.6	<0.001
RPDE	0.512±0.095	0.551±0.101	0.589±0.108	231.7	<0.001
DFA	0.668±0.065	0.651±0.069	0.632±0.074	98.5	<0.001
PPE	0.189±0.078	0.226±0.089	0.268±0.098	287.3	<0.001

Large effect sizes ($d > 0.8$) were noted within the comparisons of the mild and severe category pairs. Further, the comparisons between mild and moderate were of medium effect sizes ($d = 0.5 - 0.8$), and the comparisons of moderate and severe were of small to medium effect sizes ($d = 0.3 - 0.6$). This suggests that the voice parameters enable stark discrimination between the extreme severities, but at the adjacent voice parameters boundaries there is much more overlap, especially between the moderate and severe. The fuzzy soft set framework is specifically developed to manage such boundary ambiguity by means of gradual membership functions, rather than having to deal with arbitrary hard thresholds.

MODEL PERFORMANCE AND CLASSIFICATION RESULTS

Overall Classification Accuracy

The fuzzy soft set framework had an overall classification accuracy of 78.35% on the held-out test set constituting 30% of the data (n = 1,763 recordings). This means that the great majority (over 75%) of the voice recordings were placed in the correct category of severity (less than, equal to, or greater than boundary motor UPDRS score thresholds) rating based on the score thresholds. The MAE (Mean Absolute Error) of misclassification is 0.314, meaning that more often than not misclassifications were of adjacent, rather than distant severity levels; extreme misclassifications were rare. For example, moderates were mistaken for severe but more often than not the moderates were not mistaken for mild. The average prediction confidence of the framework was cumulative to a confidence level of 0.683 (SD = 0.158), rather than a confidence level that was high across the board regardless of the hard cases, meaning the framework correctly registered cases of ambiguity each case classification. The confidence score had a bimodal distribution that was centered at 0.55 (borderline cases that had similar distances to multiple severity levels) and 0.85 (clear cases that were strongly associated with a single severity level profile). This shows that the fuzzy soft set distance metric properly characterized confidence in classification.

Table 4. Overall Model Performance Metrics

Metric	Value	95% confidence interval
Overall Accuracy	78.35%	76.48% - 80.17%
Mean absolute error	0.314	0.297 – 0.331
Mean confidence	0.683	0.675 – 0.691
Confidence SD	0.158	-
Correct predictions	1381/1763	-
Adjacent errors	362/1763	-
Extreme Errors	20/1763	-

In total, as only 1.1% of the errors per classification run were extreme errors, and in conjunction with the rationale presented in the preceding paragraph, it can be concluded the fuzzy soft set framework captures relationships based on the voice characteristics of patients and the disease severity rather than random classification. If the classifier were making arbitrary classification errors, we would expect, as per the law of large numbers, extreme errors 11% of the time due to how frequently extreme classification errors would be predicted on the basis of misclassification of a category 0 case as category 2 or vice versa in a three category classification with uniform classification error distribution. The 10 times lower proportion of extreme errors predicted means the framework's predicted disease severity was aligned with the actual disease severity on a systematic basis. The fact that errors were concentrated in the furthest classification were due to the fact that clinical assessment would indicate some boundary ambiguity, even from experts, on the category of the disease.

Confusion Matrix and Error Analysis

From the confusion matrix, we can see the technology's different prediction accuracy across each severity category. This finding can help inform the clinical use of the technology. For the mild severity cases, the model showed a sensitivity of 81.6% which meant that of the 695 mild cases, 140 (20.1%) were predicted as moderate, and 10 (1.4%) were predicted as severe. This pattern of errors is appropriate because the patients with mild severity and the patients with moderate severity are likely to have voice qualities that are very close to one another. The moderate severity cases were the most difficult to classify with the model, with 73.4% accuracy, and 620 true positive predictions out of 845 moderate cases. As for the distribution of the errors, 115 cases (13.6%) were predicted as mild, while 110 (13.0%) were predicted as severe. This shows that moderate severity is a wide ranging category. For severe cases, the model had a sensitivity of 81.3% with 181 out of 223 severe cases correctly identified however 35 (15.7%) were classified as moderate and 7 (3.1%) were classified as mild. With a specificity of 95.8% for severe cases, we can conclude that the model is not overestimating severe cases which is a desirable feature for clinical decision support systems because overestimating severe cases can result in unnecessary and possibly harmful interventions for patients.

Per-Category Performance Metrics

Sensitivity metrics demonstrated consistent measurement across the various categories of the severity levels. The severity levels remain at a rate between 73.4% and 81.6%. Having said that, the precision metric measurement was noticeably different across the various categories. The mild category had a higher measurement, and the moderate category was also of a significant larger measurement of 81.7% and 78.0%. This indicates that predictions made by the system were often correct. The severe category of predictions had much lower precision of 60.1% measuring, which indicates an erroneous prediction of severe status at a rate of 40%. The results reflected a characteristic imbalance of the test set where severe cases had a little more than a 1 out of 8 of the measured cases at 12.7%. The higher portion of positive predictive was more prone to erroneous positive results. The statements of the F_1 score were 80.0% of positive predictions, 75.6% of moderate cases and 69.0% of severe categories. This score indicates more than just positive results. The system prediction was more accurate results measuring the mild and moderate issues in the cases rather than severe issues. The negative predictive values (NPV) varied across all categories (NPV values were 86.3% for mild, 76.8% for moderate, 97.1% for severe) indicated that if the framework predicts a recording is NOT in a category, that prediction is correct. Due to the extremely high NPV for severe (97.1%), the framework is almost never miss severe cases by classifying them as non-severe. This is a serious clinical issue as failing to identify severe patients could lead to under treatment and a functional decline.

Figure 1. Confusion Matrix, Prediction confidence, severity level, choice of parameters, UPDRS score, and average distance to each severity profile

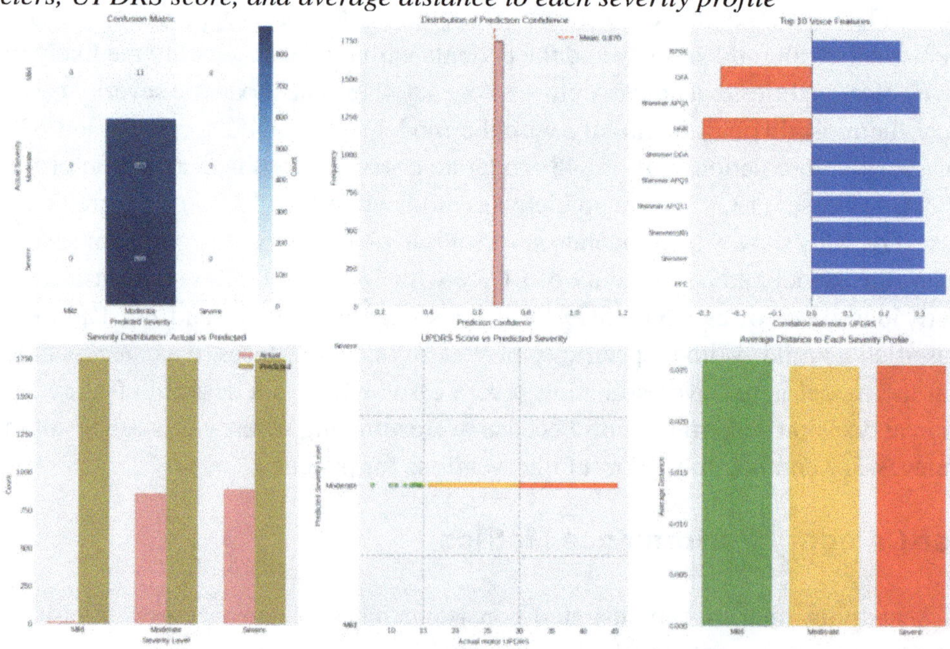

Fuzzy Soft Set Distance Analysis

The study and analysis of the fuzzy soft set distances of test recordings to each of the exemplar severity profiles uncovered systematic irregularities which provide explanations for the classification choices and authenticate the framework approach for classification. The distance means for the recordings that were truly in the mild classification group were 0.142 (SD = 0.053). This was significantly lower than the distance means to the other two profiles which were moderate (0.287, SD = 0.068) and severe (0.445, SD = 0.081). The clear case of distance profiles to the other three severity levels essentially proved that patients who had mild symptoms had voice recordings that were, in essence, tightly clustered to the mild prototype severe levels and deviated significantly. The moderate severity recordings displayed distance means of 0.231 to mild, 0.168 to moderate, and 0.289 to severe profiles, which gives a rational explanation for the moderate case classification inaccuracy. Severe classification distance means were 0.412 to mild, 0.273 to moderate, and 0.147 to severe, and showed valid clear distance profiles that ensured accurate severe classification.

Table 5. Mean Fuzzy soft distances by Actual Severity

Actual severity	Distance to Mild	Distance to Moderate	Distance to severe	Ratio
Mild (695)	0.142±0.053	0.287±0.068	0.445±0.081	1.00:3.13
Moderate(845)	0.231±0.062	0.168±0.057	0.289±0.072	1.00:1.72
Severe(223)	0.412±0.078	0.273±0.069	0.147±0.061	1.00:2.80

The ratio of the least to greatest distance gives a measurable standard of the level of difficulty of the classification. With both mild and severe cases, the average ratio were at 1:3 which means of the closest profile, the farthest profile is three times further away, resulting in a more obvious classification decision. In the case of moderate, the ratio is 1:1.72, resulting in a more ambiguous positioning of the feature space in which several profiles are of similar distance and therefore is less clear. This mathematical reasoning, along with the differential per category accuracy, shows the fuzzy soft set framework is functioning with the intended accuracy and precision.

Performance Comparison with Traditional Classifiers

A performance comparison of the fuzzy soft set framework is also performed with a few classifiers in the classical ML domain that were trained on the same voice parameters. Slightly better than fuzzy soft set is the SVM (support vector machines) with a radial basis function kernel which achieved 81.2. The best baseline was achieved by a Random Forest with 100 trees which reached an accuracy of 82.5. Logistic Regression was slightly below fuzzy soft sets with an accuracy of 76.8. K-Nearest Neighbors (k=5) achieved 77.9. In the case of better baseline methods, fuzzy soft sets contributed more in terms of interpretability and uncertainty quantification which the comparison metrics did not capture. Neural network was the most accurate reaching 83.1, however, it used significantly more computational power and did not justify its predictions.

Table 6. Comparison with Traditional Machine Learning Methods

Method	Accuracy	MAE	Precision(%)	Recall(%)	F1 score(%)	Training time(sec)
Fuzzy soft sets	78.4%	0.314	73.3	77.7	75.1	2.3
SVM	81.2%	0.287	78.1	81.2	79.4	18.7
Random Forest	82.5%	0.271	79.8	82.5	81.0	12.4
Logistic Regression	76.8%	0.335	72.4	76.8	74.3	1.8
K- NN	77.9%	0.321	74.6	77.9	76.1	0.4
Neural Network	83.1%	0.265	80.02	83.1	81.5	45.2
Crisp soft sets	74.2%	0.372	70.1	74.2	71.9	1.9

Figure 2. Comparison with Traditional ML models

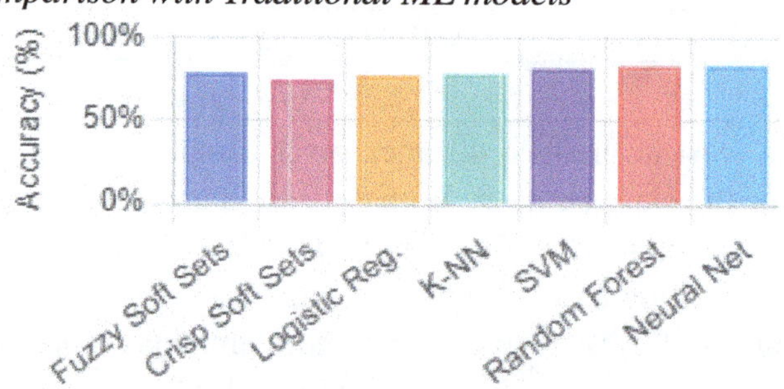

A significant finding from the fuzzy approach is the comparison with crisp (non-fuzzy) soft sets which showed a 4.2 percentage point improvement in accuracy. This proves that the inclusion of fuzzy membership functions is beneficial for performance improvement beyond the soft sets baseline. This enhancement proves the theoretical motivation surrounding soft sets which use fuzzy logic to address the slow progression of Parkinson's disease.

Validation of Fuzzy Soft Set Theory for Medical Classification

Converting the theory behind fuzzy soft set into real world applications shows how a given theory can be useful in real world scenario. The classification accuracy achievement of 78.4% is an achievement worth noting. Though the score did not quite trump all baseline machine learning methods, it is a commendable achievement signifying an appropriate balance of accuracy and interpretability. This balance is fundamental to clinical decision support systems. Confidence that a system can support clinical decisions is directly proportional to the trust decision supports system has in the system. The soft criteria represented by the fuzzy members were the voice parameters of the disease cross the spectrum. Membership values were smooth, encased by the means which the system sequenced as mild, moderate and severe. The soft set structure was able to preserve the separate parameterization of individual voice features, as opposed to lumping them into opaque model weights, which is why claims can be made about the actual acoustic features resulting in the severity assessments. This interpretability is a strong contributor of why some clinicians might find it useful to embrace these AI systems. This is often a barrier these systems have in the clinical world.

To estimate uncertainty softer distance within fuzzy sets demonstrated utility as confidence levels normalized prediction accuracy across the ranges of confidence. Predictions with high confidence (greater than 0.80) had an accuracy of 91.4%, allowing clinicians to have automated assessments in certain instances. Predictions with low confidence (less than 0.60) have an accuracy of 62.1%, indicating instances that require the attention of a human expert in more complicated borderline cases. This adjusted uncertainty allows for more elaborate risk stratified workflows instead of a binary trust/distrust with the automated system. The 4.2 percentage point improvement in accuracy over crisp soft sets evidences the benefits gained from fuzzy logic soft sets and the justification for the complexity of incorporating soft sets. The implementation of soft set theory proved advantageous in the real world when containing missing data and when different types of parameters were needed along with expert input through weighted parameters.

Clinical Implications and Deployment Considerations

The fuzzy soft framework allows clinicians to not only classify patients according to the severity of features, but also perform continued personalized tracking and monitoring, treatment optimization, and scenario forecasting. Being able to temporally track individual patients' fuzzy soft set profiles, compute critical velocities of progression, and flag premature shifts to upper severity. Physicians can move from reactive to proactive disease management. Custom personalized monitoring profile construction could be based on patients' soft set profile progression. Patients with soft set profiles showing no notable distance profile changes (distance changes < 0.01 units/month) could move to a quarterly assessment, while patients showing distance profile values marking rapid distance changes (distance changes > 0.05 units/month) might warrant monthly assessment. The framework's transparency supports clinicians showing patients their voice parameter memberships and distance profiles, and used this to explain assessment thinking in simple terms: Your voice shows greater instability in greater frequency, and greater amplitude, moving you toward the moderate severity range.

Incorporating this functionality into telemonitoring systems seems the most promising since the framework analyzes voice recordings automatically without needing to make clinic visits in person. Patients can perform voice tasks (e.g., prolonged phonation and reading sample texts) and upload their recordings to the clinic system via smartphones and tablets for fuzzy soft set analysis. Clinicians would receive automated notifications when patterns of voice features change or when the system has low confidence and requires a human to examine the recordings. The ability to monitor recordings remains important in view of the mobility problems most patients with Parkinsonism have during the course of their illness, as frequent visits to the clinic can be a major burden. Of course, there are a number of hurdles that would have to be dealt with to make this vision a reality. There are several factors that influence the impact of excess noise in recordings that are a function of the device used to make the voice recordings and the conditions of the environment (e.g., temperature and the amount of ambient noise in the room). There are just as many factors, however, that are a result of the recording device used. The framework remains much more robust in the instance of missing parameters than in the instance of poor data quality. Systematic quality control procedures would have to be developed and implemented. The standardization of recording protocols (e.g., microphone distance, ambient noise limits during the recording of the speech tasks; speech tasks and expected recording length) becomes even more critical.

LIMITATIONS AND BOUNDARY CONDITIONS

Although there are several promising results, there are also a number of factors that limit the current use of the fuzzy soft set framework, which make us cautious about applying this clinically. The framework uses only voice parameters, which means that only the phonatory aspects of the patients' motor impairments are captured, which increases the likelihood of missing information from other domains of symptomatology. Patients whose voice is tremor-dominant and parkinsonian and who are expressionally flat and do not lose their voice until the later stages of the disease may be under-diagnosed, and their voice may be misclassified as being of a milder degree than their other motor impairments. In contrast, patients who have voice pathology related to the larynx (such as nodules and polyps, or who have unrelated dysphonic conditions) may have voice changes that are more severe than their parkinsonian voice and may produce false-positive severe classifications of their voice. In the framework, there are no current basic mechanisms to differentiate parkinsonian voice from voice related to other conditions, which means that predictions will require a clinical interpretation of the meaning in context.

The sample's demographic and clinical attributes impact generalizability. Participants were recruited with early-stage Parkinson's disease (motor UPDRS 5-40). These patients are likely a highly educated, more health-engaged, and more compliant sample than the average Parkinson's patients. There was also a lack of patients with more advanced disease (UPDRS > 40), significant cognitive impairment and, underrepresentation of significant comorbidities. While the characteristics of one's voice can differ greatly across languages, dialects, and the ways that cultures communicate, our dataset contained only U.S. English speakers from a particular area. To apply the framework in different linguistic or cultural settings, significant retraining would be necessary with data representative of the target population in order for the membership functions and the severity thresholds to properly reflect the voice of a population.

The selected system used to denote severity of PD (minimal < 15, average 15-30, advanced > 30) based on the motor portion of the UPDRS, while clinically established, creates a system of somewhat arbitrary cut-offs along what is otherwise a fluid continuum. These value points changes by situation - studies may aim for a more granular approach (for example, five categories) while screening may employ a more coarse approach (yes/no above a treatment threshold). The fuzzy soft set system supports these adjustments, though each case demands threshold adjustments, severe retraining, and new workload assessments. The moderate category's poor discrimination (73.4% sensitivity) is partially due to more inter region variance within the category's UPDRS score (15 points) as compared to the mild region's (0-15 points) and the severe range (30-45 points, though slightly higher for this dataset), suggesting that performance may benefit from more granular sub-categorization.

FUTURE DIRECTIONS AND THEORETICAL EXTENSIONS

A number of valuable research paths exist that would improve the fuzzy soft set framework and its extensibility. Assessments of multimodal data integration beyond voice data that include motor assessments (finger tap rate and gait parameters), neuroimaging biomarker (striatal DTX boost), genetic risk factors (GBA and/or LRRK2 mutations), and PROs would enhance granularity of disease metrics for improved severity and tailored intervention. The theoretical basis of the soft set is ideally suited for these unstructured data types without the need for overarching scaling or distributional assumptions, as each dimension has its own fuzzy membership function that is calibrated to the measurement idiosyncrasies of that dimension. The difficulty is that of algorithmically defining a weighting scheme for the integration of softer and more reliable data. Fuzzy soft set operations could enhance the Parkinson's Disease (PD) symptoms ontology developed into the motor/non-motor domains, coupled with the severity assessments within subdomains, and the entire hierarchy aggregating into an overall disease severity metric. Such hierarchies would permit the implementation of more refined (laser-focused) and aggressive therapies. For instance, patients with motor symptomatology and mild cognitive impairment may be commenced on aggressive dopaminergic without the risk of developing delirium, while those on the opposite end of the spectrum (i.e., mild motor, severe cognitive) would require meticulous titration of medications. Incorporating the type-2 fuzzy sets, designed to capture the uncertainty on the membership functions themselves, would serve to model the uncertainty on severity, which, in the case of borderline scenarios, is a known area of controversy even among highly experienced clinicians, to better capture uncertainty on the range of borderline cases.

Extensions of the above to include Markov (or recurrent) structures would be able to model the dynamics of disease progression and allow the system to predict future states and the time required to transition from one state to another. Such predictions would allow the system to warn of a possible clinical deterioration, which, in turn, would help have the necessary interventions in place. For example, patients whose fuzzy soft set progression velocity suggests that they will reach severe status within six months may warrant an evaluation for deep brain stimulation, not just reactive to a loss of functional status. Causal inference approaches would allow the identification of those voice parameters that would facilitate the desired treatment outcome from those that do not, enabling the therapeutic interventions to be tailored to the specific voice dysfunction mechanisms.

Federated learning methods allow collaborative model building in different healthcare systems without breaching patient confidentiality. This practice allows the approach to benefit from the patient diversity of multiple centers without needing to transfer data to a data repository. Each center will be able to train local fuzzy soft set profiles on the data of the patients under their care, sharing only a few aggregated statistics to develop global models with full population diversity, namely average of the membership functions and their correlation weights. This approach resolves privacy regulation concerns (i.e. HIPAA and GDPR) and the common challenges of integrating different electronic health records and formats from multiple organizations to create a single de-identified dataset.

CONCLUSION

The assessment of the fuzzy soft set framework in relation to the severity of Parkinson's disease showcases the successful transfer of mathematical concepts into the realm of actionable clinical practice through 78.4% accuracy classification, albeit lower, coupled with enhanced explainability and uncertainty assessment when juxtaposed with black box machine learning models. The framework addresses the challenge of disease progression in stages and over time with fuzzy membership functions, tackles the ever-present issue of missing data through its parameterization, and offers logical and explainable frameworks that enable clinician assessment and trust in automated models. The soft set fuzzy approach, with its potential clinical utility in explainability, calibration, and incomplete data, builds the case for the integration of soft set fuzzy approaches and black box models, despite the fact that it outperformed traditional machine learning methods in accuracy (82-83%).

The correlation analysis reflected biological plausibility by establishing shimmer parameters and HNR as the strongest predictors of severity per the voice-related pathophysiology of Parkinson's disease. The individual case studies described how distance profiles and confidence scores facilitate personalized clinical decision making by differentiating borderline cases that could benefit from closer tracking from definitive cases that may be safely routed for automated review. The analysis of temporal progression validated the framework's ability to avoid reactively managing the disease by tracking the evolution of the disease and estimating the rate of disease progression. The use of fuzzy soft set theory to solve this difficult medical classification problem illustrates the potential for similar applications in other neurodegenerative diseases, and other areas of medicine characterized by uncertainty, missing data, and a need for explainability that precludes use of purely black-box machine learning.

REFERENCES

Ajagun, E. J., Asuku, A. O., Oyerinde, T. O., Sangodipe, H. A., Sanusi, W., Jayeoba, L. A., & Abdulsalam, T. A. (2024). The Ketogenic Diet and Stroke. In *Nutrition and Stroke. NutritionalNeuroscience*. Springer., DOI: 10.1007/978-981-97-6818-9¬¬_10

Alcantud, J. C. R., & Santos-García, G. (2017). A new criterion for soft set based decision problems under incomplete information. *International Journal of Computational Intelligence Systems, 10*(1), 394–404.

Ali, M. I., Feng, F., Liu, X., Min, W. K., & Shabir, M. (2009). On some new operations in soft set theory. *Computers & Mathematics with Applications (Oxford, England), 57*(9), 1547–1553.

Armstrong, M. J., & Okun, M. S. (2020). Diagnosis and treatment of Parkinson disease: A review. *Journal of the American Medical Association, 323*(6), 548–560. PMID: 32044947

Asuku A.O., Adeyemo M.B., Adeyemo R.O., Agoro S.A., Odugbesan O.A., & Ayoola S.A. (2022). Applications of stem cell therapy in neurodegenerative diseases. European Journal of Biotechnology and Bioscience. 10 (2): 17-24, 2321-9122

Asuku, A. O., Ayinla, M. T., Olajide, T. S., Oyerinde, T. O., Yusuf, J. A., Bayo-Olugbami, A. A., & Fajemidagba, G. A. (2024). Coffee and Parkinson's disease. In. Progress in Brain Research: Vol. 289. *Neuroscience of Coffee*. Elsevier., DOI: 10.1016/bs.pbr.2024.06.001

Bloem, B. R., Okun, M. S., & Klein, C. (2021). Parkinson's disease. *Lancet, 397*(10291), 2284–2303. PMID: 33848468

Cagman, N., & Enginoglu, S. (2010). Soft set theory and uni–int decision making. *European Journal of Operational Research, 207*(2), 848–855.

Chen, D., Tsang, E. C., Yeung, D. S., & Wang, X. (2005). The parameterization reduction of soft sets and its applications. *Computers & Mathematics with Applications (Oxford, England), 49*(5-6), 757–763.

Espay, A. J., Bonato, P., Nahab, F. B., Maetzler, W., Dean, J. M., & Klucken, J.& Movement Disorders Society Task Force on Technology. (2016). Technology in Parkinson's disease: Challenges and opportunities. *Movement Disorders, 31*(9), 1272–1282. PMID: 27125836

Feng, F., Jun, Y. B., Liu, X., & Li, L. (2010). An adjustable approach to fuzzy soft set based decision making. *Journal of Computational and Applied Mathematics*, *234*(1), 10–20.

Fereshtehnejad, S. M., Romenets, S. R., Anang, J. B., Latreille, V., Gagnon, J. F., & Postuma, R. B. (2015). New clinical subtypes of Parkinson disease and their longitudinal progression: A prospective cohort comparison with other phenotypes. *JAMA Neurology*, *72*(8), 863–873. PMID: 26076039

Goetz, C. G., Tilley, B. C., Shaftman, S. R., Stebbins, G. T., Fahn, S., Martinez-Martin, P., & LaPelle, N. (2008). Movement Disorder Society-sponsored revision of the Unified Parkinson's Disease Rating Scale (MDS-UPDRS): Scale presentation and clinimetric testing results. *Movement Disorders*, *23*(15), 2129–2170. PMID: 19025984

Kalia, L. V., & Lang, A. E. (2015). Parkinson's disease. *Lancet*, *386*(9996), 896–912. PMID: 25904081

Kong, Z., Gao, L., Wang, L., & Li, S. (2008). The normal parameter reduction of soft sets and its algorithm. *Computers & Mathematics with Applications (Oxford, England)*, *56*(12), 3029–3037.

Maji, P. K., Biswas, R., & Roy, A. R. (2003). Soft set theory. *Computers & Mathematics with Applications (Oxford, England)*, *45*(4-5), 555–562.

Majumdar, P., & Samanta, S. K. (2010). Generalised fuzzy soft sets. *Computers & Mathematics with Applications (Oxford, England)*, *59*(4), 1425–1432.

Marek, K., Chowdhury, S., Siderowf, A., Lasch, S., Coffey, C. S., Caspell-Garcia, C., & Foroud, T. (2018). The Parkinson's progression markers initiative (PPMI)–establishing a PD biomarker cohort. *Annals of Clinical and Translational Neurology*, *5*(12), 1460–1477. PMID: 30564614

Molodtsov, D. (1999). Soft set theory—First results. *Computers & Mathematics with Applications (Oxford, England)*, *37*(4-5), 19–31.

Obermeyer, Z., Powers, B., Vogeli, C., & Mullainathan, S. (2019). Dissecting racial bias in an algorithm used to manage the health of populations. *Science*, *366*(6464), 447–453. PMID: 31649194

Pawlak, Z. (1982). Rough sets. *International Journal of Computer & Information Sciences*, *11*(5), 341–356.

Poewe, W., Seppi, K., Tanner, C. M., Halliday, G. M., Brundin, P., Volkmann, J., & Lang, A. E. (2017). Parkinson disease. *Nature Reviews. Disease Primers, 3*(1), 1–21. PMID: 28332488

Postuma, R. B., Berg, D., Stern, M., Poewe, W., Olanow, C. W., Oertel, W., & Deuschl, G. (2015). MDS clinical diagnostic criteria for Parkinson's disease. *Movement Disorders, 30*(12), 1591–1601. PMID: 26474316

Roy, A. R., & Maji, P. K. (2007). A fuzzy soft set theoretic approach to decision making problems. *Journal of Computational and Applied Mathematics, 203*(2), 412–418.

Schapira, A. H., Chaudhuri, K. R., & Jenner, P. (2017). Non-motor features of Parkinson disease. *Nature Reviews. Neuroscience, 18*(7), 435–450. PMID: 28592904

Sidransky, E., Nalls, M. A., Aasly, J. O., Aharon-Peretz, J., Annesi, G., Barbosa, E. R., & Ziegler, S. G. (2009). Multicenter analysis of glucocerebrosidase mutations in Parkinson's disease. *The New England Journal of Medicine, 361*(17), 1651–1661. PMID: 19846850

Zadeh, L. A. (1965). Fuzzy sets. *Information and Control, 8*(3), 338–353.

Chapter 13
The Road Ahead:
Current Clinical Trials, Challenges, and Recommendations for Parkinson's Disease Therapies in Under-Resourced Settings

Christopher Oloruntoba Akintayo
http://orcid.org/0009-0008-3446-466X
Obafemi Awolowo University Teaching Hospital Complex, Ile-Ife, Nigeria

Samuel Onyekweli
http://orcid.org/0000-0002-4715-7932
Lagos University Teaching Hospital, Idi-Araba, Nigeria

Gloria Osayamen Omoruyi
Obafemi Awolowo University Teaching Hospital Complex, Ile-Ife, Nigeria

Joseph Oluwatomi Akintayo
University of Ibadan, Nigeria

ABSTRACT

The neurological disorder with the fastest rate of increase in the world, Parkinson's disease (PD), poses serious management challenges due to its progressive deterioration and debilitating nature, which significantly affects quality of life. The process of creating novel medical treatments, especially for neurodegenerative diseases, is drawn out and includes several testing stages before a medication is authorised for use in a clinic. As the condition worsens, treatment gets more complicated, and it is essential to have objective, straightforward instruments to identify changes in

DOI: 10.4018/979-8-3373-7437-6.ch013

patients' motor status and closely track how they respond to treatment. The available treatment aims to alleviate the symptoms caused by a deficiency of dopamine in the central nervous system, as there is no cure. The therapeutic approaches that are currently available to control the disease's early and advanced phases will be examined in this chapter.

INTRODUCTION

The fastest-growing neurological disorder in the world, Parkinson's disease (PD), is one of the most devastating psychological strains, causing serious suffering and disability that significantly impacts quality of life. The process of creating new medical treatments, particularly for neurodegenerative diseases, involves several testing phases before a medication can be approved in a clinic. The condition becomes much more complex as the disease worsens, and objective, clear instruments must be developed to measure changes in patients' motor status and to track response to treatment to accurately track what happens with these patients. It also appears that there is no cure for the symptoms of dopamine deficiency in the central nervous system. The current strategies available to control early and advanced stages of the disease will be examined in this chapter. The first stage evaluates the short-term safety of a drug, usually in healthy volunteers but occasionally in disease-infected people. The test of short-term safety and first intervention efficacy of the agent in individuals with the condition of interest is assessed during the second phase, and long-term safety and effectiveness in an extensive population of patients with the disease in the third phase. This is also a potential function of emerging technologies for providing a more comprehensive approach to disease prevention. For all these reasons, it is also noted that patients need access to multiple-disciplinary teams. New technologies are also developing, providing real-time remote monitoring in the field of escapology, which poses the problem of not being adequate to sustain such a disease. Inclusion and epidemiological context, Parkinson's disease is the fastest-growing neurological condition worldwide; age-standardized prevalence was up to 21.7% between 1990 and 2016, far ahead of the populations itself (Ray Dorsey et al., 2018) Based on demographic ageing, longevity, and potential environmental risk factor exposure, PD is a major public health challenge that will cause significant socioeconomic impacts. PD has a 2.5-fold decrease in disability adjusted life years between 1990 and 2016, suggesting the enormous individual and public costs associated with motor and nonmotor disability (Luo et al., 2024; Ray Dorsey et al., 2018). The variations in prevalence patterns and higher rates in industrialized countries suggest that complex gene-environment interactions require more research than simple demographics.

Figure 1. Prevalence trends

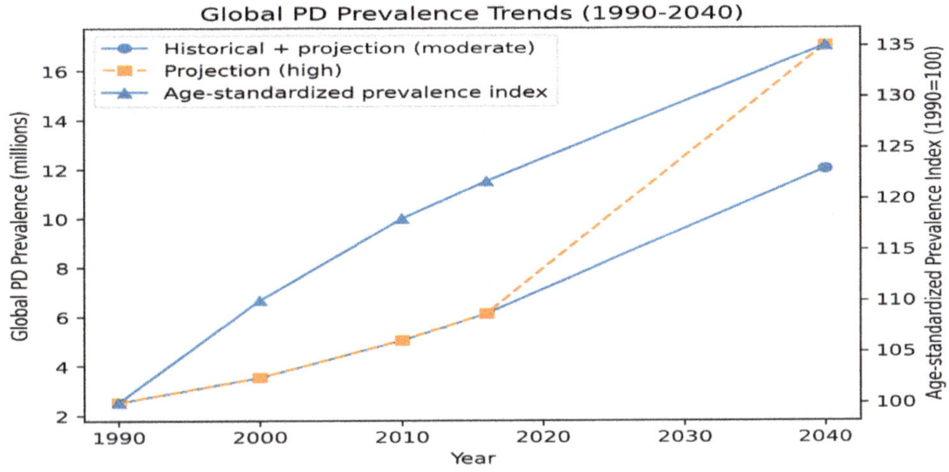

Figure 2. DALYs.

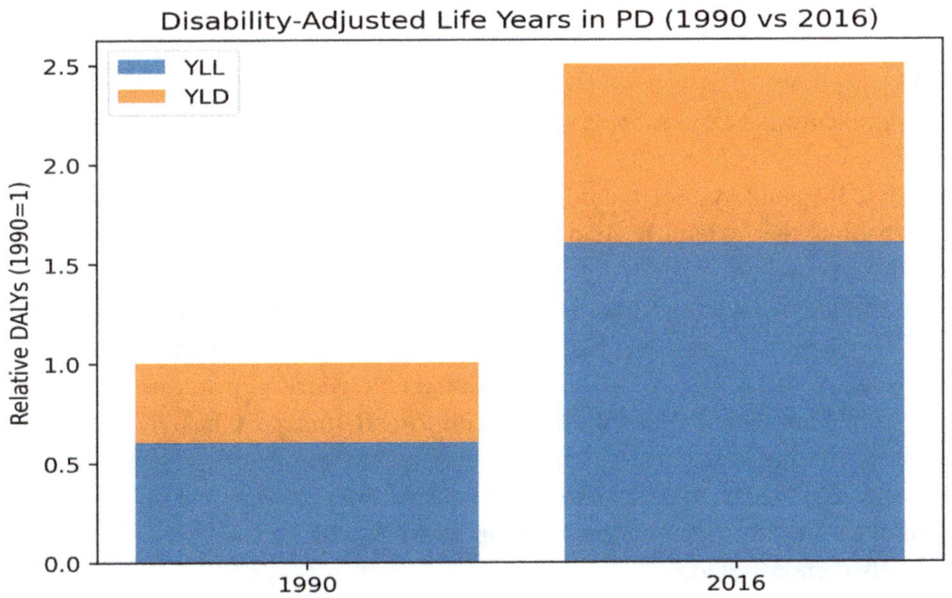

Figure 3. Geographic distribution

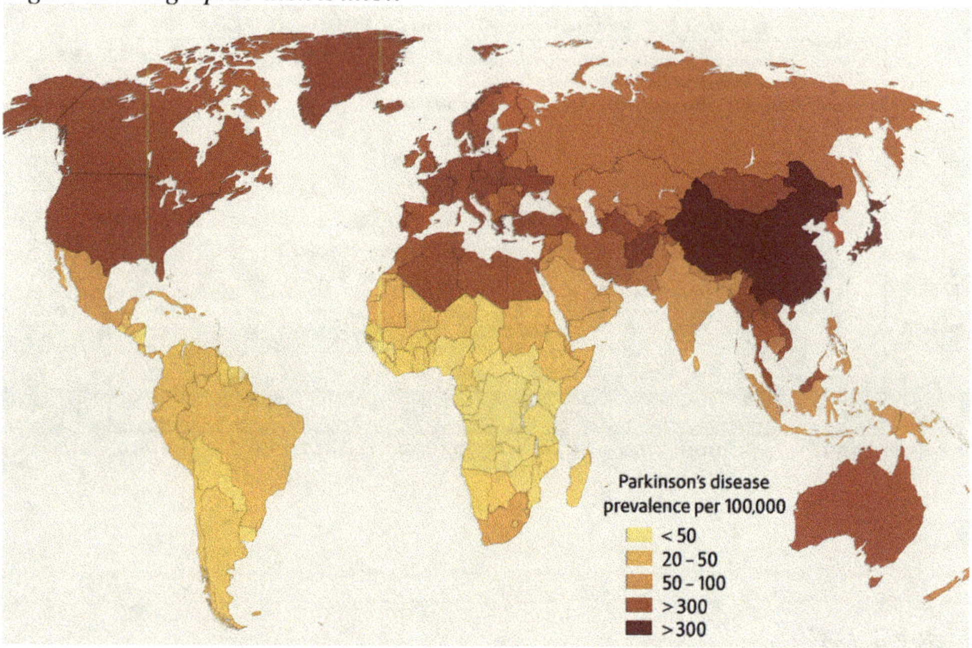

The pathophysiological substrate of PD is progressive degeneration of dopaminergic neurons in the substantia nigra pars compacta; the dopamine depletion also follows the motor manifestations that define the clinical syndrome. PD is also considered a multisystem disorder with complex molecular and cell-mediated perturbations that extend beyond the nigrostriatal pathway, but this is currently thought to be a more modern definition. As a basis for current pathogenic models, the misfolded synuclein protein is misfolded and proliferates in the Lewy bodies and Lewy neurites that constitute the neuropathological hallmark of the disease (Poewe et al., 2017). This association with the emergence of prion-like properties that permit templated misfolding and cell-to-cell transport has fundamentally redefined mechanistic constructs and opened new therapeutic avenues (Brundin & Melki, 2017). These pathogenic mechanisms interact dynamically, creating a chain of cellular dysfunction that ends up in excess compensatory capacity and is clinically demonstrated.

Table 1. Showing the pathogenesis, key mechanisms and clinical features of Parkinson's disease

Pathogenic Process	Key & Mechanisms	Clinical & References
α-Synuclein Aggregation	Lewy body/neurite formation; Templated misfolding & cell-to-cell spread	Motor progression, cognitive decline; Ref: Brundin & Melki, 2017
Mitochondrial Dysfunction	Complex I deficiency; Impaired ATP synthesis, oxidative stress, mitophagy failure	Energy depletion, oxidative damage; Ref: Kalia & Lang, 2015
Neuroinflammation	Microglial activation; Innate/adaptive immune activation & cytokine release	Disease progression, potential therapeutic target; Ref: Hirsch & Hunot, 2009
Dopaminergic Degeneration	Nigrostriatal pathway loss; Selective neuronal vulnerability	Cardinal motor symptoms

PD is characterized by the highly variable age of onset, motor phenotype, progression rate, and non-motor symptom burden. This heterogeneity is significant as genetic architecture plays a role in tens of thousands of cases. Specifically, SNCA and LRRK2 gene variants are found in SNCA, LRRK2, GBA, PRKN, PINK1, and DJ-1 and suggest causality among molecular perturbations and Parkinsonian characteristics (Billingsley et al., 2018; Asuku et al., 2025). Genome-wide association studies have identified 90 independent risk loci related to polygenic susceptibility, including lysosomal function, immune regulation, and synaptic vesicle dynamics (Nalls et al., 2019). The clinical heterogeneity is characterized by distinct motor subtypes of tremor-dominant, postural instability-gait difficulty predominant and indeterminate related to differential progression trajectories and non-motor profiles (Fereshtehnejad & Postuma, 2017). Further stratification schemas with potential therapeutic implications might be available after recent conceptual approaches that differentiate "body-first" versus "brain-first" PD subtypes of synuclein propagation patterns from peripheral autonomic structure rather than first central nervous system involvement, as reflected in current conceptual models of "body-first" and "brain-first" PD subtypes.

Figure 4. Disease heterogeneity framework

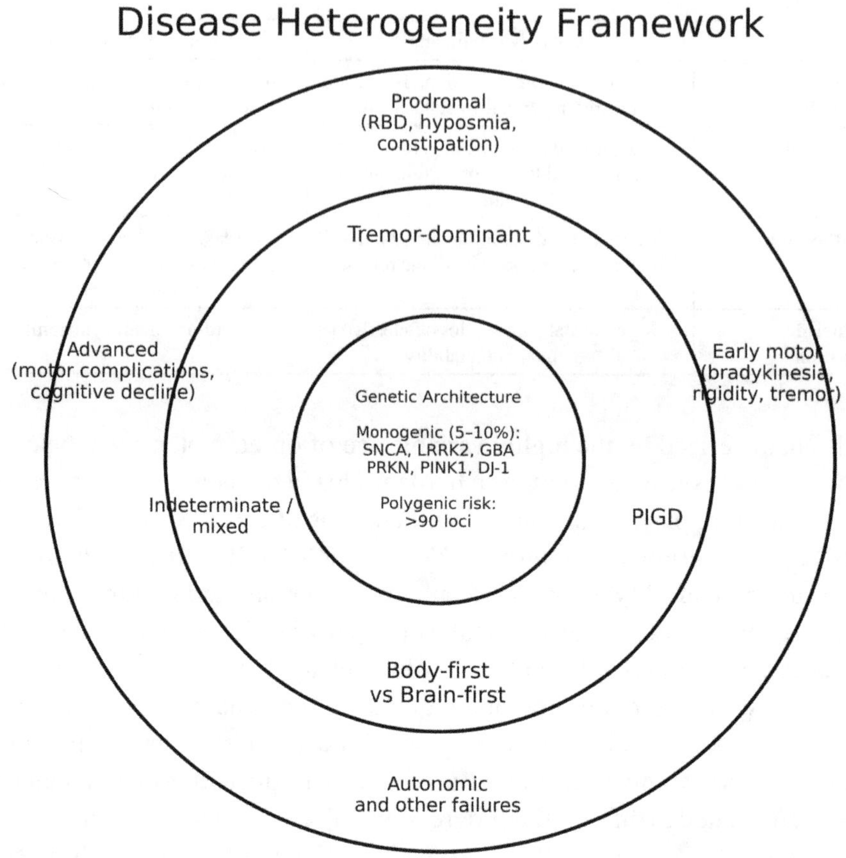

PD spans the clinical spectrum of bradykinesia, rigidity, tremor, and postural instabilities. Not only that, but many non-motor disabilities, which rarely characterize disability at advanced stages, can be seen on the diagnostic spectrum. To date, cognitive impairment is reported to affect over 19-25% of patients at the diagnostic age; dementia occurs in over 88% of patients at 30 years of age, especially in the first 20 years (Aarsland et al., 2017). They have severe impairment in quality of life and caregiver burden, resulting in neuropsychiatric symptoms such as depression, anxiety, apathy, and psychosis. Autonomic dysfunction consists of orthostatic hypotension, neurogenic bladder, constipation, and sexual dysfunction. While it is only morbid, sleep architecture disruption, particularly REM sleep behaviour disorder, has the potential to be prodromal, with approximately 74% of idiopathic RBD patients transmuting from -synuclein Pathy within 12 years (Postuma et al., 2019).

This prodromal phase also included hyposmia, constipation and subtle motor signs, which has led to the development of research criteria for prodromal PD enabling earlier intervention windows (Berg et al, 2015).

Figure 5. Prodromal to clinical PD timeline

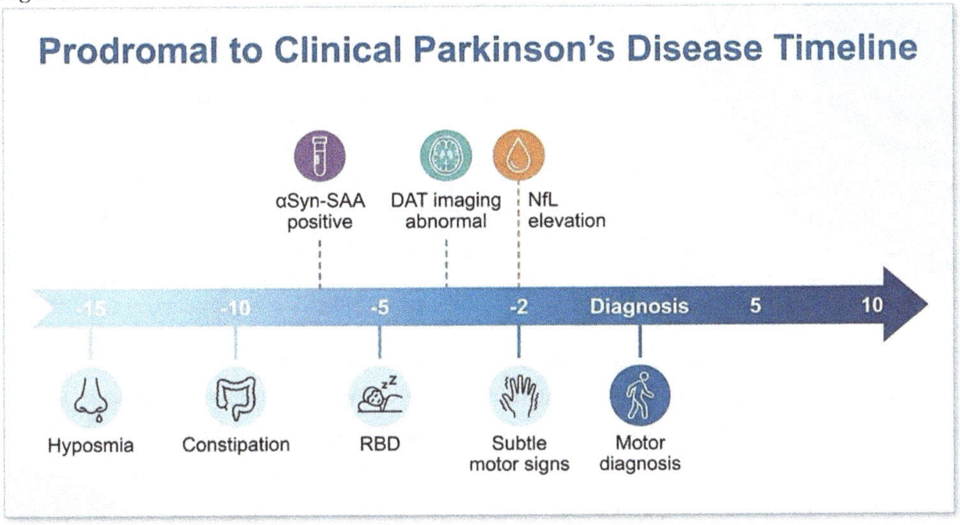

But diagnostic approaches are changing from diagnostic recognition for clinical syndromes to validation for biomarker validation. Foreclosing and supporting features were exclusionary for diagnostic accuracy, adapted to the Movement Disorder Society clinical diagnostic criteria established in 2015, whereas clinical assessment was the gold (Postuma et al., 2015). In particular, dopamine transporter single-photon emission computed tomography (SPECT and PET with 18F-DOPA demonstrate terminal integrity of presynaptic dopaminergic terminals at high sensitivity (85-95%) and specificity (90-100%) in the presence of nigrostriatal degeneration, but cannot distinguish PD from atypical parkinsonian syndromes (Politis, 2014). This newer innovation involves synuclein seed amplification assays, ostensibly ultrasensitive techniques that detect pathological synuclein aggregates in the cerebrospinal fluid, which detect diagnostic and specificity of 87.7% based on diagnosis accuracy and 96.3%, respectively – perhaps able to allow pathological confirmation during life (Siderowf et al. 2023). Additional fluid biomarkers, such as neurofilament light chain (NfL), a marker of axonal degeneration, are prognostic markers for disease progression and experimental magnetic resonance imaging techniques, such as free-water diffusion imaging and neuromelanin-sensitive sequences, provide microstructural data in the past before macroscopic atrophy (Hansson et al., 2017; Ofori et al., 2015a).

Table 2. Showing the Biomarkers, modality and performance involved in Parkinson's disease

Biomarker	Modality & Performance	Utility & Limitations
α-Synuclein SAA	CSF fluid assay; Sens 87.7%; Spec 96.3%	Pathological confirmation, trial enrichment; Limitations: Requires lumbar puncture; Ref: Siderowf et al., 2023
DAT SPECT/PET	Neuroimaging; Sens 85–100%; Spec 70–100%	Diagnostic confirmation; Limitations: Cannot distinguish PD from atypical parkinsonism; Ref: Politis, 2014
Neurofilament light chain	Blood/CSF; Sens Variable; Spec Variable	Prognostic (predict progression); Limitations: Non-specific to PD; Ref: Hansson et al., 2017
Free-water MRI	nan	Early detection & progression monitoring; Limitations: Requires specialized MRI sequences; Ref: Ofori et al., 2015
MDS Diagnostic Criteria	Clinical assessment; Sens High; Spec High	Standard diagnostic framework; Limitations: Purely clinical, no biomarker; Ref: Postuma et al., 2015

This narrative review provides a narrative account of current research in the therapeutic context of PD: from established symptoms to emerging clinical practices that incorporate translational transfer into the clinical application. The increasing number of clinical trials by 2024 shows the intensified development of therapeutic research, but also the difficulties with having a clinically meaningful benefit in a heterogeneous, slow-moving disorder (McFarthing et al., 2024). Observing successful and failed tests provides valuable information for the refinement of future directions. This review draws together preclinical mechanistic understanding with clinical trial innovations, biomarker validation, and implementation science and envisions a model for the current practice at this critical point in research, identifying priority research directions for disease modification, precision medicine, and prevention.

REPRESENTATIVE LANDSCAPE OF TREATMENT IN THE CURRENT SYSTEM

The contemporary therapeutic armamentarium for Parkinson's disease remains fundamentally symptomatic, targeting dopaminergic neurotransmission restoration and downstream motor circuit modulation without arresting underlying neurodegeneration. Levodopa, the metabolic precursor to dopamine, administered in combination with peripheral decarboxylase inhibitors (carbidopa or benserazide), continues to represent the most efficacious pharmacological intervention for motor symptom control six decades after its introduction (Poewe et al., 2017). Clinical trials demonstrate improvements ranging from 6-15 points on the Movement Disorder Society-Unified Parkinson's Disease Rating Scale (MDS-UPDRS) Part III motor examination depending on dose and formulation, substantially exceeding the minimal clinically important difference threshold of 3.25-5.2 points established through anchor-based methodologies (Horváth et al., 2015a; Schrag et al., 2006). Multiple formulation strategies aim to optimize levodopa pharmacokinetics: immediate-release preparations require multiple daily dosing due to short plasma half-life (approximately 90 minutes), while controlled-release and extended-release formulations (notably IPX066 utilizing accordion pill technology) provide more sustained plasma concentrations, though with variable absorption profiles (Hauser et al., 2013). Orally disintegrating tablets address dysphagia in advanced disease, and intestinal gel formulations bypass gastric emptying variability altogether.

It is the most effective motor therapy, but chronic levodopa therapy also has adverse consequences that, while not measurable, further limit functional benefits as the disease progresses. The underlying phenomenon of "wearing-off" effects in end-of-dose akinesia and unpredictable "on-off" fluctuations arises in 40-50% of patients within 4-6 years of beginning to take effect, requiring complex dosing adjustments and additional agents (Ahlskog & Muenter, 2001; Aquino & Fox, 2015). By the end of the five years, about 40% of patients report spontaneous choreiform or dystonic movement, and there are complex neuroplastic changes in striatal nerve plasticity and dopaminergic receptor stimulation (Bastide et al., 2015). These associations show variable replication, while also suggesting the earlier motor complication may emerge later in age at treatment placement, higher cumulative levodopa doses and a lower cumulative dose of levodopa (Martinez-Carrasco et al. 2023; Turcano et al., 2018). These observations have created a longstanding controversy regarding optimal timing of levodopa starting, whether to delay in younger patients who prefer the first dopamine agonist monotherapy or whether to improve quality-of-life optimization with the understanding that retarding levodopa does not avoid eventual complications, but postpones maximal symptomatic benefit (Frequin et al., 2024; Ramanzini et al., 2024).

Dopamine receptor agonists such as bromocriptine, cabergoline, a potentially less common delicacy due to cardiac valvulopathy and chronic complications, and non-ergot agents such as prosminole, ropinirole, rotigotine transdermal, help direct D2/D3 receptor stimulation through the inactive precursor neuron system. Among older patients, the majority of the preliminary effects of levodopa in the first place show inadequate motor symptom control and the deterioration of the motor symptoms of their own patients was not apparent, but the magnitude of this deterioration was well documented by statistical comparisons to levodopa; 5.3–5.6% MDS-UPDRS Part III points versus placebo over 3.5 years for the most prominent gains in motor symptoms and dyskinesia in youth study (Baker et al., 2009; Fox et al., 2018a). This trade-off is highlighted by network meta-analyses, which note that 87 per cent lower risk of dyskinesia is achieved with dopamine agonist monotherapy compared to dopamine agonist monotherapy (OR = 0.13, 95% CI 0.09-0.19) at the cost of decreased immediate motor efficacy. Dopamine agonists may have the potential to have significant neuropsychiatric implications, particularly with respect to impulse control disorders, 13-17% of exposed patients who suffer from the mesolimbic dopaminergic pathway (Weintraub et al., 2010). This risk is elevated by the DOMINION cross-sectional study of 3,090 patients in which ICD prevalence reaches 17.1% in dopamine agonist-treated patients, and 6.9% in dopamine-free patients. More adverse effects, including orthostatic hypotension, peripheral oedema, and excessive daytime somnolence with sudden-onset sleep attacks, require careful patient selection and monitoring. Rotigotine delivered transdermally is an effective intravenous drug for chronic pain that could improve motor function, but the dermatologic effects are limited.

The enzymes that inhibit enzymes further extend endogenous and exogenous dopamine bioavailability through complementary mechanisms. Monoamine oxidase-B (MAO-B) inhibitors, selegiline, rasagiline, and safinamide, reduce dopamine catabolism in the synaptic cleft, suggesting modest clinical efficacy as monotherapy in early disease (2-3 MDS-UPDRS Part III) and with supplementary "wearing-off" reduction in advanced disease (Binde et al., 2018). This lack of evidence to support neuroprotection claims is reflected in these agents' mechanistic arguments based on antioxidant effects and antiapoptotic signaling, but delays in trial design used to identify symptoms between disease-modifying effects and symptoms remain contradictory results (Olanow et al., 2009a). Catechol-O-methyltransferase (COMT) inhibitors include entacapone, opicapone, and tolcapone, which inhibit peripheral levodopa metabolism by extending plasma half-life and decreasing the time spent "off" to 0.6-1.6 hours, depending on the agent and that of tolcapone (Ferreira et al., 2016). Tolcapone inhibits peripheral and central COMT, increasing levodopa area-under-curve by 60-90% compared to entacapone's 35%, but also requires hepatic function monitoring for rare fulminant hepatotoxicity after fatal incidents (Longo et al. 2016). Opicapone, a once-daily COMT inhibiter which can be withdrawn from the target and activated for longer than two hours through Phase 3 development, is effective with no hepatotoxicity observed across the Phase 3 phase, possibly contributing to a better assessment of the benefit-risk profile (Lees et al., 2017).

Trihexyphenidyl and benztropine are targeted tremor suppression agents that have high cognitive adverse effects, though they do have substantial cognitive damage in the elderly: 35 cases of neuropsychiatric complications on anticholinergics, while another 13 were on placebo among controlled trials; and it is particularly dangerous for elderly persons at baseline dementia risk. Contemporary practice limits their use to younger patients with a dominant refractory tremor to dopaminergic agents and without cognitive impairment. Amantadine, as a naturally antiparkinsonian antiviral, is widely known to have antiparkinsonian properties, and has especially high efficacy for the reduction of dyskinesia when taken during levodopa therapy. As with longer-release amantadine formulations that specifically target dyskinesia management, prolonged efficacy for treatment with dyskinesia is maintained with 12- 25 week dose-controlled trials (Oertel et al., 2017, Pahwa et al., 2017), but some of the harmful side effects include livedo reticularis, hallucinations, and peripheral edema are not found to be tolerable in some patients. Unlike the traditional treatment, standardized conventional therapies do not offer advanced delivery solutions addressing the drug pharmacokinetic limitation of oral medications. Levodopa-carbidopa intestinal gel (LCIG), administered via percutaneous endoscopic gastrojejunostomy with a portable infusion pump, is easily dispensable during sleep and maintains plasma levodopa levels at all hours of the day (Olanow et al., 2014). The major randomized controlled trial had 1,91 0.57 hours of "off" time reductions over optimized oral therapy, with quality of life improvement measured as 7-12.8-point sum index reductions over the lowest available clinically significant differences (Fernandez et al., 2015). But, complications associated with device dislodgement (24%), infection, abdominal pain and procedural safety accounts for about 20-30% of patients who are in need of significant intervention. Patients' selection should be made on the basis of enhanced cognitive function in administering devices, caregiver support, and no contraindications to percutaneous endoscopic gastrojejunostomy placement.

A second method of continuous dopaminergic stimulation, using a potent and rapidly acting non-selective dopamine agonist administered via a portable infusion pump, is subcutaneous apomorphine infusion. The TOLEDO trial demonstrated the equivalent to levodopa-carbidopa intestinal gel in effectiveness as compared to levodopa-carbidopa, in addition to its clinical efficacy, with 1.89 hours of placebo-corrected "off" time reduction and no invasive intervention required in some patients. But subcutaneous nodule formation has limited long-term tolerance. One solution is to inject subcutaneous apomorphine injections while "off" episodes do not occur at any one time and must be initiated within 10–20 minutes to become effective rescue therapy. A new regulatory ad is a sublingual apomorphine film, which, when inhaled, provides a more rapid-onset rescue medication formulation with 40% of patients achieving "off" status within 15 minutes, and inhaled levodopa is administered intracutaneously via inhalation for "off" episode management. The pharmacokinetics of the oral versus subcutaneous route of delivery, with pharmacokinetics of between oral and subcutaneous route, pending FDA approval in December 2018 based on a SPAN-PD-study data for statistically significant motor improvement at 30 minutes post-inhalation; LeWitt et al., 2019. These new formulations augment the therapeutic plan for motor volatility complexity in advanced disease.

The most common device-based treatment with over three decades of experience and reliable evidence is Deep Brain stimulation (DBS) that uses stereotactic placement of electrodes that emit high-frequency electrical stimulation to specific basal ganglia nuclei. Based on a meta-analysis of 39 STN-DBS studies with 2,035 subjects, the reduction in levodopa equivalent daily dose in 31 studies with 1,644 subjects was found in 38 STN-DBS studies (Lachenmayer et al., 2021), where 50% reduction in levodopa equivalent daily dose was achieved compared to 50.5% reduction in levodopa equivalent daily dose in 31 studies with 1,644 subjects (Lachenmayer et al., 2021). Compared to standard adherence data, STN-DBS has a slight motor benefit and a better reduction in dosages of medication, while GPi-DBS may be useful for patients with high levels of baseline dyskinesia or cognitive disabilities. Indeed, appropriate patients with sustained, robust levodopa responsiveness with > 30% motor improvement and absence of dementia (cognitive thresholds vary in centers but generally require Montreal Cognitive Assessment > 21 or Dementia Rating Scale 130), psychological stability ad eve of depression or psychosis, and motor instability over 5 years after adjusting medical treatments and motor benefits may return to baseline by 5 years after disease progression associated with DBS-unresponsive symptoms (Limousin & Foltynie, 2019).

The patient counselling needs a careful watchful eye on surgical risk. In a meta-analysis of complication rates in multiple centres, intracranial haemorrhage was reported in 2-3% of procedures (with almost 1.65% resulting in permanent neurological deficits), infection was reported in 4-5%, and hardware-associated complications such as lead migration or fracture were found to be common. Stimulation negatively affects cognitive, behavioural, and speech skills in susceptible individuals, and caution needs to be exercised regarding the necessity of preoperative neuropsychological assessment and patient selection. Recently, technology improvements have included sensing-enabled DBS systems, which record locally collected local field potentials, such as Medtronic PerceptTM PC with BrainSenseTM, FDA approved in 2020.

The non-motor symptom management area is of vital importance but historically neglected, given that non-motor burden predicts quality of life rather than motor disability, especially in advanced disease. Visual impairment and dementia were associated with 19-20% at diagnosis and a level of over 80% in long-term survivors who had experienced cognitive impairment or dementia (Aarsland et al., 2017). There is a strong evidence basis in which cholinesterase inhibitors, the most stable of drugs approved for PD dementia, offer small cognitive benefit; the results of the most widely tested EXPRESS trial yielded 2.1 points on the Alzheimer's Disease Assessment Scale-Cognitive subscale (ADAS-cog) from the pivotal EXPRESS study when compared with 0.7 points worsening with placebo when the study was led by Emre et al. in 2004 (Emre et al., 2004). Memantine does not have a significant effect on PD dementia and Alzheimer's disease. Of particular note, the danger of anticholinergic residue from bladder, tricyclic antidepressants and antihistamines is significantly amplified by the increased risk of cognitive vulnerability and should be considered minimized through a systematic review of marketed medications.

In part, depression negatively affects approximately 40% of all of the PD patients at any stage of disease and is multidirectional associated with motor disability and dopaminergic drug effects (Costello et al., 2023). SSRIs and SNRIs are first-line pharmacotherapy. The SAD-PD randomised controlled trial showed paroxetine and venlafaxine XR superior to placebo with improvements of 6.2 or 4.2 points on the Hamilton Depression Rating Scale, while placebo response rates at the same level were 44% whose estimate was 50% symptom reduction in the study (Richard et al., 2012). demonstrating the strong expectation effects of depression treatments in a study involving large, expected effects of the study. Tricyclic antidepressants have some efficacy but must be considered against the anticholinergic burden. Significantly, in the case of impulse control patients, dopamine agonist withdrawal is precipitated by dopamine agonist withdrawal syndrome, characterized by depression, anxiety, dysphoria and drug-seeking behaviour, in 15-20% of these cases (19% in prospective observational studies). These conditions, with less immediate termination accompanied by abrupt discontinuation, must be progressively tapered through alternating detention and discontinuation in more frequent cases than abrupt discontinuation (Rabinak & Nirenberg, 2010). Anxiety disorders that occur in 30-40% of patients and often alter motor states (off "period anxiety), respond differently to SSRIs, SNRIs and cognitive-behavioral therapy, though they have little evidence of evidence in the literature to treat depression.

Psychosis in Parkinson's disease, particularly in the later stages, is frequent and increases with disease duration. A cross-sectional prevalence of complex visual hallucinations is about 22–38% in cross-sectional estimates, while longitudinal cohorts tend to have significantly higher cumulative prevalence when the total psychosis spectrum is assessed through systematic clinical assessment (Ffytche et al., 2017). First steps are evaluating drugs and elimination of possible culprits, including anticholinergics, amantadine, dopamine agonists, and MAO-B inhibitors according to probability. Pimavanserin, an inverse agonist of 5-HT2A without the dopamine receptor in antagonism, has proved to be effective in the placebo-controlled trials at a 9.1 point increase on the Scale for Assessment of Positive Symptoms-Parkinson's Disease compared to 5.8 points in the placebo group and obtained FDA approval on April 29, 2016, becoming the first PD psychosis drug approved specifically in this manner (Cummings et al., 2014a). Quetiapine, commonly used although there are limited data on the use of controlled trials, and clozapine, which is relatively effective but requires haematological monitoring for agranulocytosis risk, is widely used but could be withdrawn as a substitute for pimavanserin if it is inadequate. The usual antipsychotics, and most atypical, including risperidone and olanzapine, are entirely contraindicated because severe Parkinsonism exacerbation through D2 receptor blockade occurs in very high doses.

Two examples of sleep architecture disruption include RBD, a disease that causes loss of normal REM atonia with dream-like enactment behaviours in 30% of PD patients. The recommendations for best practice are in Aurora et al. (2010 which provides evidence that clonazepam has symptomatic value, but no evidence that it has implications for pathophysiology (Aurora et al., 2010). Insomnia and fragmented sleep reflect multifactorial contributions to nocturia, pain, rigidity, and drug interactions; sleep hygiene optimization and prudent use of benzodiazepine or sedating antidepressant recompense require individualisation. Stopped or prolonged nighttime somnolence is common with Parkinson's disease and reflects the interplay between the mechanisms of disease, drug-induced dopaminergic effects, and disturbed nighttime sleep. While there are few strong evidence, recent randomized placebo-controlled studies support that modafinil and methylphenidate can improve daytime sleepiness among selected patients with overall tolerability comparable to that of carefully individualized treatment (Chitsaz et al., 2024).

In particular, autonomic dysfunction is widespread across multiple organ systems and orthostatic hypotension, which by consensus measures as sustained systolic blood pressure decline 20 mmHg or diastolic 10 mmHg within 3 minutes of standing constitutes 30% of those with poor prevalence, as measured using meta-analytic estimates, is estimated to be 30 to 50% of patients with orthostatic hypotension, according to the consensus criteria of sustained systolic blood pressure decline 20 mmHg or diastolic 10 mmHg within 3 minutes of standing, which represents a substantial determinant of fall risk and functional limitation (Goldstein 2014; Velseboer et al., 2011). Non-pharmacological interventions include compression stockings, salt and fluid intake, elevating the head of the bed, and avoiding rapid postural changes, which are first-line management. Midodrine, a adrenergic agonist, and droxidopa are weakly effective in the placebo-controlled study. In the NOH301 study, droxidopa showed efficacy with a 0.90-unit improvement in the score on the Orthostatic Hypotension Questionnaire composite score as compared to placebo ($p=0.003$), but supine hypertension often limits the ability to tolerate it. This risk-benefit assessment is important for drug review, addressing culprit agents such as antihypertensives, diuretics, and dopaminergic medications with peripheral vasodilatory effects. -3 adrenergic agonists that are considered as an alternative, -3 adrenergic antagonists can respond differently to antimuscarinic agents such as oxybutynin, tolterodine, although cognitive adverse effects are associated with cognitive risk, and mirabegron, in addition to oxybutynin, are the best adrenergic agents at present.

Although this large collection of symptoms is extensive, it still maintains fundamental limitations. This present recommendation fails to arrest, slow or reverse the neurodegenerative process, providing temporary relief but no immediate cure; all efforts provide symptomatic relief with some temporary relief in the event of pathological progression. The heterogeneity in therapeutic response, with some patients experiencing excellent symptomatic control long-term, others being slow to develop and take over and medication refractoriness, is a poorly understood pathogen heterogeneity of disease, possibly linked to genetic status, -synuclein strain diversity, or particular underlying pathogenic mechanisms (Fereshtehnejad & Postuma, 2017). It is unclear whether disease-modifying strategies for non-motor symptoms are effective in addressing non-motor symptoms, such as cognitive decline, autonomic dysfunction, and refractory neuropsychiatric symptoms, yet in the latter stages, most of the cases of non-motor symptoms, such as cognitive decline, autonomic failure, and refractory neuropsychiatric symptoms, become more common. For example, symptomatic optimization is considered to be the core of current clinical trials and is a therapeutic imperative that transcends symptoms and into treatments for disease trajectory changes—disease modification or neuroprotection-specific activities that were identified in recent sections.

Evolving Clinical Trial and Biomarker Framework

Despite the strong preclinical evidence of the current pinning point for neuroprotection trials in Parkinson's disease, these recent failures stem from fundamental challenges to the rigor of traditional model design and the need for paradigm changes in trial design and outcome assessment. By the time early efforts to show disease change failed to acknowledge the fact that putative neuroprotective agents like selegiline, rasagiline, coenzyme Q10 and creatine are often seen as symptomatic dopaminergic or motor-enhancing and are not often characterised as providing symptoms for serious slowing down neurodegeneration by traditional parallel groups, they were not sufficiently well suited to recognizing difference between symptomatic benefit and genuine slowing of neurodegeneration in this general fashion. It appears this fundamental limitation was addressed in the delayed-start design by incorporating the methodological innovation in which active treatment during a first randomized controlled trial is initiated through a second phase after the first randomized controlled trial, the hypothesis is that if the intervention stimulates the cause of disease, early-start participants should maintain better outcomes than late-start participants while in the same cohort when the treatment duration is equal to the same amount of time prescribed (D'Agostino 2009).

To prevent recovery during the delay, this model assumes irreversible neuronal loss during this delay and thus cannot recapitulate the benefits obtained through earlier intervention. But, the delayed-start paradigm, which reflects equivocally critical assumptions about washout effects, linear disease progression and failure of pharmacodynamic tolerance, may not be valid in practice and may lead to interpretive confusion arising in applying a mixed group of symptomatic and potential disease-modifying agents to mixed symptomatic and possible disease-modifying agents (Olanow et al., 2009b).

On top of that, additional barriers to interpretation have been identified in the neuroprotection trial. Over a quarter of patients in PD trials aspired to obtain 50% motor improvement; there are a lot of mechanisms involved, from expectation effects, regression to the mean, rater bias and actual changes in disease severity. Goetz et al. (2008) report substantial placebo response rates as in PD studies. Plasmodium response encompasses the concept of placebo response beyond subjective symptoms reporting to quantitative motor measurements with functional imaging, providing evidence for striatal dopamine release in PD patients to confirm neurobiological substrates for symptomatic improvement in expectation-driven improvement (De la Fuente-Fernández et al., 2001). Over longer trials, ranging from 12–24 months, to be deployed to detect progression differences, these logistical complexities, attrition rates and cost increase as they increase their exposure to confounding variables such as concurrent medication changes, concurrent illness, and temporal shifts unrelated to intervention effects (Rascol, 2009). For symptomatic rescue medication, which is likely to be temporary in progressive disease but may obscure group differences, it requires precise statistical manipulation. These methodological barriers are collectively the sobering fact that despite nearly three decades of pending trial evidence of neuroprotection trials, no intervention has been approved as definitive regulatory approval for disease-modifying claims in PD.

Adaptive Trial Designs

Modern adaptive trial designs are models designed to improve efficiency, resource utilisation, and advance promising candidate success while enabling early termination of ineffective interventions. The MAMS platform trials compare multiple experimental therapies at the same time for a common control group and for an interim analysis predicting futility-based arm discontinuation or re-estimation based on outcome data after the final analyses. NET-PD pioneered a similar approach by the Neuroprotection Exploratory Trials in Parkinson Disease (NET-PD) program and early phase trials of coenzyme Q10, GPI-1485, and other candidates, but results indicated that although statistically significant based on noneffective interventions, the challenges of translating the findings of preclinical neuroprotection to human efficacy had been ignored by early phase trials of coenzyme Q10, GPI-1485, and other potential candidates.

These multi-arm, multi-stage design systems present today's modern multi-arm, multistage models in evaluating multiple repurposed candidate therapies against a shared placebo arm, enabling them to break up futile arms and inject new ones. For candidate selection, this decision-making is guided by a system of prioritization through evidence synthesis, the Cure Parkinson's International Linked Clinical Trials initiative, and expert responses (Foltynie et al., 2023; Gonzalez-Robles et al., 2025; Wyse et al., 2024).

Seamless Phase 2/3 designs incorporate dose-finding and validation effectiveness assessment in a single, continuous phase study to minimize temporal gaps between phases, as well as being capable of more efficient resource use (Bretz et al., 2009). While the primary treatment of participants who have randomized to multiple doses and placebo will undergo some interim evaluation for optimal dosing, further enrollment in the chosen doses and control arms will continue to show effective efficacy as the final dose evaluation continues. This adaptive method reduces development time by 1–2 years on a linear sequence of phase transition despite the operational complexity of real-time data monitoring, independent monitoring committee coordination, and preservation of trial integrity during adaptation. The regulatory acceptance has risen steadily, with FDA and EMA guidance documents explicitly affirming adaptive designs as justified and statistically rigorous, although sponsor resistance persists due to perceived regulatory uncertainty and operational requirements (FDA, 2019).

α-Synuclein Seed Amplification Assays

In most PD trial designs, biomarker integration offers the most transformative change in how enrichment is done to enhance statistical power, to reduce heterogeneity, and to target interventions targeted to the population who will benefit (Asuku et al., 2024). This translational advancement was illustrated by the use of misfolded synuclein for ultra-sensitive detection of short-range amounts of pathological conformers in the brain via cyclical cycles of aggregation and fragmentation (Fairfoul et al., 2016). The diagnostic probability of pathologically confirmed Lewy body disease and control and other neurodegenerative disorders is 85%–100%, with positive predictive accuracy in clinically diagnosed PD populations as high as 95% (Siderowf et al., 2023). This ability to take advantage of in vivo pathological confirmation is fundamentally influencing trial enrolment by the elimination of non-synucleinopathy "phenocopies" estimated to represent 10–15% of clinically diagnosed PD cohorts, resulting in a decrease in noise, a reduction in the detection of effect sizes, and a determination of pathologically appropriate populations of those evaluating intervention for -synuclein. The progress in syn-sAA testing using immunoprecipitation enrichment in plasma is the first to take advantage of lumbar puncture-required parameters that could allow broader population screening and longitudinal monitoring while being possible without the use of invasive sampling (Kluge et al., 2022; Okuzumi et al., 2023).

Neuroimaging Biomarkers

Another biomarker of dopaminergic system integrity and disease progression is neuroimaging biomarkers. Dopamine transporter imaging with 123I-ioflupane or positron emission tomography with 18F-DOPA shows progressive decline rates of approximately 5–12% annually in the posterior putamen of PD patients over a linear curve in proportion to healthy controls (Simuni et al., 2018). This is particularly important in the study of advanced disease that is a diagnostically valuable tool but requires floor effects in advanced disease when the remaining terminal density approaches detection thresholds and is limited to assessment for further development. DAT expression can be expressed as a pure neurodegeneration marker, while possible incongruent measures of terminal function, and it is also questionable as a pure neurodegeneration marker in comparison to confounded levels of terminal function (Chahid et al., 2023; Guttman et al., 2001; O'Shea et al., 2024; Palermo et al., 2021). MRI measures the increase in extracellular water in the posterior substantia nigra to be used by Ofori et al. to identify neuroinflammation, glial proliferation and tissue microstructural degradation before frank atrophy (Ofori et al., 2015b). Longitudinal studies show a progression biomarker of change in free-water elevation that is significantly more sensitive to clinical progression, and this measure does have promise as a less sensitive biomarker of movement than volumetric change; standardization across scanner platforms and sequence alignment are barriers to adoption (Marek et al., 2018).

Fluid Biomarkers

There are practical applications of minimally invasive blood sampling to serial monitoring and population-level screening for fluid biomarkers, if they can be administered with relatively low doses. PD is elevated by the NfL, a cytoskeletal protein that is released into cerebrospinal fluid and blood, with levels associated with disease severity and progression rate (Hansson et al., 2017). But, NfL is overly narrowly defined, based on multiple neurodegenerative disorders including Alzheimer's disease, amyotrophic lateral sclerosis, multiple sclerosis, frontotemporal dementia, and atypical parkinsonisms and does not have specific diagnostic utility but has sufficient predictive value for the identification of early progressors who may be especially likely to benefit from disease-modifying testing. Lysosomal enzyme activity and -β-glucocerebrosidase are also novel biomarkers for targeted therapy and patient stratification via mutation-specific molecular markers (Alcalay et al., 2015; Turner et al., 2025). Extracellular vesicle profiling is the latest development that utilises neuron-derived exosomes harvested from blood with cargo containing synuclein species, mitochondrial proteins, and microRNAs, possibly suggesting central nervous system pathology through peripheral sampling. Guo et al. 2020; Zhao et al., 2019. But reproducibility concerns related to heterogeneity of isolation methodology, limited validation in independent cohorts, and uncertainty regarding the relationship between peripheral vesicle contents and brain pathology require cautionary interpretation before being standardized.

Genetic Biomarkers

Genetic biomarkers help precision medicine by augmenting mutation-specific trial enrichment and pharmaceutical intervention optimization. These genotypes of GBA that encode lysosomal enzyme glucocerebrosidase induce not only disease risk but also accelerated motor and cognitive development, earlier dementia appearance and greater hallucination severity than non-carrier variants, which are found to be correlated with all variant prevalences in PD based on population. This genotype-phenotype correlation can be used to enrich experiments with glucocerebrosidase-boosting treatments such as molecular chaperone ambroxol and investigational activators from the populations of GBA-PD that most benefit from a mechanistic rationale and may be maximised in effect sizes. In addition, the target population for LRRK2 kinase inhibitor development of LRRK2 G2019S mutation carriers, representing approximately 1% of European sporadic PD patients, 10% of Ashkenazi Jewish PD patients, and up to 41% of North African Arab-Berber populations, is identified as LRRK2 G2019S mutation carriers. The target population for LRRK2 kinase inhibitor development is the target population of CNR-G401S mutation carriers, whose large-molecule selection currently appears in Phase 1 and Phase 2 trials (Tolosa et al., 2020). In many cases, population and methodology play a role in estimating some Penetrance estimates for LRRK2 G2019S, with recent large-scale studies estimating cumulative risk for up to 9–28% by age 60 and 25–50% by 80 by age 80 (Healy et al., 2008; Kmiecik et al., 2024; Lee et al., 2017; Marder et al., 2015; Trinh et al., 2025). Examples of personalized dosing include the COMT Val158Met and selected CYP polymorphisms relevant to Parkinson therapeutics, but clinical applications are limited in their scope with prospective validation and practice guidelines in Corvol & Poewe 2016.

Patient-Reported Outcomes and Digital Health Technologies

Increasingly, patient-reported outcomes (PROs) and objective digital health technologies are identified as complements to traditional clinician-rated scales for measuring disease impact and treatment benefits at the level of patient priorities. The Movement Disorder Society-Unified Parkinson's Disease Rating Scale (MDS-UPDRS), which is widely validated, has an average score of 0–272 points and was designed by clinician assessment during discrete time periods of simulated treatment, which are not typically observed every day in nature. It is a comprehensive and validated MDS-UPDRS. Performance on summary index scores of perepezko et al. and Tu et al. regarding patient-perceived health status across mobility, activities of daily living, emotional well-being, stigma, social support, cognition, communication and bodily discomfort are correlated with response to interventions and correlation with caregiver burden (Perepezko et al., 2023; Tu et al., 2017). But, subjective PROs are highly placebo responsive and may be confounded by mood, adaptation, or response shifts. Sensor technologies such as accelerometers, gyroscopes, or other motion capture devices worn repeatedly on wrists, waists, or on multiple body sites are readily available in real-world quantification of Bradykinesia, tremor, gait, or dyskinesia outside of artificial assessment contexts (Espay et al., 2016). A smartphone-based assessment that uses finger tapping tests, voice analysis, gait measurement using embedded accelerometers and cognitive functions allows for frequent ecological momentary assessments, such as capturing the variable effects of the symptoms and respondent response in the early phases of medical therapy without being atypically scheduled clinic visits (Zhan et al., 2018).

Several machine learning algorithms used in high-dimensional wearable sensor data can distinguish motor states ("on" or "off"), predict severity of symptoms, or correlation coefficients to MDS-UPDRS subscores, and may also identify digital biomarkers of progression (Erb et al., 2020; Zhan et al., 2018). But analytical validity, namely test-retest reliability, algorithm transparency, and performance across a variety of demographic groups, needs rigorous assessment before clinical assessment. Evidence of clinical validity in detecting the attribution of meaningful digital measures to clinically relevant outcomes remain limited for most digital endpoints. During the mPower study that was conducted, about 9,500 participants who were given broad data sharing consent and observed sustained participation in approximately 11% of participants, both potential and limitations of large-scale data collection were highlighted (Bot et al., 2016). FDA and EMA guidance on Software as a Medical Device and Digital Health Technologies are based on guidance on SAM and DHT regulatory pathways, although evidentiary standards are still evolving (FDA, 2023). Issues related to digital literacy across age and social class, data privacy concerns, reimbursement uncertainty, and clinical workflow integration are tempered by enthusiasm for long-term adoption, but momentum continues to move towards being included as part of confirmation tests, albeit with a focus on supporting verified digital measures as secondary endpoints.

Persistent Methodological Gaps

But this methodological change and the persistent controversy hinder progress toward disease-modifying therapy development. Biomarker reproducibility across laboratories and platforms is problematic; interlaboratory differences in the Syn-SAA protocols for recombinant synuclein variant protocols, detection methods, and amplification conditions have produced inconsistent results with a need for standardization efforts via collaborative collaboration, such as the Parkinson's Progression Markers Initiative (PPMI) (Concha-Marambio et al., 2023). The relationship between surrogate biomarkers, imaging measures of dopaminergic terminals, fluid neurodegeneration markers and clinical outcomes for the patients—ranging from motor disability, dementia, and mortality- appears weak in intervention studies. A surrogate endpoint must not only reflect clinical outcomes in observational studies but must also include the impact that treatment has on outcomes, a requirement rarely met in PD (Fleming & Powers, 2012). As a result, regulatory agencies have not been particularly willing to accept biomarker changes as a possible basis for accelerated approval without evidence of clinical benefit.

Another problem with outcome measure sensitivity is that in early disease, with slow progression rates and compensatory mechanisms which appear to obscure neurodegeneration for a long period, the test is also difficult to determine. While reliable, the MDS-UPDRS Part III motor testing cannot detect subtle changes in early disease, with sample size calculations for hypothetical interventions decreasing by 30% at 400 to 600 participants per arm, followed by 12–18-month follow-up for a 10-year follow-up for the hypothetical intervention (Guimaraes et al., 2005). The presence of multiple outcome measures that combine motor, cognitive and functional domains to enhance sensitivity suggests that more complex outcomes will potentially be vulnerable to heterogeneity, resulting in more complex interpretations. The average MCID thresholds, the smallest change that patients perceive as beneficial, are not particularly precise, with an estimate of MDS-UPDRS Part III at 3.25 to 5.2 points depending on methodology, disease stage, and reference anchors (Horváth et al., 2015b; Mishra et al., 2024). This uncertainty complicates trial design and interpretation when significant differences in uncertainty in clinical significance emerge.

In disease-modifying studies, non-motor symptoms endpoints are not significantly associated with disease-specific quality-of-life impairment, although they are largely affected by clinically significant impairment in advanced diseases. While these cognitive outcomes are increasingly applied as secondary measures, cognitive problems include learning effects on repeated testing, global scale insensitivity to domain-specific changes, and long-runs for identification of dementia incidence differences. Autonomic function measures, sleep assessment and neuropsychiatric symptoms scales are very limited in validity as clinical trial endpoints. This emphasis on motor outcomes is a precursor to past, regulatory tradition and practical considerations regarding sample size requirements, but maintains an overlap between patient outcomes and desired priorities (Gonzalez-Robles et al. 2023; Mestre et al., 2024)

Within clinic trials, few clinical trials are available. Non-white enrollment in Parkinson disease trials, which report race/ethnicity, has been consistently low at about 6-8%, and demographic reporting is often incomplete, raising concerns about generalizability and equity. For randomized research trials of neuropsychiatric treatment in PD that show race/ethnicity as a result of race/ethnicity, pooled analyses reveal that there was a high white participant presence with approximately 98% of the study group, further emphasising the need for better representation and reporting. DI Luca et al., 2020; Schneider et al., 2009; Vaswani et al., 2020). Based on the characteristics of systemic barriers such as transport, time constraints, financial burdens, mistrust over historical research abuse, language barriers and research site geographic placement at institutions that serve predominantly white, urban, high-socioeconomic populations, this study is notable for the following reasons: This diversification of trial enrolment requires intentional mechanisms involving community participation, decentralized trial configuration where local participation is voluntary, diversified site selection, financial compensation in participation, and culturally competent recruitment strategies; but progress continues to be made incremental.

This is because progress and challenges are at stake as the clinical trial and biomarker landscape change. The emergence of adaptive designs, biomarker-driven enrichment, and digital outcome measurement has opened doors to improved, biologically grounded, disease-modifying therapy development. While reproducibility, validation, standardization, and equitable implementation remain incomplete, further research into natural history studies, biomarker qualification, and trial methodology studies is needed to realise the potential of precision medicine in PD.

Emerging Disease-Modifying and Regenerative Therapies

By accelerating mechanistic analysis of pathogens and technological advances in targeted molecular intervention, Parkinson's disease has evolved into an urgent target of treatment that focuses not on easing symptoms but on facilitating the evolution of pathologic events rather than on improving symptoms. These recent approaches to disease modification include multiple approaches to the pathology of -α-synuclein, neuroprotective mechanisms, gene corrections and cell replacement in their variants of the hypothesis of modifiable disease drivers and optimal therapeutic interventions for the neurodegenerative process.

α-Synuclein-Targeted Therapeutic Approaches

The immune response relies on the findings that pathogenic synuclein species can be obtained in extracellular compartments through multiple modes of release, through regulating secretory pathways including lysosomal exocytosis or extracellular vesicle–associated mechanism, providing an immune-accessible pool and a potential barrier mechanism to intracellular transport of seeding competent conformers(Bae et al., 2012; Surmeier et al., 2017; S. Wu & Schekman, 2024; Xie et al., 2022).

The passive immunization strategies for monoclonal antibodies involving extracellular -synuclein have gone further down in clinical application. Prasinezumab, the humanized IgG1 antibody directed against a C-terminal -synuclein epitope targeted for binding aggregated species, was demonstrated to be able to exhibit active involvement in PASADENA, reducing free serum -synuclein from its target. In PASADENA, the main endpoint was the change from baseline to Week 52 in MDS-UPDRS Parts I to III in MDS-UPDRS Parts I-III; prasinezumab had a numerical advantage at 1500 mg versus placebo with a difference between the 80% CI of 4.2 to 0.2; P = 0.24), which did not indicate statistical significance (Pagano et al., 2022).

Further secondary analyses reported potential benefits in smaller subgroups with shorter disease duration and lower baseline severity, but longer follow-up results are needed to confirm whether long treatment durations with longer follow-up confirm progressive separation from placebo in line with the aptitude hypothesis for disease modification.

It is possible that -synuclein belongs to the central nervous system, the N-terminal region of -synuclein, which favours aggregated and monomeric species and is associated with target engagement in Phase 1 studies with CSF-to-serum ratios of 0.13–0.56%, suggesting concentrations of central nervous system in Brys et al., 2019. But the Phase 2 SPARK study did not show the clinical efficacy of the treatment of MDS-UPDRS in the absence of a significant difference in progression in MDS-UPDRS amplification between cinpanemab and placebo at 52 weeks, irrespective of duration of target engagement throughout the study period (Lang et al., 2022). This dissociation between pharmacodynamic effects and measurable benefit poses basic questions concerning the pathogenic significance of synuclein and whether antibody brain penetration with CSF: serum ratios generally around 0.1–0.3% is sufficient for complete extracellular clearance.

Table 3. α-Synuclein Immunotherapy Clinical Trials Summary

Agent	Trial	Primary Outcome	Result	Reference
Prasinezumab	PASADENA Phase 2	MDS-UPDRS Part III at 52 weeks	−2.0 points (P=0.24)	Pagano 2022 NEJM
Cinpanemab	SPARK Phase 2	MDS-UPDRS Part III at 52 weeks	No significant difference	Lang 2022 NEJM
UB-312 (active)	Phase 1	Safety, immunogenicity	92% antibody response	Yu 2022 Mov Disord

Active immunization procedures, generating endogenous antibody production by vaccination with synuclein-derived peptides, may provide potential advantages such as sustained antibody titers without repeated infusion. A synthetic peptide vaccine targeting the C-terminal domain of synuclein and a carrier protein, UB-312, was safe and immunogenic for the Phase 1 trials, with antibody responses in 92% (12/13) of those vaccine subjects. Yet the historical precedent for AN1792 active immunization for Alzheimer's disease, which had ended up in meningoencephalitis, increases the risk of autoimmunity (Orgogozo et al., 2003).

Small Molecule Aggregation Inhibitors

Small molecule inhibitors that target alpha-synuclein aggregation attempt to stabilize non-toxic conformations or avoid oligomerization and fibril formation by targeting alpha-synuclein. Anle138b is a diphenyl-pyrazole compound which was derived from the phenotypic screening for oxidation inhibition of the oligomer and exhibited neuroprotection in multiple preclinical models, including A53T transgenic mice (Wagner et al., 2013). NPT200-11 is a small-molecule synuclein misfolding inhibitor, which demonstrated superior clinical efficacy in the treatment of pathological synuclein and behavioural deficits in transgenic models (Price et al., 2018).

Gene Silencing Technologies

Gene silencing technologies may remain viable for sustained synuclein expression reduction by RNA interference or antisense oligonucleotide mechanisms. The use of antisense oligonucleotides targeting SNCA mRNA for intrathecally administered SNCA vaccines found a significant reduction in -α-synuclein in preclinical and early clinical studies (Cole et al., 2021). This reasoning argues for genetic evidence from SNCA multiplication patients with gene-dosage-induced disease severity to suggest that suppression of synuclein expression might slow pathology accumulation even in rare cases. But -synuclein functions physiologically in synaptic vesicle trafficking and neurotransmitter release, which may pose theoretical concerns regarding adverse effects caused by excessive suppression (Bendor et al., 2013).

Neuroprotective and Mitochondrial Enhancement Strategies

The GLP-1 receptor agonists of the glucagon-like peptide-1 (GLP-1) receptor, and developed for diabetes therapies with pleiotropic metabolic effects, are the leading neuroprotective candidates. Exenatide had promising findings in 48 weeks of open-label study with a significant 3.5-point MDS-UPDRS Part III advantage in the medication-off state after discontinuation and continued in the relapse after drug discontinuation (Athauda et al., 2017.)

Lixisenatide, a once-daily GLP-1 receptor agonist, demonstrated great utility in the Phase 2 randomised double-blinded placebo-controlled trial. Despite significant difference of 3.08 points (95% CI: 0.86–5.30; P=0.007) for lixisenatide recipients at 12 months of follow-up, the participants receiving lixisenatide were essentially no motor improvement as measured by 0.04 point change in MDS-UPDRS Part III medication-off as measured by 3.04 point worsening in the placebo group at the same time as 3.04 point change in MDS-UPDRS Part III medication-off at a mean of 3.08. This separation proved particularly remarkable, and the disease modification claims remained strong for 2 months. Phase 3 LIXIPARK trial is continuing and will continue to test efficacy and quality of durability.

Table 4. GLP-1 Receptor Agonist Clinical Trials in Parkinson's Disease

Agent	Phase	N	Key Finding	Reference
Exenatide	2 (open-label)	60	−3.5 pt MDS-UPDRS III (P=0.03)	Athauda 2017 Lancet
Lixisenatide	2 (RCT)	156	3.08 pt difference (P=0.007)	Meissner 2024 NEJM

Ambroxol is a mucolytic drug, a pharmacological chaperone associated with the effect of GCase enzyme activity, and it addresses PD pathogenesis through GBA variant association (Migdalska-Richards et al., 2016). As evidence, oral ambroxol exposure induced a 35% increase in CSF GCase protein levels but reduced enzyme activity by 19% owing to ambroxol's inhibitory action at neutral pH (Mullin et al., 2020). AiM-PD Phase 2 study (NCT02941822) is examining ambroxol in early PD patients.

UDCA, a bile acid with mitochondrial protective properties, offered promising preclinical abrasion preclinical neuroprotection in LRRK2 G2019S patient-derived neurons (Mortiboys et al., 2015). The UP Study (NCT03840005) is testing UDCA in PD patients. The safety assessment of UDCA shows that there are few concerns regarding blood-brain barrier penetration with CSF: plasma ratios lower than 0.1, allowing for low brain concentrations.

Another mitochondrial target was nicotinamide adenine dinucleotide precursors, nicotinamide riboside. Bioavailable precursors supplementation increases the concentration of tissue NAD+ levels and has shown neuroprotection of preclinical PD models with SIRT1/3 activation and increased mitophagy (Fang et al., 2019; Schöndorf et al., 2018).

Anti-Inflammatory Strategies

NLRP3 inflammasome inhibition, targeting the complex polyprotein that regulates interleukin-1 and interleukin-18 maturation following -synuclein aggregates, showed preclinical efficacy in preventing neurodegeneration (Gordon et al., 2018). Notably, the NET-PD futility trial of minocycline was below the futility threshold; the futility test of minocycline would not necessarily indicate inefficacy (Ravina et al., 2006).

GENE THERAPY APPROACHES

Gene therapy strategies use vectors—mostly AAV serotypes—promote therapeutic transgenes directly to brain regions by way of gene therapy. The aromatic L-amino acid decarboxylase gene therapy, characterized by AAV2 vectors that encode for the human AADC enzyme, which is in combination with a human AAV2 gene in the putamen, seeks to restore dopamine synthesis capability. VY-AADC01 participated in Phase 1b studies showing safety with 18–24-month follow-up and continued PET imaging findings suggesting AADC enzyme activity and clinical improvement by 1.9 hours in the best responding cohort (Christine et al., 2022).

GCLIP-derived neurotrophic factor gene therapy promotes neuroprotection by modulating the neurotrophic support of the glial cell line. Early trials with direct recombinant GDNF protein infusion in open-label studies showed promise in open-label studies but failed in double-blind placebo-controlled studies, due to overexposure to the immediate catheter location (Lang et al., 2006). The AAV2-neurturin Phase 2b trial (CERE-120) failed to show efficacy even in the absence of open-label predecessor signals (Marks et al., 2010). AAV2-GDNF is tested for improved delivery parameters under the REGENERATE-PD study (NCT04167540).

A. Cell-Based Regenerative Medicine

In conjunction, dopamine-producing neurons are implanted into the striatum to restore dopaminergic neurotransmission. Fetal ventral mesencephalic tissue transplantation demonstrated that there was a prognosis for dyskinesias, although there was a good degree of evidence that the effects of the transplant were graft-induced dyskinesias in 15–56% of those who were receiving the transplant.

hESC-derived dopaminergic neurons are synthesized by multistep differentiation processes mimicking developmental signalling cascades through human embryonic stem cell (hESC)-derived neurons (Kirkeby et al., 2017). The first clinical case study of autologous iPSC-derived dopaminergic neuron transplantation demonstrated safety at 24-month follow-up in a single patient with relatively minimal disease severity and PET imaging findings of graft survival (Schweitzer et al., 2020). The TRANSEURO study used a refined fetal tissue protocol by standard procedures, e.g. Barker et al., 2019)

Induced pluripotent stem cell (iPSC) technology allows for the formation of autologous dopaminergic neurons, which thus cannot be rejected through allogeneic immune rejection (Takahashi & Yamanaka, 2006). There is a preliminary safety hazard period of 2 years from the Kyoto University iPSC trial in 2018 conducted by Doi et al. (2020) in the Kyoto University iPSC trial, which was opened in 2018. Translational Innovations, Preclinical Advances, and Future Therapeutic Frontiers A. Preclinical Therapeutic Landscape and Translational Readiness. Historical interest in neurodegenerative drugs is high. In clinical trials, overall success rates are usually found to be 8–14%, especially in the adult-onset neurodegenerative indication, where Alzheimer's disease is typically highly praised with extremely low approval rates (Cummings et al., 2014b; Mortberg et al., 2022).

The key to modelling validity is model validity. Classic neurotoxin models (MPTP, 6-OHDA and rotenone) capture dopaminergic vulnerability and motor-like phenotypes but tend to fail to reflect the slow and multi-system biology of sporadic PD, particularly the slow, multi-system biology of progressive synuclein pathology and non-motor trajectory. These limitations are now used not as failures but as "use-case constraints" that call for a conscious model matching to the therapeutic hypothesis (Sturchio et al., 2024).

Since disease-related -α-synuclein models are now central to disease-modifying claims, health-enhancing claims are becoming more significant. Preformed fibril paradigms and related seeding models identify templated misfolding and spreading features with better direct reference to propagation-targeted interventions (Luk et al. 2012).

The most significant clinical shift is accelerating the emergence of human disease biology within the preclinical zone. These cellular systems (iPSC-derived dopaminergic neurons, glia-inclusive co-cultures, and organoid-like platforms) and patient tissue single-cell atlases are increasingly used to identify which neurons are vulnerable, which pathways are under control, and which targets are conceivably druggable within relevant cell states. On-cell profiles for single cells are also continuing to expand the identification of selective vulnerability and intrapopulation heterogeneity in dopaminergic neurons (Agarwal et al., 2020).

B. Novel Targets: The Gut-Brain Axis

The gut–brain axis has reached an associative hypothesis and is a translational domain that encompasses prodromal biology, immune and metabolic signalling, and intervention studies. Meta-analytic review and systematic reviews consistently identify changes in gut microbial structures following PD and emphasize the small but sensitive effects (Kleine Bardenhorst et al., 2023a, 2023b; Romano et al., 2021). In particular, the field has begun to move from observational signatures to interventional evidence. A randomized clinical trial of faecal microbiota transplantation for PD provides the best "real life check" of the meaning of microbiome modification in terms of how the effects of microbiome modification can be reached, but that symptoms and potential clinical significance do not directly from microbiota change. Similarly, probiotic trials and syntheses continue to develop, suggesting potential benefits for selecting outcomes but also suggesting variability in strains, dosing, and endpoints (Jin et al. 2024a).

C. Drug Delivery and Nanotechnology

Many PD disease-modifying concepts, such as biologics, nucleic acids, and gene-regulatory agents, are now known to be limited by delivery. In the current BBB reviews, the problem with insufficient CNS exposure was primarily driven by the high prevalence of poor CNS exposure, which encouraged systematic approaches to estimating and engineering brain delivery through systematic measurement and engineering.

Most actively translated approaches are receptor-mediated transcytosis (RMT), where the therapeutic payload is designed to use endogenous BBB transport systems, such as the transferrin receptor or similar RMT classes. The current reviews highlight progress as well as persistent design obstacles such as choice of receptors, trafficking fate and a risk that BBB uptake does not provide parenchymal delivery (Haqqani et al., 2024).

Similarly, focused ultrasound-mediated BBB opening is rapidly expanding as a platform technology for spatially targeted delivery, clinical safety research with specialized populations of neurons and growing interest in extended biomarker sampling and therapeutic delivery approaches (Wang & Ren, 2024).

D. Digital and AI-Enabled Health Technologies

Digital health for PD has become more of a case study, with PD testing for the possibility of using feasibility trials to learn how to develop endpoint grade measures that improve sensitivity, variable rates of variability, and understand real-world function. WATCH-PD provides a case study of how smartphone and smartwatch-derived measures can track disease-related characteristics in early PD under structured observational conditions (Adams et al., 2024).

Two pathways are described: 1) digital biomarkers for monitoring and enrichment, 2) digital endpoints that can be proven to support clinical trial decision-making, if the arithmetic validity, clinical validity, and interpretation are rigorously established (Sun et al., 2024).

We also note that digital outcomes are increasingly likely to be extended beyond motor capture and incorporate non-motor dimensions and patient-specific function not in-clinic scales (Schalkamp et al., 2024).

E. Lifestyle and Complementary Therapies

The most highly successful adjunct intervention field is exercise, but the translational frontier is no longer simply "exercise helps motor symptoms." Rather, the focus will be a discussion in the forward, but with consideration, mechanism, and personalization of the best ways of addressing gait, balance, cognition, mood, and fatigue, scales, and modalities in a manner that combines functional benefit and utility; modalities in a way that will interact with their function; and mechanistic biomarkers that change alongside functioning to effect function. Recent research on motor improvement and the heterogeneity of protocols continues to support motor improvements while placing emphasis on heterogeneity of protocols and an urgent need for more mechanism-linked designs (Jin et al., 2024b).

CLINICAL IMPLEMENTATION, GUIDELINES, AND FUTURE OUTLOOK

International Treatment Guidelines

Rather than a fixed set of "one-time" guidelines, vignettes of information and/ or grading that have been placed in the "one-time" arena of Parkinson disease management are increasingly framed by a constantly updated version of consensus statements on Parkinson disease. Evaluation of therapeutic efficacy across stages of disease is anchored by MDS's EBM reviews, with levodopa categorized as a good predictor of therapeutic efficacy for motor symptoms control in the Movement Disorder Society (Fox et al., 2018b).

Meanwhile, new MDS EBM revisions focus on the management of complications (motor fluctuations and dyskinesias) and the increasing role of device-aided and infusion strategies, illustrating that long-term outcomes are increasingly determined by complication burden and treatment personalization than by first-time symptomatic response alone (Bouça-Machado et al., 2020).

The national bodies continue to revise initial dopaminergic therapy selection and sequencing (levodopa versus dopamine agonists versus MAO-B inhibitors), the focus of trade-offs in motor benefit, dyskinesia risk, neuropsychiatric adverse effects, age, occupation, and comorbidity profile (Goetz, Tilley et al., 2008).

The guide also agrees on the need to include non-motor symptoms and patient-set priorities before care planning in a scenario of short-term transition from "motor-first" algorithms to multidomain symptom control and function-preserving strategies (Weise et al., 2024).

Disease Staging and Stratification

A popular clinimetric component for motor, non-motor, and complication domains, MDS-UPDRS is the primary clinical support for detecting motor, non-motor, and complication domains, with the structure and measurement properties highly validated, embedded in a regulatory contex [Weise et al., 2024]. The Neuronal - Synuclein Disease Integrated Staging System (NSD-ISS) uses synuclein seed amplification assays and dopaminergic imaging to indicate biological stages in patients with synuclein disease. Braak neuropathological staging is influential, but in some cases of autopsy-confirmed PD cases, there are no differences. Interestingly, the body-first versus brain-first hypothesis may explain different patterns of progression (Borghammer & Van Den Berge, 2019a).

Multidisciplinary Care Models

As Parkinson's disease develops, more complex, multidisciplinary models continue to be positioned as "optional extras" but as a delivery infrastructure for the most effective outcome to be required, especially for advanced therapies, neuropsychiatric complications, and fragility. Contemporary synthesized models emphasize the importance of coordinated movement-disorder neurology, rehabilitation, speech-language therapy, neuropsychology, nursing and social support, and the highest argument for advanced illness or therapeutic escalation (Steendam-Oldekamp & Van Laar, 2024; Weise et al., 2024b). In particular, one of the main goals for mainstreaming hybrid care (in-person plus remote) and telemedicine integrated multidisciplinary services with telerehabilitation and remotely delivered allied health care services is to allow for the normalization of hybrid care in person and remote and telemedicine-enabled multidisciplinary programs that can improve access with clinically valid outcomes (Dou et al., 2025; Federico et al., 2024). In addition to access, these models are important for access and because the next wave of trials and treatments will increasingly require frequent, real-world monitoring of wearables, home-based testing, and remote adverse event surveillance to be embraced and maintained by management and post-authorisation evidence.

Access, Cost-Effectiveness, and Health Equity

A "future outlook" debate now revolves around economic and health-system considerations because disease-modifying and regenerative treatments in the future are likely to be costly and extremely complex. A new analysis of cost-of-illness shows that Parkinson's disease imposes substantial and variable societal costs; geographical and severity-induced differences in cost drivers such as health care use, productivity loss and patient/family burden (Chaudhuri et al., 2024; Wijers et al., 2024). A widely publicised U.S. estimate of the cumulative economic burden is tens of billion dollars annually, and it increases as populations increase.

Device-aided therapy's cost-effectiveness is not determinable by time horizon, disease stage, or comparator strategy. Studies of DBS cost-effectiveness estimates by a recent systematic review show that there is a large variety of models and settings in which data on costs of DBS vary considerably, but not all models and settings need to be simplified with standard assumptions and pragmatic comparisons with alternative advanced therapies, such as Sasidharan et al. 2024.

Equity is also "future critical." Not all recent reviews and evidence-based studies have addressed racial/ethnic and socioeconomic disparities in access to DBS assessment and implantation, so they focus on referral patterns, insurance systems, geographical access, and trust/communication barriers in comparison to patient preferences. (Bishay et al., 2024).

For example, they are directly relevant to the next decade because biomarker-guided and device-/procedure intensive intervention could otherwise increase existing gaps if the implementation and reimbursement methods do not have equity as their underlying prerequisite.

CONCLUSION

This narrative analysis identifies that the therapeutic field is now at a critical inflexion, setting it aflame in this complex narrative synthesis of Parkinson's disease therapy. Within the past decade, numerous improvements have been made regarding mechanistic interpretations of -synuclein propagation using seed amplification assays that show diagnostic accuracy higher than 90%, genetic architecture analysis that indicates over 90 risk loci, and lixisenatide that may represent potentially therapeutic potential for disease modification.

The growing number of PD cases worldwide in 2040 indicates the need to improve therapeutic practice (Ray Dorsey et al. 2018). During the 12 years of study, 73.75% phenoconversion was present in REM sleep behaviour disorder patients and is very good for prevention purposes (Postuma et al., 2015). The future state of PD therapeutics is comprised of disease-modifying interventions initiated early in the process of disease progression that can slow the progression by 30–50%, regenerative medicine practices that involve restoring the dopaminergic system, precision medicine protocols that match interventions to subgroups of patients, comprehensive symptom management and integrated multidisciplinary care delivery. The combination of rigorous scientific research with patient-centred priorities, implementation science, and equity priorities will help us to determine whether therapeutic advances are viable at the population level.

REFERENCES

Aarsland, D., Creese, B., Politis, M., Chaudhuri, K. R., Ffytche, D. H., Weintraub, D., & Ballard, C. (2017). Cognitive decline in Parkinson disease. *Nature Reviews. Neurology*, *13*(4), 217–231. DOI: 10.1038/NRNEUROL.2017.27

Adams, J. L., Kangarloo, T., Gong, Y., Khachadourian, V., Tracey, B., Volfson, D., Latzman, R. D., Cosman, J., Edgerton, J., Anderson, D., Best, A., Kostrzebski, M. A., Auinger, P., Wilmot, P., Pohlson, Y., Jensen-Roberts, S., Müller, M. L. T. M., Stephenson, D., Dorsey, E. R., & Botting, E. (2024). Using a smartwatch and smartphone to assess early Parkinson's disease in the WATCH-PD study over 12 months. *NPJ Parkinson's Disease*, *10*(1), 112. DOI: 10.1038/S41531-024-00721-2

Agarwal, D., Sandor, C., Volpato, V., Caffrey, T. M., Monzón-Sandoval, J., Bowden, R., Alegre-Abarrategui, J., Wade-Martins, R., & Webber, C. (2020). A single-cell atlas of the human substantia nigra reveals cell-specific pathways associated with neurological disorders. *Nature Communications*, *11*(1), 4183. DOI: 10.1038/S41467-020-17876-0

Ahlskog, J. E., & Muenter, M. D. (2001). Frequency of levodopa-related dyskinesias and motor fluctuations as estimated from the cumulative literature. *Movement Disorders*, *16*(3), 448–458. DOI: 10.1002/MDS.1090;WGROUP:STRING:PUBLICATION

Alcalay, R. N., Levy, O. A., Waters, C. C., Fahn, S., Ford, B., Kuo, S. H., Mazzoni, P., Pauciulo, M. W., Nichols, W. C., Gan-Or, Z., Rouleau, G. A., Chung, W. K., Wolf, P., Oliva, P., Keutzer, J., Marder, K., & Zhang, X. (2015). Glucocerebrosidase activity in Parkinson's disease with and without GBA mutations. *Brain*, *138*(Pt 9), 2648–2658. DOI: 10.1093/BRAIN/AWV179

Aquino, C. C., & Fox, S. H. (2015). Clinical spectrum of levodopa-induced complications. *Movement Disorders*, *30*(1), 80–89. DOI: 10.1002/MDS.26125

Asuku, A. O., Ayinla, M. T., Olajide, T. S., Ajagun, E. J., Ganiyu, K. O., Hamza, Y. O., Ajibare, A. J., & Abdulsalam, T. A. (2024). Diagnosis and Biomarkers of Parkinson's Disease. In: Zebrafish as a Model for Parkinson's Disease. Taylor and Francis, CRC, https://doi.org/DOI: 10.1201/9781003402893-15

Asuku, A. O., Ogungbangbe, G. O., & Fajemidagba, G. A. (2025). Gene therapy for Parkinson's disease: A new frontier in neurodegenerative diseases. *Exploration of Neuroprotective Therapy*, *5*, 1004119. DOI: 10.37349/ent.2025.1004119

Athauda, D., Maclagan, K., Skene, S. S., Bajwa-Joseph, M., Letchford, D., Chowdhury, K., Hibbert, S., Budnik, N., Zampedri, L., Dickson, J., Li, Y., Aviles-Olmos, I., Warner, T. T., Limousin, P., Lees, A. J., Greig, N. H., Tebbs, S., & Foltynie, T. (2017). Exenatide once weekly versus placebo in Parkinson's disease: A randomised, double-blind, placebo-controlled trial. *Lancet, 390*(10103), 1664–1675. DOI: 10.1016/S0140-6736(17)31585-4

Aurora, R. N., Zak, R. S., Maganti, R. K., Auerbach, S. H., Casey, K. R., Chowdhuri, S., Karippot, A., Ramar, K., Kristo, D. A., Morgenthaler, T. I., & Tracy, S. L. (2010). Best Practice Guide for the Treatment of REM Sleep Behavior Disorder (RBD). *Journal of Clinical Sleep Medicine : JCSM : Official Publication of the American Academy of Sleep Medicine, 6*(1), 85. DOI: 10.5664/jcsm.27717

Bae, E. J., Lee, H. J., Rockenstein, E., Ho, D. H., Park, E. B., Yang, N. Y., Desplats, P., Masliah, E., & Lee, S. J. (2012). Antibody-aided clearance of extracellular α-synuclein prevents cell-to-cell aggregate transmission. *The Journal ofNeuroscience : The Official Journal of the Society for Neuroscience, 32*(39), 13454–13469. DOI: 10.1523/JNEUROSCI.1292-12.2012

Baker, W. L., Silver, D., White, C. M., Kluger, J., Aberle, J., Patel, A. A., & Coleman, C. I. (2009). Dopamine agonists in the treatment of early Parkinson's disease: A meta-analysis. *Parkinsonism & Related Disorders, 15*(4), 287–294. DOI: 10.1016/j.parkreldis.2008.07.004

Barker, R. A., Farrell, K., Guzman, N. V., He, X., Lazic, S. E., Moore, S., Morris, R., Tyers, P., Wijeyekoon, R., Daft, D., Hewitt, S., Dayal, V., Foltynie, T., Kefalopoulou, Z., Mahlknecht, P., Lao-Kaim, N. P., Piccini, P., Bjartmarz, H., Björklund, A., … Winkler, C. (2019). Designing stem-cell-based dopamine cell replacement trials for Parkinson's disease. *Nature Medicine 2019 25:7, 25*(7), 1045–1053. https://doi.org/DOI: 10.1038/s41591-019-0507-2

Berg, D., Postuma, R. B., Adler, C. H., Bloem, B. R., Chan, P., Dubois, B., Gasser, T., Goetz, C. G., Halliday, G., Joseph, L., Lang, A. E., Liepelt-Scarfone, I., Litvan, I., Marek, K., Obeso, J., Oertel, W., Olanow, C. W., Poewe, W., Stern, M., & Deuschl, G. (2015). MDS research criteria for prodromal Parkinson's disease. *Movement Disorders, 30*(12), 1600–1611. DOI: 10.1002/MDS.26431

Billingsley, K. J., Bandres-Ciga, S., Saez-Atienzar, S., & Singleton, A. B. (2018). Genetic risk factors in Parkinson's disease. *Cell and Tissue Research, 373*(1), 9. DOI: 10.1007/S00441-018-2817-Y

Binde, C. D., Tvete, I. F., Gåsemyr, J., Natvig, B., & Klemp, M. (2018). A multiple treatment comparison meta-analysis of monoamine oxidase type B inhibitors for Parkinson's disease. *British Journal of Clinical Pharmacology*, *84*(9), 1917–1927. DOI: 10.1111/BCP.13651;JOURNAL:JOURNAL:13652125;PAGE:STRING:ARTICLE/CHAPTER

Bishay, A. E., Hughes, N. C., Zargari, M., Paulo, D. L., Bishay, S., Lyons, A. T., Morkos, M. N., Ball, T. J., Englot, D. J., & Bick, S. K. (2024). Disparities in Access to Deep Brain Stimulation for Parkinson's Disease and Proposed Interventions: A Literature Review. *Stereotactic and Functional Neurosurgery*, *102*(3), 179. DOI: 10.1159/000538748

Borghammer, P., & Van Den Berge, N. (2019a). Brain-First versus Gut-First Parkinson's Disease: A Hypothesis. *Journal of Parkinson's Disease*, *9*(s2), S281–S295. DOI: 10.3233/JPD-191721

Bot, B. M., Suver, C., Neto, E. C., Kellen, M., Klein, A., Bare, C., Doerr, M., Pratap, A., Wilbanks, J., Dorsey, E. R., Friend, S. H., & Trister, A. D. (2016). The mPower study, Parkinson disease mobile data collected using ResearchKit. *Scientific Data*, *3*(1), 160011-. https://doi.org/DOI: 10.1038/SDATA.2016.11

Bouça-Machado, R., Pona-Ferreira, F., Gonçalves, N., Leitão, M., Cacho, R., Castro-Caldas, A., & Ferreira, J. J., & and CNS Multidisciplinary Team. (2020). Outcome Measures for Evaluating the Effect of a Multidisciplinary Intervention on Axial Symptoms of Parkinson's Disease. *Frontiers in Neurology*, *11*, 521733. DOI: 10.3389/FNEUR.2020.00328

Bretz, F., Koenig, F., Brannath, W., Glimm, E., & Posch, M. (2009). Adaptive designs for confirmatory clinical trials. *Statistics in Medicine*, *28*(8), 1181–1217. DOI: 10.1002/SIM.3538

Brundin, P., & Melki, R. (2017). Prying into the Prion Hypothesis for Parkinson's Disease. *The Journal of Neuroscience : The Official Journal of the Society for Neuroscience*, *37*(41), 9808–9818. DOI: 10.1523/JNEUROSCI.1788-16.2017

Brys, M., Fanning, L., Hung, S., Ellenbogen, A., Penner, N., Yang, M., Welch, M., Koenig, E., David, E., Fox, T., Makh, S., Aldred, J., Goodman, I., Pepinsky, B., Liu Y. T., Graham, D., Weihofen, A., & Cedarbaum, J. M. (2019). Randomized phase I clinical trial of anti–α-synuclein antibody BIIB054. *Movement Disorders*, *34*(8), 1154–1163. DOI: 10.1002/MDS.27738

Chahid, Y., Sheikh, Z. H., Mitropoulos, M., & Booij, J. (2023). A systematic review of the potential effects of medications and drugs of abuse on dopamine transporter imaging using [123I]I-FP-CIT SPECT in routine practice. *European Journal of Nuclear Medicine and Molecular Imaging 2023 50:7, 50*(7), 1974–1987. https://doi.org/DOI: 10.1007/S00259-023-06171-X

Chaudhuri, K. R., Azulay, J. P., Odin, P., Lindvall, S., Domingos, J., Alobaidi, A., Kandukuri, P. L., Chaudhari, V. S., Parra, J. C., Yamazaki, T., Oddsdottir, J., Wright, J., & Martinez-Martin, P. (2024). Economic Burden of Parkinson's Disease: A Multinational, Real-World, Cost-of-Illness Study. *Drugs - Real World Outcomes, 11*(1), 1. DOI: 10.1007/S40801-023-00410-1

Chen, K., Sun, L., Liu, Y., & Chen, R. (2025). Safety and efficacy of fecal microbiota transplantation in the treatment of Parkinson's disease: A systematic review of clinical trials. *Frontiers in Neuroscience, 19*, 1639911. DOI: 10.3389/FNINS.2025.1639911

Chitsaz, A., Najafi, M. R., Habibi, F., & Amirhajloo, S. (2024). Comparison of the effectiveness of modafinil and methylphenidate in treatment of excessive daytime sleepiness in patients with Parkinson's disease. *Current Journal of Neurology, 23*(1), 39. DOI: 10.18502/CJN.V23I1.16431

Christine, C. W., Richardson, R. M., van Laar, A. D., Thompson, M. E., Fine, E. M., Khwaja, O. S., Li, C., Liang, G. S., Meier, A., Roberts, E. W., Pfau, M. L., Rodman, J. R., Bankiewicz, K. S., & Larson, P. S. (2022). Safety of AADC Gene Therapy for Moderately Advanced Parkinson Disease: Three-Year Outcomes from the PD-1101 Trial. *Neurology, 98*(1), E40–E50. DOI: 10.1212/WNL.0000000000012952

Cole, T. A., Zhao, H., Collier, T. J., Sandoval, I., Sortwell, C. E., Steece-Collier, K., Daley, B. F., Booms, A., Lipton, J., Welch, M., Berman, M., Jandreski, L., Graham, D., Weihofen, A., Celano, S., Schulz, E., Cole-Strauss, A., Luna, E., Quach, D., & Paumier, K. L. (2021). α-Synuclein antisense oligonucleotides as a disease-modifying therapy for Parkinson's disease. *JCI Insight, 6*(5). Advance online publication. DOI: 10.1172/JCI.INSIGHT.135633

Concha-Marambio, L., Pritzkow, S., Shahnawaz, M., Farris, C. M., & Soto, C. (2023). Seed amplification assay for the detection of pathologic alpha-synuclein aggregates in cerebrospinal fluid. *Nature Protocols 2023 18:4, 18*(4), 1179–1196. https://doi.org/DOI: 10.1038/s41596-022-00787-3

Corvol, J. C., & Poewe, W. (2016). Pharmacogenetics of Parkinson's Disease in Clinical Practice. *Movement Disorders Clinical Practice, 4*(2), 173–180. DOI: 10.1002/MDC3.12444

Costello, H., Schrag, A.-E., Howard, R., & Roiser, J. P. (2023). Dissociable effects of dopaminergic medications on depression symptom dimensions in Parkinson's disease. MedRxiv *: The Preprint Server for Health Sciences*. https://doi.org/DOI: 10.1101/2023.06.30.23292073

Cummings, J., Isaacson, S., Mills, R., Williams, H., Chi-Burris, K., Corbett, A., Dhall, R., & Ballard, C. (2014). Pimavanserin for patients with Parkinson's disease psychosis: A randomised, placebo-controlled phase 3 trial. *Lancet*, *383*(9916), 533–540. DOI: 10.1016/S0140-6736(13)62106-6

Cummings, J. L., Morstorf, T., & Zhong, K. (2014). Alzheimer's disease drug-development pipeline: Few candidates, frequent failures. *Alzheimer's Research & Therapy*, *6*(4), 37. DOI: 10.1186/ALZRT269

D'Agostino, R. B. (2009). The Delayed-Start Study Design. *The New England Journal of Medicine*, *361*(13), 1304–1306. DOI: 10.1056/NEJMSM090

De la Fuente-Fernández, R., Ruth, T. J., Sossi, V., Schulzer, M., Calne, D. B., & Stoessl, A. J. (2001). Expectation and dopamine release: Mechanism of the placebo effect in Parkinson's disease. *Science*, *293*(5532), 1164–1166. DOI: 10.1126/SCIENCE.1060937

Digital Health Technologies for Remote Data Acquisition in Clinical Investigations | FDA. (n.d.). Retrieved December 13, 2025, from https://www.fda.gov/regulatory-information/search-fda-guidance-documents/digital-health-technologies-remote-data-acquisition-clinical-investigations

Doi, D., Magotani, H., Kikuchi, T., Ikeda, M., Hiramatsu, S., Yoshida, K., Amano, N., Nomura, M., Umekage, M., Morizane, A., & Takahashi, J. (2020). Pre-clinical study of induced pluripotent stem cell-derived dopaminergic progenitor cells for Parkinson's disease. *Nature Communications 2020 11:1*, *11*(1), 3369-. https://doi.org/DOI: 10.1038/s41467-020-17165-w

Dou, J., Wang, J., Gao, X., Wang, G., Bai, Y., Liang, Y., Yang, K., Yang, Y., & Zhang, L. (2025). Effectiveness of Telemedicine Interventions on Motor and Nonmotor Outcomes in Parkinson Disease: Systematic Review and Network Meta-Analysis. *Journal of Medical Internet Research*, *27*, e71169. DOI: 10.2196/71169

Eijsvogel, P., Misra, P., Concha-Marambio, L., Boyd, J. D., Ding, S., Fedor, L., Hsieh, Y. T., Sun, Y. S., Vroom, M. M., Farris, C. M., Ma, Y., de Kam, M. L., Radanovic, I., Vissers, M. F. J. M., Mirski, D., Shareghi, G., Shahnawaz, M., Singer, W., Kremer, P., … Dodart, J. C. (2024). Target engagement and immunogenicity of an active immunotherapeutic targeting pathological α-synuclein: a phase 1 placebo-controlled trial. *Nature Medicine 2024 30:9, 30*(9), 2631–2640. https://doi.org/DOI: 10.1038/s41591-024-03101-8

Elm, J. J., Hauser, R., Tilley, B. C., Kieburtz, K., Aminoff, M. J., Augustine, E., Bennett, S., Bodis-Wollner, I. G., Cambi, F., Carter, J. H., Chou, K., Christine, C. W., Dhall, R., Dewey, R. B., Elble, R. J., Fang, J., Feigin, A., Galpern, W., Gardiner, I., & Zweig, R. (2012). Design innovations and baseline findings in a long-term parkinson's trial: The national institute of neurological disorders and stroke exploratory trials in parkinson's disease long-term study-1. *Movement Disorders*, *27*(12), 1513–1521. DOI: 10.1002/MDS.25175

Emre, M., Aarsland, D., Albanese, A., Byrne, E. J., Deuschl, G., De Deyn, P. P., Durif, F., Kulisevsky, J., van Laar, T., Lees, A., Poewe, W., Robillard, A., Rosa, M. M., Wolters, E., Quarg, P., Tekin, S., & Lane, R. (2004). Rivastigmine for Dementia Associated with Parkinson's Disease. *The New England Journal of Medicine*, *351*(24), 2509–2518. DOI: 10.1056/NEJMOA041470

Erb, M. K., Karlin, D. R., Ho, B. K., Thomas, K. C., Parisi, F., Vergara-Diaz, G. P., Daneault, J. F., Wacnik, P. W., Zhang, H., Kangarloo, T., Demanuele, C., Brooks, C. R., Detheridge, C. N., Shaafi Kabiri, N., Bhangu, J. S., & Bonato, P. (2020). mHealth and wearable technology should replace motor diaries to track motor fluctuations in Parkinson's disease. *NPJ Digital Medicine*, *3*(1), 6. DOI: 10.1038/S41746-019-0214-X

Espay, A. J., Bonato, P., Nahab, F. B., Maetzler, W., Dean, J. M., Klucken, J., Eskofier, B. M., Merola, A., Horak, F., Lang, A. E., Reilmann, R., Giuffrida, J., Nieuwboer, A., Horne, M., Little, M. A., Litvan, I., Simuni, T., Dorsey, E. R., Burack, M. A., & Papapetropoulos, S. (2016). Technology in Parkinson's disease: Challenges and opportunities. *Movement Disorders*, *31*(9), 1272–1282. DOI: 10.1002/MDS.26642

Fairfoul, G., McGuire, L. I., Pal, S., Ironside, J. W., Neumann, J., Christie, S., Joachim, C., Esiri, M., Evetts, S. G., Rolinski, M., Baig, F., Ruffmann, C., Wade-Martins, R., Hu, M. T. M., Parkkinen, L., & Green, A. J. E. (2016). Alpha-synuclein RT-QuIC in the CSF of patients with alpha-synucleinopathies. *Annals of Clinical and Translational Neurology*, *3*(10), 812–818. DOI: 10.1002/ACN3.338

Fang, E. F., Hou, Y., Palikaras, K., Adriaanse, B. A., Kerr, J. S., Yang, B., Lautrup, S., Hasan-Olive, M. M., Caponio, D., Dan, X., Rocktäschel, P., Croteau, D. L., Akbari, M., Greig, N. H., Fladby, T., Nilsen, H., Cader, M. Z., Mattson, M. P., Tavernarakis, N., & Bohr, V. A. (2019). Mitophagy inhibits amyloid-β and tau pathology and reverses cognitive deficits in models of Alzheimer's disease. *Nature Neuroscience 2019 22:3, 22*(3), 401–412. https://doi.org/DOI: 10.1038/s41593-018-0332-9

Federico, S., Cacciante, L., Cieślik, B., Turolla, A., Agostini, M., Kiper, P., & Picelli, A. (2024). Telerehabilitation for Neurological Motor Impairment: A Systematic Review and Meta-Analysis on Quality of Life, Satisfaction, and Acceptance in Stroke, Multiple Sclerosis, and Parkinson's Disease. *Journal of Clinical Medicine*, *13*(1). Advance online publication. DOI: 10.3390/JCM13010299/S1

Fereshtehnejad, S. M., & Postuma, R. B. (2017). Subtypes of Parkinson's Disease: What Do They Tell Us About Disease Progression? *Current Neurology and Neuroscience Reports*, *17*(4). Advance online publication. DOI: 10.1007/S11910-017-0738-X

Fernandez, H. H., Standaert, D. G., Hauser, R. A., Lang, A. E., Fung, V. S. C., Klostermann, F., Lew, M. F., Odin, P., Steiger, M., Yakupov, E. Z., Chouinard, S., Suchowersky, O., Dubow, J., Hall, C. M., Chatamra, K., Robieson, W. Z., Benesh, J. A., & Espay, A. J. (2015). Levodopa-carbidopa intestinal gel in advanced Parkinson's disease: Final 12-month, open-label results. *Movement Disorders*, *30*(4), 500–509. DOI: 10.1002/MDS.26123

Ferreira, J. J., Lees, A., Rocha, J. F., Poewe, W., Rascol, O., & Soares-da-Silva, P. (2016). Opicapone as an adjunct to levodopa in patients with Parkinson's disease and end-of-dose motor fluctuations: A randomised, double-blind, controlled trial. *Lancet Neurology*, *15*(2), 154–165. DOI: 10.1016/S1474-4422(15)00336-1

Ffytche, D. H., Creese, B., Politis, M., Chaudhuri, K. R., Weintraub, D., Ballard, C., & Aarsland, D. (2017). The psychosis spectrum in Parkinson disease. *Nature Reviews. Neurology*, *13*(2), 81. DOI: 10.1038/NRNEUROL.2016.200

Finberg, J. P. M. (2010). Pharmacology of Rasagiline, a New MAO-B Inhibitor Drug for the Treatment of Parkinson's Disease with Neuroprotective Potential. *Rambam Maimonides Medical Journal*, *1*(1), e0003. DOI: 10.5041/RMMJ.10003

Fleming, T. R., & Powers, J. H. (2012). Biomarkers and surrogate endpoints in clinical trials. *Statistics in Medicine*, *31*(25), 2973–2984. DOI: 10.1002/SIM.5403

Foltynie, T., Gandhi, S., Gonzalez-Robles, C., Zeissler, M. L., Mills, G., Barker, R., Carpenter, J., Schrag, A., Schapira, A., Bandmann, O., Mullin, S., Duffen, J., McFarthing, K., Chataway, J., Parmar, M., Carroll, C., Ben Shlomo, Y., Edwards, M., Whone, A., & Harris, J. (2023). Towards a multi-arm multi-stage platform trial of disease modifying approaches in Parkinson's disease. *Brain, 146*(7), 2717–2722. DOI: 10.1093/BRAIN/AWAD063

Fox, S. H., Katzenschlager, R., Lim, S. Y., Barton, B., de Bie, R. M. A., Seppi, K., Coelho, M., & Sampaio, C. (2018a). International Parkinson and movement disorder society evidence-based medicine review: Update on treatments for the motor symptoms of Parkinson's disease. *Movement Disorders, 33*(8), 1248–1266. DOI: 10.1002/MDS.27372

Fox, S. H., Katzenschlager, R., Lim, S. Y., Barton, B., de Bie, R. M. A., Seppi, K., Coelho, M., & Sampaio, C. (2018b). International Parkinson and movement disorder society evidence-based medicine review: Update on treatments for the motor symptoms of Parkinson's disease. *Movement Disorders, 33*(8), 1248–1266. DOI: 10.1002/MDS.27372

Frequin, H. L., Verschuur, C. V. M., Suwijn, S. R., Boel, J. A., Post, B., Bloem, B. R., van Hilten, J. J., van Laar, T., Tissingh, G., Munts, A. G., Dijk, J. M., Lang, A. E., Dijkgraaf, M. G. W., Hoogland, J., & de Bie, R. M. A. (2024). Long-Term Follow-Up of the LEAP Study: Early Versus Delayed Levodopa in Early Parkinson's Disease. *Movement Disorders, 39*(6), 975–982. DOI: 10.1002/MDS.29796

Gan-Or, Z., Amshalom, I., Kilarski, L. L., Bar-Shira, A., Gana-Weisz, M., Mirelman, A., Marder, K., Bressman, S., Giladi, N., & Orr-Urtreger, A. (2015). Differential effects of severe vs mild GBA mutations on Parkinson disease. *Neurology, 84*(9), 880–887. DOI: 10.1212/WNL.0000000000001315

Goetz, C. G., Tilley, B. C., Shaftman, S. R., Stebbins, G. T., Fahn, S., Martinez-Martin, P., Poewe, W., Sampaio, C., Stern, M. B., Dodel, R., Dubois, B., Holloway, R., Jankovic, J., Kulisevsky, J., Lang, A. E., Lees, A., Leurgans, S., LeWitt, P. A., Nyenhuis, D., & Zweig, R. M. (2008). Movement Disorder Society-sponsored revision of the Unified Parkinson's Disease Rating Scale (MDS-UPDRS): Scale presentation and clinimetric testing results. *Movement Disorders, 23*(15), 2129–2170. DOI: 10.1002/MDS.22340

Goetz, C. G., Wuu, J., McDermott, M. P., Adler, C. H., Fahn, S., Freed, C. R., Hauser, R. A., Olanow, W. C., Shoulson, I., Tandon, P. K., Kieburtz, K., & Leurgans, S. (2008). Placebo response in Parkinson's disease: Comparisons among 11 trials covering medical and surgical interventions. *Movement Disorders, 23*(5), 690–699. DOI: 10.1002/MDS.21894

Goldstein, D. S. (2014). Dysautonomia in Parkinson's disease: Neurocardiological abnormalities. *Comprehensive Physiology*, *4*(2), 805. DOI: 10.1002/CPHY.C130026

Gonzalez-Robles, C., Athauda, D., Barber, T. R., Barker, R. A., Dexter, D. T., Duty, S., Ellis-Doyle, R., Gandhi, S., Handley, J., Jabbari, E., Martin, K., McFarthing, K., Mills, G., Mortiboys, H., Mullin, S., Petty, R., Sammler, E., Scurfield, P., Stott, S. R. W., & Petty, R. (2025). Treatment Selection and Prioritization for the EJS ACT-PD MAMS Trial Platform. *Movement Disorders*, *40*(7), 1307–1317. DOI: 10.1002/MDS.3019

Gonzalez-Robles, C., Bartlett, M., Burnell, M., Clarke, C. S., Haar, S., Hu, M. T., Huxford, B., Jha, A., Lawton, M., Noyce, A., Piccini, P., Pushparatnam, K., Rochester, L., Siu, C., van Wamelen, D., Williams-Gray, C. H., Zeissler, M. L., Zetterberg, H., Carroll, C. B., & Schrag, A. (2023). Embedding Patient Input in Outcome Measures for Long-Term Disease-Modifying Parkinson Disease Trials. *Movement Disorders*, *39*(2), 433–438. DOI: 10.1002/MDS.29691

Gordon, R., Albornoz, E. A., Christie, D. C., Langley, M. R., Kumar, V., Mantovani, S., Robertson, A. A. B., Butler, M. S., Rowe, D. B., O'Neill, L. A., Kanthasamy, A. G., Schroder, K., Cooper, M. A., & Woodruff, T. M. (2018). Inflammasome inhibition prevents α-synuclein pathology and dopaminergic neurodegeneration in mice. *Science Translational Medicine*, *10*(465). Advance online publication. DOI: 10.1126/SCITRANSLMED.AAH4066

Guimaraes, P., Kieburtz, K., Goetz, C. G., Elm, J. J., Palesch, Y. Y., Huang, P., Ravina, B., Tanner, C. M., & Tilley, B. C. (2005). Non-linearity of Parkinson's disease progression: Implications for sample size calculations in clinical trials. *Clinical Trials*, *2*(6), 509–518. DOI: 10.1191/1740774505CN125OA

Guo, M., Wang, J., Zhao, Y., Feng, Y., Han, S., Dong, Q., Cui, M., & Tieu, K. (2020). Microglial exosomes facilitate α-synuclein transmission in Parkinson's disease. *Brain*, *143*(5), 1476–1497. DOI: 10.1093/BRAIN/AWAA090

Guttman, M., Stewart, D., Hussey, D., Wilson, A., Houle, S., & Kish, S. (2001). Influence of L-dopa and pramipexole on striatal dopamine transporter in early PD. *Neurology*, *56*(11), 1559–1564. DOI: 10.1212/WNL.56.11.1559

Hansson, O., Janelidze, S., Hall, S., Magdalinou, N., Lees, A. J., Andreasson, U., Norgren, N., Linder, J., Forsgren, L., Constantinescu, R., Zetterberg, H., & Blennow, K. (2017). Blood-based NfL: A biomarker for differential diagnosis of parkinsonian disorder. *Neurology*, *88*(10), 930–937. DOI: 10.1212/WNL.0000000000003680

Haqqani, A. S., Bélanger, K., & Stanimirovic, D. B. (2024). Receptor-mediated transcytosis for brain delivery of therapeutics: Receptor classes and criteria. *Frontiers in Drug Delivery*, *4*, 1360302. DOI: 10.3389/FDDEV.2024.1360302

Hauser, R. A., Hsu, A., Kell, S., Espay, A. J., Sethi, K., Stacy, M., Ondo, W., O'Connell, M., & Gupta, S. (2013). Extended-release carbidopa-levodopa (IPX066) compared with immediate-release carbidopa-levodopa in patients with Parkinson's disease and motor fluctuations: A phase 3 randomised, double-blind trial. *Lancet Neurology*, *12*(4), 346–356. DOI: 10.1016/S1474-4422(13)70025-5

Healy, D. G., Falchi, M., O'Sullivan, S. S., Bonifati, V., Durr, A., Bressman, S., Brice, A., Aasly, J., Zabetian, C. P., Goldwurm, S., Ferreira, J. J., Tolosa, E., Kay, D. M., Klein, C., Williams, D. R., Marras, C., Lang, A. E., Wszolek, Z. K., Berciano, J., & Wood, N. W. (2008). Phenotype, genotype, and worldwide genetic penetrance of LRRK2-associated Parkinson's disease: A case-control study. *Lancet Neurology*, *7*(7), 583–590. DOI: 10.1016/S1474-4422(08)70117-0

Hirsch, E. C., & Hunot, S. (2009). Neuroinflammation in Parkinson's disease: A target for neuroprotection? *Lancet Neurology*, *8*(4), 382–397. DOI: 10.1016/S1474-4422(09)70062-6

Horváth, K., Aschermann, Z., Ács, P., Deli, G., Janszky, J., Komoly, S., Balázs, É., Takács, K., Karádi, K., & Kovács, N. (2015a). Minimal clinically important difference on the Motor Examination part of MDS-UPDRS. *Parkinsonism & Related Disorders*, *21*(12), 1421–1426. DOI: 10.1016/j.parkreldis.2015.10.006

Horváth, K., Aschermann, Z., Ács, P., Deli, G., Janszky, J., Komoly, S., Balázs, É., Takács, K., Karádi, K., & Kovács, N. (2015b). Minimal clinically important difference on the Motor Examination part of MDS-UPDRS. *Parkinsonism & Related Disorders*, *21*(12), 1421–1426. DOI: 10.1016/j.parkreldis.2015.10.006

Jin, X., Dong, W., Chang, K., Yan, Y., & Liu, X. (2024a). Efficacy of probiotic supplements on Parkinson's disease: A systematic review and meta-analysis. *Complementary Therapies in Medicine*, *82*, 103045. DOI: 10.1016/J.CTIM.2024.103045

Jin, X., Dong, W., Chang, K., Yan, Y., & Liu, X. (2024b). Efficacy of probiotic supplements on Parkinson's disease: A systematic review and meta-analysis. *Complementary Therapies in Medicine*, *82*, 103045. DOI: 10.1016/J.CTIM.2024.103045

Kalia, L. V., & Lang, A. E. (2015). Parkinson's disease. *Lancet*, *386*(9996), 896–912. DOI: 10.1016/S0140-6736(14)61393-3

Kirkeby, A., Nolbrant, S., Tiklova, K., Heuer, A., Kee, N., Cardoso, T., Ottosson, D. R., Lelos, M. J., Rifes, P., Dunnett, S. B., Grealish, S., Perlmann, T., & Parmar, M. (2017). Predictive Markers Guide Differentiation to Improve Graft Outcome in Clinical Translation of hESC-Based Therapy for Parkinson's Disease. *Cell Stem Cell, 20*(1), 135–148. DOI: 10.1016/j.stem.2016.09.004

Kleine Bardenhorst, S., Cereda, E., Severgnini, M., Barichella, M., Pezzoli, G., Keshavarzian, A., Desideri, A., Pietrucci, D., Aho, V. T. E., Scheperjans, F., Hildebrand, F., Weis, S., Egert, M., Karch, A., Vital, M., & Rübsamen, N. (2023a). Gut microbiota dysbiosis in Parkinson disease: A systematic review and pooled analysis. *European Journal of Neurology, 30*(11), 3581–3594. DOI: 10.1111/ENE.15671

Kleine Bardenhorst, S., Cereda, E., Severgnini, M., Barichella, M., Pezzoli, G., Keshavarzian, A., Desideri, A., Pietrucci, D., Aho, V. T. E., Scheperjans, F., Hildebrand, F., Weis, S., Egert, M., Karch, A., Vital, M., & Rübsamen, N. (2023b). Gut microbiota dysbiosis in Parkinson disease: A systematic review and pooled analysis. *European Journal of Neurology, 30*(11), 3581–3594. DOI: 10.1111/ENE.15671

Kluge, A., Bunk, J., Schaeffer, E., Drobny, A., Xiang, W., Knacke, H., Bub, S., Lückstädt, W., Arnold, P., Lucius, R., Berg, D., & Zunke, F. (2022). Detection of neuron-derived pathological α-synuclein in blood. *Brain, 145*(9), 3058–3071. DOI: 10.1093/BRAIN/AWAC115

Kmiecik, M. J., Micheletti, S., Coker, D., Heilbron, K., Shi, J., Stagaman, K., Sonmez, T. F., Fontanillas, P., Shringarpure, S., Wetzel, M., Rowbotham, H. M., Cannon, P., Shelton, J. F., Hinds, D. A., Tung, J. Y., Holmes, M. V., Aslibekyan, S., Norcliffe-Kaufmann, L., Auton, A., & Wong, C. D. (2024). Genetic analysis and natural history of Parkinson's disease due to the LRRK2 G2019S variant. *Brain, 147*(6), 1996. DOI: 10.1093/BRAIN/AWAE073

Lachenmayer, M. L., Mürset, M., Antih, N., Debove, I., Muellner, J., Bompart, M., Schlaeppi, J. A., Nowacki, A., You, H., Michelis, J. P., Dransart, A., Pollo, C., Deuschl, G., & Krack, P. (2021). Subthalamic and pallidal deep brain stimulation for Parkinson's disease—meta-analysis of outcomes. *Npj Parkinson's Disease 2021 7:1, 7*(1), 77-. https://doi.org/DOI: 10.1038/s41531-021-00223-5

Lang, A. E., Gill, S., Patel, N. K., Lozano, A., Nutt, J. G., Penn, R., Brooks, D. J., Hotton, G., Moro, E., Heywood, P., Brodsky, M. A., Burchiel, K., Kelly, P., Dalvi, A., Scott, B., Stacy, M., Turner, D., Wooten, V. G. F., Elias, W. J., & Traub, M. (2006). Randomized controlled trial of intraputamenal glial cell line-derived neurotrophic factor infusion in Parkinson disease. *Annals of Neurology, 59*(3), 459–466. DOI: 10.1002/ANA.20737

Lang, A. E., Siderowf, A. D., Macklin, E. A., Poewe, W., Brooks, D. J., Fernandez, H. H., Rascol, O., Giladi, N., Stocchi, F., Tanner, C. M., Postuma, R. B., Simon, D. K., Tolosa, E., Mollenhauer, B., Cedarbaum, J. M., Fraser, K., Xiao, J., Evans, K. C., Graham, D. L., & Dam, T. (2022). Trial of Cinpanemab in Early Parkinson's Disease. *The New England Journal of Medicine*, *387*(5), 408–420. DOI: 10.1056/NEJMOA2203395

Lee, A. J., Wang, Y., Alcalay, R. N., Mejia-Santana, H., Saunders-Pullman, R., Bressman, S., Corvol, J. C., Brice, A., Lesage, S., Mangone, G., Tolosa, E., Pont-Sunyer, C., Vilas, D., Schüle, B., Kausar, F., Foroud, T., Berg, D., Brockmann, K., Goldwurm, S., & Marder, K. (2017). Penetrance estimate of LRRK2 p.G2019S mutation in individuals of non-Ashkenazi Jewish ancestry. *Movement Disorders*, *32*(10), 1432–1438. DOI: 10.1002/MDS.27059

Lees, A. J., Ferreira, J., Rascol, O., Poewe, W., Rocha, J. F., McCrory, M., & Soares-Da-Silva, P. (2017). Opicapone as Adjunct to Levodopa Therapy in Patients With Parkinson Disease and Motor Fluctuations: A Randomized Clinical Trial. *JAMA Neurology*, *74*(2), 197–206. DOI: 10.1001/JAMANEUROL.2016.4703

LeWitt, P. A., Hauser, R. A., Pahwa, R., Isaacson, S. H., Fernandez, H. H., Lew, M., Saint-Hilaire, M., Pourcher, E., Lopez-Manzanares, L., Waters, C., Rudzínska, M., Sedkov, A., Batycky, R., & Oh, C. (2019). Safety and efficacy of CVT-301 (levodopa inhalation powder) on motor function during off periods in patients with Parkinson's disease: A randomised, double-blind, placebo-controlled phase 3 trial. *Lancet Neurology*, *18*(2), 145–154. DOI: 10.1016/S1474-4422(18)30405-8

Limousin, P., & Foltynie, T. (2019). Long-term outcomes of deep brain stimulation in Parkinson disease. *Nature Reviews Neurology 2019 15:4*, *15*(4), 234–242. https://doi.org/DOI: 10.1038/s41582-019-0145-9

Longo, D. M., Yang, Y., Watkins, P. B., Howell, B. A., & Siler, S. Q. (2016). Elucidating Differences in the Hepatotoxic Potential of Tolcapone and Entacapone With DILIsym(®), a Mechanistic Model of Drug-Induced Liver Injury. *CPT: Pharmacometrics & Systems Pharmacology*, *5*(1), 31–39. DOI: 10.1002/PSP4.12053

Luca, DI, D. G., Sambursky, J. A., Margolesky, J., Cordeiro, J. G., DIaz, A., Shpiner, D. S., Moore, H. P., Singer, C., & Luca, C. (2020). Minority Enrollment in Parkinson's Disease Clinical Trials: Meta-Analysis and Systematic Review of Studies Evaluating Treatment of Neuropsychiatric Symptoms. *Journal of Parkinson's Disease*, *10*(4), 1709–1716. DOI: 10.3233/JPD-202045

Luk, K. C., Kehm, V., Carroll, J., Zhang, B., O'Brien, P., Trojanowski, J. Q., & Lee, V. M. Y. (2012). Pathological α-Synuclein Transmission Initiates Parkinson-like Neurodegeneration in Non-transgenic Mice. *Science, 338*(6109), 949. DOI: 10.1126/SCIENCE.1227157

Luo, Y., Qiao, L., Li, M., Wen, X., Zhang, W., & Li, X. (2024). Global, regional, national epidemiology and trends of Parkinson's disease from 1990 to 2021: Findings from the Global Burden of Disease Study 2021. *Frontiers in Aging Neuroscience, 16*, 1498756. DOI: 10.3389/FNAGI.2024.1498756

Marder, K., Wang, Y., Alcalay, R. N., Mejia-Santana, H., Tang, M. X., Lee, A., Raymond, D., Mirelman, A., Saunders-Pullman, R., Clark, L., Ozelius, L., Orr-Urtreger, A., Giladi, N., & Bressman, S. (2015). Age-specific penetrance of LRRK2 G2019S in the Michael J. Fox Ashkenazi Jewish LRRK2 Consortium. *Neurology, 85*(1), 89–95. DOI: 10.1212/WNL.0000000000001708

Marek, K., Chowdhury, S., Siderowf, A., Lasch, S., Coffey, C. S., Caspell-Garcia, C., Simuni, T., Jennings, D., Tanner, C. M., Trojanowski, J. Q., Shaw, L. M., Seibyl, J., Schuff, N., Singleton, A., Kieburtz, K., Toga, A. W., Mollenhauer, B., Galasko, D., Chahine, L. M., & Taucher, J. (2018). The Parkinson's progression markers initiative (PPMI) – establishing a PD biomarker cohort. *Annals of Clinical and Translational Neurology, 5*(12), 1460–1477. DOI: 10.1002/ACN3.644;JOURNAL:-JOURNAL:23289503

Marks, W. J., Bartus, R. T., Siffert, J., Davis, C. S., Lozano, A., Boulis, N., Vitek, J., Stacy, M., Turner, D., Verhagen, L., Bakay, R., Watts, R., Guthrie, B., Jankovic, J., Simpson, R., Tagliati, M., Alterman, R., Stern, M., Baltuch, G., & Olanow, C. W. (2010). Gene delivery of AAV2-neurturin for Parkinson's disease: A double-blind, randomised, controlled trial. *Lancet Neurology, 9*(12), 1164–1172. DOI: 10.1016/S1474-4422(10)70254-4

Martinez-Carrasco, A., Real, R., Lawton, M., Iwaki, H., Tan, M. M. X., Wu, L., Williams, N. M., Carroll, C., Hu, M. T. M., Grosset, D. G., Hardy, J., Ryten, M., Foltynie, T., Ben-Shlomo, Y., Shoai, M., & Morris, H. R. (2023). Genetic meta-analysis of levodopa induced dyskinesia in Parkinson's disease. *Npj Parkinson's Disease 2023 9:1, 9*(1), 128-. https://doi.org/DOI: 10.1038/s41531-023-00573-2

McFarthing, K., Buff, S., Rafaloff, G., Pitzer, K., Fiske, B., Navangul, A., Beissert, K., Pilcicka, A., Fuest, R., Wyse, R. K., & Stott, S. R. W. (2024). Parkinson's Disease Drug Therapies in the Clinical Trial Pipeline: 2024 Update. *Journal of Parkinson's Disease, 14*(5), 899–912. DOI: 10.3233/JPD-240272

Medtronic earns U.S. FDA approval for the world's first Adaptive deep brain stimulation system for people with Parkinson's - Feb 24, 2025. (n.d.). Retrieved December 12, 2025, from https://news.medtronic.com/2025-02-24-Medtronic-earns-U-S-FDA-approval-for-the-worlds-first-Adaptive-deep-brain-stimulation-system-for-people-with-Parkinsons

Meissner, W. G., Remy, P., Giordana, C., Maltête, D., Derkinderen, P., Houéto, J.-L., Anheim, M., Benatru, I., Boraud, T., Brefel-Courbon, C., Carrière, N., Catala, H., Charif, M., Colin, O., Corvol, J.-C., Damier, P., Dellapina, E., Devos, D., Drapier, S., & Rascol, O. (2024). Trial of Lixisenatide in Early Parkinson's Disease. *The New England Journal of Medicine, 390*(13), 1176–1185. DOI: 10.1056/NEJMOA231232

Mestre, T. A., Stebbins, G. T., Stephenson, D., Dexter, D., Lee, K. K., Xiao, Y., Dam, T., Kopil, C. M., & Simuni, T. (2024). Patient-centered development of clinical outcome assessments in early Parkinson disease: key priorities and advances. *Npj Parkinson's Disease 2024 10:1, 10*(1), 101-. https://doi.org/DOI: 10.1038/s41531-024-00716-z

Migdalska-Richards, A., Daly, L., Bezard, E., & Schapira, A. H. V. (2016). Ambroxol effects in glucocerebrosidase and α-synuclein transgenic mice. *Annals of Neurology, 80*(5), 766–775. DOI: 10.1002/ANA.24790

Mishra, B., Sudheer, P., Rajan, R., Agarwal, A., Srivastava, M. V. P., Nilima, N., & Vishnu, V. Y. (2024). Bridging the gap between statistical significance and clinical relevance: A systematic review of minimum clinically important difference (MCID) thresholds of scales reported in movement disorders research. *Heliyon, 10*(5). Advance online publication. DOI: 10.1016/j.heliyon.2024.e26479

Mortberg, M. A., Vallabh, S. M., & Minikel, E. V. (2022). Disease stages and therapeutic hypotheses in two decades of neurodegenerative disease clinical trials. *Scientific Reports, 12*(1), 17708. DOI: 10.1038/S41598-022-21820-1

Mortiboys, H., Furmston, R., Bronstad, G., Aasly, J., Elliott, C., & Bandmann, O. (2015). UDCA exerts beneficial effect on mitochondrial dysfunction in LRRK2 G2019S carriers and in vivo. *Neurology, 85*(10), 846–852. DOI: 10.1212/WNL.0000000000001905

Mullin, S., Smith, L., Lee, K., D'Souza, G., Woodgate, P., Elflein, J., Hällqvist, J., Toffoli, M., Streeter, A., Hosking, J., Heywood, W. E., Khengar, R., Campbell, P., Hehir, J., Cable, S., Mills, K., Zetterberg, H., Limousin, P., Libri, V., & Schapira, A. H. V. (2020). Ambroxol for the Treatment of Patients With Parkinson Disease With and Without Glucocerebrosidase Gene Mutations: A Nonrandomized, Noncontrolled Trial. *JAMA Neurology, 77*(4), 427–434. DOI: 10.1001/JAMANEUROL.2019.4611

Nalls, M. A., Blauwendraat, C., Vallerga, C. L., Heilbron, K., Bandres-Ciga, S., Chang, D., Tan, M., Kia, D. A., Noyce, A. J., Xue, A., Bras, J., Young, E., von Coelln, R., Simón-Sánchez, J., Schulte, C., Sharma, M., Krohn, L., Pihlstrøm, L., Siitonen, A., & Zhang, F. (2019). Identification of novel risk loci, causal insights, and heritable risk for Parkinson's disease: A meta-analysis of genome-wide association studies. *Lancet Neurology*, *18*(12), 1091–1102. DOI: 10.1016/S1474-4422(19)30320-5

O'Shea, D. M., Arkhipenko, A., Galasko, D., Goldman, J. G., Sheikh, Z. H., Petrides, G., Toledo, J. B., & Galvin, J. E. (2024). Practical use of DAT SPECT imaging in diagnosing dementia with Lewy bodies: A US perspective of current guidelines and future directions. *Frontiers in Neurology*, *15*, 1395413. DOI: 10.3389/FNEUR.2024.1395413

Oertel, W., Eggert, K., Pahwa, R., Tanner, C. M., Hauser, R. A., Trenkwalder, C., Ehret, R., Azulay, J. P., Isaacson, S., Felt, L., & Stempien, M. J. (2017). Randomized, placebo-controlled trial of ADS-5102 (amantadine) extended-release capsules for levodopa-induced dyskinesia in Parkinson's disease (EASE LID 3). *Movement Disorders*, *32*(12), 1701–1709. DOI: 10.1002/MDS.2713

Ofori, E., Pasternak, O., Planetta, P. J., Burciu, R., Snyder, A., Febo, M., Golde, T. E., Okun, M. S., & Vaillancourt, D. E. (2015a). Increased free water in the substantia nigra of Parkinson's disease: A single-site and multi-site study. *Neurobiology of Aging*, *36*(2), 1097–1104. DOI: 10.1016/j.neurobiolaging.2014.10.029

Ofori, E., Pasternak, O., Planetta, P. J., Burciu, R., Snyder, A., Febo, M., Golde, T. E., Okun, M. S., & Vaillancourt, D. E. (2015b). Increased free water in the substantia nigra of Parkinson's disease: A single-site and multi-site study. *Neurobiology of Aging*, *36*(2), 1097–1104. DOI: 10.1016/J.NEUROBIOLAGING.2014.10.029

Okuzumi, A., Hatano, T., Matsumoto, G., Nojiri, S., Ueno, S. ichi, Imamichi-Tatano, Y., Kimura, H., Kakuta, S., Kondo, A., Fukuhara, T., Li, Y., Funayama, M., Saiki, S., Taniguchi, D., Tsunemi, T., McIntyre, D., Gérardy, J. J., Mittelbronn, M., Kruger, R., … Hattori, N. (2023). Propagative α-synuclein seeds as serum biomarkers for synucleinopathies. *Nature Medicine 2023 29:6*, *29*(6), 1448–1455. https://doi.org/ DOI: 10.1038/s41591-023-02358-9

Olanow, C. W., Kieburtz, K., Odin, P., Espay, A. J., Standaert, D. G., Fernandez, H. H., Vanagunas, A., Othman, A. A., Widnell, K. L., Robieson, W. Z., Pritchett, Y., Chatamra, K., Benesh, J., Lenz, R. A., & Antonini, A. (2014). Continuous intrajejunal infusion of levodopa-carbidopa intestinal gel for patients with advanced Parkinson's disease: A randomised, controlled, double-blind, double-dummy study. *Lancet Neurology*, *13*(2), 141–149. DOI: 10.1016/S1474-4422(13)70293-X

Olanow, C. W., Rascol, O., Hauser, R., Feigin, P. D., Jankovic, J., Lang, A., Langston, W., Melamed, E., Poewe, W., Stocchi, F., & Tolosa, E. (2009a). A double-blind, delayed-start trial of rasagiline in Parkinson's disease. *The New England Journal of Medicine, 361*(13), 1268–1278. DOI: 10.1056/NEJMOA0809335

Olanow, C. W., Rascol, O., Hauser, R., Feigin, P. D., Jankovic, J., Lang, A., Langston, W., Melamed, E., Poewe, W., Stocchi, F., & Tolosa, E. (2009b). A double-blind, delayed-start trial of rasagiline in Parkinson's disease. *The New England Journal of Medicine, 361*(13), 1268–1278. DOI: 10.1056/NEJMOA0809335

Orgogozo, J. M., Gilman, S., Dartigues, J. F., Laurent, B., Puel, M., Kirby, L. C., Jouanny, P., Dubois, B., Eisner, L., Flitman, S., Michel, B. F., Boada, M., Frank, A., & Hock, C. (2003). Subacute meningoencephalitis in a subset of patients with AD after Aβ42 immunization. *Neurology, 61*(1), 46–54. DOI: 10.1212/01.WNL.0000073623.84

Pagano, G., Taylor, K. I., Anzures-Cabrera, J., Marchesi, M., Simuni, T., Marek, K., Postuma, R. B., Pavese, N., Stocchi, F., Azulay, J.-P., Mollenhauer, B., López-Manzanares, L., Russell, D. S., Boyd, J. T., Nicholas, A. P., Luquin, M. R., Hauser, R. A., Gasser, T., Poewe, W., & Bonni, A. (2022). Trial of Prasinezumab in Early-Stage Parkinson's Disease. *The New England Journal of Medicine, 387*(5), 421–432. DOI: 10.1056/NEJMOA2202867

Pahwa, R., Tanner, C. M., Hauser, R. A., Isaacson, S. H., Nausieda, P. A., Truong, D. D., Agarwal, P., Hull, K. L., Lyons, K. E., Johnson, R., & Stempien, M. J. (2017). ADS-5102 (Amantadine) Extended-Release Capsules for Levodopa-Induced Dyskinesia in Parkinson Disease (EASE LID Study): A Randomized Clinical Trial. *JAMA Neurology, 74*(8), 941–949. DOI: 10.1001/JAMANEUROL.2017.0943

Palermo, G., Giannoni, S., Bellini, G., Siciliano, G., & Ceravolo, R. (2021). Dopamine Transporter Imaging, Current Status of a Potential Biomarker: A Comprehensive Review. *International Journal of Molecular Sciences 2021, Vol. 22, Page 11234, 22*(20), 11234. https://doi.org/DOI: 10.3390/IJMS222011234

Perepezko, K., Hinkle, J. T., Forbes, E. J., Pontone, G. M., Mills, K. A., & Gallo, J. J. (2023). The impact of caregiving on quality of life in Parkinson's disease: A systematic review. *International Journal of Geriatric Psychiatry, 38*(1), e5870. DOI: 10.1002/GPS.5870

Poewe, W., Seppi, K., Tanner, C. M., Halliday, G. M., Brundin, P., Volkmann, J., Schrag, A. E., & Lang, A. E. (2017). Parkinson disease. *Nature Reviews. Disease Primers, 3*, 1–21. DOI: 10.1038/NRDP.2017.13

Politis, M. (2014). Neuroimaging in Parkinson disease: From research setting to clinical practice. *Nature Reviews. Neurology, 10*(12), 708–722. DOI: 10.1038/NRNEUROL.2014.205

Postuma, R. B., Berg, D., Stern, M., Poewe, W., Olanow, C. W., Oertel, W., Obeso, J., Marek, K., Litvan, I., Lang, A. E., Halliday, G., Goetz, C. G., Gasser, T., Dubois, B., Chan, P., Bloem, B. R., Adler, C. H., & Deuschl, G. (2015). MDS clinical diagnostic criteria for Parkinson's disease. *Movement Disorders, 30*(12), 1591–1601. DOI: 10.1002/MDS.26424

Postuma, R. B., Iranzo, A., Hu, M., Högl, B., Boeve, B. F., Manni, R., Oertel, W. H., Arnulf, I., Ferini-Strambi, L., Puligheddu, M., Antelmi, E., Cochen De Cock, V., Arnaldi, D., Mollenhauer, B., Videnovic, A., Sonka, K., Jung, K. Y., Kunz, D., Dauvilliers, Y., & Pelletier, A. (2019). Risk and predictors of dementia and parkinsonism in idiopathic REM sleep behaviour disorder: A multicentre study. *Brain, 142*(3), 744–759. DOI: 10.1093/BRAIN/AWZ030

Price, D. L., Koike, M. A., Khan, A., Wrasidlo, W., Rockenstein, E., Masliah, E., & Bonhaus, D. (2018). The small molecule alpha-synuclein misfolding inhibitor, NPT200-11, produces multiple benefits in an animal model of Parkinson's disease. *Scientific Reports 2018 8:1, 8*(1), 16165-. https://doi.org/DOI: 10.1038/s41598-018-34490-9

Rabinak, C. A., & Nirenberg, M. J. (2010). Dopamine Agonist Withdrawal Syndrome in Parkinson Disease. *Archives of Neurology, 67*(1), 58–63. DOI: 10.1001/ARCHNEUROL.2009.294

Ramanzini, L. G., Frare, J. M., Camargo, L. F. M., Silveira, J. O. F., & Jankovic, J. (2024). Does Delaying Levodopa Prevent Motor Complications in Parkinson's Disease? A Meta-Analysis. *Movement Disorders Clinical Practice, 11*(10), 1195–1202. DOI: 10.1002/MDC3.14198

Rascol, O. (2009). "disease-modification" trials in Parkinson disease: Target populations, endpoints and study design. *Neurology, 72*(7, SUPPL. 2), S51–S58. DOI: 10.1212/WNL.0B013E318199049E

Rasiah, N. P., Maheshwary, R., Kwon, C. S., Bloomstein, J. D., & Girgis, F. (2023). Complications of Deep Brain Stimulation for Parkinson Disease and Relationship between Micro-electrode tracks and hemorrhage: Systematic Review and Meta-Analysis. *World Neurosurgery, 171*, e8–e23. DOI: 10.1016/j.wneu.2022.10.034

Ravina, B., Kieburtz, K., Tilley, B., Shannon, K., Tanner, C., Frederick Wooten, G., Racette, B., Deppen, P., Dewey, R. B., Hayward, B., Scott, B., Field, J., Carter, J., Brodsky, M., Andrews, P., Manyam, B., Whetteckey, J., Rao, J., Cook, M., & Fagan, S. (2006). A randomized, double-blind, futility clinical trial of creatine and minocycline in early Parkinson disease. *Neurology*, *66*(5), 664–671. DOI: 10.1212/01.WNL.0000201252.57661.E1

Ray Dorsey, E., Elbaz, A., Nichols, E., Abd-Allah, F., Abdelalim, A., Adsuar, J. C., Ansha, M. G., Brayne, C., Choi, J. Y. J., Collado-Mateo, D., Dahodwala, N., Do, H. P., Edessa, D., Endres, M., Fereshtehnejad, S. M., Foreman, K. J., Gankpe, F. G., Gupta, R., Hankey, G. J., & Murray, C. J. L. (2018). Global, regional, and national burden of Parkinson's disease, 1990–2016: A systematic analysis for the Global Burden of Disease Study 2016. *Lancet Neurology*, *17*(11), 939–953. DOI: 10.1016/S1474-4422(18)30295-3

Richard, I. H., McDermott, M. P., Kurlan, R., Lyness, J. M., Como, P. G., Pearson, N., Factor, S. A., Juncos, J., Ramos, C. S., Brodsky, M., Manning, C., Marsh, L., Shulman, L., Fernandez, H. H., Black, K. J., Panisset, M., Christine, C. W., Jiang, W., Singer, C., & McDonald, W. (2012). A randomized, double-blind, placebo-controlled trial of antidepressants in Parkinson disease. *Neurology*, *78*(16), 1229–1236. DOI: 10.1212/WNL.0B013E318251624

Romano, S., Savva, G. M., Bedarf, J. R., Charles, I. G., Hildebrand, F., & Narbad, A. (2021). Meta-analysis of the Parkinson's disease gut microbiome suggests alterations linked to intestinal inflammation. *Npj Parkinson's Disease 2021 7:1, 7*(1), 27-. https://doi.org/DOI: 10.1038/s41531-021-00156-z

Sasidharan, A., Bagepally, B. S., & Kumar, S. S. (2024). Cost Effectiveness of Deep Brain Stimulation for Parkinson's Disease: A Systematic Review. *Applied Health Economics and Health Policy*, *22*(2), 181–192. DOI: 10.1007/S40258-023-00848-Y

Schalkamp, A. K., Harrison, N. A., Peall, K. J., & Sandor, C. (2024). Digital outcome measures from smartwatch data relate to non-motor features of Parkinson's disease. *Npj Parkinson's Disease 2024 10:1, 10*(1), 110-. https://doi.org/DOI: 10.1038/s41531-024-00719-w

Schneider, M. G., Swearingen, C. J., Shulman, L. M., Ye, J., Baumgarten, M., & Tilley, B. C. (2009). Minority enrollment in Parkinson's disease clinical trials. *Parkinsonism & Related Disorders*, *15*(4), 258–262. DOI: 10.1016/j.parkreldis.2008.06.005

Schöndorf, D. C., Ivanyuk, D., Baden, P., Sanchez-Martinez, A., De Cicco, S., Yu, C., Giunta, I., Schwarz, L. K., Di Napoli, G., Panagiotakopoulou, V., Nestel, S., Keatinge, M., Pruszak, J., Bandmann, O., Heimrich, B., Gasser, T., Whitworth, A. J., & Deleidi, M. (2018). The NAD+ Precursor Nicotinamide Riboside Rescues Mitochondrial Defects and Neuronal Loss in iPSC and Fly Models of Parkinson's Disease. *Cell Reports*, *23*(10), 2976–2988. DOI: 10.1016/j.celrep.2018.05.009

Schrag, A., Sampaio, C., Counsell, N., & Poewe, W. (2006). Minimal clinically important change on the Unified Parkinson's Disease Rating Scale. *Movement Disorders*, *21*(8), 1200–1207. DOI: 10.1002/MDS.20914

Schweitzer, J. S., Song, B., Herrington, T. M., Park, T.-Y., Lee, N., Ko, S., Jeon, J., Cha, Y., Kim, K., Li, Q., Henchcliffe, C., Kaplitt, M., Neff, C., Rapalino, O., Seo, H., Lee, I.-H., Kim, J., Kim, T., Petsko, G. A., & Kim, K.-S. (2020). Personalized iPSC-Derived Dopamine Progenitor Cells for Parkinson's Disease. *The New England Journal of Medicine*, *382*(20), 1926–1932. DOI: 10.1056/NEJMOA1915872

Siderowf, A., Concha-Marambio, L., Lafontant, D. E., Farris, C. M., Ma, Y., Urenia, P. A., Nguyen, H., Alcalay, R. N., Chahine, L. M., Foroud, T., Galasko, D., Kieburtz, K., Merchant, K., Mollenhauer, B., Poston, K. L., Seibyl, J., Simuni, T., Tanner, C. M., Weintraub, D., & Soto, C. (2023). Assessment of heterogeneity among participants in the Parkinson's Progression Markers Initiative cohort using α-synuclein seed amplification: A cross-sectional study. *Lancet Neurology*, *22*(5), 407–417. DOI: 10.1016/S1474-4422(23)00109-6

Simuni, T., Siderowf, A., Lasch, S., Coffey, C. S., Caspell-Garcia, C., Jennings, D., Tanner, C. M., Trojanowski, J. Q., Shaw, L. M., Seibyl, J., Schuff, N., Singleton, A., Kieburtz, K., Toga, A. W., Mollenhauer, B., Galasko, D., Chahine, L. M., Weintraub, D., Foroud, T., & Marek, K. (2018). Longitudinal Change of Clinical and Biological Measures in Early Parkinson's Disease: Parkinson's Progression Markers Initiative Cohort. *Movement Disorders*, *33*(5), 771–782. DOI: 10.1002/MDS.27361

Steendam-Oldekamp, E., & Van Laar, T. (2024). The Effectiveness of Inpatient Rehabilitation in Parkinson's Disease: A Systematic Review of Recent Studies. *Journal of Parkinson's Disease*, *14*(Suppl 1), S93. DOI: 10.3233/JPD-230271

Sturchio, A., Rocha, E. M., Kauffman, M. A., Marsili, L., Mahajan, A., Saraf, A. A., Vizcarra, J. A., Guo, Z., & Espay, A. J. (2024). Recalibrating the Why and Whom of Animal Models in Parkinson Disease: A Clinician's Perspective. *Brain Sciences 2024, Vol. 14,14*(2). https://doi.org/DOI: 10.3390/BRAINSCI14020151

Sun, Y. M., Wang, Z. Y., Liang, Y. Y., Hao, C. W., & Shi, C. H. (2024). Digital biomarkers for precision diagnosis and monitoring in Parkinson's disease. *Npj Digital Medicine 2024 7:1, 7*(1), 218-. https://doi.org/DOI: 10.1038/s41746-024-01217-2

Surmeier, J., Obeso, J. A., Halliday, G. M., Brundin, P., & Melki, R. (2017). Prying into the Prion Hypothesis for Parkinson's Disease. *The Journal of Neuroscience : The Official Journal of the Society for Neuroscience, 37*(41), 9808–9818. DOI: 10.1523/JNEUROSCI.1788-16.2017

Takahashi, K., & Yamanaka, S. (2006). Induction of Pluripotent Stem Cells from Mouse Embryonic and Adult Fibroblast Cultures by Defined Factors. *Cell, 126*(4), 663–676. DOI: 10.1016/j.cell.2006.07.024

Tolosa, E., Vila, M., Klein, C., & Rascol, O. (2020). LRRK2 in Parkinson disease: challenges of clinical trials. *Nature Reviews Neurology 2020 16:2, 16*(2), 97–107. https://doi.org/DOI: 10.1038/s41582-019-0301-2

Trinh, J., Farrer, M., Ross, O. A., & Guella, I. (2025). LRRK2-Related Parkinson Disease. *GeneReviews®*. https://www.ncbi.nlm.nih.gov/books/NBK1208/

Tu, X. J., Hwang, W. J., Hsu, S. P., & Ma, H. I. (2017). Responsiveness of the short-form health survey and the Parkinson's disease questionnaire in patients with Parkinson's disease. *Health and Quality of Life Outcomes, 15*(1), 75. DOI: 10.1186/S12955-017-0642-8

Turcano, P., Mielke, M. M., Bower, J. H., Parisi, J. E., Cutsforth-Gregory, J. K., Ahlskog, J. E., & Savica, R. (2018). Levodopa-induced dyskinesia in Parkinson disease. *Neurology, 91*(24), e2238–e2243. DOI: 10.1212/WNL.0000000000006643

Turner, M. R., Thompson, A. G., & Teunissen, C. E. (2025). Blood level of neurofilament light chain as a biomarker for neurological disorders. *BMJ Medicine, 4*(1), e000958. DOI: 10.1136/BMJMED-2024-000958

Vaswani, P. A., Tropea, T. F., & Dahodwala, N. (2020). Overcoming Barriers to Parkinson Disease Trial Participation: Increasing Diversity and Novel Designs for Recruitment and Retention. *Neurotherapeutics; the Journal of the American Society for Experimental NeuroTherapeutics, 17*(4), 1724–1735. DOI: 10.1007/S13311-020-00960-0

Velseboer, D. C., de Haan, R. J., Wieling, W., Goldstein, D. S., & de Bie, R. M. A. (2011). Prevalence of orthostatic hypotension in Parkinson's disease: A systematic review and meta-analysis. *Parkinsonism & Related Disorders, 17*(10), 724–729. DOI: 10.1016/j.parkreldis.2011.04.016

Wagner, J., Ryazanov, S., Leonov, A., Levin, J., Shi, S., Schmidt, F., Prix, C., Pan-Montojo, F., Bertsch, U., Mitteregger-Kretzschmar, G., Geissen, M., Eiden, M., Leidel, F., Hirschberger, T., Deeg, A. A., Krauth, J. J., Zinth, W., Tavan, P., Pilger, J., … Giese, A. (2013). Anle138b: a novel oligomer modulator for disease-modifying therapy of neurodegenerative diseases such as prion and Parkinson's disease. *Acta Neuropathologica 2013 125:6, 125*(6), 795–813. https://doi.org/DOI: 10.1007/S00401-013-1114-9

Wang, C., & Ren, J. (2024). Ultrasound blood–brain barrier opening: A new era of treatment for Alzheimer's disease? *Aging Medicine (Milton, N.S.W.), 7*(6), 673–675. DOI: 10.1002/AGM2.12371

Weintraub, D., Koester, J., Potenza, M. N., Siderowf, A. D., Stacy, M., Voon, V., Whetteckey, J., Wunderlich, G. R., & Lang, A. E. (2010). Impulse Control Disorders in Parkinson Disease: A Cross-Sectional Study of 3090 Patients. *Archives of Neurology, 67*(5), 589–595. DOI: 10.1001/ARCHNEUROL.2010.65

Weise, D., Claus, I., Dresel, C., Kalbe, E., Liepelt-Scarfone, I., Lorenzl, S., Redecker, C., & Urban, P. P. (2024a). Multidisciplinary care in Parkinson's disease. *Journal of Neural Transmission (Vienna, Austria), 131*(10), 1217. DOI: 10.1007/S00702-024-02807-W

Weise, D., Claus, I., Dresel, C., Kalbe, E., Liepelt-Scarfone, I., Lorenzl, S., Redecker, C., & Urban, P. P. (2024b). Multidisciplinary care in Parkinson's disease. *Journal of Neural Transmission (Vienna, Austria), 131*(10), 1217. DOI: 10.1007/S00702-024-02807-W

Wijers, A., Ravi, A., Evers, S. M. A. A., Tissingh, G., & van Mastrigt, G. A. P. G. (2024). Systematic Review of the Cost of Illness of Parkinson's Disease from a Societal Perspective. *Movement Disorders, 39*(11), 1938–1951. DOI: 10.1002/MDS.29995

Wu, D., Chen, Q., Chen, X., Han, F., Chen, Z., & Wang, Y. (2023). The blood–brain barrier: structure, regulation, and drug delivery. *Signal Transduction and Targeted Therapy, 8*(1), 217-. https://doi.org/DOI: 10.1038/S41392-023-01481

Wu, S., & Schekman, R. W. (2024). Intercellular transmission of alpha-synuclein. *Frontiers in Molecular Neuroscience, 17*, 1470171. DOI: 10.3389/FNMOL.2024.1470171

Wyse, R. K., Isaacs, T., Barker, R. A., Cookson, M. R., Dawson, T. M., Devos, D., Dexter, D. T., Duffen, J., Federoff, H., Fiske, B., Foltynie, T., Fox, S., Greenamyre, J. T., Kieburtz, K., Kordower, J. H., Krainc, D., Matthews, H., Moore, D. J., Mursaleen, L., & Brundin, P. (2024). Twelve Years of Drug Prioritization to Help Accelerate Disease Modification Trials in Parkinson's Disease: The International Linked Clinical Trials Initiative. *Journal of Parkinson's Disease*, *14*(4), 657–666. DOI: 10.3233/JPD-230363

Xie, Y. X., Naseri, N. N., Fels, J., Kharel, P., Na, Y., Lane, D., Burré, J., & Sharma, M. (2022). Lysosomal exocytosis releases pathogenic α-synuclein species from neurons in synucleinopathy models. *Nature Communications 2022 13:1*, *13*(1), 4918-. https://doi.org/DOI: 10.1038/s41467-022-32625-1

Zhan, A., Mohan, S., Tarolli, C., Schneider, R. B., Adams, J. L., Sharma, S., Elson, M. J., Spear, K. L., Glidden, A. M., Little, M. A., Terzis, A., Ray Dorsey, E., & Saria, S. (2018). Using Smartphones and Machine Learning to Quantify Parkinson Disease Severity: The Mobile Parkinson Disease Score. *JAMA Neurology*, *75*(7), 876–880. DOI: 10.1001/JAMANEUROL.2018.0809

Zhao, Z. H., Chen, Z. T., Zhou, R. L., Zhang, X., Ye, Q. Y., & Wang, Y. Z. (2019). Increased DJ-1 and α-Synuclein in Plasma Neural-Derived Exosomes as Potential Markers for Parkinson's Disease. *Frontiers in Aging Neuroscience*, *10*(JAN), 438. DOI: 10.3389/FNAGI.2018.00438

Compilation of References

Aarsland, D., Andersen, K., Larsen, J. P., Lolk, A., & Kragh-Sørensen, P. (2003). Prevalence and characteristics of dementia in Parkinson disease: An 8-year prospective study. *Archives of Neurology*, *60*(3), 387–392. PMID: 12633150

Aarsland, D., Brønnick, K., Larsen, J. P., & Alves, G. (2021). Parkinson disease-associated cognitive impairment. *Nature Reviews. Disease Primers*, *7*, 61.

Aarsland, D., Creese, B., Politis, M., Chaudhuri, K. R., Ffytche, D. H., Weintraub, D., & Ballard, C. (2017). Cognitive decline in Parkinson disease. *Nature Reviews. Neurology*, *13*(4), 217–231. DOI: 10.1038/NRNEUROL.2017.27

Abbaszadeh, H., Ghorbani, F., Derakhshani, M., Movassaghpour, A., & Yousefi, M. (2020). Human umbilical cord mesenchymal stem cell-derived extracellular vesicles: A novel therapeutic paradigm. *Journal of Cellular Physiology*, *235*(2), 706–717. PMID: 31254289

Abbott, A. (2010). Levodopa: The story so far. *Nature*, *466*(7310), S6–S7. PMID: 20739934

Abdel-Bari, S. H., Amer, H., Ayoub, B. M., & Kamel, R. (2021). Surgical management of Parkinson's disease: The role of lesioning procedures in developing countries in the modern era. *Open Access Macedonian Journal of Medical Sciences*, *9*, 1241. DOI: 10.3889/oamjms.2021.6649

Adams, J. L., Dinesh, K., Snyder, C. W., Xiong, M., Tarolli, C. G., Sharma, S., Dorsey, E. R., & Sharma, G. (2021). A real-world study of wearable sensors in Parkinson's disease. *NPJ Parkinson's Disease*, *7*(1). Advance online publication. DOI: 10.1038/s41531-021-00248-w PMID: 34845224

Adams, J. L., Kangarloo, T., Gong, Y., Khachadourian, V., Tracey, B., Volfson, D., Latzman, R. D., Cosman, J., Edgerton, J., Anderson, D., Best, A., Kostrzebski, M. A., Auinger, P., Wilmot, P., Pohlson, Y., Jensen-Roberts, S., Müller, M. L. T. M., Stephenson, D., Dorsey, E. R., & Botting, E. (2024). Using a smartwatch and smartphone to assess early Parkinson's disease in the WATCH-PD study over 12 months. *NPJ Parkinson's Disease, 10*(1), 112. DOI: 10.1038/S41531-024-00721-2

Adelson, P. D., Bratton, S. L., Carney, N., Chesnut, R. M., du Coudray, H. E. M., & Goldstein, B.. (2003). Chapter 1: Introduction. *Pediatric Critical Care Medicine, 4*. Advance online publication. DOI: 10.1097/01.ccm.0000066600.71233.01 PMID: 12847337

Adetunji, C. O., Olaniyan, O. T., Adeyomoye, O., Dare, A., Adeniyi, M. J., & Alex, E. (2022a). *Classification of neurodegenerative disorders using machine learning techniques. In book: ARTIFICIAL INTELLIGENCE FOR NEUROLOGICAL DISORDERS. Publisher*. Elsevier., DOI: 10.1016/B978-0-323-90277-9.00028-6

Adetunji, C. O., Olaniyan, O. T., Adeyomoye, O., Dare, A., Adeniyi, M. J., & Alex, E. (2022b). *An intelligent diagnostic approach for epileptic seizure detection and classification using machine learning. In book: ARTIFICIAL INTELLIGENCE FOR NEUROLOGICAL DISORDERS. Publisher*. Elsevier., DOI: 10.1016/B978-0-323-90277-9.00011-0

Agapov, S. N., Bulanov, V. A., Zakharov, A. V., & Sergeeva, M. S. (2017). Comparison of classifiers in the tasks of the single-trial vep classification. *Zhurnal Vysshei Nervnoi Deyatelnosti Imeni IP Pavlova, 67*(4), Article 4.

Agarwal, D., Sandor, C., Volpato, V., Caffrey, T. M., Monzón-Sandoval, J., Bowden, R., Alegre-Abarrategui, J., Wade-Martins, R., & Webber, C. (2020). A single-cell atlas of the human substantia nigra reveals cell-specific pathways associated with neurological disorders. *Nature Communications, 11*(1), 4183. DOI: 10.1038/S41467-020-17876-0

Ahlskog, J. E., & Muenter, M. D. (2001). Frequency of levodopa-related dyskinesias and motor fluctuations as estimated from the cumulative literature. *Movement Disorders, 16*(3), 448–458. DOI: 10.1002/MDS.1090;WGROUP:STRING:PUBLICATION

Ajagun, E. J., Asuku, A. O., Ayinla, M. T., Abdulsalam, T. A., Ajibare, A. J., Olajide, T. S., Hamza, Y. O., & Ganiyu, K. O. (2024). Pharmacotherapy of Parkinson's Disease and their Limitations. In: Zebrafish as a Model for Parkinson's Disease. Taylor and Francis, CRC, https://doi.org/DOI: 10.1201/9781003402893-17

Ajagun, E. J., Asuku, A. O., Oyerinde, T. O., Sangodipe, H. A., Sanusi, W., Jayeoba, L. A., & Abdulsalam, T. A. (2024). The Ketogenic Diet and Stroke. In *Nutrition and Stroke. Nutritional Neuroscience*. Springer., DOI: 10.1007/978-981-97-6818-9¬¬_10

Ajibare, A. J., Akintoye, O. O., Aransi-Ola, K. T., Adejumo, M. O., Folarin, E. O. A., & Asuku, A. O. (2026). Nanoformulations of Plant Compounds for Metabolic Syndrome: A Multitarget Approach. In Gosh, V., Bhardwaj, A. K., & Maddela, N. R. (Eds.), *Applications of Plant Bioactive Compounds-Based Nanoformulations. Nanotechnology in the Life Sciences*. Springer., DOI: 10.1007/978-3-032-13086-0_17

Akinyemi, R. O., & Owolabi, M. O. (2023). Neurology in Africa: Bridging the gap between burden and resources. *The Lancet. Global Health, 11*(7), e1125–e1134. PMID: 37349038

Alassaf, Y. (2024). Comprehensive review of the advancements, benefits, challenges, and design integration of energy-efficient materials for sustainable buildings. *Buildings (Basel, Switzerland), 14*(9), 2994.

Albin, R. L., Young, A. B., & Penney, J. B. (1989). The functional anatomy of basal ganglia disorders. *Trends in Neurosciences, 12*(10), 366–375. PMID: 2479133

Alcalay, R. N., Levy, O. A., Waters, C. C., Fahn, S., Ford, B., Kuo, S. H., Mazzoni, P., Pauciulo, M. W., Nichols, W. C., Gan-Or, Z., Rouleau, G. A., Chung, W. K., Wolf, P., Oliva, P., Keutzer, J., Marder, K., & Zhang, X. (2015). Glucocerebrosidase activity in Parkinson's disease with and without GBA mutations. *Brain, 138*(Pt 9), 2648–2658. DOI: 10.1093/BRAIN/AWV179

Alcantud, J. C. R., & Santos-García, G. (2017). A new criterion for soft set based decision problems under incomplete information. *International Journal of Computational Intelligence Systems, 10*(1), 394–404.

Ali, M. I., Feng, F., Liu, X., Min, W. K., & Shabir, M. (2009). On some new operations in soft set theory. *Computers & Mathematics with Applications (Oxford, England), 57*(9), 1547–1553.

Al-Jaber, H., Biswas, K. H., & Al-Mansoori, L. (2025). Advancing targeted therapy for colorectal cancer: Harnessing ligand-directed enzyme prodrug therapy for highly specific interventions. *Frontiers in Oncology, 15*. Advance online publication. DOI: 10.3389/fonc.2025.1570712 PMID: 40510154

Antonini, A., Benti, R., De Notaris, R., Tesei, S., Zecchinelli, A., Sacilotto, G., Meucci, N., Canesi, M., Mariani, C., Pezzoli, G., & Gerundini, P. (2003). 123I-Ioflupane/SPECT binding to striatal dopamine transporter (DAT) uptake in patients with Parkinson's disease, multiple system atrophy, and progressive supranuclear palsy. *Neurological Sciences, 24*(3), 149–150. DOI: 10.1007/s10072-003-0103-5 PMID: 14598060

Antonini, A., De Notaris, R., Benti, R., De Gaspari, D., & Pezzoli, G. (2001). Perfusion ECD/SPECT in the characterization of cognitive deficits in Parkinson's disease. *Neurological Sciences, 22*(1), 45–46. DOI: 10.1007/s100720170039 PMID: 11487194

Aquino, C. C., & Fox, S. H. (2015). Clinical spectrum of levodopa-induced complications. *Movement Disorders, 30*(1), 80–89. DOI: 10.1002/MDS.26125

Armstrong, M. J., Litvan, I., Lang, A. E., Bak, T. H., Bhatia, K. P., Borroni, B., Boxer, A. L., Dickson, D. W., Grossman, M., Hallett, M., Josephs, K. A., Kertesz, A., Lee, S. E., Miller, B. L., Reich, S. G., Riley, D. E., Tolosa, E., Tröster, A. I., Vidailhet, M., & Weiner, W. J. (2013). Criteria for the diagnosis of corticobasal degeneration. *Neurology, 80*(5), 496–503. DOI: 10.1212/WNL.0b013e31827f0fd1 PMID: 23359374

Armstrong, M. J., & Okun, M. S. (2020). Diagnosis and treatment of Parkinson disease: A review. *Journal of the American Medical Association, 323*(6), 548–560. PMID: 32044947

Arya, R., Haque, A. A., Shakya, H., Billah, M. M., Parvin, A., Rahman, M. M., Sakib, K. M., Faruquee, H. M., Kumar, V., & Kim, J. J. (2024). Parkinson's disease: Biomarkers for diagnosis and disease progression. *International Journal of Molecular Sciences, 25*(22), 12379. PMID: 39596444

Asci, F., Vivacqua, G., Zampogna, A., D'onofrio, V., Mazzeo, A., & Suppa, A. (2022). Wearable Electrochemical Sensors in Parkinson's Disease. *Sensors (Basel), 22*(3). Advance online publication. DOI: 10.3390/s22030951 PMID: 35161694

Asija, S., Pahwa, B., Agarwal, A., Patil, Y., & Chaurasia, B. (2024). Status of functional neurosurgery in lower middle-income countries (LMICs): A multinational cross sectional survey based analysis of exposure, utilization and perceived barriers. *Clinical Neurology and Neurosurgery, 245*, 108411. PMID: 39089202

Aslam, S., Sharrief, A. Z., Holden, S. K., Fullard, M., Holtrop, J. S., Maw, A. M., & Amara, A. W. (2025). The future of Parkinson's care: A need to expand access. *Frontiers in Neurology, 16*, 1622283. PMID: 40612798

Asuku A.O., Adeyemo M.B., Adeyemo R.O., Agoro S.A., Odugbesan O.A., & Ayoola S.A. (2022). Applications of stem cell therapy in neurodegenerative diseases. European Journal of Biotechnology and Bioscience. 10 (2): 17-24, 2321-9122

Asuku, A. O., Ayinla, M. T., Olajide, T. S., Ajagun, E. J., Ganiyu, K. O., Hamza, Y. O., Ajibare, A. J., & Abdulsalam, T. A. (2024). Diagnosis and Biomarkers of Parkinson's Disease. In: Zebrafish as a Model for Parkinson's Disease. Taylor and Francis, CRC, https://doi.org/DOI: 10.1201/9781003402893-15

Asuku, A. O., Ajagun, E. J., & Oyinlola Ogungbangbe, G. (2025b). *Non-Pharmacological Interventions for Dementia: A Comprehensive Approach* (1st ed.). CRC Press., DOI: 10.1201/9781003516033

Asuku, A. O., Ayinla, M. T., Aransiola, S. A., Ajibare, A. J., Adeyemo, M. B., & Adeyemo, R. O. (2024). Chitosan-Based Nanoparticles to bypass the Blood-Brain Barrier for the Treatment of Neurological Diseases: A Review. *Pakistan Journal of Medical Sciences*, *25*(1), 2072–1625.

Asuku, A. O., Ayinla, M. T., Olajide, T. S., Oyerinde, T. O., Yusuf, J. A., Bayo-Olugbami, A. A., & Fajemidagba, G. A. (2024). Coffee and Parkinson's disease. In. Progress in Brain Research: Vol. 289. *Neuroscience of Coffee*. Elsevier., DOI: 10.1016/bs.pbr.2024.06.001

Asuku, A. O., Ogungbangbe, G. O., & Fajemidagba, G. A. (2025). Gene therapy for Parkinson's disease: A new frontier in neurodegenerative diseases. *Exploration of Neuroprotective Therapy*, *5*, 1004119. DOI: 10.37349/ent.2025.1004119

Atewologun, F. A., Okesanya, O. J., Okon, I. I., Kayode, H. H., Ukoaka, B. M., Olaleke, N. O., Ogaya, J. B., Okikiola, L. A., Manirambona, E., & Lucero-Prisno, D. E.III. (2024). Examining the potentials of stem cell therapy in reducing the burden of selected non-communicable diseases in Africa. *Stem Cell Research & Therapy*, *15*(1), 253. PMID: 39135088

Athauda, D., Maclagan, K., Skene, S. S., Bajwa-Joseph, M., Letchford, D., Chowdhury, K., Hibbert, S., Budnik, N., Zampedri, L., Dickson, J., Li, Y., Aviles-Olmos, I., Warner, T. T., Limousin, P., Lees, A. J., Greig, N. H., Tebbs, S., & Foltynie, T. (2017). Exenatide once weekly versus placebo in Parkinson's disease: A randomised, double-blind, placebo-controlled trial. *Lancet*, *390*(10103), 1664–1675. DOI: 10.1016/S0140-6736(17)31585-4

Aubignat, M., Tir, M., & Krystkowiak, P. (2021). Non-motor symptoms of Parkinson's disease from pathophysiology to early diagnosis. *Revue de Médecine Interne*, *42*(4), 251–257. DOI: 10.1016/j.revmed.2020.06.019 PMID: 32680717

Aureli, F., Gaudiano, M. C., Raimondo, M., Maccelli, A., Di Giorgio, D., Gramazio, M., & Bartolomei, M. (2025). Quality assessment of" naturally occurring" high percentage L-dopa commercial products proposed as dietary supplements by Internet: From labelling to analytical findings. *Frontiers in Chemistry*, *13*, 1597784. PMID: 41169659

Aurora, R. N., Zak, R. S., Maganti, R. K., Auerbach, S. H., Casey, K. R., Chowdhuri, S., Karippot, A., Ramar, K., Kristo, D. A., Morgenthaler, T. I., & Tracy, S. L. (2010). Best Practice Guide for the Treatment of REM Sleep Behavior Disorder (RBD). *Journal of Clinical Sleep Medicine : JCSM : Official Publication of the American Academy of Sleep Medicine*, *6*(1), 85. DOI: 10.5664/jcsm.27717

Bacanoiu, M. V., Rusu, L., Marin, M. I., Piele, D., Rusu, M. R., Danoiu, R., & Danoiu, M. (2025). Digital Health in Parkinson's Disease and Atypical Parkinsonism—New Frontiers in Motor Function and Physical Activity Assessment [Review]. *Journal of Clinical Medicine*, *2025*(14), 4140. DOI: 10.3390/jcm14124140 PMID: 40565895

Bae, E. J., Lee, H. J., Rockenstein, E., Ho, D. H., Park, E. B., Yang, N. Y., Desplats, P., Masliah, E., & Lee, S. J. (2012). Antibody-aided clearance of extracellular α-synuclein prevents cell-to-cell aggregate transmission. *The Journal of Neuroscience : The Official Journal of the Society for Neuroscience*, *32*(39), 13454–13469. DOI: 10.1523/JNEUROSCI.1292-12.2012

Bagrodia, V., Vikram, V.H., Nitish, L.K., Pramod, K.P., & Ravi, Y. (2022). Parkinson's Disease and Wearable Technology: An Indian Perspective. Annals of Indian Academy of Neurology | Published by Wolters Kluwer – Medknow. Vol 25(5). 817-820. DOI: .DOI: 10.4103/aian.aian_653_22

Baguet, C., Larghero, J., & Mebarki, M. (2023). Early predictive factors of failure in autologous CAR T-cell manufacturing and/or efficacy in hematologic malignancies. *Blood Advances*, *8*, 337. DOI: 10.1182/bloodadvances.2023011992 PMID: 38052048

Baker, W. L., Silver, D., White, C. M., Kluger, J., Aberle, J., Patel, A. A., & Coleman, C. I. (2009). Dopamine agonists in the treatment of early Parkinson's disease: A meta-analysis. *Parkinsonism & Related Disorders*, *15*(4), 287–294. DOI: 10.1016/j.parkreldis.2008.07.004

Balakrishnan, A., Medikonda, J., Namboothiri, P. K., & Natarajan, M. (2022). Role of Wearable Sensors with Machine Learning Approaches in Gait Analysis for Parkinson's Disease Assessment: A Review. *Engineering and Science*, *19*, 5–19. DOI: 10.30919/es8e622

Balakrishnan, R., Azam, S., Cho, D. Y., Su-Kim, I., & Choi, D. K. (2021). Natural Phytochemicals as Novel Therapeutic Strategies to Prevent and Treat Parkinson's Disease: Current Knowledge and Future Perspectives. *Oxidative Medicine and Cellular Longevity, 6680935*. Advance online publication. DOI: 10.1155/2021/6680935 PMID: 34122727

Balzanelli, M. G., Distratis, P., Lazzaro, R., Pham, V. H., Tran, T. C., Dipalma, G., Inchingolo, F., Serlenga, E. M., Aityan, S. K., Ballini, A., Nguyen, K. C. D., & Isacco, C. G. (2023). The Anti-Viral Activity of Stem Cells: A Rational Explanation for their Use in Clinical Application. *Endocrine, Metabolic & Immune Disorders Drug Targets*, *23*(6), 739–747. PMID: 37254275

Bange, M., Rick, C.G.H, Aparna, A. W. S, Günther, D. & Muthuraman, M. (2025). Non-invasive brain stimulation to modulate neural activity in Parkinson's disease. npj | parkinson's disease. (2025) 11:68. https://doi.org/.DOI: 10.1038/s41531-025-00908-1

Baradaran, N., Tan, S. N., Liu, A., Ashoori, A., Palmer, S. J., Wang, Z. J., Oishi, M. M., & McKeown, M. J. (2013). Parkinson's disease rigidity: Relation to brain connectivity and motor performance. *Frontiers in Neurology*, *4*, 67. PMID: 23761780

Barber, D., Wijeratne, T., Singh, L., Barnham, K., & Masters, C. L. (2025). The search for disease modification in Parkinson's disease: A review of the literature. *Life (Chicago, Ill.), 15*. Advance online publication. DOI: 10.3390/life15081169 PMID: 40868817

Barker, R. A., Farrell, K., Guzman, N. V., He, X., Lazic, S. E., Moore, S., Morris, R., Tyers, P., Wijeyekoon, R., Daft, D., Hewitt, S., Dayal, V., Foltynie, T., Kefalopoulou, Z., Mahlknecht, P., Lao-Kaim, N. P., Piccini, P., Bjartmarz, H., Björklund, A., … Winkler, C. (2019). Designing stem-cell-based dopamine cell replacement trials for Parkinson's disease. *Nature Medicine 2019 25:7, 25*(7), 1045–1053. https://doi.org/DOI: 10.1038/s41591-019-0507-2

Barker, R. A., Björklund, A., & Parmar, M. (2024). The history and status of dopamine cell therapies for Parkinson's disease. *BioEssays*, *46*(12), 2400118. PMID: 39058892

Barker, R. A., Carpenter, M. K., Forbes, S., Goldman, S. A., Jamieson, C., Murry, C. E., & Weir, G. (2018). The challenges of first-in-human stem cell clinical trials: What does this mean for ethics and institutional review boards? *Stem Cell Reports*, *10*(5), 1429–1431. PMID: 29742388

Barker, R. A., & Parmar, M. (2025). Stem cell-derived dopamine cell therapies for Parkinson's disease: What have the first trials shown? *Brain, 148*(10), 3428–3430. PMID: 40898774

Barrachina-Fernández, M., Maitín, A. M., Sánchez-ávila, C., & Romero, J. P. (2021). Wearable technology to detect motor fluctuations in parkinson's disease patients: Current state and challenges. *Sensors (Basel), 21*(12). Advance online publication. DOI: 10.3390/s21124188 PMID: 34207198

Barretto, M., & D'souza, N. (2023). Conceptualizing a Rehabilitation 'Model of Care'for Improving the Quality of Life of People with Parkinson's in India. *Annals of Indian Academy of Neurology, 26*(4), 387–394. PMID: 37970321

Bátiz, L. F., Castro, M. A., Burgos, P. V., Velásquez, Z. D., Muñoz, R. I., Lafourcade, C. A., Troncoso-Escudero, P., & Wyneken, U. (2016). Exosomes as Novel Regulators of Adult Neurogenic Niches. *Frontiers in Cellular Neuroscience, 9*, 501. PMID: 26834560

Beach, T. G., Adler, C. H., Sue, L. I., Vedders, L., Lue, L., White, C. L.III, Akiyama, H., Caviness, J. N., Shill, H. A., Sabbagh, M. N., & Walker, D. G.Arizona Parkinson's Disease Consortium. (2010). Multi-organ distribution of phosphorylated alpha-synuclein histopathology in subjects with Lewy body disorders. *Acta Neuropathologica, 119*(6), 689–702. DOI: 10.1007/s00401-010-0664-3 PMID: 20306269

Bello-Mojeed, M. A., Ani, C., Lagunju, I., & Omigbodun, O. (2016). Feasibility of parent-mediated behavioural intervention for behavioural problems in children with autism spectrum disorder in Nigeria: A pilot study. *Child and Adolescent Psychiatry and Mental Health, 10*. Advance online publication. DOI: 10.1186/s13034-016-0117-4 PMID: 27594900

Benninger, D. H., Lomarev, M., Lopez, G., Wassermann, E. M., Li, X., Considine, E., & Hallett, M. (2010). Transcranial direct current stimulation for the treatment of Parkinson's disease. *Journal of Neurology, Neurosurgery, and Psychiatry, 81*(10), 1105–1111. DOI: 10.1136/jnnp.2009.202556 PMID: 20870863

Ben-Shlomo, Y., Darweesh, S., Llibre-Guerra, J., Marras, C., San Luciano, M., & Tanner, C. (2024). The epidemiology of Parkinson's disease. *Lancet, 403*(10423), 283–292. PMID: 38245248

Berardelli, A., Sabra, A. F., & Hallett, M. (1983). Physiological mechanisms of rigidity in Parkinson's disease. *Journal of Neurology, Neurosurgery, and Psychiatry, 46*(1), 45–53. DOI: 10.1136/jnnp.46.1.45 PMID: 6842199

Berg, D., Postuma, R. B., Adler, C. H., Bloem, B. R., Chan, P., Dubois, B., Gasser, T., Goetz, C. G., Halliday, G., Joseph, L., Lang, A. E., Liepelt-Scarfone, I., Litvan, I., Marek, K., Obeso, J., Oertel, W., Olanow, C. W., Poewe, W., Stern, M., & Deuschl, G. (2015). MDS research criteria for prodromal Parkinson's disease. *Movement Disorders*, *30*(12), 1600–1611. DOI: 10.1002/MDS.26431

Bezard, E., Brotchie, J. M., & Gross, C. E. (2001). Pathophysiology of levodopa-induced dyskinesia: Potential for new therapies. *Nature Reviews. Neuroscience*, *2*(8), 577–588. DOI: 10.1038/35086062 PMID: 11484001

Bhidayasiri, R., Virameteekul, S., Sukoandari, B., Tran, T. N., & Lim, T. T. (2021). Challenges of Parkinson's disease care in Southeast Asia. https://doi.org/DOI: 10.1007/978-3-319-56015-1_442-1

Bhidayasiri, R. (2005). Differential diagnosis of common tremor syndromes. *Postgraduate Medical Journal*, *81*(962), 756–762. PMID: 16344298

Bhidayasiri, R. (2024). Old problems, new solutions: Harnessing technology and innovation in Parkinson's disease—Evidence and experiences from Thailand. *Journal of Neural Transmission (Vienna, Austria)*, *131*, 721. DOI: 10.1007/s00702-023-02727-1 PMID: 38189972

Bhidayasiri, R., Sringean, J., Phumphid, S., Anan, C., Thanawattano, C., Deoisres, S., & Bunnag, T. (2024). The rise of Parkinson's disease is a global challenge, but efforts to tackle this must begin at a national level: A protocol for national digital screening and "eat, move, sleep" lifestyle interventions to prevent or slow the rise of non-communicable diseases in Thailand. *Frontiers in Neurology*, *15*, 1386608. PMID: 38803644

Bhusal, C. K., Uti, D. E., Mukherjee, D., Alqahtani, T., Alqahtani, S., Bhattacharya, A., & Akash, S. (2023). Unveiling Nature's potential: Promising natural compounds in Parkinson's disease management. *Parkinsonism & Related Disorders*, *115*, 105799. DOI: 10.1016/j.parkreldis.2023.105799 PMID: 37633805

Bianco, L., Linardi, A., & Stilhano, R. S. (2024). Effect of the anti-inflammatory action of β-carbolines on SH-SY5Y cell line (human neuroblastoma) and modulation of TMPRSS11 and Furin receptors. *Arquivos de Neuro-Psiquiatria*, *1*. Advance online publication. DOI: 10.5327/cbn240003

Billingsley, K. J., Bandres-Ciga, S., Saez-Atienzar, S., & Singleton, A. B. (2018). Genetic risk factors in Parkinson's disease. *Cell and Tissue Research*, *373*(1), 9. DOI: 10.1007/S00441-018-2817-Y

Binde, C. D., Tvete, I. F., Gåsemyr, J., Natvig, B., & Klemp, M. (2018). A multiple treatment comparison meta-analysis of monoamine oxidase type B inhibitors for Parkinson's disease. *British Journal of Clinical Pharmacology*, *84*(9), 1917–1927. DOI: 10.1111/BCP.13651;JOURNAL:JOURNAL:13652125;PAGE:STRING:ARTICLE/CHAPTER

Bishay, A. E., Hughes, N. C., Zargari, M., Paulo, D. L., Bishay, S., Lyons, A. T., Morkos, M. N., Ball, T. J., Englot, D. J., & Bick, S. K. (2024). Disparities in Access to Deep Brain Stimulation for Parkinson's Disease and Proposed Interventions: A Literature Review. *Stereotactic and Functional Neurosurgery*, *102*(3), 179. DOI: 10.1159/000538748

Bloem, B. R., Henderson, E. J., Dorsey, E. R., Okun, M. S., Okubadejo, N., & Chan, P.. (2020). Integrated and patient-centred management of Parkinson's disease: A network model for reshaping chronic neurological care. *Lancet Neurology*, *19*, 623. DOI: 10.1016/S1474-4422(20)30064-8 PMID: 32464101

Bloem, B. R., Okun, M. S., & Klein, C. (2021). Parkinson's disease. *Lancet*, *397*(10291), 2284–2303. DOI: 10.1016/S0140-6736(21)00218-X PMID: 33848468

Bloem, B. R., Rompen, L., Vries, N. M. D., Klink, A., Munneke, M., & Jeurissen, P. (2017). ParkinsonNet: A low-cost health care innovation with a systems approach from the Netherlands. *Health Affairs*, *36*(11), 1987–1996. PMID: 29137501

Bond, A. E., Shah, B. B., Huss, D. S., Dallapiazza, R. F., Warren, A., Harrison, M. B., Sperling, S. A., Wang, X.-Q., Gwinn, R., Witt, J., Ro, S., & Elias, W. J.International Essential Tremor Stereotactic Radiofrequency Ablation (ESTRA) Study Group. (2017). Safety and efficacy of focused ultrasound thalamotomy for patients with medication-refractory, tremor-dominant Parkinson disease: A randomized clinical trial. *JAMA Neurology*, *74*(12), 1412–1418. DOI: 10.1001/jamaneurol.2017.3098 PMID: 29084313

Bonnechère, B., Kossi, O., Mapinduzi, J., Panda, J., Rintala, A., Guidetti, S., Spooren, A., & Feys, P. (2023). Mobile health solutions: An opportunity for rehabilitation in low- and middle income countries? *Frontiers in Public Health*, *10*, 1072322. DOI: 10.3389/fpubh.2022.1072322 PMID: 36761328

Borghammer, P., & Van Den Berge, N. (2019a). Brain-First versus Gut-First Parkinson's Disease: A Hypothesis. *Journal of Parkinson's Disease*, *9*(s2), S281–S295. DOI: 10.3233/JPD-191721

Bot, B. M., Suver, C., Neto, E. C., Kellen, M., Klein, A., Bare, C., Doerr, M., Pratap, A., Wilbanks, J., Dorsey, E. R., Friend, S. H., & Trister, A. D. (2016). The mPower study, Parkinson disease mobile data collected using ResearchKit. *Scientific Data, 3*(1), 160011-. https://doi.org/DOI: 10.1038/SDATA.2016.11

Botello-Villagrana, F., & Martinez-Ramirez, D. (2021). Mucuna pruriens as adjunct therapy to levodopa in advanced Parkinson's disease. Revista mexicana de neurociencia, 22(5), 180-183.

Bouça-Machado, R., Pona-Ferreira, F., Gonçalves, N., Leitão, M., Cacho, R., Castro-Caldas, A., & Ferreira, J. J., & and CNS Multidisciplinary Team. (2020). Outcome Measures for Evaluating the Effect of a Multidisciplinary Intervention on Axial Symptoms of Parkinson's Disease. *Frontiers in Neurology, 11*, 521733. DOI: 10.3389/FNEUR.2020.00328

Bougea, A. (2025). Application of Wearable Sensors in Parkinson's Disease: State of the Art. *J. Sens. Actuator Netw., 2025*(14), 23. DOI: 10.3390/jsan14020023

Braak, H., Del Tredici, K., Rüb, U., de Vos, R. A., Jansen Steur, E. N., & Braak, E. (2003). Staging of brain pathology related to sporadic Parkinson's disease. *Neurobiology of Aging*, *24*(2), 197–211. PMID: 12498954

Bray, F., Laversanne, M., Sung, H., Ferlay, J., Siegel, R. L., & Soerjomataram, I.. (2024). Global cancer statistics 2022: GLOBOCAN estimates of incidence and mortality worldwide for 36 cancers in 185 countries. *CA: a Cancer Journal for Clinicians*, *74*, 229. DOI: 10.3322/caac.21834 PMID: 38572751

Bretz, F., Koenig, F., Brannath, W., Glimm, E., & Posch, M. (2009). Adaptive designs for confirmatory clinical trials. *Statistics in Medicine*, *28*(8), 1181–1217. DOI: 10.1002/SIM.3538

Bright-Ohaeri, F. C., Ihebuzo, N. G., Ejeta, K. O., Odimegwu, N., & Militus, I. O. (2024). Cell Culture and Laboratory Contaminants, Prevention and Recovery Strategy- A Review. *European Journal of Biology and Medical Science Research*, *12*(2), 32–51.

Bril, E., Fedorova, N. D., Кулуа, T. K., & Zimnyakova, O. S. (2024). Treatment of the early stages of Parkinson's disease. Differences in approaches to the choice of therapy in different countries. *Neurology Neuropsychiatry Psychosomatics*, *16*, 130–135. DOI: 10.14412/2074-2711-2024-3-130-135

Brummer, T., Zipp, F., & Bittner, S. (2022). T cell–neuron interaction in inflammatory and progressive multiple sclerosis biology. *Current Opinion in Neurobiology*, *75*, 102588. PMID: 35732103

Brundin, P., & Melki, R. (2017). Prying into the Prion Hypothesis for Parkinson's Disease. *The Journal of Neuroscience : The Official Journal of the Society for Neuroscience, 37*(41), 9808–9818. DOI: 10.1523/JNEUROSCI.1788-16.2017

Bruno, B. G., Gabriel, D. A., Daniel, G. Q., Vanessa, M. H., Thiago, J., & Marcelo, B. T. (2019). Parkinson's disease and wearable devices, new perspectives for a public health issue: An integrative literature review. *Revista da Associação Médica Brasileira, 65*(11), 1413–1420. DOI: 10.1590/1806-9282.65.11.1413 PMID: 31800906

Brys, M., Fanning, L., Hung, S., Ellenbogen, A., Penner, N., Yang, M., Welch, M., Koenig, E., David, E., Fox, T., Makh, S., Aldred, J., Goodman, I., Pepinsky, B., Liu, Y. T., Graham, D., Weihofen, A., & Cedarbaum, J. M. (2019). Randomized phase I clinical trial of anti–α-synuclein antibody BIIB054. *Movement Disorders, 34*(8), 1154–1163. DOI: 10.1002/MDS.27738

Burns, M. R., Shannon, Y. C., Bhavana, P., Sotiris, G. M., Joshua, K. W., & Ramirez-Zamora, A. (2021). Advances and Future Directions of Neuromodulation in Neurologic Disorders. *Neurologic Clinics, 39*, 71–85. DOI: 10.1016/j.ncl.2020.09.004 PMID: 33223090

Busch, J.L., Jonathan, K, Jennifer, K.B, Victoria, S.W, Luisa, D, Jeroen, G.V.H & Andrea, A.K. (2025). Chronic adaptive deep brain stimulation for Parkinson's disease: clinical outcomes and programming strategies. (2025) 11:264.

Cagman, N., & Enginoglu, S. (2010). Soft set theory and uni–int decision making. *European Journal of Operational Research, 207*(2), 848–855.

Cao, X.-Y., Lu, J.-M., Zhao, Z.-Q., Li, M.-C., Lu, T., An, X.-S., & Xue, L.-J. (2017). MicroRNA biomarkers of Parkinson's disease in serum exosome-like microvesicles. *Neuroscience Letters, 644*, 94–99. DOI: 10.1016/j.neulet.2017.02.045 PMID: 28223160

Carina, F., Rafael, B. C., Juliete, M. D., Renato, P. M., & Rubens, G. C. (2022). Deep brain stimulation in Parkinson's disease: State of the art and future perspectives. DBS in Parkinson's disease. *Arquivos de Neuro-Psiquiatria, 80*(5, Suppl. 1), 105–115. DOI: 10.1590/0004-282X-ANP-2022-S133 PMID: 35976323

Caronni, S., Del Sorbo, F., Barichella, M., Fothergill-Misbah, N., & Denne, T., Laguna, & Cilia, R. (2024). Mucuna pruriens to treat Parkinson's disease in low-income countries: Recommendations and practical guidelines from the farmer to clinical trials. Paving the way for future use in clinical practice. *Parkinsonism & Related Disorders, 124*, 106983. PMID: 38797572

Castelli Gattinara Di Zubiena, F., Menna, G., Mileti, I., Zampogna, A., Asci, F., Paoloni, M., Suppa, A., Del Prete, Z., & Palermo, E. (2022). Machine Learning and Wearable Sensors for the Early Detection of Balance Disorders in Parkinson's Disease. *Sensors (Basel)*, *22*(24). Advance online publication. DOI: 10.3390/s22249903 PMID: 36560278

Cerneckis, J., Cai, H., & Shi, Y. (2024). Induced pluripotent stem cells (iPSCs): Molecular mechanisms of induction and applications. *Signal Transduction and Targeted Therapy*, *9*(1), 112. PMID: 38670977

Chahid, Y., Sheikh, Z. H., Mitropoulos, M., & Booij, J. (2023). A systematic review of the potential effects of medications and drugs of abuse on dopamine transporter imaging using [123I]I-FP-CIT SPECT in routine practice. *European Journal of Nuclear Medicine and Molecular Imaging 2023 50:7, 50*(7), 1974–1987. https://doi.org/DOI: 10.1007/S00259-023-06171-X

Channa, A., Nirvana, P., & Vlad, C. (2020). Wearable Solutions for Patients with Parkinson's Disease and Neurocognitive Disorder: A Systematic Review. *Sensors (Basel)*, *2020*(20), 2713. DOI: 10.3390/s20092713 PMID: 32397516

Channa, A., Ruggeri, G., Ifrim, R. C., Mammone, N., Iera, A., & Popescu, N. (2024). Cloud-Connected Bracelet for Continuous Monitoring of Parkinson's Disease Patients: Integrating Continuous Wavelet Transform and AlexNet Network. *Electronics (Basel)*, *2024*(13), 1002. DOI: 10.3390/electronics13061002

Chatzaki, C., Skaramagkas, V., Tachos, N., Christodoulakis, G., Maniadi, E., Kefalopoulou, Z., Fotiadis, D. I., & Tsiknakis, M. (2021). The smart-insole dataset: Gait analysis using wearable sensors with a focus on elderly and parkinson's patients. *Sensors (Basel)*, *21*(8). Advance online publication. DOI: 10.3390/s21082821 PMID: 33923809

Chaudhary, S., Chaudhary, S., & Rawat, S. (2025). Understanding Parkinson's disease: Current trends and its multifaceted complications. *Frontiers in Aging Neuroscience*, *17*. Advance online publication. DOI: 10.3389/fnagi.2025.1617106 PMID: 41049533

Chaudhuri, K. R., Azulay, J. P., Odin, P., Lindvall, S., Domingos, J., Alobaidi, A., Kandukuri, P. L., Chaudhari, V. S., Parra, J. C., Yamazaki, T., Oddsdottir, J., Wright, J., & Martinez-Martin, P. (2024). Economic Burden of Parkinson's Disease: A Multinational, Real-World, Cost-of-Illness Study. *Drugs - Real World Outcomes*, *11*(1), 1. DOI: 10.1007/S40801-023-00410-1

Chaudhuri, K. R., Azulay, J., Odin, P., Lindvall, S., Domingos, J., & Alobaidi, A.. (2024). Economic burden of Parkinson's disease: A multinational, real-world, cost-of-illness study. *Drugs - Real World Outcomes, 11*, 1. DOI: 10.1007/s40801-023-00410-1 PMID: 38193999

Chaudhuri, K. R., & Batzu, L. (2023). Can continuous levodopa delivery be achieved in the absence of Intrajejunal Levodopa Infusion? Implications for India and Underserved Countries. *Movement Disorders Clinical Practice, 11*(1), 21–29. PMID: 38291849

Cha, Y., Park, T. Y., Leblanc, P., & Kim, K. S. (2023). Current Status and Future Perspectives on Stem Cell-Based Therapies for Parkinson's Disease. *Journal of Movement Disorders, 16*(1), 22–41. PMID: 36628428

Chen, D., Tsang, E. C., Yeung, D. S., & Wang, X. (2005). The parameterization reduction of soft sets and its applications. *Computers & Mathematics with Applications (Oxford, England), 49*(5-6), 757–763.

Chen, K., Sun, L., Liu, Y., & Chen, R. (2025). Safety and efficacy of fecal microbiota transplantation in the treatment of Parkinson's disease: A systematic review of clinical trials. *Frontiers in Neuroscience, 19*, 1639911. DOI: 10.3389/FNINS.2025.1639911

Chen, Q., Cheng, H. J., Bian, Z. X., Lyu, A. P., Yang, Y., & Chan, K. W. (2025). Regulatory frameworks and evidence requirements for traditional, complementary and integrative medicines. *Bulletin of the World Health Organization, 103*(11), 696–707C. PMID: 41180280

Chilvery, A., Palwai, S., Guggilla, P., Wren, K., & Edinburgh, D. (2020). Perovskite materials: Recent advancements and challenges. In *Perovskite materials, devices and integration*. IntechOpen., DOI: 10.5772/intechopen.88500

Chirra, M., Marsili, L., Wattley, L., Sokol, L. L., Keeling, E., Maule, S., & Merola, A. (2019). Telemedicine in neurological disorders: Opportunities and challenges. *Telemedicine Journal and e-Health, 25*(7), 541–550. PMID: 30136898

Chitsaz, A., Najafi, M. R., Habibi, F., & Amirhajloo, S. (2024). Comparison of the effectiveness of modafinil and methylphenidate in treatment of excessive daytime sleepiness in patients with Parkinson's disease. *Current Journal of Neurology, 23*(1), 39. DOI: 10.18502/CJN.V23I1.16431

Cho, I. H. (2012). Effects of Panax ginseng in Neurodegenerative Diseases. *Journal of Ginseng Research, 36*(4), 342–353. DOI: 10.5142/jgr.2012.36.4.342 PMID: 23717136

Christine, C. W., Richardson, R. M., van Laar, A. D., Thompson, M. E., Fine, E. M., Khwaja, O. S., Li, C., Liang, G. S., Meier, A., Roberts, E. W., Pfau, M. L., Rodman, J. R., Bankiewicz, K. S., & Larson, P. S. (2022). Safety of AADC Gene Therapy for Moderately Advanced Parkinson Disease: Three-Year Outcomes from the PD-1101 Trial. *Neurology*, *98*(1), E40–E50. DOI: 10.1212/WNL.0000000000012952

Cilia, R., Akpalu, A., Sarfo, F. S., Cham, M., Amboni, M., Cereda, E., Fabbri, M., Adjei, P., Akassi, J., Bonetti, A., & Pezzoli, G. (2014). The modern pre-levodopa era of Parkinson's disease: Insights into motor complications from sub-Saharan Africa. *Brain*, *137*(10), 2731–2742. DOI: 10.1093/brain/awu195 PMID: 25034897

Cilia, R., Laguna, J., Cassani, E., Cereda, E., Pozzi, N. G., Isaias, I. U., & Pezzoli, G. (2017). Mucuna pruriens in Parkinson disease: A double-blind, randomized, controlled, crossover study. *Neurology*, *89*(5), 432–438. PMID: 28679598

Cole, T. A., Zhao, H., Collier, T. J., Sandoval, I., Sortwell, C. E., Steece-Collier, K., Daley, B. F., Booms, A., Lipton, J., Welch, M., Berman, M., Jandreski, L., Graham, D., Weihofen, A., Celano, S., Schulz, E., Cole-Strauss, A., Luna, E., Quach, D., & Paumier, K. L. (2021). α-Synuclein antisense oligonucleotides as a disease-modifying therapy for Parkinson's disease. *JCI Insight*, *6*(5). Advance online publication. DOI: 10.1172/JCI.INSIGHT.135633

Concha-Marambio, L., Pritzkow, S., Shahnawaz, M., Farris, C. M., & Soto, C. (2023). Seed amplification assay for the detection of pathologic alpha-synuclein aggregates in cerebrospinal fluid. *Nature Protocols 2023 18:4, 18*(4), 1179–1196. https://doi.org/DOI: 10.1038/s41596-022-00787-3

Contini, N., Martins, W. A., & Schilling, L. P. (2024). Unsteadiness of gait in terminal renal failure: Miller Fisher syndrome triggered by haemodialysis. *Arquivos de Neuro-Psiquiatria*, *481*. Advance online publication. DOI: 10.5327/cbn241718

Corvol, J. C., & Poewe, W. (2016). Pharmacogenetics of Parkinson's Disease in Clinical Practice. *Movement Disorders Clinical Practice*, *4*(2), 173–180. DOI: 10.1002/MDC3.12444

Costello, H., Schrag, A.-E., Howard, R., & Roiser, J. P. (2023). Dissociable effects of dopaminergic medications on depression symptom dimensions in Parkinson's disease. MedRxiv *: The Preprint Server for Health Sciences*. https://doi.org/DOI: 10.1101/2023.06.30.23292073

Cubo, E., & Delgado-López, P. D. (2022). Telemedicine in the management of Parkinson's disease: Achievements, challenges, and future perspectives. *Brain Sciences*, *12*(12), 1735. PMID: 36552194

Cueva, E., Wiesheu, A., Sordo, Z., González, J., Falconi, S., Rodas, J. A., & Leon-Rojas, J. E. (2025). Tissue Stem Cell-Based Therapies in Parkinson's Disease: A Scoping Review of Therapeutic Mechanisms and Translational Outcomes. *Cells, 14*(11), 822. PMID: 40497998

Cummings, J. L., Morstorf, T., & Zhong, K. (2014). Alzheimer's disease drug-development pipeline: Few candidates, frequent failures. *Alzheimer's Research & Therapy*, *6*(4), 37. DOI: 10.1186/ALZRT269

Cummings, J., Isaacson, S., Mills, R., Williams, H., Chi-Burris, K., Corbett, A., Dhall, R., & Ballard, C. (2014). Pimavanserin for patients with Parkinson's disease psychosis: A randomised, placebo-controlled phase 3 trial. *Lancet*, *383*(9916), 533–540. DOI: 10.1016/S0140-6736(13)62106-6

D'Agostino, R. B. (2009). The Delayed-Start Study Design. *The New England Journal of Medicine*, *361*(13), 1304–1306. DOI: 10.1056/NEJMSM090

Daneault, J. F., Vergara-Diaz, G., Parisi, F., Admati, C., Alfonso, C., Bertoli, M., Bonizzoni, E., Carvalho, G. F., Costante, G., Fabara, E. E., Fixler, N., Golabchi, F. N., Growdon, J., Sapienza, S., Snyder, P., Shpigelman, S., Sudarsky, L., Daeschler, M., Bataille, L., & Bonato, P. (2021). Accelerometer data collected with a minimum set of wearable sensors from subjects with Parkinson's disease. *Scientific Data*, *8*(1). Advance online publication. DOI: 10.1038/s41597-021-00830-0 PMID: 33547309

Das, S., & Ramteke, H. (2024). A comprehensive review of the role of biomarkers in early diagnosis of Parkinson's disease. *Cureus*, *16*(2). PMID: 38500934

Davidsona, B., Luka, M., Laura, K., Lorraine, V. K., & Suneil, K. K. (2024). Neuroscience fundamentals relevant to neuromodulation: Neurobiology of deep brain stimulation in Parkinson's disease. *Neurotherapeutics; the Journal of the American Society for Experimental NeuroTherapeutics*, *21*, e00348. PMID: 38579455

de Graaf, D., de Vries, N. M., van de Zande, T., Schimmel, J. J. P., Shin, S., Kowahl, N., Barman, P., Kapur, R., Marks, W. J., Jr., van 't Hul, A., & Bloem, B. R. (2024). Measuring Physical Functioning Using Wearable Sensors in Parkinson Disease and Chronic Obstructive Pulmonary Disease (the Accuracy of Digital Assessment of Performance Trial Study): Protocol for a Prospective Observational Study JMIR Res Protoc 2024; 13: e55452 URL: https://www.researchprotocols.org/2024/1/e55452 doi: DOI: 10.2196/55452

de Heer, J. A., Buijtenhuijs, D., & de Wit-Bos, L. (2024). Risk assessment of herbal preparations containing seed extracts of Mucana pruriens.

De la Fuente-Fernández, R., Ruth, T. J., Sossi, V., Schulzer, M., Calne, D. B., & Stoessl, A. J. (2001). Expectation and dopamine release: Mechanism of the placebo effect in Parkinson's disease. *Science*, *293*(5532), 1164–1166. DOI: 10.1126/SCIENCE.1060937

Deb, S., Retzer, A., Roy, M., Acharya, R., Limbu, B., & Roy, A. (2020). The effectiveness of parent training for children with autism spectrum disorder: A systematic review and meta-analyses. *BMC Psychiatry*, *20*. Advance online publication. DOI: 10.1186/s12888-020-02973-7 PMID: 33287762

Degli Esposti, L., Piccinni, C., Sangiorgi, D., Nobili, F., & Buda, S. (2016). Prescribing pattern and resource utilization of monoamine oxidase-B inhibitors in Parkinson treatment: Comparison between rasagiline and selegiline. *Neurological Sciences*, *37*(2), 227–234. PMID: 26474874

Dekker, M. C. J., Coulibaly, T., Bardien, S., Ross, O. A., Carr, J., & Komolafe, M. (2020). Parkinson's disease research on the African continent: Obstacles and opportunities. *Frontiers in Neurology*, *11*. Advance online publication. DOI: 10.3389/fneur.2020.00512 PMID: 32636796

Del Din, S., Kirk, C., Yarnall, A. J., Rochester, L., & Hausdorff, J. M. (2021). Body-worn sensors for remote monitoring of Parkinson's disease motor symptoms: Vision, state of the art, and challenges ahead. *Journal of Parkinson's Disease*, *11*(s1), S35–S47. PMID: 33523020

Del Tredici, K., Hawkes, C. H., Ghebremedhin, E., & Braak, H. (2010). Lewy pathology in the submandibular gland of individuals with incidental Lewy body disease and sporadic Parkinson's disease. *Acta Neuropathologica*, *119*(6), 703–713. DOI: 10.1007/s00401-010-0665-2 PMID: 20229352

DeMaagd, G., & Philip, A. (2015). Parkinson's disease and its management: Part 1—Disease entity, risk factors, pathophysiology, clinical presentation, and diagnosis. *P&T : a Peer-Reviewed Journal for Formulary Management*, *40*(8), 504–532. PMID: 26236139

Denaro, F., Worthington, M., Williams, S., Benedetti, E., Zealand, D., & Davis, H.. (2022). Identification of increased blood–brain barrier permeability in the substantia nigra of HIV-1 transgenic rat. *Microscopy and Microanalysis*, *28*, 3214–3215. DOI: 10.1017/S1431927622011953

Deuschl, G., Beghi, E., Fazekas, F., Varga, T., Christoforidi, K. A., Sipido, E., Bassetti, C. L., Vos, T., & Feigin, V. L. (2020). The burden of neurological diseases in Europe: An analysis for the Global Burden of Disease Study 2017. *The Lancet. Public Health*, *5*(10), e551–e567. DOI: 10.1016/S2468-2667(20)30190-0 PMID: 33007212

Deuschl, G., Schade-Brittinger, C., Krack, P., Volkmann, J., Schäfer, H., Bötzel, K., Daniels, C., Deutschländer, A., Dillmann, U., Eisner, W., Gruber, D., Hamel, W., Herzog, J., Hilker, R., Klebe, S., Kloß, M., Koy, J., Krause, M., Kupsch, A., & Voges, J. (2006). A Randomized Trial of Deep-Brain Stimulation for Parkinson's Disease. *The New England Journal of Medicine*, *355*(9), 896–908. DOI: 10.1056/NEJMoa060281 PMID: 16943402

Dias, J., García, J., Agliardi, G., & Roddie, C. (2024). CAR-T cell manufacturing landscape—Lessons from the past decade and considerations for early clinical development. *Molecular Therapy. Methods & Clinical Development*, *32*, 101250. DOI: 10.1016/j.omtm.2024.101250 PMID: 38737799

Dickson, D. W., Braak, H., Duda, J. E., Duyckaerts, C., Gasser, T., Halliday, G. M., Hardy, J., Leverenz, J. B., Del Tredici, K., Wszolek, Z. K., & Litvan, I. (2009). Neuropathological assessment of Parkinson's disease: Refining the diagnostic criteria. *Lancet Neurology*, *8*(12), 1150–1157. DOI: 10.1016/S1474-4422(09)70238-8 PMID: 19909913

Digital Health Technologies for Remote Data Acquisition in Clinical Investigations | FDA. (n.d.). Retrieved December 13, 2025, from https://www.fda.gov/regulatory-information/search-fda-guidance-documents/digital-health-technologies-remote-data-acquisition-clinical-investigations

Dilsiz, N. (2024). A comprehensive review on recent advances in exosome isolation and characterization: Toward clinical applications. *Translational Oncology*, *50*, 102121. DOI: 10.1016/j.tranon.2024.102121 PMID: 39278189

Dirkx, M., & Bologna, M. (2022). The pathophysiology of Parkinson's disease tremor. *Journal of the Neurological Sciences*, *435*, 120196. DOI: 10.1016/j.jns.2022.120196 PMID: 35240491

Doi, D., Magotani, H., Kikuchi, T., Ikeda, M., Hiramatsu, S., Yoshida, K., Amano, N., Nomura, M., Umekage, M., Morizane, A., & Takahashi, J. (2020). Pre-clinical study of induced pluripotent stem cell-derived dopaminergic progenitor cells for Parkinson's disease. *Nature Communications 2020 11:1*, *11*(1), 3369-. https://doi.org/DOI: 10.1038/s41467-020-17165-w

Donaghy, P. C., Firbank, M. J., Thomas, A. J., Lloyd, J., Petrides, G., Barnett, N., Olsen, K., Taylor, J.-P., & O'Brien, J. T. (2020). Amyloid imaging and longitudinal clinical progression in dementia with lewy bodies. *The American Journal of Geriatric Psychiatry*, *28*(5), 573–577. DOI: 10.1016/j.jagp.2019.12.009 PMID: 31953009

Dong, W., Liu, S., Li, S., & Wang, Z. (2024). Cell reprogramming therapy for Parkinson's disease. *Neural Regeneration Research*, *19*(11), 2444–2455. PMID: 38526281

Dorsey, E. R.. (2018). Global, regional, and national burden of Parkinson's disease, 1990–2016. *Lancet Neurology, 17*(11), 939–953. PMID: 30287051

Dorsey, E. R., Elbaz, A., Nichols, E., Abbasi, N., Abd-Allah, F., & Abdelalim, A.. (2018). Global, regional, and national burden of Parkinson's disease, 1990–2016: A systematic analysis for the Global Burden of Disease Study 2016. *Lancet Neurology, 17*, 939. DOI: 10.1016/S1474-4422(18)30295-3 PMID: 30287051

Dorsey, E. R., Papapetropoulos, S., Xiong, M., & Kieburtz, K. (2017). The first frontier: Digital biomarkers for neurodegenerative disorders. *Digital Biomarkers, 1*(1), 6–13. DOI: 10.1159/000477383 PMID: 32095743

Dorsey, E. R., Sherer, T., Okun, M. S., & Bloem, B. R. (2018). The emerging evidence of the Parkinson pandemic. *Journal of Parkinson's Disease, 8*(s1), S3–S8. DOI: 10.3233/JPD-181474 PMID: 30584159

Dou, J., Wang, J., Gao, X., Wang, G., Bai, Y., Liang, Y., Yang, K., Yang, Y., & Zhang, L. (2025). Effectiveness of Telemedicine Interventions on Motor and Nonmotor Outcomes in Parkinson Disease: Systematic Review and Network Meta-Analysis. *Journal of Medical Internet Research, 27*, e71169. DOI: 10.2196/71169

Duecker, F., & Sack, A. T. (2015). Rethinking the role of sham TMS. *Frontiers in Psychology, 6*. Advance online publication. DOI: 10.3389/fpsyg.2015.00210 PMID: 25767458

Dutta, S., Hornung, S., Kruayatidee, A., Maina, K. N., del Rosario, I., Paul, K. C., Wong, D. Y., Duarte Folle, A., & Bitan, G. (2021). α-Synuclein in blood exosomes immunoprecipitated using neuronal and oligodendroglial markers distinguishes Parkinson's disease from multiple system atrophy. *Acta Neuropathologica, 142*(3), 495–511. DOI: 10.1007/s00401-021-02324-0 PMID: 33991233

Edison, P., Rowe, C. C., Rinne, J. O., Ng, S., Ahmed, I., Kemppainen, N., Villemagne, V. L., O'Keefe, G., Någren, K., Chaudhury, K. R., Masters, C. L., & Brooks, D. J. (2008). Amyloid load in Parkinson's disease dementia and Lewy body dementia measured with [11C]PIB positron emission tomography. *Journal of Neurology, Neurosurgery, and Psychiatry, 79*(12), 1331–1338. DOI: 10.1136/jnnp.2007.127878 PMID: 18653550

Eggers, C., Kahraman, D., Fink, G. R., Schmidt, M., & Timmermann, L. (2011). Akinetic-rigid and tremor-dominant Parkinson's disease patients show different patterns of FP-CIT single photon emission computed tomography. *Movement Disorders, 26*(3), 416–423. PMID: 21264942

Eggers, C., Pedrosa, D. J., Kahraman, D., Maier, F., Lewis, C. J., Fink, G. R., Schmidt, M., & Timmermann, L. (2012). Parkinson subtypes progress differently in clinical course and imaging pattern. *PLoS One*, *7*(10), e46813. PMID: 23056463

Eijsvogel, P., Misra, P., Concha-Marambio, L., Boyd, J. D., Ding, S., Fedor, L., Hsieh, Y. T., Sun, Y. S., Vroom, M. M., Farris, C. M., Ma, Y., de Kam, M. L., Radanovic, I., Vissers, M. F. J. M., Mirski, D., Shareghi, G., Shahnawaz, M., Singer, W., Kremer, P., … Dodart, J. C. (2024). Target engagement and immunogenicity of an active immunotherapeutic targeting pathological α-synuclein: a phase 1 placebo-controlled trial. *Nature Medicine 2024 30:9, 30*(9), 2631–2640. https://doi.org/DOI: 10.1038/s41591-024-03101-8

Elefante, C., Brancaster, G. E., Bacciardi, S., Mazzucchi, S., Del Prete, E., & Palermo, G.. (2021). Prevalence and clinical correlates of comorbid anxiety and panic disorders in patients with Parkinson's disease. *Journal of Clinical Medicine*, *10*, 2302. PMID: 34070549

Elm, J. J., Hauser, R., Tilley, B. C., Kieburtz, K., Aminoff, M. J., Augustine, E., Bennett, S., Bodis-Wollner, I. G., Cambi, F., Carter, J. H., Chou, K., Christine, C. W., Dhall, R., Dewey, R. B., Elble, R. J., Fang, J., Feigin, A., Galpern, W., Gardiner, I., & Zweig, R. (2012). Design innovations and baseline findings in a long-term parkinson's trial: The national institute of neurological disorders and stroke exploratory trials in parkinson's disease long-term study-1. *Movement Disorders*, *27*(12), 1513–1521. DOI: 10.1002/MDS.25175

El-Shorbagi, A.-N., Chaudhary, S., Alshemali, K. A., Alabdulrazzaq, R. F., & Alqahtani, F. Y. (2020). A comprehensive review on management of Parkinson's disease, inclusive of drug discovery and pharmacological approaches. *Journal of Applied Pharmaceutical Science*, *10*(10), 130–150.

Emilio, A. R., & Portes, J. R. M. (2024). Modelo híbrido de entrenamiento parental para madres de niños en edad preescolar con trastorno del espectro autista basado en el análisis de comportamiento aplicado para reducir el estrés parental. *Ciencias Psicológicas (Montevideo)*, *18*. Advance online publication. DOI: 10.22235/cp.v18i2.3285

Emre, M., Aarsland, D., Albanese, A., Byrne, E. J., Deuschl, G., De Deyn, P. P., Durif, F., Kulisevsky, J., van Laar, T., Lees, A., Poewe, W., Robillard, A., Rosa, M. M., Wolters, E., Quarg, P., Tekin, S., & Lane, R. (2004). Rivastigmine for Dementia Associated with Parkinson's Disease. *The New England Journal of Medicine*, *351*(24), 2509–2518. DOI: 10.1056/NEJMOA041470

Erb, M. K., Karlin, D. R., Ho, B. K., Thomas, K. C., Parisi, F., Vergara-Diaz, G. P., Daneault, J. F., Wacnik, P. W., Zhang, H., Kangarloo, T., Demanuele, C., Brooks, C. R., Detheridge, C. N., Shaafi Kabiri, N., Bhangu, J. S., & Bonato, P. (2020). mHealth and wearable technology should replace motor diaries to track motor fluctuations in Parkinson's disease. *NPJ Digital Medicine*, *3*(1), 6. DOI: 10.1038/S41746-019-0214-X

Eruaga, M. A., Itua, E. O. and Bature, J. T. (2024). Exploring herbal medicine regulation in Nigeria: Balancing traditional practices with modern standards. GSC Advanced Research and Reviews. 18(3): 083–090.

Espay, A. J., Bonato, P., Nahab, F. B., Maetzler, W., Dean, J. M., & Klucken, J.& Movement Disorders Society Task Force on Technology. (2016). Technology in Parkinson's disease: Challenges and opportunities. *Movement Disorders*, *31*(9), 1272–1282. PMID: 27125836

Etukudoh, N., & Ejinaka, O. (2024). Advancements, challenges, and opportunities in physical systems.

Evarts, E. V., Teräväinen, H., & Calne, D. B. (1981). Reaction time in Parkinson's disease. *Brain*, *104*(1), 167–186. PMID: 7470841

Ezike, T., Okpala, U., Onoja, U., & Nwike, C. (2023). Advances in drug delivery systems: Challenges and future directions. *Heliyon*. PMID: 37416680

Faghri, F., Hashemi, S. H., Leonard, H., Scholz, S. W., Campbell, R. H., Nalls, M. A., & Singleton, A. B. (2018). Predicting onset, progression, and clinical subtypes of Parkinson disease using machine learning [Preprint]. *bioRxiv*. https://doi.org/ DOI: 10.1101/338913

Fagiani, F., Marino, D. D., Romagnoli, A., Travelli, C., Voltan, D., & Mannelli, L. D. C.. (2022). Molecular regulations of circadian rhythm and implications for physiology and diseases. *Signal Transduction and Targeted Therapy*, *7*, 41. DOI: 10.1038/s41392-022-00899-y PMID: 35136018

Fahn, S. (2011). Classification of movement disorders. *Movement Disorders*, *26*(6), 947–957. PMID: 21626541

Fairfoul, G., McGuire, L. I., Pal, S., Ironside, J. W., Neumann, J., Christie, S., Joachim, C., Esiri, M., Evetts, S. G., Rolinski, M., Baig, F., Ruffmann, C., Wade-Martins, R., Hu, M. T. M., Parkkinen, L., & Green, A. J. E. (2016). Alpha-synuclein RT-QuIC in the CSF of patients with alpha-synucleinopathies. *Annals of Clinical and Translational Neurology*, *3*(10), 812–818. DOI: 10.1002/ACN3.338

Fanciulli, A., & Wenning, G. K. (2015). Multiple-system atrophy. *The New England Journal of Medicine, 372*(3), 249–263. DOI: 10.1056/NEJMra1311488 PMID: 25587949

Fang, E. F., Hou, Y., Palikaras, K., Adriaanse, B. A., Kerr, J. S., Yang, B., Lautrup, S., Hasan-Olive, M. M., Caponio, D., Dan, X., Rocktäschel, P., Croteau, D. L., Akbari, M., Greig, N. H., Fladby, T., Nilsen, H., Cader, M. Z., Mattson, M. P., Tavernarakis, N., & Bohr, V. A. (2019). Mitophagy inhibits amyloid-β and tau pathology and reverses cognitive deficits in models of Alzheimer's disease. *Nature Neuroscience 2019 22:3, 22*(3), 401–412. https://doi.org/DOI: 10.1038/s41593-018-0332-9

Fang, J. Y., & Tolleson, C. (2017). The role of deep brain stimulation in Parkinson's disease: An overview and update on new developments. *Neuropsychiatric Disease and Treatment, 2017*(13), 723–732. PMID: 28331322

Fan, Y., Winanto, & Ng, S. Y. (2020). Replacing what's lost: A new era of stem cell therapy for Parkinson's disease. *Translational Neurodegeneration, 9*(1), 2. PMID: 31911835

Farkouh, R. A., Wilson, M. R., Tarrants, M. L., Castelli-Haley, J., & Armand, C. (2012). Cost-effectiveness of rasagiline compared with first-line early Parkinson disease therapies. *The American Journal of Pharmacy Benefits, 4*(3), 99–107.

Faruqui, N., Yousuf, M. A., Whaiduzzaman, M., Azad, A., Barros, A., & Moni, M. A. (2021). LungNet: A hybrid deep-CNN model for lung cancer diagnosis using CT and wearable sensor-based medical IoT data. *Computers in Biology and Medicine, 139*, 104961. DOI: 10.1016/j.compbiomed.2021.104961 PMID: 34741906

Federico, S., Cacciante, L., Cieślik, B., Turolla, A., Agostini, M., Kiper, P., & Picelli, A. (2024). Telerehabilitation for Neurological Motor Impairment: A Systematic Review and Meta-Analysis on Quality of Life, Satisfaction, and Acceptance in Stroke, Multiple Sclerosis, and Parkinson's Disease. *Journal of Clinical Medicine, 13*(1). Advance online publication. DOI: 10.3390/JCM13010299/S1

Feng, F., Jun, Y. B., Liu, X., & Li, L. (2010). An adjustable approach to fuzzy soft set based decision making. *Journal of Computational and Applied Mathematics, 234*(1), 10–20.

Fereshtehnejad, S. M., & Postuma, R. B. (2017). Subtypes of Parkinson's Disease: What Do They Tell Us About Disease Progression? *Current Neurology and Neuroscience Reports, 17*(4). Advance online publication. DOI: 10.1007/S11910-017-0738-X

Fereshtehnejad, S. M., Romenets, S. R., Anang, J. B., Latreille, V., Gagnon, J. F., & Postuma, R. B. (2015). New clinical subtypes of Parkinson disease and their longitudinal progression: A prospective cohort comparison with other phenotypes. *JAMA Neurology*, *72*(8), 863–873. PMID: 26076039

Fereshtehnejad, S.-M., Zeighami, Y., Dagher, A., & Postuma, R. B. (2017). Clinical criteria for subtyping Parkinson's disease: Biomarkers and longitudinal progression. *Brain*, *140*(7), 1959–1976. DOI: 10.1093/brain/awx118 PMID: 28549077

Fernandez, H. H., Standaert, D. G., Hauser, R. A., Lang, A. E., Fung, V. S. C., Klostermann, F., Lew, M. F., Odin, P., Steiger, M., Yakupov, E. Z., Chouinard, S., Suchowersky, O., Dubow, J., Hall, C. M., Chatamra, K., Robieson, W. Z., Benesh, J. A., & Espay, A. J. (2015). Levodopa-carbidopa intestinal gel in advanced Parkinson's disease: Final 12-month, open-label results. *Movement Disorders*, *30*(4), 500–509. DOI: 10.1002/MDS.26123

Ferreira, J. J., Lees, A., Rocha, J. F., Poewe, W., Rascol, O., & Soares-da-Silva, P. (2016). Opicapone as an adjunct to levodopa in patients with Parkinson's disease and end-of-dose motor fluctuations: A randomised, double-blind, controlled trial. *Lancet Neurology*, *15*(2), 154–165. DOI: 10.1016/S1474-4422(15)00336-1

Fezeu, F., Ramesh, A., Melmer, P. D., Moosa, S., Larson, P., & Henderson, F. (2018). Challenges and solutions for functional neurosurgery in developing countries. *Cureus*. Advance online publication. DOI: 10.7759/cureus.3314 PMID: 30473947

Ffytche, D. H., Creese, B., Politis, M., Chaudhuri, K. R., Weintraub, D., Ballard, C., & Aarsland, D. (2017). The psychosis spectrum in Parkinson disease. *Nature Reviews. Neurology*, *13*(2), 81. DOI: 10.1038/NRNEUROL.2016.200

Finberg, J. P. M. (2010). Pharmacology of Rasagiline, a New MAO-B Inhibitor Drug for the Treatment of Parkinson's Disease with Neuroprotective Potential. *Rambam Maimonides Medical Journal*, *1*(1), e0003. DOI: 10.5041/RMMJ.10003

Finberg, J. P. M., Lamensdorf, I., Commissiong, J. W., & Youdim, M. B. H. (1996). Pharmacology and neuroprotective properties of rasagiline. In Deprenyl—Past and Future [Vienna: Springer Vienna.]. *Journal of Neural Transmission. Supplementum*, *48*, 95–101. PMID: 8988465

Firbank, M. J., Molloy, S., McKeith, I. G., Burn, D. J., & O'Brien, J. T. (2005). Longitudinal change in 99mTcHMPAO cerebral perfusion SPECT in Parkinson's disease over one year. *Journal of Neurology, Neurosurgery, and Psychiatry*, *76*(10), 1448–1451. DOI: 10.1136/jnnp.2004.058685 PMID: 16170094

Fleming, T. R., & Powers, J. H. (2012). Biomarkers and surrogate endpoints in clinical trials. *Statistics in Medicine, 31*(25), 2973–2984. DOI: 10.1002/SIM.5403

Foltynie, T., Gandhi, S., Gonzalez-Robles, C., Zeissler, M. L., Mills, G., Barker, R., Carpenter, J., Schrag, A., Schapira, A., Bandmann, O., Mullin, S., Duffen, J., McFarthing, K., Chataway, J., Parmar, M., Carroll, C., Ben Shlomo, Y., Edwards, M., Whone, A., & Harris, J. (2023). Towards a multi-arm multi-stage platform trial of disease modifying approaches in Parkinson's disease. *Brain, 146*(7), 2717–2722. DOI: 10.1093/BRAIN/AWAD063

Foote, A., de Waal, E., Caiado, F., Samman, A., & Ukolov, A. (2025). A comprehensive review of deep brain stimulation for Parkinson's disease: The history, current state of the art and future possibilities. *Medicine in Novel Technology and Devices, 26*, 100362.

Formaggio, E., Tonellato, M., Antonini, A., Castiglia, L., Gallo, L., Manganotti, P., Masiero, S., & Del Felice, A. (2023). Oscillatory EEG-TMS Reactivity in Parkinson Disease. *Journal of Clinical Neurophysiology, 40*(3), 263–268. DOI: 10.1097/WNP.0000000000000881 PMID: 34280941

Fornari, A., Lanza, M., Guastafierro, E., Marcassoli, A., Sismondo, P., Curatoli, C., & Leonardi, M. (2025). Inequities in neurological care: Access to services, care gaps, and other barriers—A systematic review. *European Journal of Neurology, 32*(1), e16553. PMID: 39582360

Forsaa, E. B., Larsen, J. P., Wentzel-Larsen, T., & Alves, G. (2010). What predicts mortality in Parkinson disease? A prospective population-based long-term study. *Neurology, 75*(14), 1270–1276. PMID: 20921512

Foster, E. R., Campbell, M. C., Burack, M. A., Hartlein, J., Flores, H. P., Cairns, N. J., Hershey, T., & Perlmutter, J. S. (2010). Amyloid imaging of Lewy body-associated disorders. *Movement Disorders, 25*(15), 2516–2523. DOI: 10.1002/mds.23393 PMID: 20922808

Fothergill-Misbah, N., Cataldi, R., Stothard, M., Chowdhary, N., Okubadejo, N., Cappello, B., & Dua, T. (2025). Parkinson disease treatments on national essential medicines lists, African Region. *Bulletin of the World Health Organization, 103*(10), 626–634. PMID: 41035551

Fothergill-Misbah, N., Hooker, J., Kwasa, J., & Walker, R. (2024). Access to medicines for Parkinson's disease in Kenya: A qualitative exploration. *Movement Disorders Clinical Practice, 11*(11), 1373–1378. PMID: 39166895

Fox, M. D., Liu, H., & Pascual-Leone, A. (2013). Identification of reproducible individualized targets for treatment of depression with TMS based on intrinsic connectivity. *NeuroImage*, *66*, 151–160. DOI: 10.1016/j.neuroimage.2012.10.082 PMID: 23142067

Fox, S. H., Katzenschlager, R., Lim, S. Y., Barton, B., de Bie, R. M. A., Seppi, K., Coelho, M., & Sampaio, C. (2018a). International Parkinson and movement disorder society evidence-based medicine review: Update on treatments for the motor symptoms of Parkinson's disease. *Movement Disorders*, *33*(8), 1248–1266. DOI: 10.1002/MDS.27372

Franzoi, A. E. A., Bonchoski, A. B., & Koerbel, A. (2018). The advances of Deep Brain Stimulation (DBS) for treatment of Parkinson's Disease (PD). *Clinical & Biomedical Research*, *38*(4).

Fregni, F., Boggio, P. S., Nitsche, M. A., Marcolin, M. A., Rigonatti, S. P., & Pascual-Leone, A. (2006). Treatment of major depression with transcranial direct current stimulation. *Bipolar Disorders*, *8*(2), 203–204. DOI: 10.1111/j.1399-5618.2006.00291.x PMID: 16542193

Frequin, H. L., Verschuur, C. V. M., Suwijn, S. R., Boel, J. A., Post, B., Bloem, B. R., van Hilten, J. J., van Laar, T., Tissingh, G., Munts, A. G., Dijk, J. M., Lang, A. E., Dijkgraaf, M. G. W., Hoogland, J., & de Bie, R. M. A. (2024). Long-Term Follow-Up of the LEAP Study: Early Versus Delayed Levodopa in Early Parkinson's Disease. *Movement Disorders*, *39*(6), 975–982. DOI: 10.1002/MDS.29796

Friedman, L. M., Furberg, C. D., DeMets, D. L., Reboussin, D. M., & Granger, C. B. (2015). *Fundamentals of clinical trials*. Springer.

Frolov, N., Pitsik, E., Grubov, V., Badarin, A., Maksimenko, V., Zakharov, A., Kurkin, S., & Hramov, A. (2023). Perceptual Integration Compensates for Attention Deficit in Elderly during Repetitive Auditory-Based Sensorimotor Task. *Sensors, 23*(14). *Scopus*. Advance online publication. DOI: 10.3390/s23146420 PMID: 37514714

Fumimura, Y., Ikemura, M., Saito, Y., Sengoku, R., Kanemaru, K., Sawabe, M., Arai, T., Ito, G., Iwatsubo, T., Fukayama, M., & Hattori, N. (2007). Analysis of the adrenal gland is useful for evaluating pathology of the peripheral autonomic nervous system in lewy body disease. *Journal of Neuropathology and Experimental Neurology*, *66*(5), 354–362. DOI: 10.1097/nen.0b013e3180517454 PMID: 17483692

Gage, F. H. (2000). Mammalian neural stem cells. *Science*, *287*(5457), 1433–1438. PMID: 10688783

Galvin, J. E., Lee, V. M.-Y., & Trojanowski, J. Q. (2001). Synucleinopathies: Clinical and pathological implications. *Archives of Neurology, 58*(2), 186–190. DOI: 10.1001/archneur.58.2.186 PMID: 11176955

Gan-Or, Z., Amshalom, I., Kilarski, L. L., Bar-Shira, A., Gana-Weisz, M., Mirelman, A., Marder, K., Bressman, S., Giladi, N., & Orr-Urtreger, A. (2015). Differential effects of severe vs mild GBA mutations on Parkinson disease. *Neurology, 84*(9), 880–887. DOI: 10.1212/WNL.0000000000001315

Gao, C., Liu, J., Tan, Y., & Chen, S. (2020). Freezing of gait in Parkinson's disease: Pathophysiology, risk factors and treatments. *Translational Neurodegeneration, 9*(1), 12. DOI: 10.1186/s40035-020-00191-5 PMID: 32322387

García, S. F. R., Morón-Duarte, L. S., Arango, G., López, C. L. M., & González, N. Y. (2025). Generadores de pulso implantable recargables y no recargables para la estimulación cerebral profunda en pacientes con enfermedad de Parkinson. *Acta Neurologica Colombiana, 41*. Advance online publication. DOI: 10.22379/anc.v41i1.1861

Geranmayeh, M. H., Nourazarian, A., Avci, Ç. B., Rahbarghazi, R., & Farhoudi, M. (2017). Stem cells as a promising tool for the restoration of brain neurovascular unit and angiogenic orientation. *Molecular Neurobiology, 54*, 7689–7705. PMID: 27844280

Getz, K. A., & Campo, R. A. (2018). New benchmarks characterizing growth in protocol design complexity. *Therapeutic Innovation & Regulatory Science, 52*, 22–28. DOI: 10.1177/2168479017713039 PMID: 29714620

Gibbons, C. H., Levine, T., Adler, C., Bellaire, B., Wang, N., Stohl, J., Agarwal, P., Aldridge, G. M., Barboi, A., Evidente, V. G. H., Galasko, D., Geschwind, M. D., Gonzalez-Duarte, A., Gil, R., Gudesblatt, M., Isaacson, S. H., Kaufmann, H., Khemani, P., Kumar, R., & Freeman, R. (2024). Skin Biopsy Detection of Phosphorylated α-Synuclein in Patients With Synucleinopathies. *Journal of the American Medical Association, 331*(15), 1298. DOI: 10.1001/jama.2024.0792 PMID: 38506839

Gilbert, E. A. B., Lakshman, N., Lau, K. S. K., & Morshead, C. M. (2022). Regulating Endogenous Neural Stem Cell Activation to Promote Spinal Cord Injury Repair. *Cells, 11*(5), 846. PMID: 35269466

Gilman, S., Wenning, G. K., Low, P. A., Brooks, D. J., Mathias, C. J., Trojanowski, J. Q., Wood, N. W., Colosimo, C., Dürr, A., Fowler, C. J., Kaufmann, H., Klockgether, T., Lees, A., Poewe, W., Quinn, N., Revesz, T., Robertson, D., Sandroni, P., Seppi, K., & Vidailhet, M. (2008). Second consensus statement on the diagnosis of multiple system atrophy. *Neurology*, *71*(9), 670–676. DOI: 10.1212/01.wnl.0000324625.00404.15 PMID: 18725592

Goetz, C. G., Tilley, B. C., Shaftman, S. R., Stebbins, G. T., Fahn, S., Martinez-Martin, P., & LaPelle, N. (2008). Movement Disorder Society-sponsored revision of the Unified Parkinson's Disease Rating Scale (MDS-UPDRS): Scale presentation and clinimetric testing results. *Movement Disorders*, *23*(15), 2129–2170. PMID: 19025984

Goetz, C. G., Wuu, J., McDermott, M. P., Adler, C. H., Fahn, S., Freed, C. R., Hauser, R. A., Olanow, W. C., Shoulson, I., Tandon, P. K., Kieburtz, K., & Leurgans, S. (2008). Placebo response in Parkinson's disease: Comparisons among 11 trials covering medical and surgical interventions. *Movement Disorders*, *23*(5), 690–699. DOI: 10.1002/MDS.21894

Golchin, A., Chatziparasidou, A., Ranjbarvan, P., Niknam, Z., & Ardeshirylajimi, A. (2021). Embryonic Stem Cells in Clinical Trials: Current Overview of Developments and Challenges. *Advances in Experimental Medicine and Biology*, *1312*, 19–37. PMID: 33159303

Goldman, J. G., Volpe, D., Ellis, T. D., Hirsch, M. A., Johnson, J., Wood, J., & Wallock, K. (2024). Delivering multidisciplinary rehabilitation care in Parkinson's disease: An international consensus statement. *Journal of Parkinson's Disease*, *14*(1), 135–166. PMID: 38277303

Goldstein, D. S. (2014). Dysautonomia in Parkinson's disease: Neurocardiological abnormalities. *Comprehensive Physiology*, *4*(2), 805. DOI: 10.1002/CPHY.C130026

Golovanova, K. A., Skorokhodov, A. P., & Torubarova, I. I. (2013). Patients with neurological disorders: Specifics of communication. *Youth Innovation Bulletin*, *2*(1), 251.

Gomperts, S. N., Locascio, J. J., Marquie, M., Santarlasci, A. L., Rentz, D. M., Maye, J., Johnson, K. A., & Growdon, J. H. (2012). Brain amyloid and cognition in Lewy body diseases. *Movement Disorders*, *27*(8), 965–973. DOI: 10.1002/mds.25048 PMID: 22693110

Gonçalves, J., & Caliceti, P. (2024). Optimizing pharmacological and immunological properties of therapeutic proteins through PEGylation: Investigating key parameters and their impact. *Drug Design, Development and Therapy, 5041*. Advance online publication. DOI: 10.2147/DDDT.S481420 PMID: 39529843

Gonzalez-Robles, C., Athauda, D., Barber, T. R., Barker, R. A., Dexter, D. T., Duty, S., Ellis-Doyle, R., Gandhi, S., Handley, J., Jabbari, E., Martin, K., McFarthing, K., Mills, G., Mortiboys, H., Mullin, S., Petty, R., Sammler, E., Scurfield, P., Stott, S. R. W., & Petty, R. (2025). Treatment Selection and Prioritization for the EJS ACT-PD MAMS Trial Platform. *Movement Disorders*, *40*(7), 1307–1317. DOI: 10.1002/MDS.3019

Gonzalez-Robles, C., Bartlett, M., Burnell, M., Clarke, C. S., Haar, S., Hu, M. T., Huxford, B., Jha, A., Lawton, M., Noyce, A., Piccini, P., Pushparatnam, K., Rochester, L., Siu, C., van Wamelen, D., Williams-Gray, C. H., Zeissler, M. L., Zetterberg, H., Carroll, C. B., & Schrag, A. (2023). Embedding Patient Input in Outcome Measures for Long-Term Disease-Modifying Parkinson Disease Trials. *Movement Disorders*, *39*(2), 433–438. DOI: 10.1002/MDS.29691

Gordon, R., Albornoz, E. A., Christie, D. C., Langley, M. R., Kumar, V., Mantovani, S., Robertson, A. A. B., Butler, M. S., Rowe, D. B., O'Neill, L. A., Kanthasamy, A. G., Schroder, K., Cooper, M. A., & Woodruff, T. M. (2018). Inflammasome inhibition prevents α-synuclein pathology and dopaminergic neurodegeneration in mice. *Science Translational Medicine*, *10*(465). Advance online publication. DOI: 10.1126/SCITRANSLMED.AAH4066

Greene, B. R., Premoli, I., McManus, K., McGrath, D., & Caulfield, B. (2022). Predicting fall counts using wearable sensors: A novel digital biomarker for parkinson's disease. *Sensors (Basel)*, *22*(1). Advance online publication. DOI: 10.3390/s22010054 PMID: 35009599

Groiss, S.J.L., Wojtecki, M., Su¨dmeyer, & Schnitzler, A. (2009). Deep brain stimulation in Parkinson's disease. Ther Adv Neurol Disord (2009) 2(6) 379 391 DOI: .DOI: 10.1177/ 1756285609339382

Guerra, A., Rocchi, L., Grego, A., Berardi, F., Luisi, C., & Ferreri, F. (2021). Contribution of TMS and TMS-EEG to the Understanding of Mechanisms Underlying Physiological Brain Aging. *Brain Sciences*, *11*(3), 405. DOI: 10.3390/brainsci11030405 PMID: 33810206

Guevremont, D., Roy, J., Cutfield, N. J., & Williams, J. M. (2023). MicroRNAs in Parkinson's disease: A systematic review and diagnostic accuracy meta-analysis. *Scientific Reports*, *13*, 16272. DOI: 10.1038/s41598-023-43463-6 PMID: 37770507

Gugliandolo, A., Bramanti, P., & Mazzon, E. (2019). Mesenchymal Stem Cells: A Potential Therapeutic Approach for Amyotrophic Lateral Sclerosis? *Stem Cells International, 2019*, 3675627. PMID: 30956667

Guimaraes, P., Kieburtz, K., Goetz, C. G., Elm, J. J., Palesch, Y. Y., Huang, P., Ravina, B., Tanner, C. M., & Tilley, B. C. (2005). Non-linearity of Parkinson's disease progression: Implications for sample size calculations in clinical trials. *Clinical Trials*, *2*(6), 509–518. DOI: 10.1191/1740774505CN125OA

Gui, Y., Liu, H., Zhang, L., Lv, W., & Hu, X. (2015). Altered microRNA profiles in cerebrospinal fluid exosome in Parkinson disease and Alzheimer disease. *Oncotarget*, *6*(35), 37043–37053. DOI: 10.18632/oncotarget.6158 PMID: 26497684

Guo, M., Wang, J., Zhao, Y., Feng, Y., Han, S., Dong, Q., Cui, M., & Tieu, K. (2020). Microglial exosomes facilitate α-synuclein transmission in Parkinson's disease. *Brain*, *143*(5), 1476–1497. DOI: 10.1093/BRAIN/AWAA090

Guttman, M., Stewart, D., Hussey, D., Wilson, A., Houle, S., & Kish, S. (2001). Influence of L-dopa and pramipexole on striatal dopamine transporter in early PD. *Neurology*, *56*(11), 1559–1564. DOI: 10.1212/WNL.56.11.1559

Hajzer, Z. E., Alibrahem, W., Helu, N. K., Oláh, C., & Prokisch, J. (2025). Functional foods in clinical trials and future research directions. *Foods*, *14*, 2675. DOI: 10.3390/foods14152675 PMID: 40807611

Hammoud, F., Ismail, A., Zaher, R., El Majzoub, R., & Abou-Abbas, L. (2025). Mucuna pruriens Treatment for Parkinson Disease: A Systematic Review of Clinical Trials. *Parkinson's Disease*, *2025*(1), 1319419. PMID: 40860042

Hamood, H. M., Alsaedi, M. A. Z., Al-Qrimli, A. F., & Jawad, A. Q. (2024). Parkinson Disease Pharmacological and Herbal Management: A Review. *South Asian Research Journal of Applied Medical Sciences.*, *6*(1), 1–9.

Hanson, E., Nwakile, C., & Hammed, V. (2025). Carbon capture, utilization, and storage (CCUS) technologies: Evaluating the effectiveness of advanced CCUS solutions for reducing CO_2 emissions. *Results in Surfaces and Interfaces*.

Hansson, O., Janelidze, S., Hall, S., Magdalinou, N., Lees, A. J., Andreasson, U., Norgren, N., Linder, J., Forsgren, L., Constantinescu, R., Zetterberg, H., & Blennow, K. (2017). Blood-based NfL: A biomarker for differential diagnosis of parkinsonian disorder. *Neurology*, *88*(10), 930–937. DOI: 10.1212/WNL.0000000000003680

Han, Y., Liu, X., Zhang, N., Zhang, X., Zhang, B., Wang, S., Liu, T., & Yi, J. (2023). Automatic Assessments of Parkinsonian Gait with Wearable Sensors for Human Assistive Systems. *Sensors (Basel), 23*(4). Advance online publication. DOI: 10.3390/s23042104 PMID: 36850705

Han, Y., Yang, J., Fang, J., Zhou, Y., Candi, E., Wang, J., Hua, D., Shao, C., & Shi, Y. (2022). The secretion profile of mesenchymal stem cells and potential applications in treating human diseases. *Signal Transduction and Targeted Therapy, 7*(1), 92. PMID: 35314676

Haqqani, A. S., Bélanger, K., & Stanimirovic, D. B. (2024). Receptor-mediated transcytosis for brain delivery of therapeutics: Receptor classes and criteria. *Frontiers in Drug Delivery, 4*, 1360302. DOI: 10.3389/FDDEV.2024.1360302

Harding, A. J., & Halliday, G. M. (2001). Cortical Lewy body pathology in the diagnosis of dementia. *Acta Neuropathologica, 102*(4), 355–363. DOI: 10.1007/s004010100390 PMID: 11603811

Hartmann, C.J., Sabine, F., Stefan, J.G, Lars, W. & Alfons, S. (2019). An update on best practice of deep brain stimulation in Parkinson's disease. Therapeutic Advances in Neurological Disorders. 2019, Vol. 12: 1–20 https://doi.org/ https://doi.org/.DOI: 10.1177/1756286419838096

Hassan, A., Khan, H., Ali, A., Din, I. U., Sajid, A., & Husain, M.. (2024). An enhanced lung cancer identification and classification based on advanced deep learning and convolutional neural network. *Bulletin of Business and Economics, 13*, 136. DOI: 10.61506/01.00308

Hauser, R. A., Hsu, A., Kell, S., Espay, A. J., Sethi, K., Stacy, M., Ondo, W., O'Connell, M., & Gupta, S. (2013). Extended-release carbidopa-levodopa (IPX066) compared with immediate-release carbidopa-levodopa in patients with Parkinson's disease and motor fluctuations: A phase 3 randomised, double-blind trial. *Lancet Neurology, 12*(4), 346–356. DOI: 10.1016/S1474-4422(13)70025-5

Hauser, R. A., Skarpaas, T. C., Merriam, A., Rivera, J., Hoxhaj, V., Barbato, L. M., & Baladi, M. (2025). Burden of tremor in Parkinson's disease: A survey study. *Journal of Parkinson's Disease, 15*(3), 541–551. PMID: 40123351

Haxhiu, H., Hoxha, M., Zela, I., & Zappacosta, B. (2025). An Overview of the Role of Medicinal Plants in Parkinson's Disease: A Semi-Systematic Review. *Biomedicines, 13*(8), 2008. PMID: 40868260

Healy, D. G., Falchi, M., O'Sullivan, S. S., Bonifati, V., Durr, A., Bressman, S., Brice, A., Aasly, J., Zabetian, C. P., Goldwurm, S., Ferreira, J. J., Tolosa, E., Kay, D. M., Klein, C., Williams, D. R., Marras, C., Lang, A. E., Wszolek, Z. K., Berciano, J., & Wood, N. W. (2008). Phenotype, genotype, and worldwide genetic penetrance of LRRK2-associated Parkinson's disease: A case-control study. *Lancet Neurology*, *7*(7), 583–590. DOI: 10.1016/S1474-4422(08)70117-0

Helmer, R. S., Merscher, M. N., Lobo, C. C., de Souza, V. M., de Jesus, M. A., & Ganho, T.. (2024). A rare case of hemichorea secondary to giant perivascular space: A case report. *Arquivos de Neuro-Psiquiatria*, *13*. Advance online publication. DOI: 10.5327/cbn240046

Helmers, A.-K., Stieglitz, L. H., & Werner, B. (2025). Focused Ultrasound in Parkinson's Disease. In E. Ch. Wolters & C. R. Baumann (Eds.), *International Compendium of Movement Disorders* (pp. 328–338). Cambridge University Press. Cambridge Core. https://doi.org/DOI: 10.1017/9781108989855.029

Helmich, R. C., Hallett, M., Deuschl, G., Toni, I., & Bloem, B. R. (2012). Cerebral causes and consequences of parkinsonian resting tremor: A tale of two circuits? *Brain*, *135*(Pt 11), 3206–3226. PMID: 22382359

Helmich, R. C., Janssen, M. J. R., Oyen, W. J. G., Bloem, B. R., & Toni, I. (2011). Pallidal dysfunction drives a cerebellothalamic circuit into Parkinson tremor. *Annals of Neurology*, *69*(2), 269–281. PMID: 21387372

He, Q., Wang, Q., Yuan, C., & Wang, Y. (2017). Downregulation of miR-7116-5p in microglia by MPP+ sensitizes TNF-alpha production to induce dopaminergic neuron damage. *Glia*, *65*(8), 1251–1263. DOI: 10.1002/glia.23153 PMID: 28543680

Heris, R. M., Shirvaliloo, M., Abbaspour-Aghdam, S., Hazrati, A., Shariati, A., Youshanlouei, H. R., Niaragh, F. J., Valizadeh, H., & Ahmadi, M. (2022). The potential use of mesenchymal stem cells and their exosomes in Parkinson's disease treatment. *Stem Cell Research & Therapy*, *13*(1), 371. PMID: 35902981

Hess, D. C., Wechsler, L. R., & Clark, W. M.. (2017). Safety and efficacy of multipotent adult progenitor cells in acute ischaemic stroke (MASTERS): A randomised, double-blind, placebo-controlled, phase 2 trial. *Lancet Neurology*, *16*(5), 360–368. PMID: 28320635

Hirczy, S., Zabetian, C., & Lin, Y. H. (2024). The current state of wearable device uses in Parkinson's disease: A survey of individuals with Parkinson's. *Frontiers in Digital Health*, *6*, 1472691. DOI: 10.3389/fdgth.2024.1472691 PMID: 39764207

Hirsch, E. C., & Hunot, S. (2009). Neuroinflammation in Parkinson's disease: A target for neuroprotection? *Lancet Neurology*, *8*(4), 382–397. DOI: 10.1016/S1474-4422(09)70062-6

Horváth, K., Aschermann, Z., Ács, P., Deli, G., Janszky, J., Komoly, S., Balázs, É., Takács, K., Karádi, K., & Kovács, N. (2015a). Minimal clinically important difference on the Motor Examination part of MDS-UPDRS. *Parkinsonism & Related Disorders*, *21*(12), 1421–1426. DOI: 10.1016/j.parkreldis.2015.10.006

Huang, Y.-Z., Edwards, M. J., Rounis, E., Bhatia, K. P., & Rothwell, J. C. (2005). Theta Burst Stimulation of the Human Motor Cortex. *Neuron*, *45*(2), 201–206. DOI: 10.1016/j.neuron.2004.12.033 PMID: 15664172

Hughes, A. J., Daniel, S. E., Kilford, L., & Lees, A. J. (1992). Accuracy of clinical diagnosis of idiopathic Parkinson's disease: A clinico-pathological study of 100 cases. *Journal of Neurology, Neurosurgery, and Psychiatry*, *55*(3), 181–184. PMID: 1564476

Hussen, B. M., Taheri, M., Yashooa, R. K., Abdullah, G. H., Abdullah, S. R., Kheder, R. K., & Mustafa, S. A. (2024). Revolutionizing medicine: Recent developments and future prospects in stem-cell therapy. *International Journal of Surgery*, *110*(12), 8002–8024. PMID: 39497543

Huynh, P. D., Tran, Q. X., Nguyen, S. T., Nguyen, V. Q., & Vu, N. B. (2022). Mesenchymal stem cell therapy for wound healing: An update to 2022. *Biomedical Research and Therapy*, *9*(12), 5437–5449.

Hwang, S., Gill, S., Pathak, S., & Subramanian, S. (2018). A Comparison of Stem Cell Therapies for Parkinson Disease. *Georgetown Medical Review, 2*(1).

Iansek, R., & Danoudis, M. (2017). Freezing of Gait in Parkinson's Disease: Its Pathophysiology and Pragmatic Approaches to Management. *Movement Disorders Clinical Practice*, *4*(3), 290–297. DOI: 10.1002/mdc3.12463 PMID: 30868095

Iemmi, V., Blanchet, K., Gibson, L. J., Kumar, K. S., Rath, S., Hartley, S., & Kuper, H. (2016). Community-based rehabilitation for people with physical and mental disabilities in low-and middle-income countries: A systematic review and meta-analysis. *Journal of Development Effectiveness*, *8*(3), 368–387.

Iemmi, V., Kumar, K. S., Blanchet, K., Gibson, L., Hartley, S., Murthy, G. V., & Kuper, H. (2017). Community-based rehabilitation for people with physical and mental disabilities in low-and middle-income countries. *Cochrane Database of Systematic Reviews*, *2017*(3), CD010617.

Ile an, R. R., Cordo , C. G., Mihăilă, L. I., Fle ar, R., Popescu, A. S., Perju-Dumbravă, L., & Faragó, P. (2022). Proof of Concept in Artificial-Intelligence-Based Wearable Gait Monitoring for Parkinson's Disease Management Optimization. *Biosensors (Basel), 12*(4). Advance online publication. DOI: 10.3390/bios12040189 PMID: 35448249

Irwin, D. J., White, M. T., Toledo, J. B., Xie, S. X., Robinson, J. L., Van Deerlin, V., Lee, V. M.-Y., Leverenz, J. B., Montine, T. J., Duda, J. E., Hurtig, H. I., & Trojanowski, J. Q. (2012). Neuropathologic substrates of Parkinson disease dementia. *Annals of Neurology, 72*(4), 587–598. DOI: 10.1002/ana.23659 PMID: 23037886

Ishiguro, M., Li, Y., & Yoshino, H.. (2021). Clinical manifestations of Parkinson's disease harboring VPS35 retromer complex component p.D620N with long-term follow-up. *Parkinsonism & Related Disorders, 84*, 139–143. PMID: 33611076

Jahanshahi, M., Jenkins, I. H., Brown, R. G., Marsden, C. D., Passingham, R. E., & Brooks, D. J. (1995). Self-initiated versus externally triggered movements. I. An investigation using measurement of regional cerebral blood flow with PET and movement-related potentials in normal and Parkinson's disease subjects. *Brain, 118*(Pt 4), 913–933. DOI: 10.1093/brain/118.4.913 PMID: 7655888

Jaiswal, V., Alquraish, D., & Sandra, Z.. (2021). The influence of COVID-19 on Parkinson's disease: An updated systematic review. *Journal of Primary Care & Community Health, 12*, 21501327211039708. PMID: 34404266

Jankovic, J., McDermott, M., Carter, J., Gauthier, S., Goetz, C., Golbe, L., Huber, S., Koller, W., Olanow, C., Shoulson, I., Stern, M., Tanner, C., & Weiner, W. (1990). Variable expression of Parkinson's disease: A base-line analysis of the DATATOP cohort. *Neurology, 40*(10), 1529–1534. PMID: 2215943

Janssen Daalen, J. M., Schootemeijer, S., Richard, E., Darweesh, S. K., & Bloem, B. R. (2022). Lifestyle interventions for the prevention of Parkinson disease: A recipe for action. *Neurology, 99*(7), 42–51. PMID: 35970584

Jellinger, K. A. (2012). Neuropathology of sporadic Parkinson's disease: Evaluation and changes of concepts. *Movement Disorders, 27*(1), 8–30. DOI: 10.1002/mds.23795 PMID: 22081500

Jeong, J. Y., Lee, H. J., Kim, N., Li, Y., Rah, J. C., & Oh, W. J. (2023). Impaired neuronal activity as a potential factor contributing to the underdeveloped cerebrovasculature in a young Parkinson's disease mouse model. *Scientific Reports, 13*(1), 22613. PMID: 38114623

Jiang, C., Hopfner, F., Berg, D., Hu, M. T., Pilotto, A., Borroni, B., Davis, J. J., & Tofaris, G. K. (2021). Validation of alpha-synuclein in L1CAM-immunocaptured exosomes as a biomarker for the stratification of parkinsonian syndromes. *Movement Disorders*, *36*(11), 2663–2669. DOI: 10.1002/mds.28591 PMID: 33826157

Jin, C., Cho, K.-H., Kwon, S., Lee, H.-G., Kim, T.-H., Jung, W.-S., Moon, S.-K., Cho, S.-Y., Kang, B.-K., Park, J.-M., Park, H.-J., & Ko, C.-N. (2022). Effectiveness and safety of herbal medicine Ukgansan for clinical symptoms in Parkinson's disease: A pilot, randomized, assessor-blinded clinical trial. *Frontiers in Neurology*, *13*, 1025269. DOI: 10.3389/fneur.2022.1025269 PMID: 36438946

Jin, X., Dong, W., Chang, K., Yan, Y., & Liu, X. (2024a). Efficacy of probiotic supplements on Parkinson's disease: A systematic review and meta-analysis. *Complementary Therapies in Medicine*, *82*, 103045. DOI: 10.1016/J.CTIM.2024.103045

John-Stuart, B., & Hayriye, C. (2018). Recent Trends in the Use of Electrical Neuromodulation in Parkinson's Disease. *Current Behavioral Neuroscience Reports*, *2018*(5), 170–178. DOI: 10.1007/s40473-018-0154-9 PMID: 29862163

Jost, S. T., Salima, A., Julian, E., Keyoumars, A., Anna, S., Alexandra, R., Jan, N. P. S., Alexandra, G., & Gereon, R. F. V. (2024). Visser-Vandewalle, Angelo, A., Monty, S., Lars, T.P., Martinez-Martin, K. R., Chaudhuri, Haidar, S., & Dafsari, M. (2024). Neurostimulation for Advanced Parkinson Disease and Quality of Life at 5 Years A Non-Randomized Controlled Trial. *JAMA Network Open*, *7*(1), e2352177. DOI: 10.1001/jamanetworkopen.2023.52177 PMID: 38236600

Jun, P., Zhao, H., Jung, I. C., Kwon, O., Han, C. H., Won, J., & Jang, J. H. (2023). Efficacy of herbal medicine treatment based on syndrome differentiation for Parkinson's disease: A systematic review and meta-analysis of randomized placebo-controlled clinical trials. *Frontiers in Pharmacology*, *14*, 1108407. DOI: 10.3389/fphar.2023.1108407 PMID: 36925641

Kalinderi, K., Papaliagkas, V., & Fidani, L. (2019). Pharmacogenetics and levodopa induced motor complications. *The International Journal of Neuroscience*, *129*(4), 384–392. DOI: 10.1080/00207454.2018.1538993 PMID: 30359152

Kalluri, R., & LeBleu, V. S. (2020). The biology, function, and biomedical applications of exosomes. *Science*, *367*(6478), eaau6977. Advance online publication. DOI: 10.1126/science.aau6977 PMID: 32029601

Kanungo, J., Sorkin, B. C., Krzykwa, J., Mitchell, C. A., Embry, M., Spencer, P., Harry, G. J., Cannon, J., Liu, F., McPherson, C. A., Gafner, S., & Westerink, R. H. S. (2024). Screening tools to evaluate the neurotoxic potential of botanicals: Building a strategy to assess safety. *Expert Opinion on Drug Metabolism & Toxicology, 20*(7), 629–646. PMID: 38984683

Kassubek, J., Juengling, F. D., Hellwig, B., Spreer, J., & Lücking, C. H. (2002). Thalamic gray matter changes in unilateral Parkinsonian resting tremor: A voxel-based morphometric analysis of 3-dimensional magnetic resonance imaging. *Neuroscience Letters, 323*(1), 29–32. PMID: 11911983

Katzenschlager, R., Evans, A., Manson, A., Patsalos, P. N., Ratnaraj, N., Watt, H., & Lees, A. J. (2004). Mucuna pruriens in Parkinson's disease: A double blind clinical and pharmacological study. *Journal of Neurology, Neurosurgery, and Psychiatry, 75*(12), 1672–1677. PMID: 15548480

Kaur, M., & Gupta, M. (2025). Role and mechanism of herbal bioactives in treatment of Parkinson's disease: A promising therapeutic approach. *South African Journal of Botany, 181*, 315–338.

Kaur, R., Mehan, S., & Singh, S. (2019). Understanding multifactorial architecture of Parkinson's disease: Pathophysiology to management. *Neurological Sciences.* PMID: 30267336

Kehnemouyi, Y. M., Coleman, T. P., & Tass, P. A. (2024). Emerging wearable technologies for multisystem monitoring and treatment of Parkinson's disease: A narrative review. *Frontiers in Network Physiology, 4*, 1354211. DOI: 10.3389/fnetp.2024.1354211 PMID: 38414636

Kelly, V. E., Eusterbrock, A. J., & Shumway-Cook, A. (2012). The Effects of Instructions on Dual-Task Walking and Cognitive Task Performance in People with Parkinson's Disease. *Parkinson's Disease, 2012*, 1–9. DOI: 10.1155/2012/671261 PMID: 23326758

Kenny, L., Moore, K., O' Riordan, C., Fox, S., Barton, J., Tedesco, S., Sica, M., Crowe, C., Alamäki, A., Condell, J., Nordström, A., & Timmons, S. (2022). The Views and Needs of People with Parkinson Disease Regarding Wearable Devices for Disease Monitoring: Mixed Methods Exploration. *JMIR Formative Research, 6*(1), e27418. https://formative.jmir.org/2022/1/e27418. DOI: 10.2196/27418 PMID: 34989693

Keus, S. H. J., Oude Nijhuis, L. B., Nijkrake, M. J., Bloem, B. R., & Munneke, M. (2012). Improving Community Healthcare for Patients with Parkinson′ s Disease: The Dutch Model. *Parkinson's Disease, 2012*(1), 543426. PMID: 22496990

Khalid, T., Malik, A., Rasool, N., Kanwal, A., Nawaz, H., & Almas, I. (2025). Cracking the code: The clinical and molecular impact of aminopyridines; A review (2019–2024). *RSC Advances*, *15*, 688. DOI: 10.1039/D4RA07438F PMID: 39781020

Khazdair, M. R., Kianmehr, M., & Anaeigoudari, A. (2021). Effects of Medicinal Plants and Flavonoids on Parkinson's Disease: A Review on Basic and Clinical Evidence. *Advanced Pharmaceutical Bulletin*, *11*(2), 224–232. PMID: 33880344

Kim, C. K., Lee, Y. R., Ong, L., Gold, M., Kalali, A., & Sarkar, J. (2022). Alzheimer's Disease: Key Insights from Two Decades of Clinical Trial Failures. *Journal of Alzheimer's Disease*, *87*, 83–100. PMID: 35342092

Kim, T. W. (2026). Human stem cell–based cell replacement therapy for Parkinson's disease: Enhancing the survival of postmitotic dopamine neuron grafts. *Neural Regeneration Research*, *21*(2), 689–690. PMID: 40326986

Kim, T.-H., Cho, K.-H., Jung, W.-S., & Lee, M. S. (2012). Herbal Medicines for Parkinson's Disease: A Systematic Review of Randomized Controlled Trials. *PLoS One*, *7*(5), e35695. DOI: 10.1371/journal.pone.0035695 PMID: 22615738

Kim, Y. W., Shin, I.-S., Moon, H. I., Lee, S. C., & Yoon, S. Y. (2019). Effects of non-invasive brain stimulation on freezing of gait in parkinsonism: A systematic review with meta-analysis. *Parkinsonism & Related Disorders*, *64*, 82–89. DOI: 10.1016/j.parkreldis.2019.02.029 PMID: 30902526

Kirkeby, A., Main, H., & Carpenter, M. (2025). Pluripotent stem-cell-derived therapies in clinical trial: A 2025 update. *Cell Stem Cell*, *32*(1), 10–37. PMID: 39753110

Kirkeby, A., Nolbrant, S., Tiklova, K., Heuer, A., Kee, N., Cardoso, T., Ottosson, D. R., Lelos, M. J., Rifes, P., Dunnett, S. B., Grealish, S., Perlmann, T., & Parmar, M. (2017). Predictive Markers Guide Differentiation to Improve Graft Outcome in Clinical Translation of hESC-Based Therapy for Parkinson's Disease. *Cell Stem Cell*, *20*(1), 135–148. DOI: 10.1016/j.stem.2016.09.004

Kirmani, M. A., & Afaq, Y. (2024). Developments in deep learning approaches for apple leaf Alternaria disease identification: A review. *Computers and Electronics in Agriculture*, *227*, 109593. DOI: 10.1016/j.compag.2024.109593

Kish, S. J., Shannak, K., & Hornykiewicz, O. (1988). Uneven pattern of dopamine loss in the striatum of patients with idiopathic Parkinson's disease: Pathophysiologic and clinical implications. *The New England Journal of Medicine*, *318*(14), 876–880. PMID: 3352672

Kleine Bardenhorst, S., Cereda, E., Severgnini, M., Barichella, M., Pezzoli, G., Keshavarzian, A., Desideri, A., Pietrucci, D., Aho, V. T. E., Scheperjans, F., Hildebrand, F., Weis, S., Egert, M., Karch, A., Vital, M., & Rübsamen, N. (2023a). Gut microbiota dysbiosis in Parkinson disease: A systematic review and pooled analysis. *European Journal of Neurology*, *30*(11), 3581–3594. DOI: 10.1111/ENE.15671

Kluge, A., Bunk, J., Schaeffer, E., Drobny, A., Xiang, W., Knacke, H., Bub, S., Lückstädt, W., Arnold, P., Lucius, R., Berg, D., & Zunke, F. (2022). Detection of neuron-derived pathological α-synuclein in blood. *Brain*, *145*(9), 3058–3071. DOI: 10.1093/BRAIN/AWAC115

Kmiecik, M. J., Micheletti, S., Coker, D., Heilbron, K., Shi, J., Stagaman, K., Sonmez, T. F., Fontanillas, P., Shringarpure, S., Wetzel, M., Rowbotham, H. M., Cannon, P., Shelton, J. F., Hinds, D. A., Tung, J. Y., Holmes, M. V., Aslibekyan, S., Norcliffe-Kaufmann, L., Auton, A., & Wong, C. D. (2024). Genetic analysis and natural history of Parkinson's disease due to the LRRK2 G2019S variant. *Brain*, *147*(6), 1996. DOI: 10.1093/BRAIN/AWAE073

Koehn, S., Drummond, N., Jasper, L., Pham, A. N., Leung, K., Cloutier, D., & Jones, C. A. (2025). Mechanisms of inequitable access to Parkinson's disease care: A critical interpretive synthesis. *International Journal for Equity in Health*, *24*(1), 250. PMID: 41039438

Koirala, N., Manuel, B., Aparna, W.S. & Muthuraman, M. (2025). Advancements in invasive and non-invasive neuromodulation for Parkinson's disease: current findings and future directions. | (2025) 11:221. https://doi.org/.DOI: 10.1038/s41531-025-01071-3

Komarova, Y., Zakharov, A., Sergeeva, M., Romanchuk, N., Vladimirova, T., & Shirolapov, I. (2025). Modeling Working Memory in Neurodegeneration: A Focus on EEG Methods. *Diagnostics (Basel)*, *15*(23), 2992. DOI: 10.3390/diagnostics15232992 PMID: 41374372

Kong, Z., Gao, L., Wang, L., & Li, S. (2008). The normal parameter reduction of soft sets and its algorithm. *Computers & Mathematics with Applications (Oxford, England)*, *56*(12), 3029–3037.

Kordower, J. H., Olanow, C. W., Dodiya, H. B., Chu, Y., Beach, T. G., Adler, C. H., Halliday, G. M., & Bartus, R. T. (2013). Disease duration and the integrity of the nigrostriatal system in Parkinson's disease. *Brain*, *136*(8), 2419–2431. DOI: 10.1093/brain/awt192 PMID: 23884810

Kotyal, K., Nautiyal, P., & Singh, M. (2024). Advancements and challenges in artificial intelligence applications: A comprehensive review. *Journal of Scientific Research*.

Kouli, A., Torsney, K. M., & Kuan, W. L. (2018). Parkinson's Disease: Etiology, Neuropathology, and Pathogenesis. In: Stoker TB, Greenland JC, editors. Parkinson's Disease: Pathogenesis and Clinical Aspects [Internet]. Brisbane (AU): Codon Publications. Chapter 1.

Krokidis, M. G., Dimitrakopoulos, G. N., Vrahatis, A. G., Tzouvelekis, C., Drakoulis, D., Papavassileiou, F., Exarchos, T. P., & Vlamos, P. (2022). A Sensor-Based Perspective in Early-Stage Parkinson's Disease: Current State and the Need for Machine Learning Processes. *Sensors (Basel), 22*(2). Advance online publication. DOI: 10.3390/s22020409 PMID: 35062370

Kumar, G. (2023). Editorial: Neuroprotective mechanisms by phytochemicals in neurological disorders. *Frontiers in Neuroscience, 17*, 1149639. DOI: 10.3389/fnins.2023.1149639 PMID: 37008215

Kumar, L., Malhotra, M., Sharma, A., & Singh, A. P. (2024). A holistic approach to Parkinson's disease: Integrating advances in pathophysiology, diagnosis, and therapy. *Journal of Drug Delivery and Therapeutics, 14*, 141. DOI: 10.22270/jddt.v14i5.6558

Kumar, L., Malhotra, M., Singh, A., & Singh, A. P. (2024). Comprehensive Review on Parkinson's Disease: Insights into Prevalence, Pathophysiology, Diagnosis, and Multifaceted Treatment Approaches. *Journal of Drug Delivery and Therapeutics, 14*(6). Advance online publication. DOI: 10.22270/jddt.v14i6.6637

Kumar, M., & Sathiya, P. (2021). Methods and materials for additive manufacturing: A critical review on advancements and challenges. *Thin-walled Structures*.

Kwok, J. Y., Kwan, J. C., Auyeung, M., Mok, V. C., Lau, C. K., Choi, K. C., & Chan, H. Y. (2019). Effects of mindfulness yoga vs stretching and resistance training exercises on anxiety and depression for people with Parkinson disease: A randomized clinical trial. *JAMA Neurology, 76*(7), 755–763. PMID: 30958514

Laar, A., Silva de Lima, A. L., Maas, B. R., Bloem, B. R., & de Vries, N. M. (2023). Successful implementation of technology in the management of Parkinson's disease: Barriers and facilitators. *Clinical Parkinsonism & Related Disorders*.

Lachenal, G., Pernet-Gallay, K., Chivet, M., Hemming, F. J., Belly, A., Bodon, G., Blot, B., Haase, G., Goldberg, Y., & Sadoul, R. (2011). Release of exosomes from differentiated neurons and its regulation by synaptic glutamatergic activity. *Molecular and Cellular Neurosciences, 46*(2), 409–418. DOI: 10.1016/j.mcn.2010.11.004 PMID: 21111824

Lachenmayer, M. L., Mürset, M., Antih, N., Debove, I., Muellner, J., Bompart, M., Schlaeppi, J. A., Nowacki, A., You, H., Michelis, J. P., Dransart, A., Pollo, C., Deuschl, G., & Krack, P. (2021). Subthalamic and pallidal deep brain stimulation for Parkinson's disease—meta-analysis of outcomes. *Npj Parkinson's Disease 2021 7:1, 7*(1), 77-. https://doi.org/DOI: 10.1038/s41531-021-00223-5

Lang, A. E., & Espay, A. J. (2018). Disease modification in Parkinson's disease: Current approaches, challenges, and future considerations. *Movement Disorders, 33*, 660–677. DOI: 10.1002/mds.27360 PMID: 29644751

Lang, A. E., Gill, S., Patel, N. K., Lozano, A., Nutt, J. G., Penn, R., Brooks, D. J., Hotton, G., Moro, E., Heywood, P., Brodsky, M. A., Burchiel, K., Kelly, P., Dalvi, A., Scott, B., Stacy, M., Turner, D., Wooten, V. G. F., Elias, W. J., & Traub, M. (2006). Randomized controlled trial of intraputamenal glial cell line-derived neurotrophic factor infusion in Parkinson disease. *Annals of Neurology, 59*(3), 459–466. DOI: 10.1002/ANA.20737

Lang, A. E., Siderowf, A. D., Macklin, E. A., Poewe, W., Brooks, D. J., Fernandez, H. H., Rascol, O., Giladi, N., Stocchi, F., Tanner, C. M., Postuma, R. B., Simon, D. K., Tolosa, E., Mollenhauer, B., Cedarbaum, J. M., Fraser, K., Xiao, J., Evans, K. C., Graham, D. L., & Dam, T. (2022). Trial of Cinpanemab in Early Parkinson's Disease. *The New England Journal of Medicine, 387*(5), 408–420. DOI: 10.1056/NEJMOA2203395

Lavano, A., Attilio, D.T. & Giusy, G. (2016). Directional Deep Brain Stimulation. Brain Disord The 2016, 5:3. 1000220. DOI: .DOI: 10.4172/2168-975X.1000220

Lee, A. J., Wang, Y., Alcalay, R. N., Mejia-Santana, H., Saunders-Pullman, R., Bressman, S., Corvol, J. C., Brice, A., Lesage, S., Mangone, G., Tolosa, E., Pont-Sunyer, C., Vilas, D., Schüle, B., Kausar, F., Foroud, T., Berg, D., Brockmann, K., Goldwurm, S., & Marder, K. (2017). Penetrance estimate of LRRK2 p.G2019S mutation in individuals of non-Ashkenazi Jewish ancestry. *Movement Disorders, 32*(10), 1432–1438. DOI: 10.1002/MDS.27059

Lee, J., Lim, J., Kang, S., Kim, S., Jung, S. Y., & Kim, S.. (2024). Mobile app–assisted parent training intervention for behavioral problems in children with autism spectrum disorder: Pilot randomized controlled trial. *JMIR Human Factors, 11*. Advance online publication. DOI: 10.2196/52295 PMID: 39466295

Lees, A. J., Ferreira, J., Rascol, O., Poewe, W., Rocha, J. F., McCrory, M., & Soares-Da-Silva, P. (2017). Opicapone as Adjunct to Levodopa Therapy in Patients With Parkinson Disease and Motor Fluctuations: A Randomized Clinical Trial. *JAMA Neurology, 74*(2), 197–206. DOI: 10.1001/JAMANEUROL.2016.4703

Lee, Y., Chang, Y. Y., Chen, Y. F., Lin, T. K., Hung, C. F., & Chiou, Y. J.. (2022). Prevalence and risk factors of depression between patients with Parkinson's disease and their caregivers: A one-year prospective study. *Health Care*, *10*, 1305. PMID: 35885832

Lefaucheur, J.-P., Aleman, A., Baeken, C., Benninger, D. H., Brunelin, J., Di Lazzaro, V., Filipović, S. R., Grefkes, C., Hasan, A., Hummel, F. C., Jääskeläinen, S. K., Langguth, B., Leocani, L., Londero, A., Nardone, R., Nguyen, J.-P., Nyffeler, T., Oliveira-Maia, A. J., Oliviero, A., & Ziemann, U. (2020). Evidence-based guidelines on the therapeutic use of repetitive transcranial magnetic stimulation (rTMS): An update (2014–2018). *Clinical Neurophysiology*, *131*(2), 474–528. DOI: 10.1016/j.clinph.2019.11.002 PMID: 31901449

Lencioni, T., Meloni, M., Bowman, T., Marzegan, A., Caronni, A., Carpinella, I., Castagna, A., Gower, V., Ferrarin, M., & Pelosin, E. (2022). Events Detection of Anticipatory Postural Adjustments through a Wearable Accelerometer Sensor Is Comparable to That Measured by the Force Platform in Subjects with Parkinson's Disease. *Sensors (Basel)*, *22*(7). Advance online publication. DOI: 10.3390/s22072668 PMID: 35408282

Leon-Rojas, J. E. (2025). The global rise in Parkinson's disease: A critical analysis of causes and future directions. *Frontiers in Public Health*, *13*, 1606732. PMID: 40535452

Lerose, V., Ponticelli, M., Benedetto, N., Carlucci, V., Lela, L., Tzvetkov, N. T., & Milella, L. (2024). *Withania somnifera* (L.) Dunal, a Potential Source of Phytochemicals for Treating Neurodegenerative Diseases: A Systematic Review. *Plants*, *13*(6), 771. DOI: 10.3390/plants13060771 PMID: 38592845

Lewis, S. J. G., Foltynie, T., Blackwell, A. D., Robbins, T. W., Owen, A. M., & Barker, R. A. (2005). Heterogeneity of Parkinson's disease in the early clinical stages using a data driven approach. *Journal of Neurology, Neurosurgery, and Psychiatry*, *76*(3), 343–348. PMID: 15716523

LeWitt, P. A., Hauser, R. A., Pahwa, R., Isaacson, S. H., Fernandez, H. H., Lew, M., Saint-Hilaire, M., Pourcher, E., Lopez-Manzanares, L., Waters, C., Rudzínska, M., Sedkov, A., Batycky, R., & Oh, C. (2019). Safety and efficacy of CVT-301 (levodopa inhalation powder) on motor function during off periods in patients with Parkinson's disease: A randomised, double-blind, placebo-controlled phase 3 trial. *Lancet Neurology*, *18*(2), 145–154. DOI: 10.1016/S1474-4422(18)30405-8

Liang, X., Ding, Y., Zhang, Y., Tse, H. F., & Lian, Q. (2014). Paracrine mechanisms of mesenchymal stem cell-based therapy: Current status and perspectives. *Cell Transplantation*, *23*(9), 1045–1059. PMID: 23676629

Li, D., Yang, H., Ma, J., Luo, S., Chen, S., & Gu, Q. (2018). MicroRNA-30e regulates neuroinflammation in MPTP model of Parkinson's disease by targeting Nlrp3. *Human Cell*, *31*(2), 106–115. DOI: 10.1007/s13577-017-0187-5 PMID: 29274035

Li, J., Mi, T.-M., Zhu, B., Ma, J.-H., Han, C., Li, Y., Yang, W.-M., & Chan, P. (2020). High-frequency repetitive transcranial magnetic stimulation over the primary motor cortex relieves musculoskeletal pain in patients with Parkinson's disease: A randomized controlled trial. *Parkinsonism & Related Disorders*, *80*, 113–119. DOI: 10.1016/j.parkreldis.2020.07.006 PMID: 32980772

Li, M., Jiang, Y., Hou, Q., Zhao, Y., Zhong, L., & Fu, X. (2022). Potential pre-activation strategies for improving therapeutic efficacy of mesenchymal stem cells: Current status and future prospects. *Stem Cell Research & Therapy*, *13*(1), 146. PMID: 35379361

Limousin, P., & Foltynie, T. (2019). Long-term outcomes of deep brain stimulation in Parkinson disease. *Nature Reviews Neurology 2019 15:4*, *15*(4), 234–242. https://doi.org/DOI: 10.1038/s41582-019-0145-9

Lim, S. Y., Moro, E., & Lang, A. E. (2009). *Non-motor symptoms of Parkinson's disease and the effects of deep brain stimulation. Non Motor Symptoms of Parkinson's Disease*. Oxford University Press.

Lin, C.-H., Chiu, H. E., Wu, S.-Y., Tseng, S.-T., Wu, T.-C., Hung, Y.-C., Hsu, C. Y., Chen, H.-J., Hsu, S.-F., Kuo, C. E., & Hu, W.-L. (2021). Chinese Herbal Products for Non-Motor Symptoms of Parkinson's Disease in Taiwan: A Population-Based Study. *Frontiers in Pharmacology*, *11*, 615657. DOI: 10.3389/fphar.2020.615657 PMID: 33584294

Lindvall, O., & Kokaia, Z. (2011). Stem cell research in stroke: How far from the clinic? *Stroke*, *42*(8), 2369–2375. PMID: 21757669

Ling, H., Kovacs, G. G., Vonsattel, J. P. G., Davey, K., Mok, K. Y., Hardy, J., Morris, H. R., Warner, T. T., Holton, J. L., & Revesz, T. (2016). Astrogliopathy predominates the earliest stage of corticobasal degeneration pathology. *Brain*, *139*(12), 3237–3252. DOI: 10.1093/brain/aww256 PMID: 27797812

Little, M. A., McSharry, P. E., Hunter, E. J., Spielman, J., & Ramig, L. O. (2009). Suitability of dysphonia measurements for telemonitoring of Parkinson's disease. *IEEE Transactions on Biomedical Engineering*, *56*(4), 1015–1022. DOI: 10.1109/TBME.2008.2005954 PMID: 21399744

Little, S., Alex, P., Spencer, N., Baltazar, Z., Ludvic, Z., Marwan, H., Thomas, F., Patricia, L., Keyoumars, A., James, F., Alexander, L. G., Tipu, Z. A., & Peter, B. (2013). Adaptive Deep Brain Stimulation in Advanced Parkinson Disease. *Annals of Neurology*, *74*, 449–457. PMID: 23852650

Liu, Z., & Cheung, H. H. (2020). Stem cell-based therapies for Parkinson disease. *International Journal of Molecular Sciences*, *21*(21), 8060. PMID: 33137927

Li, Y., Lv, Z., Dai, Y., Yu, L., Zhang, L., & Wang, K.. (2025). The global, regional, and national burden of Parkinson's disease in 204 countries and territories, 1990–2021: A systematic analysis for the Global Burden of Disease Study 2021. *BMC Public Health,* Liu, B., Zhou, H., Tan, L., Siu, K. T. H., & Guan, X. (2024). Exploring treatment options in cancer: Tumor treatment strategies. *Signal Transduction and Targeted Therapy*, *9*, 175. DOI: 10.1038/s41392-024-01856-7

Lobotesis, K., Fenwick, J. D., Phipps, A., Ryman, A., Swann, A., Ballard, C., McKeith, I. G., & O'Brien, J. T. (2001). Occipital hypoperfusion on SPECT in dementia with Lewy bodies but not AD. *Neurology*, *56*(5), 643–649. DOI: 10.1212/wnl.56.5.643 PMID: 11245717

Lolekha, P., & Jieamanukulkit, P. (2025). Diagnostic Delays in Parkinson's Disease in Thailand: Clinical Pitfalls and Health System Barriers. *Life (Chicago, Ill.)*, *15*(10), 1513. PMID: 41157185

Longo, D. M., Yang, Y., Watkins, P. B., Howell, B. A., & Siler, S. Q. (2016). Elucidating Differences in the Hepatotoxic Potential of Tolcapone and Entacapone With DILIsym(®), a Mechanistic Model of Drug-Induced Liver Injury. *CPT: Pharmacometrics & Systems Pharmacology*, *5*(1), 31–39. DOI: 10.1002/PSP4.12053

Lo, R. Y., Tanner, C. M., Albers, K. B., Leimpeter, A. D., Fross, R. D., Bernstein, A. L., McGuire, V., Quesenberry, C. P., Nelson, L. M., Van Den Eeden, S. K., & Tanner, C. M. (2009). Clinical features in early Parkinson disease and survival. *Archives of Neurology*, *66*(11), 1353–1358. PMID: 19901166

Louis, E. D., Levy, G., Côte, L. J., Mejia, H., Fahn, S., & Marder, K. (2001). Clinical correlates of action tremor in Parkinson disease. *Archives of Neurology*, *58*(10), 1630–1634. PMID: 11594921

Louis, E. D., Tang, M. X., Cote, L., Alfaro, B., Mejia, H., & Marder, K. (1999). Progression of parkinsonian signs in Parkinson disease. *Archives of Neurology, 56*(3), 334–337. PMID: 10190824

Lozano, A. M., Lipsman, N., Bergman, H., Brown, P., Chabardes, S., Chang, J. W., Matthews, K., McIntyre, C. C., Schlaepfer, T. E., Schulder, M., Temel, Y., Volkmann, J., & Krauss, J. K. (2019). Deep brain stimulation: Current challenges and future directions. *Nature Reviews. Neurology, 15*(3), 148–160. DOI: 10.1038/s41582-018-0128-2 PMID: 30683913

Luca, DI, D. G., Sambursky, J. A., Margolesky, J., Cordeiro, J. G., DIaz, A., Shpiner, D. S., Moore, H. P., Singer, C., & Luca, C. (2020). Minority Enrollment in Parkinson's Disease Clinical Trials: Meta-Analysis and Systematic Review of Studies Evaluating Treatment of Neuropsychiatric Symptoms. *Journal of Parkinson's Disease, 10*(4), 1709–1716. DOI: 10.3233/JPD-202045

Luk, K. C., Kehm, V., Carroll, J., Zhang, B., O'Brien, P., Trojanowski, J. Q., & Lee, V. M. Y. (2012). Pathological α-Synuclein Transmission Initiates Parkinson-like Neurodegeneration in Non-transgenic Mice. *Science, 338*(6109), 949. DOI: 10.1126/SCIENCE.1227157

Lund University. (2024, May 6). *Update on STEM-PD clinical trial* - stem cell based transplant for parkinson's disease. Lund University; Accessed on November, 2025.

Luo, Y., Qiao, L., Li, M., Wen, X., Zhang, W., & Li, X. (2024). Global, regional, national epidemiology and trends of Parkinson's disease from 1990 to 2021: Findings from the Global Burden of Disease Study 2021. *Frontiers in Aging Neuroscience, 16*, 1498756. DOI: 10.3389/FNAGI.2024.1498756

Lv, R., Du, L., Zhou, F., Yuan, X., Liu, X., & Zhang, L. (2020). Rosmarinic Acid Alleviates Inflammation, Apoptosis, and Oxidative Stress through Regulating miR-155-5p in a Mice Model of Parkinson's Disease. *ACS Chemical Neuroscience, 11*(20), 3259–3266. DOI: 10.1021/acschemneuro.0c00425 PMID: 32946211

Lyu, S., Zhang, C. S., Mao, Z., Guo, X., Li, Z., Luo, X., Sun, J., & Su, Q. (2024). Real-world Chinese herbal medicine for Parkinson's disease: A hospital-based retrospective analysis of electronic medical records. *Frontiers in Aging Neuroscience, 16*, 1362948. DOI: 10.3389/fnagi.2024.1362948 PMID: 38756536

Magrinelli, F., Picelli, A., & Tocco, P. (2016). Pathophysiology of motor dysfunction in Parkinson's disease as the rationale for drug treatment and rehabilitation. *Parkinson's Disease, 9832839.* Advance online publication. DOI: 10.1155/2016/9832839 PMID: 27366343

Mahlknecht, P., Seppi, K., & Poewe, W. (2015). The Concept of Prodromal Parkinson's Disease. *Journal of Parkinson's Disease*, *5*(4), 681–697. DOI: 10.3233/JPD-150685 PMID: 26485429

Maini Rekdal, V., Bess, E. N., Bisanz, J. E., Turnbaugh, P. J., & Balskus, E. P. (2019). Discovery and inhibition of an interspecies gut bacterial pathway for Levodopa metabolism. *Science*, *364*(6445), eaau6323. Advance online publication. DOI: 10.1126/science.aau6323 PMID: 31196984

Maji, P. K., Biswas, R., & Roy, A. R. (2003). Soft set theory. *Computers & Mathematics with Applications (Oxford, England)*, *45*(4-5), 555–562.

Majumdar, P., & Samanta, S. K. (2010). Generalised fuzzy soft sets. *Computers & Mathematics with Applications (Oxford, England)*, *59*(4), 1425–1432.

Makanjuola, A., Taiwo, F., Yaria, J., Akinyemi, R., & Ogunniyi, A. (2021). Parkinson's disease – A review of pathogenesis, recent advances in management, and challenges of care in sub-Saharan Africa. *Journal of Global Medicine*. https://doi.org/DOI: 10.51496/jogm.v1.35

Malek, N. (2019). Deep Brain Stimulation in Parkinson's Disease. *Neurology India*, *67*, 968–978. PMID: 31512617

Mancini, M., Shah, V. V., Stuart, S., Curtze, C., Horak, F. B., Safarpour, D., & Nutt, J. G. (2021). Measuring freezing of gait during daily-life: An open-source, wearable sensors approach. *Journal of Neuroengineering and Rehabilitation*, *18*(1). Advance online publication. DOI: 10.1186/s12984-020-00774-3 PMID: 33397401

Manna, I., De Benedittis, S., Quattrone, A., Maisano, D., Iaccino, E., & Quattrone, A. (2021). Exosomal miRNA as peripheral biomarkers in Parkinson's disease and progressive supranuclear palsy: A pilot study. *Parkinsonism & Related Disorders*, *93*, 77–84. DOI: 10.1016/j.parkreldis.2021.11.020 PMID: 34839044

Mao, A. S., Özkale, B., Shah, N. J., Vining, K. H., Descombes, T., Zhang, L., Tringides, C. M., Wong, S. W., Shin, J. W., Scadden, D. T., Weitz, D. A., & Mooney, D. J. (2019). Programmable microencapsulation for enhanced mesenchymal stem cell persistence and immunomodulation. *Proceedings of the National Academy of Sciences of the United States of America*, *116*(31), 15392–15397. PMID: 31311862

Mao, Q., Qin, W. Z., Zhang, A., & Ye, N. (2020). Recent advances in dopaminergic strategies for the treatment of Parkinson's disease. *Acta Pharmacologica Sinica*, *41*(4), 471–482. PMID: 32112042

Marder, K., Wang, Y., Alcalay, R. N., Mejia-Santana, H., Tang, M. X., Lee, A., Raymond, D., Mirelman, A., Saunders-Pullman, R., Clark, L., Ozelius, L., Orr-Urtreger, A., Giladi, N., & Bressman, S. (2015). Age-specific penetrance of LRRK2 G2019S in the Michael J. Fox Ashkenazi Jewish LRRK2 Consortium. *Neurology*, *85*(1), 89–95. DOI: 10.1212/WNL.0000000000001708

Marei, H. E. (2025). Stem cell therapy: A revolutionary cure or a pandora's box. *Stem Cell Research & Therapy*, *16*(1), 255. PMID: 40405306

Marek, K., Chowdhury, S., Siderowf, A., Lasch, S., Coffey, C. S., Caspell-Garcia, C., & Foroud, T. (2018). The Parkinson's progression markers initiative (PPMI)–establishing a PD biomarker cohort. *Annals of Clinical and Translational Neurology*, *5*(12), 1460–1477. PMID: 30564614

Marek, K., Chowdhury, S., Siderowf, A., Lasch, S., Coffey, C. S., Caspell-Garcia, C., Simuni, T., Jennings, D., Tanner, C. M., Trojanowski, J. Q., Shaw, L. M., Seibyl, J., Schuff, N., Singleton, A., Kieburtz, K., Toga, A. W., Mollenhauer, B., Galasko, D., Chahine, L. M., & Taucher, J. (2018). The Parkinson's progression markers initiative (PPMI) – establishing a PD biomarker cohort. *Annals of Clinical and Translational Neurology*, *5*(12), 1460–1477. DOI: 10.1002/ACN3.644;JOURNAL:-JOURNAL:23289503

Marino, B. L. B., de Souza, L. R., Sousa, K. P. A., Ferreira, J. V., Padilha, E. C., & da Silva, C. H. T. P.. (2020). Parkinson's disease: A review from pathophysiology to treatment. *Mini-Reviews in Medicinal Chemistry*, *20*, 754–767. DOI: 10.2174/1389557519666191104110908 PMID: 31686637

Marino, F., Failla, C., Chilà, P., Minutoli, R., Puglisi, A., & Arnao, A. A.. (2021). The effect of acceptance and commitment therapy for improving psychological well-being in parents of individuals with autism spectrum disorders: A randomized controlled trial. *Brain Sciences*, *11*, 880. DOI: 10.3390/brainsci11070880 PMID: 34209171

Marks, W. J., Bartus, R. T., Siffert, J., Davis, C. S., Lozano, A., Boulis, N., Vitek, J., Stacy, M., Turner, D., Verhagen, L., Bakay, R., Watts, R., Guthrie, B., Jankovic, J., Simpson, R., Tagliati, M., Alterman, R., Stern, M., Baltuch, G., & Olanow, C. W. (2010). Gene delivery of AAV2-neurturin for Parkinson's disease: A double-blind, randomised, controlled trial. *Lancet Neurology*, *9*(12), 1164–1172. DOI: 10.1016/S1474-4422(10)70254-4

Marras, C., & Lang, A. (2013). Parkinson's disease subtypes: Lost in translation? *Journal of Neurology, Neurosurgery, and Psychiatry*, *84*(4), 409–415. DOI: 10.1136/jnnp-2012-303455 PMID: 22952329

Martinez-Carrasco, A., Real, R., Lawton, M., Iwaki, H., Tan, M. M. X., Wu, L., Williams, N. M., Carroll, C., Hu, M. T. M., Grosset, D. G., Hardy, J., Ryten, M., Foltynie, T., Ben-Shlomo, Y., Shoai, M., & Morris, H. R. (2023). Genetic meta-analysis of levodopa induced dyskinesia in Parkinson's disease. *Npj Parkinson's Disease 2023 9:1, 9*(1), 128-. https://doi.org/DOI: 10.1038/s41531-023-00573-2

Martínez-Fernández, R., Rodríguez-Rojas, R., Del Álamo, M., Hernández-Fernández, F., Pineda-Pardo, J. A., Dileone, M., Alonso-Frech, F., Foffani, G., Obeso, I., Gasca-Salas, C., de Luis-Pastor, E., Vela, L., & Obeso, J. A. (2018). Focused ultrasound subthalamotomy in patients with asymmetric Parkinson's disease: A pilot study. *Lancet Neurology, 17*(1), 54–63. DOI: 10.1016/S1474-4422(17)30403-9 PMID: 29203153

Martinez-Nunez, A. E., Maria, B. J., Michael, S. O., & Alfonso, F. (2024). Emerging therapies for neuromodulation in Parkinson's disease. *Neurotherapeutics; the Journal of the American Society for Experimental NeuroTherapeutics, 21*, e00310.

Martinez-Ramirez, D., Wei, H., Alberto, R. B., Michael, S. O., & Aparna, W. S. (2015). Update on deep brain stimulation in Parkinson's disease. *Translational Neurodegeneration, 2015*(4), 12. DOI: 10.1186/s40035-015-0034-0 PMID: 26257895

Mass General Brigham. (2025, March 6). Clinical trial tests novel stem-cell treatment for parkinson's disease; Accessed on November, 2025. http://www.massgeneralbrigham.org/en/about/newsroom/press-releases/clinical-trial-novel-stem-cell-treatment-for-parkinson's

Matsuda, H., Imabayashi, E., Kuji, I., Seto, A., Ito, K., Kikuta, D., & Yamada, M. (2010). Evaluation of both perfusion and atrophy in multiple system atrophy of the cerebellar type using brain SPECT alone. *BMC Medical Imaging, 10*, 17. DOI: 10.1186/1471-2342-10-17 PMID: 20701753

Matsui, H., Udaka, F., Miyoshi, T., Hara, N., Tamura, A., Oda, M., Kubori, T., & Nishinaka, K. (2005). Brain perfusion differences between Parkinson's disease and multiple system atrophy with predominant parkinsonian features. *Parkinsonism & Related Disorders, 11*(4), 227–232. DOI: 10.1016/j.parkreldis.2005.01.001 PMID: 15878583

McFall, S. L., Yerkes, A. M., & Cowan, L. D. (2000). Outcomes of a small group educational intervention for urinary incontinence. *Journal of Aging and Health, 12*, 301. DOI: 10.1177/089826430001200302 PMID: 11067699

McFarthing, K., Buff, S., Rafaloff, G., Pitzer, K., Fiske, B., Navangul, A., Beissert, K., Pilcicka, A., Fuest, R., Wyse, R. K., & Stott, S. R. W. (2024). Parkinson's Disease Drug Therapies in the Clinical Trial Pipeline: 2024 Update. *Journal of Parkinson's Disease*, *14*(5), 899–912. DOI: 10.3233/JPD-240272

McGhee, D. J. M., Ritchie, C. W., Zajicek, J. P., & Counsell, C. E. (2016). Clinical trial designs used to detect disease-modifying effects in Alzheimer's and Parkinson's disease. *BMC Neurology*, *16*, 92. DOI: 10.1186/s12883-016-0606-3 PMID: 27312378

Medtronic earns U.S. FDA approval for the world's first Adaptive deep brain stimulation system for people with Parkinson's - Feb 24, 2025. (n.d.). Retrieved December 12, 2025, from https://news.medtronic.com/2025-02-24-Medtronic-earns-U-S-FDA-approval-for-the-worlds-first-Adaptive-deep-brain-stimulation-system-for-people-with-Parkinsons

Meissner, W. G., Remy, P., Giordana, C., Maltête, D., Derkinderen, P., Houéto, J.-L., Anheim, M., Benatru, I., Boraud, T., Brefel-Courbon, C., Carrière, N., Catala, H., Charif, M., Colin, O., Corvol, J.-C., Damier, P., Dellapina, E., Devos, D., Drapier, S., & Rascol, O. (2024). Trial of Lixisenatide in Early Parkinson's Disease. *The New England Journal of Medicine*, *390*(13), 1176–1185. DOI: 10.1056/NEJMOA231232

Meloni, M., Agliardi, C., Guerini, F. R., Zanzottera, M., Bolognesi, E., Picciolini, S., Marano, M., Magliozzi, A., Di Fonzo, A., Arighi, A., Fenoglio, C., Scarpini, E., Parnetti, L., & Clerici, M. (2023). Oligomeric alpha-synuclein and tau aggregates in NDEVs differentiate Parkinson's disease from atypical parkinsonisms. *Neurobiology of Disease*, *176*, 105947. DOI: 10.1016/j.nbd.2022.105947 PMID: 36481435

Mendoza, M. M. (2022). Is Extended-Release Amantadine Effective at Treating Levodopa-Induced Dyskinesia in Parkinson's Disease Patients?.

Merello, M. (2018). The dark side of globalization: Lack of universal levodopa availability. *Movement Disorders Clinical Practice*, *6*(1), 7–8. PMID: 30746409

Mestre, T. A., Stebbins, G. T., Stephenson, D., Dexter, D., Lee, K. K., Xiao, Y., Dam, T., Kopil, C. M., & Simuni, T. (2024). Patient-centered development of clinical outcome assessments in early Parkinson disease: key priorities and advances. *Npj Parkinson's Disease 2024 10:1*, *10*(1), 101-. https://doi.org/DOI: 10.1038/s41531-024-00716-z

Metman, L. V., Del Dotto, P., LePoole, K., Konitsiotis, S., Fang, J., & Chase, T. N. (1999). Amantadine for levodopa-induced dyskinesias: A 1-year follow-up study. *Archives of Neurology*, *56*(11), 1383–1386. PMID: 10555659

Metman, L. V., Del Dotto, P., Van Den Munckhof, P., Fang, J., Mouradian, M. M., & Chase, T. N. (1998). Amantadine as treatment for dyskinesias and motor fluctuations in Parkinson's disease. *Neurology, 50*(5), 1323–1326. PMID: 9595981

Migdalska-Richards, A., Daly, L., Bezard, E., & Schapira, A. H. V. (2016). Ambroxol effects in glucocerebrosidase and α-synuclein transgenic mice. *Annals of Neurology, 80*(5), 766–775. DOI: 10.1002/ANA.24790

Miller, D. B., & O'Callaghan, J. P. (2015). Biomarkers of Parkinson's disease: Present and future. *Metabolism: Clinical and Experimental, 64*(3, Suppl 1), S40–S46. PMID: 25510818

Misch, M. R., Mitchell, S., Francis, P. L., Sherborn, K., Meradje, K., McNeely, A. A., Chen, J. J., & Tang-Wai, D. F. (2019). Differentiating between visual hallucination-free dementia with Lewy bodies and corticobasal syndrome on the basis of neuropsychology and perfusion single-photon emission computed tomography. *Alzheimer's Research & Therapy, 11*(1), 9. DOI: 10.1186/s13195-018-0456-x PMID: 30658705

Mishra, B., Sudheer, P., Rajan, R., Agarwal, A., Srivastava, M. V. P., Nilima, N., & Vishnu, V. Y. (2024). Bridging the gap between statistical significance and clinical relevance: A systematic review of minimum clinically important difference (MCID) thresholds of scales reported in movement disorders research. *Heliyon, 10*(5). Advance online publication. DOI: 10.1016/j.heliyon.2024.e26479

Mitchell, C. L., & Kurouski, D. (2024). Novel strategies in Parkinson's disease treatment: A review. *Frontiers in Molecular Neuroscience, 17*, 1431079. PMID: 39183754

Mokhtari, Y. G., Varnava, I., Kyrgiannis, K., Ampatsidou, V., & Giakoumettis, D. (2025). Stem cell therapy for Parkinson's disease: A new hope for neural regeneration. *World Journal of Biological Chemistry, 16*(2), 106850. PMID: 40476258

Molodtsov, D. (1999). Soft set theory—First results. *Computers & Mathematics with Applications (Oxford, England), 37*(4-5), 19–31.

Mondal, B., Choudhury, S., Banerjee, R., Roy, A., Chatterjee, K., Basu, P., Singh, R., Halder, S., Shubham, S., Baker, S. N., Baker, M. R., & Kumar, H. (2024). Effects of non-invasive vagus nerve stimulation on clinical symptoms and molecular biomarkers in Parkinson's disease. *Frontiers in Aging Neuroscience, 15*, 1331575. DOI: 10.3389/fnagi.2023.1331575 PMID: 38384731

Moreau, C., Rouaud, T., Grabli, D., Benatru, I., Remy, P., Marques, A. R., & Fabbri, M. (2023). Overview on wearable sensors for the management of Parkinson's disease. *NPJ Parkinson's Disease*, *9*(1), 153. PMID: 37919332

Moreau, C., Tiphaine, R., David, G., Isabelle, B., Philippe, R., Ana-Raquel, M. S. D., Louise-Laure, M., Emmanuel, R., David, D., Gwendoline, D. M. B., & Margherita, F. (2023). Overview on wearable sensors for the management of Parkinson's disease. npj. *Parkinson's Disease*, *2023*(9), 153. DOI: 10.1038/s41531-023-00585-y PMID: 37919332

More, S. V., Kumar, H., Kang, S. M., Song, S. Y., Lee, K., & Choi, D. K. (2013). Advances in neuroprotective ingredients of medicinal herbs by using cellular and animal models of Parkinson's disease. *Evidence-Based Complementary and Alternative Medicine : eCAM*, *957875*. Advance online publication. DOI: 10.1155/2013/957875 PMID: 24073012

Morgante, F., Espay, A. J., Gunraj, C., Lang, A. E., & Chen, R. (2006). Motor cortex plasticity in Parkinson's disease and levodopa-induced dyskinesias. *Brain*, *129*(4), 1059–1069. DOI: 10.1093/brain/awl031 PMID: 16476674

Morizane, A. (2023). Cell therapy for Parkinson's disease with induced pluripotent stem cells. *Inflammation and Regeneration*, *43*(1), 16. PMID: 36843101

Mortberg, M. A., Vallabh, S. M., & Minikel, E. V. (2022). Disease stages and therapeutic hypotheses in two decades of neurodegenerative disease clinical trials. *Scientific Reports*, *12*(1), 17708. DOI: 10.1038/S41598-022-21820-1

Mortiboys, H., Furmston, R., Bronstad, G., Aasly, J., Elliott, C., & Bandmann, O. (2015). UDCA exerts beneficial effect on mitochondrial dysfunction in LRRK2 G2019S carriers and in vivo. *Neurology*, *85*(10), 846–852. DOI: 10.1212/WNL.0000000000001905

Moscovich, M., Camila, H. de A., Murilo, M. M., Lorena, B. B., André, C. F., Matthew, H., Clement, H., Henrique, B. F., & Munhoz, R. P. (2024). Fundamentals of deep brain stimulation for Parkinson's disease in clinical practice: part2. *Arquivos de Neuro-Psiquiatria*, *82*(4), s00441786037. PMID: 38653486

Moshayedi, A.J., & Mokhtari, T., & Emadi, Andani, M. (2025). Brain Stimulation Techniques in Research and Clinical Practice: A Comprehensive Review of Applications and Therapeutic Potential in Parkinson's Disease. *Brain Sciences*, *2025*(15), 20. DOI: 10.3390/brainsci15010020 PMID: 39851388

Mousaei Ghasroldasht, M., Seok, J., Park, H. S., Liakath Ali, F. B., & Al-Hendy, A. (2022). Stem cell therapy: From idea to clinical practice. *International Journal of Molecular Sciences*, *23*(5), 2850. PMID: 35269990

Mponda, J. S., Muula, A. S., Choko, A., Ajuwon, A. J., & Moody, J. O. (2025). Traditional medicine regulation status and challenges in Malawi and Nigeria. *BMC Complementary Medicine and Therapies*, *25*(1), 53. PMID: 39953523

Mughal, H., Abdul, R. J., Muhammad, R., Ahmads, A., & Natalia, K. (2022). *Parkinson's Disease Management via Wearable Sensors: A Systematic Review. IEEE Access. VOLUME 10, 35219- 35237.* Digital Object Identifier., DOI: 10.1109/ACCESS.2022.3162844

Mughal, H., Javed, A. R., Rizwan, M., Almadhor, A. S., & Kryvinska, N. (2022). Parkinson's disease management via wearable sensors: A systematic review. *IEEE Access : Practical Innovations, Open Solutions*, *10*, 35219–35237.

Mullin, S., Smith, L., Lee, K., D'Souza, G., Woodgate, P., Elflein, J., Hällqvist, J., Toffoli, M., Streeter, A., Hosking, J., Heywood, W. E., Khengar, R., Campbell, P., Hehir, J., Cable, S., Mills, K., Zetterberg, H., Limousin, P., Libri, V., & Schapira, A. H. V. (2020). Ambroxol for the Treatment of Patients With Parkinson Disease With and Without Glucocerebrosidase Gene Mutations: A Nonrandomized, Noncontrolled Trial. *JAMA Neurology*, *77*(4), 427–434. DOI: 10.1001/JAMANEUROL.2019.4611

Mure, H., Hirano, S., Tang, C. C., Isaias, I. U., Antonini, A., Ma, Y., Dhawan, V., & Eidelberg, D. (2011). Parkinson's disease tremor-related metabolic network: Characterization, progression, and treatment effects. *NeuroImage*, *54*(2), 1244–1253. PMID: 20851193

Mythri, R. B., & Bharath, M. M. S. (2012). Mitochondrial dysfunction and oxidative stress in Parkinson's disease. *Molecular Neurobiology*, *46*(1), 194–214. PMID: 22821186

Nahar, L., Charoensup, R., Kalieva, K., Habibi, E., Guo, M., Wang, D., Kvasnica, M., Onder, A., & Sarker, S. D. (2025). Natural products in neurodegenerative diseases: Recent advances and future outlook. *Frontiers in Pharmacology*, *16*, 1529194. DOI: 10.3389/fphar.2025.1529194 PMID: 40176910

Nalls, M. A., Blauwendraat, C., Vallerga, C. L., Heilbron, K., Bandres-Ciga, S., Chang, D., Tan, M., Kia, D. A., Noyce, A. J., Xue, A., Bras, J., Young, E., von Coelln, R., Simón-Sánchez, J., Schulte, C., Sharma, M., Krohn, L., Pihlstrøm, L., Siitonen, A., & Zhang, F. (2019). Identification of novel risk loci, causal insights, and heritable risk for Parkinson's disease: A meta-analysis of genome-wide association studies. *Lancet Neurology*, *18*(12), 1091–1102. DOI: 10.1016/S1474-4422(19)30320-5

Nims, R. W., & Price, P. J. (2017). Best practices for detecting and mitigating the risk of cell culture contaminants. *In Vitro Cellular & Developmental Biology. Animal, 53*(10), 872–879. PMID: 29197027

O'Shea, D. M., Arkhipenko, A., Galasko, D., Goldman, J. G., Sheikh, Z. H., Petrides, G., Toledo, J. B., & Galvin, J. E. (2024). Practical use of DAT SPECT imaging in diagnosing dementia with Lewy bodies: A US perspective of current guidelines and future directions. *Frontiers in Neurology, 15*, 1395413. DOI: 10.3389/FNEUR.2024.1395413

Obermeyer, Z., Powers, B., Vogeli, C., & Mullainathan, S. (2019). Dissecting racial bias in an algorithm used to manage the health of populations. *Science, 366*(6464), 447–453. PMID: 31649194

Obeso, J. A.. (2017). Past, present, and future of Parkinson's disease. *Movement Disorders, 32*(9), 1264–1310. PMID: 28887905

Oertel, W. H., Depboylu, C., Krenzer, M., Vadasz, D., Ries, V., Sixel-Döring, F., & Mayer, G. (2014). REM sleep behavior disorder as a prodromal stage of alpha-synucleinopathies: Symptoms, epidemiology, pathophysiology, diagnosis and therapy. *Der Nervenarzt, 85*(1), 19–25. DOI: 10.1007/s00115-013-3870-0 PMID: 24399499

Oertel, W., Eggert, K., Pahwa, R., Tanner, C. M., Hauser, R. A., Trenkwalder, C., Ehret, R., Azulay, J. P., Isaacson, S., Felt, L., & Stempien, M. J. (2017). Randomized, placebo-controlled trial of ADS-5102 (amantadine) extended-release capsules for levodopa-induced dyskinesia in Parkinson's disease (EASE LID 3). *Movement Disorders, 32*(12), 1701–1709. DOI: 10.1002/MDS.2713

Oertel, W., Eggert, K., Pahwa, R., Tanner, C. M., Hauser, R. A., Trenkwalder, C., & Stempien, M. J. (2017). Randomized, placebo-controlled trial of ADS-5102 (amantadine) extended-release capsules for levodopa-induced dyskinesia in Parkinson's disease (EASE LID 3). *Movement Disorders, 32*(12), 1701–1709. PMID: 28833562

Oertel, W., & Schulz, J. B. (2016). Current and experimental treatments of Parkinson disease: A guide for neuroscientists. *Journal of Neurochemistry, 139*(Suppl 1), 325–337. DOI: 10.1111/jnc.13750 PMID: 27577098

Ofori, E., Pasternak, O., Planetta, P. J., Burciu, R., Snyder, A., Febo, M., Golde, T. E., Okun, M. S., & Vaillancourt, D. E. (2015a). Increased free water in the substantia nigra of Parkinson's disease: A single-site and multi-site study. *Neurobiology of Aging, 36*(2), 1097–1104. DOI: 10.1016/j.neurobiolaging.2014.10.029

Okunoye, O., Zewde, Y. Z., Azar, J., Ayele, B. A., Dindayal, S., & Moustafa, A.. (2023). The state of play of Parkinson's disease in Africa: A systematic review and point of view. *bioRxiv.* https://doi.org/DOI: 10.1101/2023.07.07.23292392

Okuzumi, A., Hatano, T., Matsumoto, G., Nojiri, S., Ueno, S. ichi, Imamichi-Tatano, Y., Kimura, H., Kakuta, S., Kondo, A., Fukuhara, T., Li, Y., Funayama, M., Saiki, S., Taniguchi, D., Tsunemi, T., McIntyre, D., Gérardy, J. J., Mittelbronn, M., Kruger, R., … Hattori, N. (2023). Propagative α-synuclein seeds as serum biomarkers for synucleinopathies. *Nature Medicine 2023 29:6, 29*(6), 1448–1455. https://doi.org/DOI: 10.1038/s41591-023-02358-9

Olaniyan, O.T., Adetunji, C.O., Dare, A., Adeyomoye, O., Adeniyi, M.J., & Alex, E. (2022a). Clinical applications of deep learning in neurology and its enhancements with future predictions. In book: ARTIFICIAL INTELLIGENCE FOR NEUROLOGICAL DISORDERS. Publisher: Elsevier. September 2022. DOI: .DOI: 10.1016/B978-0-323-90277-9.00016-X

Olaniyan, O. T., Adetunji, C. O., Adeyomoye, O., Dare, A., Adeniyi, M. J., & Alex, E. (2022a). *Ensemble sparse intelligent mining techniques for cognitive disease. In book: ARTIFICIAL INTELLIGENCE FOR NEUROLOGICAL DISORDERS. Publisher.* Elsevier., DOI: 10.1016/B978-0-323-90277- 9.00027-4

Olaniyan, O. T., Adetunji, C. O., Adeyomoye, O., Dare, A., Adeniyi, M. J., & Alex, E. (2022e). *Cognitive therapy for brain diseases using deep learning models. In book: ARTIFICIAL INTELLIGENCE FOR NEUROLOGICAL DISORDERS. Publisher.* Elsevier., DOI: 10.106/B978-0-323-90277-9.00017-1

Olaniyan, O. T., Adetunji, C. O., Adeyomoye, O., Dare, A., Adeniyi, M. J., & Alex, E. (2022f). *Clinical applications of deep learning in neurology and its enhancements with future directions. In book: ARTIFICIAL INTELLIGENCE FOR NEUROLOGICAL DISORDERS. Publisher.* Elsevier., DOI: 10.1016/B978-0-323-90277-9.00026-2

Olaniyan, O. T., Adetunji, C. O., Dare, A., Adeyomoye, O., Adeniyi, M. J., & Alex, E. (2022b). *Cognitive therapy for brain diseases using artificial intelligence models. In book: ARTIFICIAL INTELLIGENCE FOR NEUROLOGICAL DISORDERS. Publisher.* Elsevier., DOI: 10.1016/B978-0-323-90277-9.00013-4

Olaniyan, O. T., Adetunji, C. O., Dare, A., Adeyomoye, O., Adeniyi, M. J., & Alex, E. (2022b). *Neural signaling and communication using machine learning. In book: ARTIFICIAL INTELLIGENCE FOR NEUROLOGICAL DISORDERS. Publisher.* Elsevier., DOI: 10.1016/B978-0-323-90277-9.00010-9

Olaniyan, O. T., Adetunji, C. O., Dare, A., Adeyomoye, O., Adeniyi, M. J., & Alex, E. (2022c). *Artificial intelligence-based early detection of neurological disease using noninvasive method based on speech analysis. In book: ARTIFICIAL INTELLIGENCE FOR NEUROLOGICAL DISORDERS. Publisher*. Elsevier., DOI: 10.1016/B978-0-323-90277-9.00008-0

Olaniyan, O. T., Adetunji, C. O., Dare, A., Adeyomoye, O., Adeniyi, M. J., & Alex, E. (2022c). *New trends in deep learning for neuroimaging analysis and disease prediction. In book: ARTIFICIAL INTELLIGENCE FOR NEUROLOGICAL DISORDERS. Publisher*. Elsevier., DOI: 10.1016/B978-0-323-90277-9.00012-2

Olaniyan, O. T., Adetunji, C. O., Dare, A., Adeyomoye, O., Adeniyi, M. J., & Alex, E. (2022d). *Prevention and diagnosis of neurodegenerative diseases using machine learning models. In book: ARTIFICIAL INTELLIGENCE FOR NEUROLOGICAL DISORDERS. Publisher*. Elsevier., DOI: 10.1016/B978-0-323-90277-9.00009-2

Olaniyan, O., Adetunji, C. O., Adeyomoye, O., Dare, A., Adeniyi, M. J., & Enoch, A. (2022g). *Computational methods for translational brain-behavior analysis. In book: ARTIFICIAL INTELLIGENCE FOR NEUROLOGICAL DISORDERS. Publisher*. Elsevier., DOI: 10.1016/B978-0-323-90277-9.00025-0

Olanow, C. W., Kieburtz, K., Odin, P., Espay, A. J., Standaert, D. G., Fernandez, H. H., Vanagunas, A., Othman, A. A., Widnell, K. L., Robieson, W. Z., Pritchett, Y., Chatamra, K., Benesh, J., Lenz, R. A., & Antonini, A. (2014). Continuous intrajejunal infusion of levodopa-carbidopa intestinal gel for patients with advanced Parkinson's disease: A randomised, controlled, double-blind, double-dummy study. *Lancet Neurology*, *13*(2), 141–149. DOI: 10.1016/S1474-4422(13)70293-X

Olanow, C. W., Rascol, O., Hauser, R., Feigin, P. D., Jankovic, J., Lang, A., Langston, W., Melamed, E., Poewe, W., Stocchi, F., & Tolosa, E. (2009a). A double-blind, delayed-start trial of rasagiline in Parkinson's disease. *The New England Journal of Medicine*, *361*(13), 1268–1278. DOI: 10.1056/NEJMOA0809335

Olanow, C. W., Stern, M. B., & Sethi, K. (2009). The scientific and clinical basis for the treatment of Parkinson disease. *Neurology*, *72*(21, Suppl 4), S1–S136. PMID: 19470958

Olugbemi, T., Olaniyan, C. O., Adetunji, A. D., Olorunsola, A., Mayowa, J., & Adeniyi, A. E. (2023). Prevention and diagnosis of neurodegenerative diseases using machine learning models. In *Artificial Intelligence for Neurological Disorders* (pp. 289–304). Academic Press.

Oluwole, O. G., Kuivaniemi, H., Carr, J. A., Ross, O. A., Olaogun, M. O. B., Bardien, S., & Komolafe, M. A. (2019). Parkinson's disease in Nigeria: A review of published studies and recommendations for future research. *Parkinsonism & Related Disorders*, *62*, 36–43. PMID: 30573414

Opuni, K. F. M., Kretchy, J-P., Agyabeng, K., Boadu, J. A., Adanu, T., Ankamah, S., Appiah, A., Amoah, G. B., Baidoo, M. and Kretchy, I. A. (2023). Contamination of herbal medicinal products in low-and-middle-income countries: A systematic review. Heliyon. 9: 9. e19370. https://doi.org/.DOI: 10.1016/j.heliyon.2023.e19370

Orgogozo, J. M., Gilman, S., Dartigues, J. F., Laurent, B., Puel, M., Kirby, L. C., Jouanny, P., Dubois, B., Eisner, L., Flitman, S., Michel, B. F., Boada, M., Frank, A., & Hock, C. (2003). Subacute meningoencephalitis in a subset of patients with AD after Aβ42 immunization. *Neurology*, *61*(1), 46–54. DOI: 10.1212/01.WNL.0000073623.84

Orhan, N., Gafner, S., & Blumenthal, M. (2024). Estimating the extent of adulteration of the popular herbs black cohosh, echinacea, elder berry, ginkgo, and turmeric – its challenges and limitations. *Natural Product Reports*, *41*(10). Advance online publication. DOI: 10.1039/d4np00014e PMID: 39108221

Ortega-Pinazo, J., Pacheco-Rodríguez, M. J., Serrano-Castro, P. J., Martínez, B., Pinto-Medel, M. J., Gómez-Zumaquero, J. M., Lago-Sampedro, A., García-Díaz, B., Estivill-Torrús, G., & Emilio Ferro Gallego, P. (2023). Comparing RNA extraction methods to face the variations in RNA quality using two human biological matrices. *Molecular Biology Reports*, *50*(11), 9263–9271. DOI: 10.1007/s11033-023-08809-3 PMID: 37812354

Osborn, T. M., Hallett, P. J., Schumacher, J. M., & Isacson, O. (2020). Advantages and recent developments of autologous cell therapy for Parkinson's disease patients. *Frontiers in Cellular Neuroscience*, *14*, 58. PMID: 32317934

Ovallath, S., & Sulthana, B. (2017). Levodopa: History and therapeutic applications. *Annals of Indian Academy of Neurology*, *20*(3), 185–189. PMID: 28904446

Owen, A. M. (2004). Cognitive Dysfunction in Parkinson's Disease: The Role of Frontostriatal Circuitry. *The Neuroscientist*, *10*(6), 525–537. DOI: 10.1177/1073858404266776 PMID: 15534038

Paccoud, I., Valero, M. M., Marín, L. C., Bontridder, N., Ibrahim, A., Winkler, J., Fomo, M., Sapienza, S., Khoury, F., Corvol, J. C., Fröhlich, H., & Klucken, J. (2024). Patient perspectives on the use of digital medical devices and health data for AI-driven personalised medicine in Parkinson's Disease. *Frontiers in Neurology*, *15*, 1453243. DOI: 10.3389/fneur.2024.1453243 PMID: 39697442

Padma, V. V. (2024). An overview of targeted cancer therapy. *Biomedicine (Taipei), 5*. Advance online publication. DOI: 10.37796/2211-8039.1512 PMID: 26613930

Paff, M., Aaron, L., Can, S., Andres, M. L., & Alfonso, F. (2020). Update on Current Technologies for Deep Brain Stimulation in Parkinson's Disease. *Journal of Movement Disorders, 13*(3), 185–198. DOI: 10.14802/jmd.20052 PMID: 32854482

Pagano, G., Taylor, K. I., Anzures-Cabrera, J., Marchesi, M., Simuni, T., Marek, K., Postuma, R. B., Pavese, N., Stocchi, F., Azulay, J.-P., Mollenhauer, B., López-Manzanares, L., Russell, D. S., Boyd, J. T., Nicholas, A. P., Luquin, M. R., Hauser, R. A., Gasser, T., Poewe, W., & Bonni, A. (2022). Trial of Prasinezumab in Early-Stage Parkinson's Disease. *The New England Journal of Medicine, 387*(5), 421–432. DOI: 10.1056/NEJMOA2202867

Pahwa, R., Tanner, C. M., Hauser, R. A., Isaacson, S. H., Nausieda, P. A., Truong, D. D., Agarwal, P., Hull, K. L., Lyons, K. E., Johnson, R., & Stempien, M. J. (2017). ADS-5102 (Amantadine) Extended-Release Capsules for Levodopa-Induced Dyskinesia in Parkinson Disease (EASE LID Study): A Randomized Clinical Trial. *JAMA Neurology, 74*(8), 941–949. DOI: 10.1001/JAMANEUROL.2017.0943

Pahwa, R., Tanner, C. M., Hauser, R. A., Isaacson, S. H., Nausieda, P. A., Truong, D. D., & Stempien, M. J. (2017). ADS-5102 (amantadine) extended-release capsules for levodopa-induced dyskinesia in Parkinson disease (EASE LID study): A randomized clinical trial. *JAMA Neurology, 74*(8), 941–949. PMID: 28604926

Palermo, G., Giannoni, S., Bellini, G., Siciliano, G., & Ceravolo, R. (2021). Dopamine Transporter Imaging, Current Status of a Potential Biomarker: A Comprehensive Review. *International Journal of Molecular Sciences 2021, Vol. 22, Page 11234, 22*(20), 11234. https://doi.org/DOI: 10.3390/IJMS222011234

Palmer, M., Tarver, J., Perez, J. P., Cawthorne, T., Romeo, R., & Stringer, D.. (2019). A novel group parenting intervention to reduce emotional and behavioural difficulties in young autistic children: Protocol for the Autism Spectrum Treatment and Resilience pilot randomised controlled trial. *BMJ Open, 9*. Advance online publication. DOI: 10.1136/bmjopen-2019-029959 PMID: 31248932

Parastarfeizabadi, M., & Kouzani, A. Z. (2017). Advances in closed-loop deep brain stimulation devices. *Journal of Neuroengineering and Rehabilitation, 2017*(14), 79. DOI: 10.1186/s12984-017-0295-1 PMID: 28800738

Park, S., Park, C. W., Eom, J. H., Jo, M. Y., Hur, H. J., Choi, S. K., Lee, J. S., Nam, S. T., Jo, K. S., Oh, Y. W., & Kim, D. W. (2024). Preclinical and dose-ranging assessment of hESC-derived dopaminergic progenitors for a clinical trial on Parkinson's disease. *Cell Stem Cell, 31*(1), 25–38. PMID: 38086390

Pastana Ramos, L. F., Vilacorta-Pereira, T. D. C. S., Duarte, J. D. S., Yamada, E. S., & Santos-Lobato, B. L. (2023). Feasibility and effectiveness of a remote individual rehabilitation program for people with Parkinson's disease living in the Brazilian Amazon: A randomized clinical trial. *Frontiers in Neurology*, *14*, 1244661. PMID: 37693755

Pawlak, Z. (1982). Rough sets. *International Journal of Computer & Information Sciences*, *11*(5), 341–356.

Peng, S., Liu, P., Wang, X., & Li, K. (2025). Global, regional and national burden of Parkinson's disease in people over 55 years of age: A systematic analysis of the Global Burden of Disease Study, 1991–2021. *BMC Neurology*, *25*, 178. DOI: 10.1186/s12883-025-04191-8 PMID: 40269818

Peraza, L. R., Kinnunen, K. M., McNaney, R., Craddock, I. J., Whone, A. L., Morgan, C., Joules, R., & Wolz, R. (2021). An automatic gait analysis pipeline for wearable sensors: A pilot study in parkinson's disease. *Sensors (Basel)*, *21*(24). Advance online publication. DOI: 10.3390/s21248286 PMID: 34960379

Pereira, G. M., dos Santos, D. T., Soares, N. M., Marconi, G. A., Friedrich, D. C., & Awad, P. S.. (2024). A systematic review and meta-analysis of the prevalence of Parkinson's disease in lower- to upper-middle-income countries. *npj. Parkinson's Disease*, *10*. Advance online publication. DOI: 10.1038/s41531-024-00779-y PMID: 39349513

Perepezko, K., Hinkle, J. T., Forbes, E. J., Pontone, G. M., Mills, K. A., & Gallo, J. J. (2023). The impact of caregiving on quality of life in Parkinson's disease: A systematic review. *International Journal of Geriatric Psychiatry*, *38*(1), e5870. DOI: 10.1002/GPS.5870

Petrou, M., Bohnen, N. I., Müller, M. L. T. M., Koeppe, R. A., Albin, R. L., & Frey, K. A. (2012). Aβ-Amyloid deposition in patients with Parkinson disease at risk for development of dementia. *Neurology*, *79*(11), 1161–1167. DOI: 10.1212/WNL.0b013e3182698d4a PMID: 22933741

Picillo, M., Andres, M. L., Nancy, K., Renato, P. M., & Alfonso, F. (2016). Programming Deep Brain Stimulation for Parkinson's Disease: The Toronto Western Hospital Algorithms. *Brain Stimulation*, *9*, 425–437. PMID: 26968806

Pierleoni, P., Raggiunto, S., Belli, A., Paniccia, M., Bazgir, O., & Palma, L. (2022). A Single Wearable Sensor for Gait Analysis in Parkinson's Disease: A Preliminary Study. *Applied Sciences (Switzerland)*, *12*(11). Advance online publication. DOI: 10.3390/app12115486

Pirtošek, Z. (2024). Breaking barriers in Parkinson's care: The multidisciplinary team approach. *Journal of Neural Transmission (Vienna, Austria)*, *131*(11), 1349–1361. PMID: 39417880

Poewe, W. (2008). Non-motor symptoms in Parkinson's disease. *European Journal of Neurology*, *15*(s1), 14–20. DOI: 10.1111/j.1468-1331.2008.02056.x PMID: 18353132

Poewe, W., Seppi, K., Marini, K., & Mahlknecht, P. (2020). New hopes for disease modification in Parkinson's Disease. *Neuropharmacology*, *171*, 108085. DOI: 10.1016/j.neuropharm.2020.108085 PMID: 32298705

Poewe, W., Seppi, K., Tanner, C. M., Halliday, G. M., Brundin, P., Volkmann, J., & Lang, A. E. (2017). Parkinson disease. *Nature Reviews. Disease Primers*, *3*(1), 1–21. PMID: 28332488

Poletti, M., Frosini, D., Pagni, C., Baldacci, F., Nicoletti, V., Tognoni, G., Lucetti, C., Del Dotto, P., Ceravolo, R., & Bonuccelli, U. (2012). Mild cognitive impairment and cognitive-motor relationships in newly diagnosed drug-naive patients with Parkinson's disease. *Journal of Neurology, Neurosurgery, and Psychiatry*, *83*(6), 601–606. PMID: 22492216

Politis, M. (2014). Neuroimaging in Parkinson disease: From research setting to clinical practice. *Nature Reviews. Neurology*, *10*(12), 708–722. DOI: 10.1038/NRNEUROL.2014.205

Polvorinos-Fernández, C., Sigcha, L., Centeno-Cerrato, M., de Arcas, G., Grande, M., Marín, M., Pareés, I., Martínez-Castrillo, J. C., & Pavón, I. (2025). Evaluation of Free-Living Motor Symptoms in Patients With Parkinson Disease Through Smartwatches: Protocol for Defining Digital Biomarkers JMIR Res Protoc 2025;14: e72820 URL: https://www.researchprotocols.org/2025/1/e72820 doi: DOI: 10.2196/72820

Polvorinos-Fernández, C., Sigcha, L., Borzì, L., Olmo, G., Asensio, C., López, J. M., de Arcas, G., & Pavón, I. (2024). Evaluating Motor Symptoms in Parkinson's Disease Through Wearable Sensors: A Systematic Review of Digital Biomarkers. *Applied Sciences (Basel, Switzerland)*, *2024*(14), 10189. DOI: 10.3390/app142210189

Posadzki, P., Watson, L., & Ernst, E. (2013). Contamination and adulteration of herbal medicinal products (HMPs): An overview of systematic reviews. *European Journal of Clinical Pharmacology*, *69*(3), 295–307. PMID: 22843016

Postuma, R. B., & Berg, D. (2016). Advances in markers of prodromal Parkinson disease. *Nature Reviews. Neurology*, *12*(11), 622–634. DOI: 10.1038/nrneurol.2016.152 PMID: 27786242

Postuma, R. B., Berg, D., Stern, M., Poewe, W., Olanow, C. W., Oertel, W., & Deuschl, G. (2015). MDS clinical diagnostic criteria for Parkinson's disease. *Movement Disorders, 30*(12), 1591–1601. PMID: 26474316

Postuma, R. B., Iranzo, A., Hu, M., Högl, B., Boeve, B. F., Manni, R., Oertel, W. H., Arnulf, I., Ferini-Strambi, L., Puligheddu, M., Antelmi, E., Cochen De Cock, V., Arnaldi, D., Mollenhauer, B., Videnovic, A., Sonka, K., Jung, K. Y., Kunz, D., Dauvilliers, Y., & Pelletier, A. (2019). Risk and predictors of dementia and parkinsonism in idiopathic REM sleep behaviour disorder: A multicentre study. *Brain, 142*(3), 744–759. DOI: 10.1093/BRAIN/AWZ030

Price, D. L., Koike, M. A., Khan, A., Wrasidlo, W., Rockenstein, E., Masliah, E., & Bonhaus, D. (2018). The small molecule alpha-synuclein misfolding inhibitor, NPT200-11, produces multiple benefits in an animal model of Parkinson's disease. *Scientific Reports 2018 8:1, 8*(1), 16165-. https://doi.org/DOI: 10.1038/s41598-018-34490-9

Pringsheim, T., Jette, N., Frolkis, A., & Steeves, T. D. (2014). The prevalence of Parkinson's disease: A systematic review and meta-analysis. *Movement Disorders, 29*(13), 1583–1590. DOI: 10.1002/mds.25945 PMID: 24976103

Prodoehl, J., Planetta, P. J., Kurani, A. S., Comella, C. L., Corcos, D. M., & Vaillancourt, D. E. (2013). Differences in brain activation between tremor- and nontremor-dominant Parkinson disease. *JAMA Neurology, 70*(1), 100–106. PMID: 23318516

Pulgar, V. (2019). Transcytosis to cross the blood–brain barrier: New advancements and challenges. *Frontiers in Neuroscience*. PMID: 30686985

Pycroft, L., John, S., & Tipu, A. (2018). Deep brain stimulation: An overview of history, methods, and future developments. *Brain and Neuroscience Advances, 2*, 1–6. DOI: 10.1177/2398212818816017 PMID: 32166163

Rabey, J. M., Vered, Y., Shabtai, H., Graff, E., Harsat, A., & Korczyn, A. D. (1993). Broad bean (Vicia faba) consumption and Parkinson's disease. *Advances in Neurology, 60*, 681–684. PMID: 8420210

Rabey, J. M., Vered, Y., Shabtai, H., Graff, E., & Korczyn, A. D. (1992). Improvement of parkinsonian features correlate with high plasma levodopa values after broad bean (Vicia faba) consumption. *Journal of Neurology, Neurosurgery, and Psychiatry, 55*(8), 725–727. PMID: 1527547

Rabinak, C. A., & Nirenberg, M. J. (2010). Dopamine Agonist Withdrawal Syndrome in Parkinson Disease. *Archives of Neurology, 67*(1), 58–63. DOI: 10.1001/ARCHNEUROL.2009.294

Radad, K., Moldzio, R., Krewenka, C., Kranner, B., & Rausch, W. D. (2017). Pathophysiology of non-motor signs in parkinson's disease: Some recent updating with brief presentation. Explor Neuroprotective Ther 2023; 3: 24-46. *Journal of Neurology, Neurosurgery, and Psychiatry*, *88*(8), 653–662. PMID: 28554959

Radad, K., Moldzio, R., Krewenka, C., Kranner, B., & Rausch, W. D. (2023). Pathophysiology of non-motor signs in Parkinsons disease: Some recent updating with brief presentation. *Exploration of Neuroprotective Therapy*, *3*(1), 24–46.

Radhakrishnan, D. M., & Goyal, V. (2018). Parkinson's disease: A review. *Neurology India*, *66*(Suppl 1), S26–S35. PMID: 29503325

Rajagopalan, R., Tang, Y., & Ji, X. (2020). Advancements and challenges in potassium ion batteries: A comprehensive review. *Advanced Functional Materials*.

Ramanzini, L. G., Frare, J. M., Camargo, L. F. M., Silveira, J. O. F., & Jankovic, J. (2024). Does Delaying Levodopa Prevent Motor Complications in Parkinson's Disease? A Meta-Analysis. *Movement Disorders Clinical Practice*, *11*(10), 1195–1202. DOI: 10.1002/MDC3.14198

Ramírez-Moreno, J. M., Bodes, I. S., Romaskevych, O., & Duran-Herrera, M. C. (2015). Broad bean (Vicia faba) consumption and Parkinson's disease: A natural source of L-dopa to consider. *Neurologia (Barcelona, Spain)*, *30*(6), 375–376. PMID: 24332774

Ramirez-Zamora, A., Giordano, J. J., Gunduz, A., Brown, P., Sanchez, J. C., Foote, K. D., Almeida, L., Starr, P. A., Bronte-Stewart, H. M., Hu, W., McIntyre, C., Goodman, W., Kumsa, D., Grill, W. M., Walker, H. C., Johnson, M. D., Vitek, J. L., Greene, D., Rizzuto, D. S., & Deeb, M. S. (2018). Evolving Applications, Technological Challenges and Future Opportunities in Neuromodulation: Proceedings of the Fifth Annual Deep Brain Stimulation Think Tank. *Frontiers in Neuroscience*, *11*, 734. DOI: 10.3389/fnins.2017.00734 PMID: 29416498

Rascol, O. (2009). "disease-modification" trials in Parkinson disease: Target populations, endpoints and study design. *Neurology*, *72*(7, SUPPL. 2), S51–S58. DOI: 10.1212/WNL.0B013E318199049E

Rascol, O., Payoux, P., Orym, F., Ferreira, J. J., Brefel-Courbon, C., & Montastruc, J. L. (2003). Limitations of Current Parkinson's Disease Therapy. *Annals of Neurology*, *53*(Suppl 3), S3–S12. PMID: 12666094

Rashidi Fakari, F., Hajian, S., Darvish, S., & Alavi Majd, H. (2021). Explaining factors affecting help-seeking behaviors in women with urinary incontinence: A qualitative study. *BMC Health Services Research, 21*, 60. DOI: 10.1186/s12913-020-06047-y PMID: 33435931

Rashid, M. R. A., Korim, M. A. E., Hasan, M., Ali, M. S., Islam, M. M., & Jabid, T.. (2025). An ensemble learning framework with explainable AI for interpretable leaf disease detection. *Array (New York, N.Y.), 26*, 100386. DOI: 10.1016/j.array.2025.100386

Rasiah, N. P., Maheshwary, R., Kwon, C. S., Bloomstein, J. D., & Girgis, F. (2023). Complications of Deep Brain Stimulation for Parkinson Disease and Relationship between Micro-electrode tracks and hemorrhage: Systematic Review and Meta-Analysis. *World Neurosurgery, 171*, e8–e23. DOI: 10.1016/j.wneu.2022.10.034

Ravina, B., Kieburtz, K., Tilley, B., Shannon, K., Tanner, C., Frederick Wooten, G., Racette, B., Deppen, P., Dewey, R. B., Hayward, B., Scott, B., Field, J., Carter, J., Brodsky, M., Andrews, P., Manyam, B., Whetteckey, J., Rao, J., Cook, M., & Fagan, S. (2006). A randomized, double-blind, futility clinical trial of creatine and minocycline in early Parkinson disease. *Neurology, 66*(5), 664–671. DOI: 10.1212/01.WNL.0000201252.57661.E1

Regensburger, M., Ip, C. W., Kohl, Z., Schrader, C., Urban, P. P., Kassubek, J., & Jost, W. H. (2023). Clinical benefit of MAO-B and COMT inhibition in Parkinson's disease: Practical considerations. *Journal of Neural Transmission (Vienna, Austria), 130*(6), 847–861. PMID: 36964457

Reichmann, H., Lisa, K., & Jonas, B. (2023). The use of wearables for the diagnosis and treatment of Parkinson's disease. *Journal of Neural Transmission (Vienna, Austria), 2023*(130), 783–791. DOI: 10.1007/s00702-022-02575-5 PMID: 36609737

Reid, K., Emily, B., Johnny, T., Alexander, S., Dawn, L., Judy, N., David, P., Jonathan, N., Siddharthan, C., & Suvankar, P. (2024). Perceptions of digital technology use for monitoring health in people living with neurological disorders. JournaloftheNeurologicalSciences462(2024)123072.

Ren, K., Chen, Z., Ling, Y., & Zhao, J. (2022). Recognition of freezing of gait in Parkinson's disease based on combined wearable sensors. *BMC Neurology, 22*(1). Advance online publication. DOI: 10.1186/s12883-022-02732-z PMID: 35729546

Ren, Y., Li, H., Xie, W., Wei, N., & Liu, M. (2019). MicroRNA-195 triggers neuroinflammation in Parkinson's disease in a Rho-associated kinase 1-dependent manner. *Molecular Medicine Reports, 19*(6), 5153–5161. DOI: 10.3892/mmr.2019.10178 PMID: 31059087

Richard, I. H., McDermott, M. P., Kurlan, R., Lyness, J. M., Como, P. G., Pearson, N., Factor, S. A., Juncos, J., Ramos, C. S., Brodsky, M., Manning, C., Marsh, L., Shulman, L., Fernandez, H. H., Black, K. J., Panisset, M., Christine, C. W., Jiang, W., Singer, C., & McDonald, W. (2012). A randomized, double-blind, placebo-controlled trial of antidepressants in Parkinson disease. *Neurology, 78*(16), 1229–1236. DOI: 10.1212/WNL.0B013E318251624

Riederer, P., Youdim, M. B. H., Rausch, W. D., Birkmayer, W., Jellinger, K., & Seemann, D. (1978). On the mode of action of L-deprenyl in the human central nervous system. *Journal of Neural Transmission (Vienna, Austria), 43*(3), 217–226. PMID: 745014

Roda, A. R., Serra-Mir, G., Montoliu-Gaya, L., Tiessler, L., & Villegas, S. (2022). Amyloid-beta peptide and tau protein crosstalk in Alzheimer's disease. *Neural Regeneration Research, 17*(8), 1666–1674. PMID: 35017413

Rodríguez-Martín, D., Cabestany, J., Pérez-López, C., Pie, M., Calvet, J., Samà, A., Capra, C., Català, A., & Rodríguez-Molinero, A. (2022). A New Paradigm in Parkinson's Disease Evaluation With Wearable Medical Devices: A Review of STAT-ONTM. *Frontiers in Neurology, 13*, 912343. DOI: 10.3389/fneur.2022.912343 PMID: 35720090

Rodriguez-Oroz, M. C., Jahanshahi, M., Krack, P., Litvan, I., Macias, R., Bezard, E., & Obeso, J. A. (2009). Initial clinical manifestations of Parkinson's disease: Features and pathophysiological mechanisms. *Lancet Neurology, 8*(12), 1128–1139. PMID: 19909911

Rodríguez-Pallares, J., García-Garrote, M., Parga, J. A., & Labandeira-García, J. L. (2023). Combined cell-based therapy strategies for the treatment of Parkinson's disease: Focus on mesenchymal stromal cells. *Neural Regeneration Research, 18*(3), 478–484. PMID: 36018150

Romano, S., Savva, G. M., Bedarf, J. R., Charles, I. G., Hildebrand, F., & Narbad, A. (2021). Meta-analysis of the Parkinson's disease gut microbiome suggests alterations linked to intestinal inflammation. *Npj Parkinson's Disease 2021 7:1, 7*(1), 27-. https://doi.org/DOI: 10.1038/s41531-021-00156-z

Rosenberg-Katz, K., Herman, T., Jacob, Y., Giladi, N., Hendler, T., & Hausdorff, J. M. (2013). Gray matter atrophy distinguishes between Parkinson disease motor subtypes. *Neurology, 80*(16), 1476–1484. PMID: 23516323

Rossi, C., Volterrani, D., Nicoletti, V., Manca, G., Frosini, D., Kiferle, L., Palumbo, B., Bonuccelli, U., & Ceravolo, R. (2009). "Parkinson-dementia" diseases: A comparison by double tracer SPECT studies. *Parkinsonism & Related Disorders, 15*(10), 762–766. DOI: 10.1016/j.parkreldis.2009.05.012 PMID: 19553153

Rossi, C., Volterrani, D., Nicoletti, V., Mugnaini, M., Frosini, D., Kiferle, L., Unti, E., De Feo, P., Bonuccelli, U., & Ceravolo, R. (2010). "Parkinson-dementia" diseases: From pathogenetic mechanisms to possible treatment strategies. *Journal of Alzheimer's Disease, 21*(1), 3–23. PMID: 20378955

Roy, A. R., & Maji, P. K. (2007). A fuzzy soft set theoretic approach to decision making problems. *Journal of Computational and Applied Mathematics, 203*(2), 412–418.

Ruirui, L., Yan, X., Xiaohui, L., Yongli, F., Weiqi, Z., Yang, T., Kang, R., Wenwu, C., & Xuebing, C. (2020). Evaluation of Wearable Sensor Devices in Parkinson's Disease: A Review of Current Status and Future Prospects. Hindawi Parkinson's Disease Volume 2020, Article ID 4693019, 8 pages https://doi.org/DOI: 10.1155/2020/4693019

Saji, C. V., Mohanakumar, K. P., & Shenoi, R. A. (2025). Phytomedicine nanoformulations for Parkinson's disease. *Phytomedicine Plus : International Journal of Phytotherapy and Phytopharmacology, 5*(1), 100704.

Sampaio, F., Nystrand, C., Feldman, I., & Mihalopoulos, C. (2022). Evidence for investing in parenting interventions aiming to improve child health: A systematic review of economic evaluations. *European Child & Adolescent Psychiatry, 33*, 323. DOI: 10.1007/s00787-022-01969-w PMID: 35304645

Sancho-Bielsa, F. J. (2022). Parkinson's disease: Present and future of cell therapy. *Neurology Perspectives, 2*(1), 58–68.

Sandoval-Pistorius, S.S., Nicole, R., Provenza, Coralie, de H., Mallory, L., Hacker, Allison, C.W., Kara, A.J., Jing, W., Melanie, A.M., & Stephanie, C. (2023). Advances in Deep Brain Stimulation: From Mechanisms to Applications. The Journal of Neuroscience, November 8, 2023. 43(45):7575–7586. 7575.

Santos, D. T., Camelo, D. M. F., Strelow, M. Z., Silva, M. T. S., Führ, P., Marins, L. W., & Schumacher-Schuh, A. F. (2022). Feasibility of telemedicine for patients with parkinsonism in the Brazilian public health system. *Arquivos de Neuro-Psiquiatria, 80*(09), 914–921. PMID: 36261128

Sasidharan, A., Bagepally, B. S., & Kumar, S. S. (2024). Cost Effectiveness of Deep Brain Stimulation for Parkinson's Disease: A Systematic Review. *Applied Health Economics and Health Policy, 22*(2), 181–192. DOI: 10.1007/S40258-023-00848-Y

Sawamoto, N., Doi, D., Nakanishi, E., Sawamura, M., Kikuchi, T., Yamakado, H., Taruno, Y., Shima, A., Fushimi, Y., Okada, T., & Takahashi, J. (2025). Phase I/II trial of iPS-cell-derived dopaminergic cells for Parkinson's disease. *Nature*, •••, 1–7. PMID: 40240591

Schalkamp, A. K., Harrison, N. A., Peall, K. J., & Sandor, C. (2024). Digital outcome measures from smartwatch data relate to non-motor features of Parkinson's disease. *Npj Parkinson's Disease 2024 10:1, 10*(1), 110-. https://doi.org/DOI: 10.1038/s41531-024-00719-w

Schapira, A. H. (2009). Neurobiology and treatment of Parkinson's disease. *Trends in Pharmacological Sciences, 30*(1), 41–47. PMID: 19042040

Schapira, A. H., Chaudhuri, K. R., & Jenner, P. (2017). Non-motor features of Parkinson disease. *Nature Reviews. Neuroscience, 18*(7), 435–450. PMID: 28592904

Schiess, N., Cataldi, R., Okun, M. S., Fothergill-Misbah, N., Dorsey, E. R., Bloem, B. R., & Dua, T. (2022). Six action steps to address global disparities in Parkinson disease: A World Health Organization priority. *JAMA Neurology, 79*(9), 929–936. PMID: 35816299

Schneider, M. G., Swearingen, C. J., Shulman, L. M., Ye, J., Baumgarten, M., & Tilley, B. C. (2009). Minority enrollment in Parkinson's disease clinical trials. *Parkinsonism & Related Disorders, 15*(4), 258–262. DOI: 10.1016/j.parkreldis.2008.06.005

Schnitzler, A., Pablo, M., Matthew, A. B., Leonard, V., Sergiu, G., Andrew, E., Ramiro, A., Marta, B., Julie, G. P., & Sean, N. M. (2022). Pötter-Nerger, Winona, T., Leonardo, A., Jimenez-Shahed, J., Nestor, T., Witold, L., Fatima, C., Christian, J.H., Stefan, J.G., Martin, G., Florence, D., Edward, K., Binith, C., & Jan, V., (2022). Directional Deep Brain Stimulation for Parkinson's Disease: Results of an International Crossover Study With Randomized, Double-Blind Primary Endpoint. Neuromodulation: Technology at the Neural Interface. *Neuromodulation, 25*, 817–828. DOI: 10.1111/ner.13407 PMID: 34047410

Schöndorf, D. C., Ivanyuk, D., Baden, P., Sanchez-Martinez, A., De Cicco, S., Yu, C., Giunta, I., Schwarz, L. K., Di Napoli, G., Panagiotakopoulou, V., Nestel, S., Keatinge, M., Pruszak, J., Bandmann, O., Heimrich, B., Gasser, T., Whitworth, A. J., & Deleidi, M. (2018). The NAD+ Precursor Nicotinamide Riboside Rescues Mitochondrial Defects and Neuronal Loss in iPSC and Fly Models of Parkinson's Disease. *Cell Reports, 23*(10), 2976–2988. DOI: 10.1016/j.celrep.2018.05.009

Schrag, A.. (2000). What contributes to quality of life in Parkinson's disease? *Journal of Neurology, Neurosurgery, and Psychiatry, 69*(3), 308–312. PMID: 10945804

Schrag, A., Sampaio, C., Counsell, N., & Poewe, W. (2006). Minimal clinically important change on the Unified Parkinson's Disease Rating Scale. *Movement Disorders, 21*(8), 1200–1207. DOI: 10.1002/MDS.20914

Schweitzer, J. S., Song, B., Herrington, T. M., Park, T. Y., Lee, N., Ko, S., Jeon, J., Cha, Y., & Kim, K. S. (2020). Personalized iPSC-derived dopamine progenitor cells for Parkinson's disease. *The New England Journal of Medicine, 382*(20), 1926–1932. PMID: 32402162

Schweitzer, J. S., Song, B., Herrington, T. M., Park, T.-Y., Lee, N., Ko, S., Jeon, J., Cha, Y., Kim, K., Li, Q., Henchcliffe, C., Kaplitt, M., Neff, C., Rapalino, O., Seo, H., Lee, I.-H., Kim, J., Kim, T., Petsko, G. A., & Kim, K.-S. (2020). Personalized iPSC-Derived Dopamine Progenitor Cells for Parkinson's Disease. *The New England Journal of Medicine, 382*(20), 1926–1932. DOI: 10.1056/NEJMOA1915872

Serrano, M., Elías, M., Llorens, M., Bolasell, M., Vall-Roqué, H., & Villalta, L. (2024). Early treatment for children with mental health problems and genetic conditions through a parenting intervention (The GAP): Study protocol for a pragmatic randomized controlled trial. *Trials, 25*. Advance online publication. DOI: 10.1186/s13063-024-08278-4 PMID: 39033111

Shahed, J., & Jankovic, J. (2007). Exploring the relationship between essential tremor and Parkinson's disease. *Parkinsonism & Related Disorders, 13*(2), 67–76. DOI: 10.1016/j.parkreldis.2006.05.033 PMID: 16887374

Shaheen, N., Shaheen, A., Osama, M., Nashwan, A. J., Bharmauria, V., & Flouty, O. (2024). MicroRNAs regulation in Parkinson's disease, and their potential role as diagnostic and therapeutic targets. *npj. Parkinson's Disease, 10*(1), 186. DOI: 10.1038/s41531-024-00810-2 PMID: 39369002

Shah, H., Omer, U., Habib, U. R., Sharan, J., Chaithanya, A., Kamran, H., Hamza, I., & Sailesh, I. S. K. (2022). Deep Brain Stimulation in the Treatment of Parkinson's Disease. *Cureus, 14*(9), e28760. DOI: 10.7759/cureus.28760 PMID: 36211107

Shah, N., Frey, K. A., Müller, M. L. T. M., Petrou, M., Kotagal, V., Koeppe, R. A., Scott, P. J. H., Albin, R. L., & Bohnen, N. I. (2016). Striatal and cortical β-amyloidopathy and cognition in Parkinson's disease. *Movement Disorders, 31*(1), 111–117. DOI: 10.1002/mds.26369 PMID: 26380951

Shalash, A., Spindler, M., & Cubo, E. (2021). Global perspective on telemedicine for Parkinson's disease. *Journal of Parkinson's Disease, 11*(s1), S11–S18. PMID: 33579872

Shang, R., Lee, S., Senavirathne, G., & Lai, E. C. (2023). microRNAs in action: Biogenesis, function and regulation. *Nature Reviews. Genetics*, *24*(12), 816–833. DOI: 10.1038/s41576-023-00611-y PMID: 37380761

Sharma, A., Verwilst, P., Li, M., Ma, D., Singh, N., & Yoo, J.. (2024). Theranostic fluorescent probes. *Chemical Reviews*, *124*, 2699. DOI: 10.1021/acs.chemrev.3c00778 PMID: 38422393

Sharma, N. K., Robbins, K., Wagner, K., & Colgrove, Y. M. (2015). A randomized controlled pilot study of the therapeutic effects of yoga in people with Parkinson's disease. *International Journal of Yoga*, *8*(1), 74–79. PMID: 25558138

Shirolapov, I. V., Gribkova, O. V., Kovalev, A. M., Shafigullina, L. R., Ulivanova, V. A., Kozlov, A. V., Ereshchenko, A. A., Lyamin, A. V., & Zakharov, A. V. (2024). The Role of Interactions along the Brain–Gut–Microbiome Axis in the Regulation of Circadian Rhythms, Sleep Mechanisms, and Their Disorders. *Neuroscience and Behavioral Physiology*, *54*(8), 1177–1183. DOI: 10.1007/s11055-024-01712-9

Shirolapov, I. V., Zakharov, A. V., Smirnova, D. A., Lyamin, A. V., & Gayduk, A. Ya. (2023). The significance of the glymphatic pathway in the relationship between the sleep—Wake cycle and neurodegenerative diseases. *Zhurnal Nevrologii i Psikhiatrii Imeni S. S. Korsakova*, *123*(9), 9. Advance online publication. DOI: 10.17116/jnevro202312309131 PMID: 37796065

Shirolapov, I., Zakharov, A., Gochhait, S., Pyatin, V., Sergeeva, M., Romanchuk, N., Komarova, Y., Kalinin, V., Pavlova, O., & Khivintseva, E. (2023). Aquaporin-4 as the Main Element of the Glymphatic System for Clearance of Abnormal Proteins and Prevention of Neurodegeneration: A Review. *WSEAS TRANSACTIONS ON BIOLOGY AND BIOMEDICINE*, *20*, 110–118. DOI: 10.37394/23208.2023.20.11

Shirolapov, Igor V., Zakharov, A. V., Bulgakova, S. V., Khivintseva, E. V., Sergeeva, M. S., Romanchuk, N. P., Pavlova, O. N., & Kazantsev, V. B. (2023). Glymphatic dysfunction in the pathogenesis of neurodegenerative diseases and pathological aging. *Genes to Cells*, *18*(4), 309–322. DOI: 10.23868/gc546022

Shirvan, J., Clement, N., Ye, R., Katz, S., Schultz, A., Johnson, K. A., Gomez-Isla, T., Frosch, M. P., Growdon, J. H., & Gomperts, S. N. (2019). Neuropathologic correlates of amyloid and dopamine transporter imaging in Lewy body disease. *Neurology*, *93*(5), e476–e484. DOI: 10.1212/WNL.0000000000007855 PMID: 31243072

Shi, Y., Inoue, H., Wu, J. C., & Yamanaka, S. (2017). Induced pluripotent stem cell technology: A decade of progress. *Nature Reviews. Drug Discovery*, *16*(2), 115–130. PMID: 27980341

Shlisky, J., Mandlik, R., Askari, S., Abrams, S. A., Belizán, J. M., & Bourassa, M. W.. (2022). Calcium deficiency worldwide: Prevalence of inadequate intakes and associated health outcomes. *Annals of the New York Academy of Sciences, 1512*, 10. DOI: 10.1111/nyas.14758 PMID: 35247225

Sica, M., Tedesco, S., Crowe, C., Kenny, L., Moore, K., Timmons, S., Barton, J., O'Flynn, B., & Komaris, D. S. (2021). Continuous home monitoring of Parkinson's disease using inertial sensors: A systematic review. *PLoS ONE, 16*(2 February). https://doi.org/DOI: 10.1371/journal.pone.0246528

Siderowf, A., Concha-Marambio, L., Lafontant, D. E., Farris, C. M., Ma, Y., Urenia, P. A., Nguyen, H., Alcalay, R. N., Chahine, L. M., Foroud, T., Galasko, D., Kieburtz, K., Merchant, K., Mollenhauer, B., Poston, K. L., Seibyl, J., Simuni, T., Tanner, C. M., Weintraub, D., & Soto, C. (2023). Assessment of heterogeneity among participants in the Parkinson's Progression Markers Initiative cohort using α-synuclein seed amplification: A cross-sectional study. *Lancet Neurology, 22*(5), 407–417. DOI: 10.1016/S1474-4422(23)00109-6

Sidransky, E., Nalls, M. A., Aasly, J. O., Aharon-Peretz, J., Annesi, G., Barbosa, E. R., & Ziegler, S. G. (2009). Multicenter analysis of glucocerebrosidase mutations in Parkinson's disease. *The New England Journal of Medicine, 361*(17), 1651–1661. PMID: 19846850

Sigchaa, L., Luigi, B., Federica, A., Irene, R., Ramos-Romero, C., Andrés, C., Luis, G., & Gabriella, O. (2023). Deep learning and wearable sensors for the diagnosis and monitoring of Parkinson's disease: A systematic review. *Expert Systems with Applications, 229*, 120541.

Silva-Batista, C., Jennifer, L. W., Kathleen, T. S., Margaret, S., Carlson-Kuhta, P., Siting, C., William, L., Tomas, N. G de la H., Fay, B. H., Martina, M., & Laurie, A. K. (2023). Balance telerehabilitation and wearable technology for people with Parkinson's disease (TelePD trial). *BMC Neurology, 3*, 33. DOI: 10.1186/s12883-023-03403-3 PMID: 37833645

Simon, D. K., Tanner, C. M., & Brundin, P. (2020). Parkinson disease epidemiology, pathology, genetics, and pathophysiology. *Clinics in Geriatric Medicine, 36*(1), 1–12. PMID: 31733690

Simuni, T., Siderowf, A., Lasch, S., Coffey, C. S., Caspell-Garcia, C., Jennings, D., Tanner, C. M., Trojanowski, J. Q., Shaw, L. M., Seibyl, J., Schuff, N., Singleton, A., Kieburtz, K., Toga, A. W., Mollenhauer, B., Galasko, D., Chahine, L. M., Weintraub, D., Foroud, T., & Marek, K. (2018). Longitudinal Change of Clinical and Biological Measures in Early Parkinson's Disease: Parkinson's Progression Markers Initiative Cohort. *Movement Disorders, 33*(5), 771–782. DOI: 10.1002/MDS.27361

Singh, J., & Kumar, D. (2025). *In vivo* and *in vitro* perspectives in Parkinson's disease: Mechanisms and the role of phytomedicine. *Yao Wu Shi Pin Fen Xi, 33*(3), 193–212. PMID: 41066749

Sinha, B., & Dhanalakshmi, R. (2022). Recent advancements and challenges of Internet of Things in smart agriculture: A survey. *Future Generation Computer Systems.*

Sivandzade, F., & Cucullo, L. (2021). Regenerative stem cell therapy for neurodegenerative diseases: An overview. *International Journal of Molecular Sciences, 22*(4), 2153. PMID: 33671500

Smith, J., & Zhang, L. (2021). Challenges in Natural Product Research: The Impact of Adulteration on Therapeutic Outcomes. *Phytotherapy Research, 35*(5), 2437–2446.

Song, I.-U., Yoo, I.-R., Chung, Y.-A., & Jeong, J. (2015). The value of brain perfusion SPECT for differentiation between mildly symptomatic idiopathic Parkinson's disease and the Parkinson variant of multiple system atrophy. *Nuclear Medicine Communications, 36*(10), 1049–1054. DOI: 10.1097/MNM.0000000000000354 PMID: 26087241

Sonne, J., Reddy, V., & Beato, M. R. (2024). Neuroanatomy, substantia nigra. In *StatPearls* [Internet]. StatPearls Publishing.

Sonntag, K. C., Song, B., Lee, N., Jung, J. H., Cha, Y., Leblanc, P., Neff, C., Kong, S. W., Carter, B. S., Schweitzer, J., & Kim, K. S. (2018). Pluripotent stem cell-based therapy for Parkinson's disease: Current status and future prospects. *Progress in Neurobiology, 168*, 1–20. PMID: 29653250

Sosero, Y. L., & Gan-Or, Z. (2023). LRRK2 and Parkinson's disease: From genetics to targeted therapy. *Annals of Clinical and Translational Neurology, 10*(6), 850–864. PMID: 37021623

Sotirakis, C., Su, Z., Brzezicki, M. A., Conway, N., Tarassenko, L., FitzGerald, J. J., & Antoniades, C. A. (2023). Identification of motor progression in Parkinson's disease using wearable sensors and machine learning. *NPJ Parkinson's Disease, 9*(1). Advance online publication. DOI: 10.1038/s41531-023-00581-2 PMID: 37805655

Soumyanath, A., Denne, T., Peterson, A., & Shinto, L. (2012). Assessment of commercial formulations of Mucuna pruriens seeds for Levodopa (L-DOPA) content. [Abstract from the International Research Congress on Integrative Medicine and Health]. *BMC Complementary and Alternative Medicine*, *12*(Suppl 1), 36.

Sperling, S. A., Shah, B. B., Barrett, M. J., Bond, A. E., Huss, D. S., Costa, M. G. L., & Elias, W. J. (2018). Focused ultrasound thalamotomy in Parkinson disease: Nonmotor outcomes and quality of life. *Neurology*, *91*(14), e1275–e1284. DOI: 10.1212/WNL.0000000000006279 PMID: 30158160

Spiegel, J., Hellwig, D., Samnick, S., Jost, W., Fassbender, K., Kirsch, C. M., & Dillmann, U. (2007). Striatal FP-CIT uptake differs in the subtype of early Parkinson's disease. *Journal of Nuclear Medicine*, *48*(3), 359–364. PMID: 17332612

Spillantini, M. G., & Goedert, M. (2018). Neurodegeneration and the ordered assembly of alpha-synuclein. *Cell and Tissue Research*, *373*(1), 137–152. PMID: 29119326

Srivastav, S., Fatima, M., & Mondal, A. C. (2017). Important medicinal herbs in Parkinson's disease pharmacotherapy, Biomedicine & Pharmacotherapy, Volume 92, 2017, Pages 856-863, ISSN 0753-3322, https://doi.org/DOI: 10.1016/j.biopha.2017.05.137

Steendam-Oldekamp, E., & Van Laar, T. (2024). The Effectiveness of Inpatient Rehabilitation in Parkinson's Disease: A Systematic Review of Recent Studies. *Journal of Parkinson's Disease*, *14*(Suppl 1), S93. DOI: 10.3233/JPD-230271

Stocchi, F., Bravi, D., Emmi, A., & Antonini, A. (2024). Parkinson disease therapy: Current strategies and future research priorities. *Nature Reviews. Neurology*, *20*, 695. DOI: 10.1038/s41582-024-01034-x PMID: 39496848

Sturchio, A., Rocha, E. M., Kauffman, M. A., Marsili, L., Mahajan, A., Saraf, A. A., Vizcarra, J. A., Guo, Z., & Espay, A. J. (2024). Recalibrating the Why and Whom of Animal Models in Parkinson Disease: A Clinician's Perspective. *Brain Sciences 2024, Vol. 14,14*(2). https://doi.org/DOI: 10.3390/BRAINSCI14020151

Suarez-Cedeno, G., Jessika, S., & Mya, C. S. (2017). Earlier Intervention with Deep Brain Stimulation for Parkinson's Disease. Hindawi Parkinson's Disease Volume. 2017, Article ID 9358153, 9 pages https://doi.org/DOI: 10.1155/2017/9358153

Su, D., Cui, Y., He, C., Yin, P., Bai, R., & Zhu, J.. (2025). Projections for prevalence of Parkinson's disease and its driving factors in 195 countries and territories to 2050: Modelling study of Global Burden of Disease Study 2021. *BMJ (Clinical Research Ed.)*, *388*. Advance online publication. DOI: 10.1136/bmj-2024-080952 PMID: 40044233

Sun, Q., Wang, S., Chen, J., Cai, H., Huang, W., Zhang, Y., Wang, L., & Xing, Y. (2019). MicroRNA-190 alleviates neuronal damage and inhibits neuroinflammation via Nlrp3 in MPTP-induced Parkinson's disease mouse model. *Journal of Cellular Physiology*, *234*(12), 23379–23387. DOI: 10.1002/jcp.28907 PMID: 31232472

Suppa, A., Quartarone, A., Siebner, H., Chen, R., Di Lazzaro, V., Del Giudice, P., Paulus, W., Rothwell, J. C., Ziemann, U., & Classen, J. (2017). The associative brain at work: Evidence from paired associative stimulation studies in humans. *Clinical Neurophysiology*, *128*(11), 2140–2164. DOI: 10.1016/j.clinph.2017.08.003 PMID: 28938144

Sushama, A. P., Onkar A, A., Shripad N, S., & Jyoti P, J. (2013). Biological sources of L-DOPA: An alternative approach. *Advances in Parkinson's Disease, 2013.*

Sveinbjornsdottir, S. (2016). The clinical symptoms of Parkinson's disease. *Journal of Neurochemistry*, *139*, 318–324. PMID: 27401947

Swallow, D. M. A., & Counsell, C. E. (2023). The evolution of diagnosis from symptom onset to death in progressive supranuclear palsy (PSP) and corticobasal degeneration (CBD) compared to Parkinson's disease (PD). *Journal of Neurology*, *270*(8), 4065–4076. DOI: 10.1007/s00415-023-11629-x PMID: 36971841

Tabar, V., Sarva, H., Lozano, A. M., Fasano, A., Kalia, S. K., Yu, K. K. H., & Henchcliffe, C. (2025). Phase I trial of hES cell-derived dopaminergic neurons for Parkinson's disease. *Nature*, •••, 1–6. PMID: 40240592

Takahashi, H., & Wakabayashi, K. (2001). The cellular pathology of Parkinson's disease. *Neuropathology*, *21*(4), 315–322. DOI: 10.1046/j.1440-1789.2001.00403.x PMID: 11837539

Takahashi, K., Tanabe, K., Ohnuki, M., Narita, M., Ichisaka, T., Tomoda, K., & Yamanaka, S. (2007). Induction of pluripotent stem cells from adult human fibroblasts by defined factors. *Cell*, *131*(5), 861–872. PMID: 18035408

Takahashi, K., & Yamanaka, S. (2006). Induction of Pluripotent Stem Cells from Mouse Embryonic and Adult Fibroblast Cultures by Defined Factors. *Cell*, *126*(4), 663–676. DOI: 10.1016/j.cell.2006.07.024

Tannenbaum, C., Fritel, X., Halme, A., Van Den Heuvel, E., Jutai, J., & Wagg, A. (2019). Long-term effect of community-based continence promotion on urinary symptoms, falls and healthy active life expectancy among older women: Cluster randomised trial. *Age and Ageing*, *48*, 526. DOI: 10.1093/ageing/afz038 PMID: 31220200

Terry, M.A., & Alvarez-Vazquez, E. (2017). Efficacy of Wearable Devices in Monitoring and Treating Parkinson's Disease Symptoms: A Systematic Review and Meta Analyses. Preparation of Papers for IEEE Access. 1-9. DOI DOI: 10.1109/ACCESS.2025.3569056

Thankathuraipandian, S., Walter, G., Anahita, K., Tucker, T., Binesh, B., Erika, R., & Yagna, P. (2024). Development of a remote therapeutic monitoring platform: applications for movement disorders. Scientific Reports | (2024) 14:29837 | https://doi.org/.DOI: 10.1038/s41598-024-80567-z

Thenganatt, M. A., & Louis, E. D. (2012). Distinguishing essential tremor from Parkinson's disease: Bedside tests and laboratory evaluations. *Expert Review of Neurotherapeutics*, *12*(6), 687–696. PMID: 22650171

Théry, C., Witwer, K. W., Aikawa, E., Alcaraz, M. J., Anderson, J. D., Andriantsitohaina, R., Antoniou, A., Arab, T., Archer, F., Atkin-Smith, G. K., Ayre, D. C., Bach, J.-M., Bachurski, D., Baharvand, H., Balaj, L., Baldacchino, S., Bauer, N. N., Baxter, A. A., Bebawy, M., & Zuba-Surma, E. K. (2018). Minimal information for studies of extracellular vesicles 2018 (MISEV2018): A position statement of the International Society for Extracellular Vesicles and update of the MISEV2014 guidelines. *Journal of Extracellular Vesicles*, *7*(1), 1535750. DOI: 10.1080/20013078.2018.1535750 PMID: 30637094

Thomas, S., Edwards, E., & Kobylecki, C. (2024). Parkinson's Nurses Are Crucial for the Management of Parkinson's Disease: 2007–2024. *Journal of Parkinson's Disease*, *14*(s1), S209–S217. PMID: 38578901

Thomson, J. A., Itskovitz-Eldor, J., Shapiro, S. S., Waknitz, M. A., Swiergiel, J. J., Marshall, V. S., & Jones, J. M. (1998). Embryonic stem cell lines derived from human blastocysts. *science, 282*(5391), 1145-1147.

Tibar, H., El Bayad, K., Bouhouche, A., Ait Ben Haddou, E. H., Benomar, A., Yahyaoui, M., & Regragui, W. (2018). Non-motor symptoms of Parkinson's disease and their impact on quality of life in a cohort of Moroccan patients. *Frontiers in Neurology*, *9*, 170. PMID: 29670566

Tkaczenko, H., Buyun, L., Kołodziejska, R., Kamiński, P., & Kurhaluk, N. (2025). Neuroactive Phytochemicals as Multi-Target Modulators of Mental Health and Cognitive Function: An Integrative Review. *International Journal of Molecular Sciences*, *26*(18), 8907. DOI: 10.3390/ijms26188907 PMID: 41009475

Tolosa, E., Gaig, C., Santamaría, J., & Compta, Y. (2009). Diagnosis and the premotor phase of Parkinson disease. *Neurology*, *72*(7, Suppl), S12–S20. DOI: 10.1212/WNL.0b013e318198db11 PMID: 19221308

Tolosa, E., Martí, M. J., Valldeoriola, F., & Molinuevo, J. L. (1998). History of levodopa and dopamine agonists in Parkinson's disease treatment. *Neurology*, *50*(6), S2–S10. PMID: 9633679

Tolosa, E., Vila, M., Klein, C., & Rascol, O. (2020). LRRK2 in Parkinson disease: Challenges of clinical trials. *Nature Reviews. Neurology*, *16*(2), 97–107. DOI: 10.1038/s41582-019-0301-2 PMID: 31980808

Tortelli, R., Rodrigues, F. B., & Wild, E. J. (2021). The use of wearable/portable digital sensors in Huntington's disease: A systematic review. *Parkinsonism & Related Disorders*, *83*, 93–104. DOI: 10.1016/j.parkreldis.2021.01.006 PMID: 33493786

Toshiki, T., Etsuro, N., Hiroo, S., Katsumi, S., Satoru, I., Shinji, A., Satomi, Y., Tanaka-Mizuno, S., Kayoko, M., Ryosuke, T., & Koji, K. (2024). Adherence to istradefylline in patients with Parkinson's disease: A group-based trajectory analysis. JournaloftheNeurologicalSciences462(2024)123092.

Toth, C., Rajput, A., & Rajput, A. H. (2004). Anomalies of asymmetry of clinical signs in parkinsonism. *Movement Disorders*, *19*(3), 151–157. PMID: 14978669

Treweek, S., Pitkethly, M., & Cook, J.. (2018). Strategies to improve recruitment to randomized trials. *Cochrane Database of Systematic Reviews*, *2*, MR000013. PMID: 29468635

Trinh, J., Farrer, M., Ross, O. A., & Guella, I. (2025). LRRK2-Related Parkinson Disease. *GeneReviews®*. https://www.ncbi.nlm.nih.gov/books/NBK1208/

Tufail, S., Riggs, H., Tariq, M., & Sarwat, A. (2023). Advancements and challenges in machine learning: A comprehensive review of models, libraries, applications, and algorithms. *Electronics (Basel)*.

Turcano, P., Mielke, M. M., Bower, J. H., Parisi, J. E., Cutsforth-Gregory, J. K., Ahlskog, J. E., & Savica, R. (2018). Levodopa-induced dyskinesia in Parkinson disease. *Neurology*, *91*(24), e2238–e2243. DOI: 10.1212/WNL.0000000000006643

Turner, M. R., Thompson, A. G., & Teunissen, C. E. (2025). Blood level of neurofilament light chain as a biomarker for neurological disorders. *BMJ Medicine*, *4*(1), e000958. DOI: 10.1136/BMJMED-2024-000958

Tushar, W., Yuen, C., Saha, T., & Morstyn, T. (2021). Peer-to-peer energy systems for connected communities: A review of recent advances and emerging challenges. *Applied Energy*.

Tu, X. J., Hwang, W. J., Hsu, S. P., & Ma, H. I. (2017). Responsiveness of the short-form health survey and the Parkinson's disease questionnaire in patients with Parkinson's disease. *Health and Quality of Life Outcomes*, *15*(1), 75. DOI: 10.1186/S12955-017-0642-8

Uccelli, A., Moretta, L., & Pistoia, V. (2008). Mesenchymal stem cells in health and disease. *Nature Reviews. Immunology*, *8*(9), 726–736. PMID: 19172693

Umemura, A. (2023). Deep Brain Stimulation for Parkinson's Disease. *Juntendo Medical Journal*, *69*(1), 21–29. PMID: 38854848

Valencia-Agudo, F., Urbiola, E., Romero-González, M., Navas, I., Elías, M., & Garriz, A.. (2021). Protocol for a randomized pilot study (FIRST STEPS): Implementation of the Incredible Years-ASLD® program in Spanish children with autism and preterm children with communication and/or socialization difficulties. *Trials*, *22*. Advance online publication. DOI: 10.1186/s13063-021-05229-1 PMID: 33879224

van den Bergh, R., Bloem, B. R., Meinders, M. J., & Evers, L. J. (2021). The state of telemedicine for persons with Parkinson's disease. *Current Opinion in Neurology*, *34*(4), 589–597. PMID: 33990100

van der Sande, M. A. B., Walraven, G., Milligan, P., Banya, W., Ceesay, S. M., & Nyan, O.. (2001).. . *Bulletin of the World Health Organization*, *79*, 321. PMID: 11357211

Van Kampen, J. M., Baranowski, D. B., Shaw, C. A., & Kay, D. G. (2014). Panax ginseng is neuroprotective in a novel progressive model of Parkinson's disease. *Experimental Gerontology*, *50*, 95–105. DOI: 10.1016/j.exger.2013.11.012 PMID: 24316034

Van Laar, A. D., & Jain, S. (2004). Non-motor symptoms of Parkinson disease: Update on the diagnosis and treatment. *The Neurologist*, *10*(4), 185. PMID: 15245584

van Meer, G., Voelker, D. R., & Feigenson, G. W. (2008). Membrane lipids: Where they are and how they behave. *Nature Reviews. Molecular Cell Biology*, *9*(2), 112–124. DOI: 10.1038/nrm2330 PMID: 18216768

van Munster, M., Stümpel, J., Clemens, T., Czabanowska, K., Pedrosa, D. J., & Mestre, T. A., & iCare-Pd Consortium. (2022). Telemedicine as an untapped opportunity for Parkinson's nurses training in personalized care approaches. *Journal of Personalized Medicine*, *12*(7), 1057. PMID: 35887553 van Uem, J. M. T., Tom, I., Alan, L., Eros, B., Dina, S., Alberto, J. E., Helen, M., & Walter, M. (2016). AViewpoint on Wearable Technology-Enabled Measurement of Wellbeing and Health-Related Quality of Life in Parkinson's Disease. [IOS Press.]. *Journal of Parkinson's Disease*, *6*, 279–287. DOI: 10.3233/JPD-150740 PMID: 27003779

Vaswani, P. A., Tropea, T. F., & Dahodwala, N. (2020). Overcoming Barriers to Parkinson Disease Trial Participation: Increasing Diversity and Novel Designs for Recruitment and Retention. *Neurotherapeutics; the Journal of the American Society for Experimental NeuroTherapeutics*, *17*(4), 1724–1735. DOI: 10.1007/S13311-020-00960-0

Vázquez-Vélez, G. E., & Zoghbi, H. Y. (2021). Parkinson's disease genetics and pathophysiology. *Annual Review of Neuroscience*, *44*(1), 87–108. PMID: 34236893

Velseboer, D. C., de Haan, R. J., Wieling, W., Goldstein, D. S., & de Bie, R. M. A. (2011). Prevalence of orthostatic hypotension in Parkinson's disease: A systematic review and meta-analysis. *Parkinsonism & Related Disorders*, *17*(10), 724–729. DOI: 10.1016/j.parkreldis.2011.04.016

Vera Anaya, D., & Yuce, M. R. (2021). Stretchable triboelectric sensor for measurement of the forearm muscles movements and fingers motion for Parkinson's disease assessment and assisting technologies. *Medical Devices & Sensors*, *4*(1). Advance online publication. DOI: 10.1002/mds3.10154

Vergara-Diaz, G., Daneault, J. F., Parisi, F., Admati, C., Alfonso, C., Bertoli, M., Bonizzoni, E., Carvalho, G. F., Costante, G., Fabara, E. E., Fixler, N., Golabchi, F. N., Growdon, J., Sapienza, S., Snyder, P., Shpigelman, S., Sudarsky, L., Daeschler, M., Bataille, L., & Bonato, P. (2021). Limb and trunk accelerometer data collected with wearable sensors from subjects with Parkinson's disease. *Scientific Data*, *8*(1). Advance online publication. DOI: 10.1038/s41597-021-00831-z PMID: 33547317

Wagner, J., Ryazanov, S., Leonov, A., Levin, J., Shi, S., Schmidt, F., Prix, C., Pan-Montojo, F., Bertsch, U., Mitteregger-Kretzschmar, G., Geissen, M., Eiden, M., Leidel, F., Hirschberger, T., Deeg, A. A., Krauth, J. J., Zinth, W., Tavan, P., Pilger, J., … Giese, A. (2013). Anle138b: a novel oligomer modulator for disease-modifying therapy of neurodegenerative diseases such as prion and Parkinson's disease. *Acta Neuropathologica 2013 125:6*, *125*(6), 795–813. https://doi.org/DOI: 10.1007/S00401-013-1114-9

Walker, R., Fothergill-Misbah, N., Kariuki, S., Ojo, O. O., Cilia, R., & Dekker, M.. (2023). Transforming Parkinson's care in Africa (TraPCAf): Protocol for a multimethodology National Institute for Health and Care Research Global Health Research Group project. *BMC Neurology*, *23*, 373. DOI: 10.1186/s12883-023-03414-0 PMID: 37858118

Wang, J., Zhang, S., Yuan, L., Tang, H., She, W., Zou, Y., ... (2024). Global, regional, and national burden of Parkinson's disease 1990–2021: A systematic analysis of the Global Burden of Disease Study 2021. SSRN *Electronic Journal*. https://doi.org/DOI: 10.2139/ssrn.5058486

Wang, C., & Ren, J. (2024). Ultrasound blood–brain barrier opening: A new era of treatment for Alzheimer's disease? *Aging Medicine (Milton, N.S.W.)*, *7*(6), 673–675. DOI: 10.1002/AGM2.12371

Wang, F., Sun, Z., Peng, D., Gianchandani, S., Le, W., Boltze, J., & Li, S. (2023). Cell-therapy for Parkinson's disease: A systematic review and meta-analysis. *Journal of Translational Medicine*, *21*(1), 601. PMID: 37679754

Wang, H., Chen, Y., Wang, L., Liu, Q., Yang, S., & Wang, C. (2023). Advancing herbal medicine: Enhancing product quality and safety through robust quality control practices. *Frontiers in Pharmacology*, *14*, 1265178. PMID: 37818188

Wang, K. L., Meng, F., Chen, S., Ramirez-Zamora, A., & Zhang, Y. Q. (2024). Editorial: Advances in neuromodulation treatment of Parkinson's disease and aging related movement disorders. *Frontiers in Aging Neuroscience*, *16*, 1407216. DOI: 10.3389/fnag.2024.1407216 PMID: 38659703

Wang, K., Meng, F., Zhang, Y., Ramirez-Zamora, A., & Chen, S.-Y. (Eds.). (2024). *Advances in neuromodulation treatment of Parkinson's disease and aging-related movement disorders*. Frontiers Media SA., DOI: 10.3389/978-2-8325-4818-9

Watabe, T., Hirata, K., Iima, M., Yanagawa, M., Saida, T., & Sakata, A.. (2025). Recent advances in theranostics and oncology PET: Emerging radionuclides and targets. *Annals of Nuclear Medicine*, *39*, 909. DOI: 10.1007/s12149-025-02090-z PMID: 40717183

Watson, E. D., Moosa, S., Janse Van Rensburg, D. C., Schwellnus, M., Lambert, E. V., & Stoutenberg, M. (2023). Task-shifting: Can community health workers be part of the solution to an inactive nation? *International Journal of Environmental Research and Public Health*, *20*(17), 6675. PMID: 37681815

Weerarathna, I. N., Doelakeh, E. S., Kiwanuka, L., Kumar, P., & Arora, S. (2024). Prophylactic and therapeutic vaccine development: Advancements and challenges. *Molecular Biomedicine*, *5*(1), 57. DOI: 10.1186/s43556-024-00222-x PMID: 39527305

Weintraub, D., Koester, J., Potenza, M. N., Siderowf, A. D., Stacy, M., Voon, V., Whetteckey, J., Wunderlich, G. R., & Lang, A. E. (2010). Impulse Control Disorders in Parkinson Disease: A Cross-Sectional Study of 3090 Patients. *Archives of Neurology*, *67*(5), 589–595. DOI: 10.1001/ARCHNEUROL.2010.65

Weise, D., Claus, I., Dresel, C., Kalbe, E., Liepelt-Scarfone, I., Lorenzl, S., & Urban, P. P. (2024). Multidisciplinary care in Parkinson's disease. *Journal of Neural Transmission (Vienna, Austria)*, *131*(10), 1217–1227. PMID: 39039238

Wickens, J. R., Horvitz, J. C., Costa, R. M., & Killcross, S. (2007). Dopaminergic mechanisms in actions and habits. *The Journal of Neuroscience : The Official Journal of the Society for Neuroscience*, *27*(31), 8181–8183. PMID: 17670964

Wijers, A., Ravi, A., Evers, S. M. A. A., Tissingh, G., & van Mastrigt, G. A. P. G. (2024). Systematic Review of the Cost of Illness of Parkinson's Disease from a Societal Perspective. *Movement Disorders*, *39*(11), 1938–1951. DOI: 10.1002/MDS.29995

Williams-Gray, C. H., Foltynie, T., Brayne, C. E. G., Robbins, T. W., & Barker, R. A. (2007). Evolution of cognitive dysfunction in an incident Parkinson's disease cohort. *Brain*, *130*(Pt 7), 1787–1798. PMID: 17535834

Wilson, V., & Maulik, S. K. (2019). Herb-Drug Interactions in Neurological Disorders: A Critical Appraisal. *Current Drug Metabolism*, *19*(5), 443–453. PMID: 29086684

Wójcik, R., Debska, A., Zaczkowski, K., Szmyd, B., Podstawka, M., Bobeff, E. J., Piotrowski, M., Ratajczyk, P., Jaskólski, D. J., & Wisniewski, K. (2025). Deep Brain Stimulation for Parkinson's Disease—ANarrativeReview. *Biomedicines*, *2025*(13), 2430. DOI: 10.3390/ biomedicines13102430 PMID: 41153713

Wolff, A., Schumacher, N. U., Pürner, D., Machetanz, G., Demleitner, A. F., & Feneberg, E.. (2023). Parkinson's disease therapy: What lies ahead? *Journal of Neural Transmission (Vienna, Austria)*, *130*, 793. DOI: 10.1007/s00702-023-02641-6 PMID: 37147404

Wongtrakul, J., Thongtan, T., Kumrapich, B., Saisawang, C., & Ketterman, A. J. (2021). Neuroprotective effects of *Withania somnifera* in the SH-SY5Y Parkinson cell model. *Heliyon*, *7*(10), e08172. DOI: 10.1016/j.heliyon.2021.e08172 PMID: 34765761

World Bank. Nigeria: Development News, Research, Data. World Bank. 2023. Available from: https://www.worldbank.org/en/country/nigeria

Wu, D., Chen, Q., Chen, X., Han, F., Chen, Z., & Wang, Y. (2023). The blood–brain barrier: structure, regulation, and drug delivery. *Signal Transduction and Targeted Therapy, 8*(1), 217-. https://doi.org/DOI: 10.1038/S41392-023-01481

Wu, H., Fan, Y., & Zhang, M. (2023). Advanced Progress in the Role of Adipose-Derived Mesenchymal Stromal/Stem Cells in the Application of Central Nervous System Disorders. *Pharmaceutics, 15*(11), 2637. PMID: 38004615

Wu, S., & Schekman, R. W. (2024). Intercellular transmission of alpha-synuclein. *Frontiers in Molecular Neuroscience, 17*, 1470171. DOI: 10.3389/FNMOL.2024.1470171

Wyse, R. K., Isaacs, T., Barker, R. A., Cookson, M. R., Dawson, T. M., Devos, D., Dexter, D. T., Duffen, J., Federoff, H., Fiske, B., Foltynie, T., Fox, S., Greenamyre, J. T., Kieburtz, K., Kordower, J. H., Krainc, D., Matthews, H., Moore, D. J., Mursaleen, L., & Brundin, P. (2024). Twelve Years of Drug Prioritization to Help Accelerate Disease Modification Trials in Parkinson's Disease: The International Linked Clinical Trials Initiative. *Journal of Parkinson's Disease, 14*(4), 657–666. DOI: 10.3233/JPD-230363

Xie, Y. X., Naseri, N. N., Fels, J., Kharel, P., Na, Y., Lane, D., Burré, J., & Sharma, M. (2022). Lysosomal exocytosis releases pathogenic α-synuclein species from neurons in synucleinopathy models. *Nature Communications 2022 13:1, 13*(1), 4918-. https://doi.org/DOI: 10.1038/s41467-022-32625-1

Xie, B., Chen, M., Hu, R., Han, W., & Ding, S. (2020). Therapeutic Evidence of Human Mesenchymal Stem Cell Transplantation for Cerebral Palsy: A Meta-Analysis of Randomized Controlled Trials. *Stem Cells International, 2020*(1), 5701920. PMID: 32765613

Xiong, Y., Mahmood, A., & Chopp, M. (2017). Emerging potential of exosomes for treatment of traumatic brain injury. *Neural Regeneration Research, 12*(1), 19–22. PMID: 28250732

Xu, S., Cagla, K., Keum, S.C., Rabab, R., Dylan, R., Abigail, N., Keum, S.C., Dylan, R., Albert-Smet, I., Matthew, K., Hope, C., Joy, H., Shiv, P., Jacqueline, T., Albert, Y., Aejin, S., Jessica, W., Sarah, C., Hyoyoung, J., Jong, Y.L., & Martin-Harris, B., (2025). Digital health technology for Parkinson's disease with comprehensive monitoring and artificial intelligence-enabled haptic biofeedback for bulbar dysfunction. Journal of Parkinson's Disease 2025, Vol. 15(3) 630–645 © The Author(s) 2025 Article reuse guidelines: sagepub.com/journals-permissions DOI: .DOI: 10.1177/1877718X251329354

Yamashita, K. Y., Bhoopatiraju, S., Silverglate, B. D., & Grossberg, G. T. (2023). Biomarkers in Parkinson's disease: A state of the art review. *Biomarkers in Neuropsychiatry*, *9*, 100074.

Yang, R., Sun, M., Chen, W., Feng, H., Chen, B., Liu, Y., He, Q., Wang, L., Zou, C., Luo, X., Li, Z., Fu, A., Qiao, F., Tang, H., Yang, J., & Ren, H. (2026). Global, regional and national burden of Parkinson's disease, 1990–2021: Update from the GBD 2021 study. *Journal of the Neurological Sciences*, *480*, 125703. DOI: 10.1016/j.jns.2025.125703 PMID: 41435482

Yanjie, M., Yifan, Z., Rui, L., Wenlin, C., & Fang, W. (2025). The experience and perception of wearable devices in Parkinson's disease patients: A systematic review and meta-synthesis of qualitative studies. *Journal of Neurology*, *2025*(272), 350. DOI: 10.1007/s00415-025-13085-1 PMID: 40252116

Yan, Y.-C., Xu, Z.-H., Wang, J., & Yu, W.-B. (2022). Uncovering the pharmacology of *Ginkgo biloba folium* in the cell-type specific targets of Parkinson's disease. *Frontiers in Pharmacology*, *13*, 1007556. DOI: 10.3389/fphar.2022.1007556 PMID: 36249800

Yin, R., Xue, J., Tan, Y., Fang, C., Hu, C., Yang, Q., Mei, X., & Qi, D. (2021). The Positive Role and Mechanism of Herbal Medicine in Parkinson's Disease. *Oxidative Medicine and Cellular Longevity*, *3*, 9923331. PMID: 34567415

Ymeri, G., Salvi, D., Olsson, C. M., Wassenburg, M. V., Tsanas, A., & Svenningsson, P. (2023). Quantifying Parkinson's disease severity using mobile wearable devices and machine learning: The ParkApp pilot study protocol. *BMJ Open*, *13*, e077766. DOI: 10.1136/ bmjopen-2023-077766 PMID: 38154904

Younas, M., Kong, L. L., & Bashir, M. (2016). Recent advancements, fundamental challenges, and opportunities in catalytic methanation of CO_2. *Energy*.

Yu, D., Zhang, P., Li, J., Liu, T., Zhang, Y., Wang, Q., Zhang, J., Lu, X., & Fan, X. (2021). Neuroprotective effects of *Ginkgo biloba* dropping pills in Parkinson's disease. *Journal of Pharmaceutical Analysis*, *11*(2), 220–231. PMID: 34012698

Yue-meng, S., Zhi-yun, W., Yuan-yuan, L., Chen-wei, H., & Chang-heShi, (2024). Digital biomarkers for precision diagnosis and monitoring in Parkinson's disease. npj | digital medicine. 7:218. https://doi.org/.DOI: 10.1038/s41746-024-01217-2

Yuexuan, L. (2024). *Development of Wearable Medical Devices in Parkin son's Disease. In2024InternationalConferenceonSmartHealthcareandWear able Intelligent Devices (SHWID2024), October18–20, 2024, Guangzhou, China*. ACM., DOI: 10.1145/3703847.3703874

Yu, T., & Li, X. (2023). Development of ZD2767P–carboxypeptidase G2–ultrasound therapy against cisplatin-resistant cancer. *Frontiers in Oncology, 13*, 1151613. DOI: 10.3389/fonc.2023.1151613 PMID: 37274240

Zadeh, L. A. (1965). Fuzzy sets. *Information and Control, 8*(3), 338–353.

Zafar, S., Lui, F., & Yaddanapudi, S. S. (2025). Parkinson Disease. NLB, https://www.ncbi.nlm.nih.gov/books/NBK470193/ Accessed Dec 26 2025.

Zakaria, R., Lenz, F. A., Hua, S., Avin, B. H., Liu, C. C., & Mari, Z. (2013). Thalamic physiology of intentional essential tremor is more like cerebellar tremor than postural essential tremor. *Brain Research, 1529*, 188–199. PMID: 23856324

Zakharov, A. V., Khivintseva, E. V., Pytin, V. F., Sergeeva, M. S., & Antipov, O. I. (2017). Melatonin—Known problems and perspectives of clinical usage. *Zhurnal Nevrologii i Psikhiatrii Im. S.S. Korsakova, 117*(4. Vyp. 2), 74. https://doi.org/DOI: 10.17116/jnevro20171174274-78

Zeng, X., & Qin, H. (2022). Stem cell transplantation for Parkinson's disease: Current challenges and perspectives. *Aging and Disease, 13*(6), 1652. PMID: 36465172

Zervos, T. M., Hamani, C., & Schwalb, J. M. (2018). MRIgFUS in tremor-dominant PD does not lead to substantial cognitive adverse events. *Neurology, 91*(14), 641–642. DOI: 10.1212/WNL.0000000000006241 PMID: 30158164

Zewde, Y. (2020). Health related quality of life of Ethiopian Parkinson's disease patients in Addis Ababa, Ethiopia. *Parkinsonism & Related Disorders, 79*, e82. Gavidia M. (2020). Access to Parkinson Disease Medication Affected in Low-Income Countries. [AJMC]. *The American Journal of Managed Care.*

Zhan, A., Mohan, S., Tarolli, C., Schneider, R. B., Adams, J. L., Sharma, S., Elson, M. J., Spear, K. L., Glidden, A. M., Little, M. A., Terzis, A., Ray Dorsey, E., & Saria, S. (2018). Using Smartphones and Machine Learning to Quantify Parkinson Disease Severity: The Mobile Parkinson Disease Score. *JAMA Neurology, 75*(7), 876–880. DOI: 10.1001/JAMANEUROL.2018.0809

Zhang, W., Xiao, D., Mao, Q., & Xia, H. (2023). Role of neuroinflammation in neurodegeneration development. *Signal Transduction and Targeted Therapy, 8*(1), 267. PMID: 37433768

Zhang, Y., Chopp, M., Meng, Y., Katakowski, M., Xin, H., Mahmood, A., & Xiong, Y. (2015). Effect of exosomes derived from multipluripotent mesenchymal stromal cells on functional recovery and neurovascular plasticity in rats after traumatic brain injury. *Journal of Neurosurgery, 122*(4), 856–867. PMID: 25594326

Zhao, W., Cui, H., Liu, J., Sun, H., Zhang, Z., & Ma, D. (2025). Herbal Interventions in Parkinson's Disease: A Systematic Review of Preclinical Studies. *Cellular and Molecular Neurobiology*, *45*(1), 50. PMID: 40410612

Zhao, Z. H., Chen, Z. T., Zhou, R. L., Zhang, X., Ye, Q. Y., & Wang, Y. Z. (2019). Increased DJ-1 and α-Synuclein in Plasma Neural-Derived Exosomes as Potential Markers for Parkinson's Disease. *Frontiers in Aging Neuroscience*, *10*(JAN), 438. DOI: 10.3389/FNAGI.2018.00438

Zhidu, S., Ying, T., Rui, J., & Chao, Z. (2024). Translational potential of mesenchymal stem cells in regenerative therapies for human diseases: Challenges and opportunities. *Stem Cell Research & Therapy*, *15*(1), 266. PMID: 39183341

Zhou, L., Wang, Q., Gao, H., Tan, Y. X., Xu, Q., & Zhang, J.. (2024). Trends in the global burden of Parkinson's disease 1990–2021. *Findings from the Global Burden of Disease Study*, *2021*. Advance online publication. DOI: 10.2139/ssrn.4950652

Zhou, T., Yuan, Z., Weng, J., Pei, D., & Du, X. (2021). Challenges and advances in clinical applications of mesenchymal stromal cells. *Journal of Hematology (Brossard, Quebec)*. PMID: 33579329

Zhou, Y., Lu, M., Du, R.-H., Qiao, C., Jiang, C.-Y., Zhang, K.-Z., Ding, J.-H., & Hu, G. (2016). MicroRNA-7 targets Nod-like receptor protein 3 inflammasome to modulate neuroinflammation in the pathogenesis of Parkinson's disease. *Molecular Neurodegeneration*, *11*, 28. DOI: 10.1186/s13024-016-0094-3 PMID: 27084336

Zhu, J., Cui, Y., Zhang, J., Yan, R., Su, D., Zhao, D., Wang, A., & Feng, T. (2024). Temporal trends in the prevalence of Parkinson's disease from 1980 to 2023: A systematic review and meta-analysis. *The Lancet. Healthy Longevity*, *5*(7), e464–e479. DOI: 10.1016/S2666-7568(24)00094-1 PMID: 38945129

Zhu, M., Li, M., Ye, D., Jiang, W., Lei, T., & Shu, K. (2016). Sensory symptoms in Parkinson's disease: Clinical features, pathophysiology, and treatment. *Journal of Neuroscience Research*, *94*(8), 685–692. PMID: 26948282

About the Contributors

Abraham Olufemi Asuku is a Ph.D. holder in neurophysiology in the Department of Physiology, Faculty of Basic Medical Sciences, University of Ilorin, Ilorin, Nigeria. He obtained his first degree (B.Sc.) and master's degree (M.Sc.) from the same department. Dr. Asuku is a passionate neuroscientist and medical biotechnologist. He currently works with the National Biotechnology Research and Development Agency, Nigeria, as an Assistant Chief Research Officer. His area of interest is on mitigation of neurotoxicity, neurodegenerative diseases, and neurodevelopmental disorders by phytochemicals, and also on the applications of nanotechnology for neurodegenerative disease drug delivery. He is a member of the Neuroscience Society of Nigeria, the International Parkinson and Movement Disorder Society, USA, the Physiological Society, United Kingdom. He is an award-winning researcher and has over 60 publications (More than 30 are Scopus-based), including book chapters, research and review articles of good international repute. He has served as a reviewer for many reputable journals. Dr Asuku was ranked by SCIVAL among the Top 500 authors, by Scholarly Output from 2022 to 2025 in Neuroscience as number 21 and 93 in Nigeria and Africa respectively. He has also presented seminars at many conferences, both locally and internationally. He was one of the invited guest speakers at the VII International Conference of Universidad Tecnica De Manabi, Ecuador, in 2023. Dr. Asuku was an editor of the book titled Non-pharmacological Intervention for Dementia: A Comprehensive Approach, and he is currently editing other book, Bioresources for Managing and Treating Dementiato be published by CRC Taylor and Francis Publisher. His long-term goal is to discover therapeutic targets and help create focused treatments for neurodegenerative diseases. By bridging the gap between basic and translational neuroscience, he seeks to further knowledge of neuronal health and provide insights that may result in novel treatments.

Olugbemi Tope Olaniyan had his B.Sc. Hons (Ilorin), M.Sc., and Ph.D. (Ibadan) all in Physiology, Postgraduate Diploma in Education (PGDE) (Nigeria), Certificate in Clinical Embryology & Assisted Reproductive Medicine from India, and Postdoctoral Research Fellowship from Universidad de Granada, Spain. He is currently a Senior Lecturer at the Department of Physiology,Faculty of Basic Medical Sciences, Kwara State University, Malete, Nigeria.

***

Ajoke Basirat Akinola is a distinguished public health expert, researcher, and academic leader whose work spans across Nigeria and India. She is currently recognized for her significant contributions to public health education and research, particularly in the areas of health equity, maternal health, and infectious cum non infectious disease management. Academic Background and Education Dr. Akinola's academic journey began in Nigeria, where she earned a Bachelor of Science (B.Sc.) in Cell Biology and Genetics from the University of Lagos in 2005. Driven by a passion for community well-being, she transitioned into the field of healthcare management, obtaining a Post Graduate Diploma in Hospital Management from the Central Institute of Management in New Delhi, India. She further specialized by earning a Master of Public Health (MPH) with a focus on Public Health Management, followed by a Ph.D. in Public Health from the SRM University & Research Institute in Kattankulathur,, TamilNadu State, India. Her doctoral research laid the groundwork for her career as a specialist in epidemiology and health systems. Professional Career and Leadership Dr. Akinola has held various influential roles in academia and clinical administration. Her early career included service with the Bayelsa State Government in Nigeria, where she worked on the National Program on Immunization and logistics management. She later served as a Public Health Consultant for the Ministry of Health and Family Welfare in New Delhi, contributing to the Health Management Information System (HMIS). In the academic sector, she has served several times as the Head, Department of Public Health at Noida International University (NIU), Delhi NCR India and more recently at Achievers University in Owo, Nigeria. In December 2024, she was honored with a Meritorious Award by African Institute of Public Health Professionals, Abuja for her exceptional leadership and dedication to public health education. Research Contributions As a prolific researcher, Dr. Akinola has published extensively in national and international scopus indexed journals. Her research portfolio is diverse, covering: Health Equity: Investigating the treatment-seeking behaviors and ethical health perspectives of internal migrant laborers. Maternal and Reproductive Health: Researching breastfeeding practices, the importance of colostrum, and cervical cancer screening uptake. Infectious Diseases: Contributing to studies on COVID-

19 transmission, vaccine hesitancy, and the re-emergence of human monkeypox. Gender-Based Violence: Analyzing the impact of domestic and social violence on women's mental and physical health. Philanthropy and Impact Beyond her academic duties, Dr. Akinola has been involved in community-driven initiatives. She served as a Disable Children Public Health Coordinator for the SOS Foundation-Africa, where she focused on child health advocacy. Her work is characterized by a commitment to improving healthcare quality and planning for underserved populations. Today, Dr. Ajoke Akinola remains a leading voice in the global public health community, bridging the gap between academic research, education and practical healthcare delivery to foster a more equitable world.

Athilakshmi R is currently working as an assistant professor in the Department of Computational Intelligence at SRM Institute of Science and Technology. Her research interests include artificial intelligence in signal processing.

Alvin Ben George is a final-year undergraduate student in Electronics and Computer Engineering at S.R.M. Institute of Science and Technology, Chennai, graduating in 2026. His technical interests sit at the intersection of Edge AI, Distributed Systems, and Scalable Backend Architecture. He has strong experience in bridging hardware-software gaps, with hands-on work in architecting AI-driven systems, handling high-concurrency traffic, and optimizing resource-constrained environments using Python, Node.js, and AWS. His work focuses on System Design, Machine Learning integration, and developing efficient, low-latency architectures for both intelligent edge devices and cloud platforms, demonstrated by his development of robust, production-grade applications

Daniel Biju Joseph is an undergraduate student in Electronics and Computer Engineering at SRM Institute of Science and Technology, Chennai, graduating in 2026. His technical interests center on embedded systems, robotics, and hardware–software co-design, with strong hands-on experience in PCB design, firmware development, and real-time communication protocols such as CAN, SPI, I2C, UART, and Ethernet. He has led the electronics development for multiple ABU Robocon projects, designing and integrating reliable robotic systems using microcontrollers, MicroPython, OpenCV, and NVIDIA Jetson platforms, while also gaining industry exposure through embedded firmware development on STM32 platforms.

Vibhas Mittra is a B.Pharmacy student with a strong interest in pharmacology, drug delivery systems, and pharmaceutical research. He is focused on academic excellence and developing practical skills for a career in the pharmaceutical and healthcare sector.

Samuel Onyekweli is a medical doctor (MBChB, 2022) and Medical Officer at St. Ives Specialist Hospital, Lagos, Nigeria. He serves as Clinical Head of occupational health services at New Ikeja Hospital, managing care for over 1,200 employees. His research focuses on antimicrobial resistance in hematologic malignancies and metabolic-epigenetic mechanisms in reproductive disorders, with publications examining bacterial colonization dynamics in acute leukemia patients and short-chain fatty acid interventions in polycystic ovary syndrome models. Samuel is currently pursuing PhD opportunities in translational biomedical sciences, with research interests spanning microbiome-cancer interactions, metabolic reprogramming, immunotherapy resistance mechanisms, and neuroscience.

R. Jansi completed her Ph.D. from Anna University, India, in 2022. She received her B.E. degree in Electronics and Communication Engineering from R.M.K. Engineering College, India, in 2010, and her M.E. degree in Communication Systems from SSN College of Engineering, India, in 2013. She is currently working as an assistant professor in the Department of Electronics and Communication Engineering at SRM Institute of Science and Technology. Her research interests include signal and image processing.

Debanshu Roy is a final-year undergraduate student in Electronics and Computer Engineering at S.R.M. Institute of Science and Technology, Chennai, graduating in 2026. His technical interests span Embedded Systems, Machine Learning, Automotive Systems, Electronics, Android Development, Edge AI, Circuit Design and CAD Modelling. He has strong experience in developing Proof Of Concepts and R&D-oriented engineering, with hands-on work in hardware–software co-design, digital system architecture, and low-level firmware development across microcontrollers, FPGA platforms, and edge computing devices. His work focuses on Product design, Rapid Prototyping for Software and Firmware Design Concepts and workflows.

Haarish S, a 3rd year B.Tech in Electronics and Communication Engineering (ECE) and expected to graduate in 2027 from S.R.M. Institute of Science and Technology. His primary research interests lie in AI, Machine Learning,Deep learning, Data science and the Internet of Things (IoT). He has specialized expertise in hardware-software interfacing using platforms like Raspberry Pi to create responsive monitoring environments, cloud services like AWS and GCP and professional-grade tools such as Airflow, Terraform, Databricks. His work focuses on developing automated tools and pushes the boundaries of Edge Intelligence.

Index

N

O

P

S

T

V

W

www.ingramcontent.com/pod-product-compliance
Lightning Source LLC
LaVergne TN
LVHW062333300926
849161LV00007B/1676